NURSING: MENTAL HEALTH AND COMMUNITY CONCEPTS

NURSING: MENTAL HEALTH AND COMMUNITY CONCEPTS

OPEN RESOURCES FOR NURSING (OPEN RN)

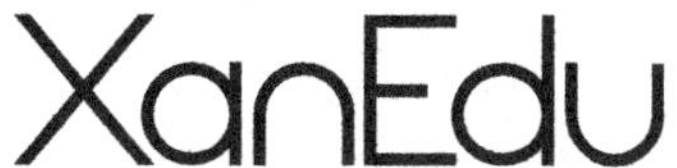

Printed in the United States of America

ISBN 13: 978-1-73491-417-7

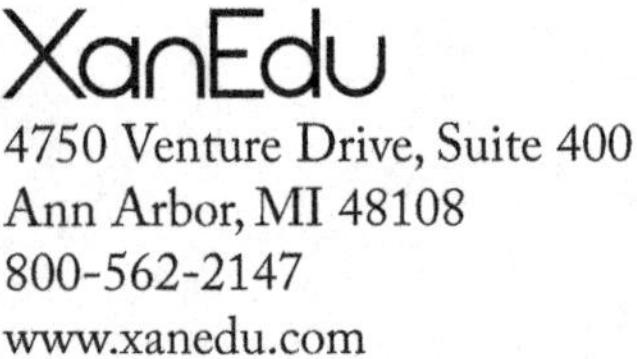

4750 Venture Drive, Suite 400
Ann Arbor, MI 48108
800-562-2147
www.xanedu.com

CONTENTS

INTRODUCTION

This textbook is an open educational resource with CC-BY licensing developed specifically for prelicensure nursing students. The e-book and downloadable versions are free. Affordable print versions are published in collaboration with XanEdu and available on Amazon and in college bookstores.

Content is based on the Wisconsin Technical College System (WTCS) statewide nursing curriculum for the Nursing Mental Health and Community Concepts course (543-110), the NCLEX-RN Test Plan[1], and the American Psychiatric Nurses Association Education Council's *Crosswalk Toolkit: Defining and Using Psychiatric-Mental Health Nursing Skills in Undergraduate Nursing Education.*[2] Mental health and community health concepts are discussed while emphasizing stress management techniques, healthy coping strategies, referrals to community resources, and other preventative interventions. Nursing care for individuals with specific mental health and substance use disorders is examined, and the nurse's role in community health needs assessments and caring for vulnerable populations is introduced.

Throughout the print version, URLs and videos are called out within blue boxes with icons. Refer to the online book for the most current URLs to access these supplementary sources. The online book is available at www.cvtc.edu/OpenRN.

View a video that provides a quick overview of how to navigate the online version: Nursing: Mental Health and Community Concepts Walkthrough https://wtcs.pressbooks.pub/nursingmhcc/?p=4#oembed-1

1 NCSBN. (n.d.). *2019 NCLEX-RN test plan.* https://www.ncsbn.org/2019_RN_TestPlan-English.htm

2 American Psychiatric Nurses Association Education Council, Undergraduate Branch. (2016). *Crosswalk toolkit: Defining and using psychiatric-mental health nursing skills in undergraduate nursing education.* https://www.apna.org/resources/undergraduate-education-toolkit/

PREFACE

The Open RN project is supported by a $2.5 million grant from the Department of Education to create five free, open-source nursing textbooks. However, this content does not necessarily represent the policy of the Department of Education, and you should not assume endorsement by the federal government. More information about the Open RN grant can be found at cvtc.edu/OpenRN. The first three textbooks of the Open RN textbook series, *Nursing Pharmacology, Nursing Skills*, and *Nursing Fundamentals*, received a Best OER Award from OE Global in 2020 and 2021.

Usage Survey and Feedback

We would love to hear if you have integrated some or all of this resource into your course. Please use this short survey to provide constructive feedback or report errors: https://cvtc.az1.qualtrics.com/jfe/form/SV_54PkuNI7Qb0ipJb.

Editors

- Kimberly Ernstmeyer, MSN, RN, CNE, CHSE, APNP-BC
- Dr. Elizabeth Christman, DNP, RN, CNE

Graphics Editor

- Nic Ashman, MLIS, Librarian, Chippewa Valley Technical College

Developing Authors

Developing authors remixed existing open educational resources and/or developed content based on evidence-based sources and experience in the mental health field:

- Dr. Elizabeth Christman, DNP, RN, CNE
- Dawn Barone, MSN, RN, Chippewa Valley Technical College
- Sue Dzubay, MSN, RN, CHSE, RN-BC, Chippewa Valley Technical College
- Kimberly Ernstmeyer, MSN, RN, CNE, CHSE, APNP-BC, Chippewa Valley Technical College
- Jeanne Green, EdS, MSN, RN, CNE, CHEP, RN-BC, Chippewa Valley Technical College
- Deb Johnson-Schuh, MSN, RN, Mid-State Technical College
- Rorey Pritchard, EdS, MEd, MSN, RN-BC, CNOR(E), CNE, Senior RN Clinical Educator, Allevant Solutions, LLC
- Dr. Miriam Sward, DNP, PMHNP, APNP, Psychiatric Mental Health Nurse Practitioner
- Alicia Tays, MS, LPC, Counselor

Contributors

Contributors assisted in creating this textbook:

- Jane Flesher, MST, Proofreader, Chippewa Valley Technical College
- Shronda Green, MSN, RN, Gateway Technical College

- Vince Mussehl, MLIS, Open RN Lead Librarian, Chippewa Valley Technical College
- Joshua Myers, Web Developer, Chippewa Valley Technical College
- Kelly Nelson, MSN, RN, Mid-State Technical College
- Amanda Olson-Komisar, CSW, Social Worker; Pupil Services Teacher Assistant, Pepin Area Schools
- Andrea Olson, MSN, RN, Trempealeau County Healthcare Center
- Meredith Pomietlo, BA, Retail Design and Marketing, University of Wisconsin – Stout
- Dominic Slauson, BA, Open RN Instructional Technologist
- Dr. Jamie Zwicky, EdD, MSN, RN, Moraine Park Technical College

Advisory Committee

The Open RN Advisory Committee consists of industry members and nursing deans who provide input for the Open RN textbooks and virtual reality scenarios:

- Jenny Bauer, MSN, RN, NPD-BC, Mayo Clinic Health System Northwest Wisconsin, Eau Claire, WI
- Lisa Cannestra, Eastern Wisconsin Healthcare Alliance
- Travis Christman, MSN, RN, Chief Nursing Officer, HSHS Sacred Heart and St. Joseph's Hospitals
- Sheri Johnson, UW Population Health Institute
- Dr. Vicki Hulback, DNP, RN, Dean of Nursing, Gateway Technical College
- Jenna Julson, MSN, RN, NPD-BC, Nursing Education Specialist, Mayo Clinic Health System Northwest Wisconsin, Eau Claire, WI
- Brian Krogh, MSN, RN, Associate Dean – Health Sciences, Northeast Wisconsin Technical College
- Hugh Leasum, MBA, MSN, RN, Nurse Manager Cardiology/ICU, Marshfield Clinic Health System, Eau Claire, WI
- Pam Maxwell, SSM Health
- Mari Kay-Nobozny, NW Wisconsin Workforce Development Board
- Dr. Amy Olson, DNP, RN, Nursing Education Specialist, Mayo Clinic Health System Northwest Wisconsin, Eau Claire, WI
- Gina Petrie, MSN, RN, Dean of Nursing, Chippewa Valley Technical College
- Rorey Pritchard, EdS, MEd, MSN, RN-BC, CNOR(E), CNE, Senior RN Clinical Educator, Allevant Solutions, LLC
- Kelly Shafaie, MSN, RN, Associate Dean of Nursing, Moraine Park Technical College
- Dr. Ernise Watson, PhD, RN, Associate Dean of Nursing, Madison Area Technical College
- Sherry Willems, HSHS St. Vincent Hospital

Reviewers

- Dr. Caryn Aleo, PhD, RN, CCRN, CEN, CNE, CNEcl, Pasco-Hernando State College
- Dawn Barone, MSN, RN, Chippewa Valley Technical College
- Lisa Bechard, MSN, RN, Mid-State Technical College
- Shanleigh Bechard, MS, LPC, Beloit Area Community Health Center
- Ginger Becker, Nursing Student, Portland Community College
- Nancy Bonard, MSN, RN-BC, St. Joseph's College of Maine
- Dr. Joan Buckley, PhD, RN, Nassau Community College
- Kathleen Capone, MS, RN, CNE, EdD, Utica College
- Lorraine Chiappetta, MSN, RN, CNE, Emeritus Washtenaw Community College
- Travis Christman, MSN, RN, Hospital Sister's Health System
- Maria Darris, MSN, RN, St. Louis Community College
- Tamara Davis, MSN, RN, Chippewa Valley Technical College
- Dr. Andrea Dobogai, DNP, RN, Moraine Park Technical College
- Dr. Judith Dornbach, DNP, MSN, RN, NEA-BC, Southwestern Oregon Community College
- Jessica Dwork, MSN-Ed, RN, Maricopa Community Colleges-Phoenix Collège
- Dr. Terri J. Farmer, PhD, PMHNP-BC, University of Arizona College of Nursing
- Dr. Rachael Farrell, EdD, MSN, CNE Howard Community College, Columbia, MD
- Dr. Vivienne Friday, EdD, MSN, RN, CNE, MSOL, Goodwin University
- Jocelyn E. Goodwin, MSN, RN, Paradise Valley Community College
- Kerry L. Hamm, MSN, RN, Lakeland University
- Julia Harelstad, MSN, RN, Mayo Clinic Health System, Eau Claire WI
- Deborah Harmon, BSN, RN, AdventHealth Zephyrhills/Dade City
- Melissa Hauge, MSN, RN, Madison College
- Camille Hernandez, MSN, APRN-Rx, ACNP/FNP, Hawaii Community College – Palamanui
- Katherine Howard, MS, RN-BC, CNE, Middlesex College New Jersey
- Susan Jepsen, MSN, RN, CNE, Lansing Community College
- Eric Johnson, MSN, RN, Chippewa Valley Technical College
- Dr. Kathi L. Johnson, DNP, MS, RN-BC, CNE, Howard Community College
- Jenna Julson, MSN, RN, NPD-RN, Mayo Clinic Health System
- Dr. Andrew D. Kehl, DNP, MSN, MPH, APRN, RN, Vermont Technical College
- Kathryn Kieran, MSN, PMHNP-BC, MGH Institute of Health Professions
- Lindsay Kuhlman, BSN, RN, HSHS Sacred Heart
- Kathy L. Loppnow, MSN, RN, WTCS Health Science Education Director (retired)
- Dawn M. Lyon, MSN, RN, Saint Clair County Community College

- Dr. Erin Micale-Sexton, DNP, MSN-RN, CNL, Lansing Community College, Madonna University, Arizona College
- Sara K. Mitchell, MSN, RN, Fox Valley Technical College
- Dr. Jamie Murphy, PhD, RN, SUNY Delhi
- Kelly Nelson, MSN, RN, Mid-State Technical College
- Tram Nguyen, Nursing Student, Portland Community College
- Dr. Tennille O'Connor, DNP, RN, CNE, College of Central Florida
- Andrea Olson, MSN, RN, Trempealeau County Health Care Center
- Amanda Olson-Komisar, CSW, Social Worker; Pupil Services Teacher Assistant, Pepin Area Schools
- Dr. Grace Paul, DNP, MPhil, RN, CNE, Glendale Community College
- Krista Polomis, MSN, RN, CNE, Nicolet College
- Mary A. Pomietlo, MSN, RN, CNE, University of Wisconsin – Eau Claire
- Cassandra Porter, MSN, RN, Lake Land College
- Rachel Potaczek, BSN, RN, Chippewa County Department of Public Health
- Rorey Pritchard, EdS, MSN, RN-BC, NPD, CNOR(E), CNE, Allevant Solutions, LLC
- Dr. Debbie Rickeard, DNP, MSN, BScN, BA, RN, CNE, CCRN, University of Windsor
- Dr. Argie Rivera, DNP, MAN, PMHNP-BC, Polara Health, Grand Canyon University, Cara Behavioral Health
- Kathleen S. Rizzo, MSN, RN, St. Louis Community College at Forest Park
- Ann K. Rosemeyer, MSN, RN, Chippewa Valley Technical College
- Brenda Scheurer, MS, PMP, Eau Claire City-County Health Department
- Cynthia Schroder, MSN, RN, FNP, Yavapai College
- Katherine A. Sell, MSN, RN, IBCLC, CNE, University of Wisconsin – Eau Claire
- Alexis Smith, MScN, RN, Western University
- Justin Spargrove, MSN, RN, Southwest Wisconsin Technical College
- Morgan Stock, MSN-Ed, RN, CNE, University of Arizona
- Dr. Miriam A. Sward, DNP, PMHNP, APNP, Northlakes Community Clinic
- Maria E. Thomas, MSN, MS, RN, CNE, Yavapai College
- Jane Trainis, MS, PMHCNS-BC, CNE, Community College of Baltimore County
- Jennie E. Ver Steeg, MLIS, AHIP, Mercy College of Health Sciences
- Emily Vergenz, MSN, RN, Lakeshore Technical College
- Devon Rice Weaver, MSN, RN, Clatsop Community College
- Dr. Nancy Whitehead, PhD, APNP, RN, Milwaukee Area Technical College

Licensing/Terms of Use

Attribution

Some of the content for this textbook was adapted from the following open educational resources. For specific reference information about what was used and/or changed in this adaptation, please refer to the footnotes at the bottom of each page of the book.

- *Nursing Fundamentals* by Chippewa Valley Technical College is licensed under CC BY 4.0
- *Nursing Management and Professional Concepts* by Chippewa Valley Technical College is licensed under CC BY 4.0
- *Nursing Pharmacology* by Chippewa Valley Technical College is licensed under CC BY 4.0
- *mhGAP Intervention Guide – Version 2.0* by World Health Organization is licensed under CC BY-NC-SA 3.0 IGO
- *Culture and Psychology* by Worthy, Lavigne, and Romero is licensed under CC BY-NC-SA 4.0
- *Human Relations* by LibreTexts is licensed under CC BY-NC-SA 4.0
- *Anatomy and Physiology* by OpenStax is licensed under CC BY 4.0. Access for free at https://openstax.org/books/anatomy-and-physiology/pages/1-introduction
- *Nursing Care at the End of Life* by Lowey is licensed under CC BY-NC-SA 4.0
- *Doing What Matters in Times of Stress: An Illustrated Guide* by World Health Organization is licensed under CC BY-NC-SA 3.0 IGO
- *StatPearls* by Orenstein & Lewis is licensed under CC BY 4.0
- *Psychology 2e* by OpenStax is licensed under CC BY 4.0. Access for free at https://openstax.org/books/psychology-2e/pages/1-introduction
- *StatPearls* by Jabbari & Rouster is licensed under CC BY 4.0

- *StatPearls* by Sheffler, Reddy, and Pillarisetty is licensed under CC BY 4.0
- *StatPearls* by Dhaliwal and Gupta is licensed under CC BY 4.0
- *StatPearls* by Shin and Saadabadi is licensed under CC BY 4.0
- *StatPearls* by Wilson and Tripp is licensed under CC BY 4.0
- *StatPearls* by Chokhawala and Stevens is licensed under CC BY 4.0
- *StatPearls* by Ahuja and Abdijadid is licensed under CC BY 4.0
- *StatPearls* by Padda and Derian is licensed under CC BY 4.0
- *Foundations of Addiction Studies* by Flori and Trytek is licensed under CC BY-NC-SA 4.0
- *StatPearls* by Vasan and Kumar is licensed under CC BY 4.0
- *StatPearls* by Kang, Galuska, & Ghassemzadeh is licensed under CC BY 4.0
- *Action Steps Using ACEs and Trauma-Informed Care: A Resilience Model* by Laurie Leitch is licensed under CC BY 4.0
- *StatPearls* by Kisling and Das is licensed under CC BY 4.0
- *Community Tool Box* by Center for Community Health and Development at the University of Kansas is licensed under CC BY NC SA 3.0
- *Daily New Confirmed COVID-19 Deaths Per Million People* by Our World in Data is licensed under CC BY 4.0
- *The Emerging Neurobiology of Bipolar Disorder* by Harrison, Geddes, & Tunbridge is licensed under CC BY 4.0
- *StatPearls* by Fisher, Hany, and Doerr is licensed under CC BY 4.0
- *StatPearls* by Lewis and O'Day is licensed under CC BY 4.0
- *StatPearls* by Vasan and Padhy is licensed under CC BY 4.0
- *The Scholarship of Writing in Nursing Education: 1st Canadian Edition* by Lapum, St-Amant, Hughes, Tan, Bogdan, Dimaranan, Frantzke, and Savicevic is licensed under CC BY-SA 4.0

Suggested attribution statement: Ernstmeyer, K., & Christman, E. (Eds.). (2022). *Nursing Mental Health and Community Concepts* by Chippewa Valley Technical College is licensed under CC BY 4.0

STANDARDS AND CONCEPTUAL APPROACH

The Open RN *Nursing Mental Health and Community Concepts* textbook is based on several external standards and uses a conceptual approach.

External Standards

American Nurses Association (ANA)

The ANA establishes Standards for Professional Nursing Practice and the Nursing Code of Ethics.[3,4,5]

- https://www.nursingworld.org/ana/about-ana/standards/

American Psychiatric Nurses Association (APNA)

The APNA advances the science and education of psychiatric-mental health nursing. The APNA is committed to the practice of psychiatric-mental health nursing, health and wellness promotion through identification of mental health issues, prevention of mental health problems, and the care and treatment of persons with mental health disorders.[6]

- https://www.apna.org/

American Psychiatric Nurses Association Education Council, Undergraduate Branch

The APNA created a toolkit to help define and integrate psychiatric-mental health nursing content into undergraduate nursing curricula.[7]

- https://www.apna.org/resources/undergraduate-education-toolkit/

Substance Abuse and Mental Health Services Administration (SAMHSA)

The Substance Abuse and Mental Health Services Administration (SAMHSA) is the agency within the U.S. Department of Health and Human Services that leads public health efforts to advance the behavioral health of the nation and to improve the lives of individuals living with mental health and substance use disorders and their

---

3 American Nurses Association. (2021). *Nursing: Scope and standards of practice* (4th ed.). American Nurses Association.

4 American Nurses Association. (2015). *Code of ethics for nurses with interpretive statements*. American Nurses Association. https://www.nursingworld.org/practice-policy/nursing-excellence/ethics/code-of-ethics-for-nurses/

5 American Nurses Association. (2014). *Psychiatric-mental health nursing: Scope and standards of practice* (2nd ed.). Nursesbooks.org.

6 American Psychiatric Nurses Association. https://www.apna.org/

7 American Psychiatric Nurses Association Education Council, Undergraduate Branch. (2016). *Crosswalk toolkit: Defining and using psychiatric-mental health nursing skills in undergraduate nursing education*. https://www.apna.org/resources/undergraduate-education-toolkit/

families. SAMHSA's mission is to reduce the impact of substance abuse and mental illness on America's communities and draws advice from public members and professionals in the field of substance abuse and mental health.[8]

- https://www.samhsa.gov/

The National Council Licensure Examination for Registered Nurses: NCLEX-RN Test Plans

The NCLEX-RN test plans are updated every three years to reflect fair, comprehensive, current, and entry-level nursing competency.[9]

- https://www.ncsbn.org/nclex.htm

The National League of Nursing (NLN): Competencies for Graduates of Nursing Programs

NLN competencies guide nursing curricula to position graduates in a dynamic health care arena with practice that is informed by a body of knowledge to help ensure the public receives safe, quality care.[10]

- https://www.nln.org/education/nursing-education-competencies/competencies-for-graduates-of-nursing-programs

American Association of Colleges of Nursing (AACN): The Essentials: Competencies for Professional Nursing Education

The AACN provides a framework for preparing individuals as members of the discipline of nursing, reflecting expectations across the trajectory of nursing education and applied experience.

- https://www.aacnnursing.org/Portals/42/AcademicNursing/pdf/Essentials-2021.pdf

Quality and Safety Education for Nurses (QSEN) Institute: Prelicensure Competencies

Quality and safety competencies include knowledge, skills, and attitudes to be developed in nursing prelicensure programs. QSEN competencies include patient-centered care, teamwork and collaboration, evidence-based practice, quality improvement, safety, and informatics.[11]

- https://qsen.org/competencies/

---

8 Substance Abuse and Mental Health Services Administration. (n.d.). *Strategic plan FY2019-FY2023*. https://www.samhsa.gov/sites/default/files/samhsa_strategic_plan_fy19-fy23_final-508.pdf

9 NCSBN. (n.d.). *2019 NCLEX-RN test plan*. https://www.ncsbn.org/2019_RN_TestPlan-English.htm

10 National League of Nursing. *Competencies for graduates of nursing programs*. https://www.nln.org/education/nursing-education-competencies/competencies-for-graduates-of-nursing-programs

11 QSEN. (n.d.). *About*. https://qsen.org/about-qsen/

Wisconsin State Legislature, Administrative Code Chapter N6

The Wisconsin Administrative Code governs the Registered Nursing and Practical Nursing professions in Wisconsin.[12]

- https://docs.legis.wisconsin.gov/code/admin_code/n/6

Healthy People 2030

Healthy People 2030 envisions a society in which all people can achieve their full potential for health and well-being across the life span. Healthy People provides objectives based on national data and includes social determinants of health.[13]

- https://health.gov/healthypeople

Conceptual Approach

The Open RN *Nursing Mental Health and Community Concepts* textbook incorporates the following concepts:

Holism. Florence Nightingale taught nurses to focus on the principles of holism, including wellness and the interrelationship of human beings and their environment. This textbook encourages holistic nursing care by addressing the impact of social determinants of health (SDOH) on mental health.

Evidence-Based Practice (EBP). Evidence-based practices are referenced by footnotes throughout the textbook. To promote the development of digital literacy, URLs are provided to credible, free online resources that supplement content. The Open RN textbooks will be updated as new EBP is established and after the release of updated NCLEX Test Plans every three years.

Clinical Judgment. Associated unfolding case studies are written to reflect the NCSBN Clinical Judgment Measurement Model used on the NCLEX-RN. Formative assessments encourage students to recognize cues, analyze cues, prioritize hypotheses, generate solutions, take action, and evaluate outcomes.[14]

Cultural Competency. Nurses have an ethical obligation to practice with cultural humility and provide culturally responsive care to the clients and communities they serve based on the ANA Code of Ethics[15] and the ANA Scope and Standards of Practice.[16]

---

12 Wisconsin State Legislature. (2018). *Chapter 6: Standards of practice for registered nurses and licensed practical nurses.* Board of Nursing. https://docs.legis.wisconsin.gov/statutes/statutes/441

13 Healthy People 2030. (n.d.). *Social determinants of health.* U.S. Department of Health and Human Services. https://health.gov/healthypeople/objectives-and-data/social-determinants-health

14 Dickison, P., Haerling, K. A., & Lasater, K. (2019). Integrating the national council of state boards of nursing clinical judgment model into nursing educational frameworks. *Journal of Nursing Education. 58*(2), 72-78. https://doi.org/10.3928/01484834-20190122-03

15 American Nurses Association. (2015). *Code of ethics for nurses with interpretive statements.* American Nurses Association. https://www.nursingworld.org/practice-policy/nursing-excellence/ethics/code-of-ethics-for-nurses/

16 American Nurses Association. (2021). *Nursing: Scope and standards of practice* (4th ed.). American Nurses Association.

Safe, Quality, Patient-Centered Care. Content reflects the priorities of safe, quality, patient-centered care.

Clear and Inclusive Language. Clear language is used based on preferences expressed by prelicensure nursing students to enhance understanding of complex concepts.[17] "They" is used as a singular pronoun to refer to a person whose gender is unknown or irrelevant to the context of the usage, as endorsed by APA style. It is inclusive of all people and helps writers avoid making assumptions about gender.[18]

Open-Source Images and Fair Use. Images are included to promote visual learning. Students and faculty can reuse open-source images by following the terms of their associated Creative Commons licensing. Some images are included based on Fair Use as described in the "Code of Best Practices for Fair Use and Fair Dealing in Open Education" presented at the OpenEd 2020 conference. Refer to the footnotes of images for source and licensing information throughout the text.

Open Pedagogy. Students are encouraged to contribute to the Open RN project in meaningful ways by reviewing content for clarity and assisting in the creation of open-source images.[19]

Supplementary Material Provided

Several supplementary resources are provided with this textbook.

Supplementary, free videos promote student understanding of concepts and procedures.

Online, interactive, and written learning activities provide formative feedback.

Critical thinking questions encourage the development of clinical judgment as students apply content to realistic patient scenarios.

Free downloadable textbook versions are available for offline use.

Affordable soft cover print versions are published by XanEdu and available on Amazon and in college bookstores based on the finding that over 65% of students prefer a print version of their textbooks.[20]

---

17 Verkuyl, M., Lapum, J., St-Amant, O., Bregstein, J., & Hughes, M. (2020). Healthcare students' use of an e-textbook open educational resource on vital sign measurement: A qualitative study. *Open Learning: The Journal of Open, Distance and e-Learning.* https://doi.org/10.1080/02680513.2020.1835623

18 American Psychological Association. (2021). *Singular "They."* https://apastyle.apa.org/style-grammar-guidelines/grammar/singular-they

19 *The Open Pedagogy Notebook* by Steel Wagstaff is licensed under CC BY 4.0

20 Verkuyl, M., Lapum, J., St-Amant, O., Bregstein, J., & Hughes, M. (2020). Healthcare students' use of an e-textbook open educational resource on vital sign measurement: A qualitative study. *Open Learning: The Journal of Open, Distance and e-Learning.* https://doi.org/10.1080/02680513.2020.1835623

Chapter 1

Foundational Mental Health Concepts

1.1 INTRODUCTION

My Notes

Learning Objectives

- Describe basic concepts related to mental health care
- Establish a safe environment for clients, nurses, and other staff
- Discuss psychiatric-mental health nursing and associated standards of care
- Apply principles of patient-centered care while considering client diversity across the life span

Mental health is an important part of everyone's overall health and well-being. Mental health includes our emotional, psychological, and social well-being. It affects how we think, feel, and act. It also helps determine how we handle stress, relate to others, and make healthy choices. Mental health is important at every stage of life, from childhood to adolescence and through adulthood.[1] This chapter will provide an overview of mental health, mental illness, and mental health nursing. As with all areas of nursing, when caring for a person with a mental health diagnosis, it is important to focus on patient-centered care and evaluate the effectiveness of care in terms of the highest level of functioning that person is able to achieve.

Reflective Questions

As we begin this chapter, reflect on the following questions:

1. How do you define mental health?
2. How do you define mental illness?
3. How do you differentiate between the two with everyday functioning?
4. Consider how you communicate with clients. Which therapeutic techniques have you found work best? What interferes with effective communication?
5. How does ineffective communication impact client care? How can it affect your nursing license or create legal implications?

1 Centers for Disease Control and Prevention. (2021, July 20). *Mental health*. https://www.cdc.gov/mentalhealth/index.htm

My Notes

1.2 MENTAL HEALTH AND MENTAL ILLNESS

Mental health is an essential component of health. The World Health Organization (WHO) defines **health** as a state of complete physical, mental, and social well-being and not merely the absence of disease or infirmity. **Mental health** is a state of well-being in which an individual realizes their own abilities, copes with the normal stresses of life, works productively, and contributes to their community. The promotion, protection, and restoration of mental health is a vital concern of individuals, nurses, communities, and societies throughout the world.[1]

According to the American Psychiatric Association, **mental illness** is a health condition involving changes in emotion, thinking, or behavior (or a combination of these) associated with emotional distress and problems functioning in social, work, or family activities.[2] Mental illness is common in the United States. Nearly one in five (19 percent) of adults experience some form of mental illness, one in twelve (8.5 percent) have a substance use disorder, and one in 24 (4 percent) have a serious mental illness.[3]

Poor mental health increases the risk of chronic physical illnesses, such as heart disease, cancer, and strokes, and can lead to thoughts and intentions of suicide. Suicide is a common symptom associated with mental illness and is the second leading cause of death in Americans aged 15-34.[4]

 View a video: The WHO Special Initiative on Mental Health (2019-2023).[5]

---

1 World Health Organization. (2018, March 30). *Mental health: Strengthening our response.* https://www.who.int/news-room/fact-sheets/detail/mental-health-strengthening-our-response

2 American Psychiatric Association. (n.d.). *What is mental illness?* https://www.psychiatry.org/patients-families/what-is-mental-illness

3 American Psychiatric Association. (n.d.). *What is mental illness?* https://www.psychiatry.org/patients-families/what-is-mental-illness

4 Centers for Disease Control and Prevention. (2021, July 20). *Mental health.* https://www.cdc.gov/mentalhealth/index.htm

5 World Health Organization (WHO). (2020, July 20). *WHO special initiative on mental health (2019-2023)* [Video]. YouTube. All rights reserved. https://youtu.be/ti7OIMq7V9I

Mental Health Continuum

My Notes

Mental health fluctuates over the course of an individual's life span and can range from well-being to emotional problems and/or mental illness as indicated on the **mental health continuum** illustrated in Figure 1.1.[6,7,8]

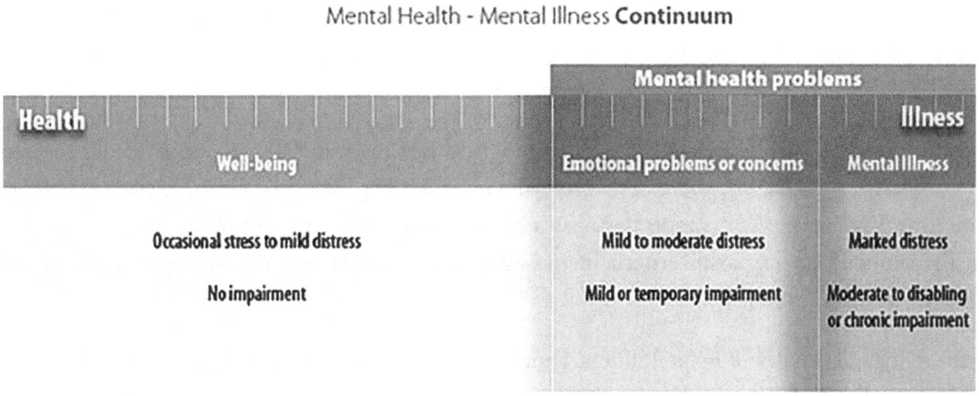

Mental Health - Mental Illness **Continuum**

Mental health problems
Health
Illness
Well-being
Emotional problems or concerns
Mental Illness
Occasional stress to mild distress
No impairment
Mild to moderate distress
Mild or temporary impairment
Marked distress
Moderate to disabling or chronic impairment

Figure 1.1 Mental Health Continuum (Used with permission.)

Well-being is on the "healthy" range of the mental health continuum in which individuals are experiencing a state of good mental and emotional health. They may experience stress and discomfort resulting from occasional problems of everyday life, but they are able to cope effectively with these stressors and experience no impairments to daily functioning.

On the other end of the mental health continuum are mental health problems where individuals have progressively more difficulty coping with serious problems and stressors. Within this range are two categories: emotional problems/concerns and mental illness. For individuals experiencing emotional problems, discomfort has risen to a level of mild to moderate distress, and they are experiencing mild or temporary impairments in functioning, such as insomnia, lack of concentration, or loss of appetite. As their level of distress increases, they may seek treatment and often start with visiting their primary health care provider.

Emotional problems become classified as "mental illness" when an individual's level of distress becomes significant, and they have moderate to severe impairment in daily functioning at work, school, or home. Mental illness includes relatively common disorders, such as depression and anxiety, as well as less common disorders such as schizophrenia. Mental illness is characterized by alterations in thinking, mood, or behavior. The term **serious**

6 "continuum.jpg" by University of Michigan is used with permission. Access the original at https://hr.umich.edu/benefits-wellness/health-well-being/mhealthy/faculty-staff-well-being/mental-emotional-health/mental-emotional-health-classes-training-events/online-tutorial-supervisors/section-1-what-you-need-know-about-mental-health-problems-substance-misuse

7 William, S. (2021, January 18). The continuum between temperament and mental illness as dynamical phases and transitions. *Frontiers in Psychiatry, 11*, 1617. https://doi.org/10.3389/fpsyt.2020.614982

8 University of Michigan Human Resources. (n.d.). *Section 1: What you need to know about mental health problems and substance misuse.* https://hr.umich.edu/benefits-wellness/health-well-being/mhealthy/faculty-staff-well-being/mental-emotional-health/mental-emotional-health-classes-training-events/online-tutorial-supervisors/section-1-what-you-need-know-about-mental-health-problems-substance-misuse

My Notes

mental illness refers to mental illness that causes disabling functional impairment that substantially interferes with one or more major life activities. The Americans With Disabilities Act defines **major life activities** as, "caring for oneself, performing manual tasks, seeing, hearing, eating, sleeping, walking, standing, lifting, bending, speaking, breathing, learning, reading, concentrating, thinking, communicating, and working."[9] Examples of serious mental illnesses that commonly interfere with major life activities include major depressive disorder, schizophrenia, and bipolar disorder.[10] Individuals with serious mental illnesses may experience long-term impairments ranging from moderate to disabling in nature, but many can lead productive lives with effective treatment. Roughly half of schizophrenia patients recovered or significantly improved over the long-term, suggesting that functional remission is possible.[11,12]

Mental health providers, such as psychiatrists, psychologists, therapists, social workers, or advanced practice mental health nurses, use the *Diagnostic and Statistical Manual of Mental Disorders, Fifth Edition (DSM-5)* published by the American Psychiatric Association to assess a client's signs and symptoms and determine a mental health diagnosis. The manual lists diagnostic criteria including feelings, behaviors, and time frames to be officially classified as a mental health disorder.[13]

There are more than 200 types of mental illness. People can experience different types of mental health disorders, and different disorders can occur at the same time or vary in intensity over time. Mental illness can be ongoing, occur over a short period of time, or be episodic (i.e., it comes and goes with discrete beginnings and ends).[14]

Read more information about specific mental health disorders at the Medline Plus Mental Health and Behavior web page.

Assessing Dysfunction and Impairment

Mental health disorders have been defined as a type of dysfunction that causes distress or impaired functioning and deviates from typical or expected behavior according to societal or cultural standards. This definition includes three components referred to as dysfunction, distress, and deviance.[15]

Dysfunction includes disturbances in a person's thinking, emotional regulation, or behavior that reflects significant dysfunction in psychological, biological, or developmental processes underlying mental functioning. In other words, dysfunction refers to a breakdown in cognition, emotion, and/or behavior. For instance, an individual

---

9 Office of Federal Contract Compliance Programs. (2009, January 1). *ADA Amendments Act of 2008 frequently asked questions.* U.S. Department of Labor. https://www.dol.gov/agencies/ofccp/faqs/americans-with-disabilities-act-amendments

10 American Psychiatric Association. (n.d.). *What is mental illness?* https://www.psychiatry.org/patients-families/what-is-mental-illness

11 Vita, A., & Barlati, S. (2018). Recovery from schizophrenia: Is it possible? *Current Opinion in Psychiatry, 31*(3), 246–255. https://doi.org/10.1097/YCO.0000000000000407

12 Rakitzi, S., Georgila, P., & Becker-Woitag, A. P. (2021). The recovery process for individuals with schizophrenia in the context of evidence-based psychotherapy and rehabilitation: A systematic review. *European Psychologist, 26*(2), 96–111. https://doi.org/10.1027/1016-9040/a000400

13 American Psychiatric Association. (2013). *Desk reference to the diagnostic criteria from DSM-5.*

14 Centers for Disease Control and Prevention. (2021, July 20). *Mental health.* https://www.cdc.gov/mentalhealth/index.htm

15 *Culture and Psychology* by Worthy, Lavigne, and Romero is licensed under CC BY-NC-SA 4.0

My Notes

experiencing a delusion that they are an omnipotent deity has a breakdown in cognition because their thought processes are not consistent with reality. An individual who is unable to experience pleasure has a breakdown in emotion, and an individual who is unable to leave home and attend work due to fear of having a panic attack is exhibiting a breakdown in behavior.[16]

Distress refers to psychological and/or physical pain. Simply put, distress refers to suffering. For example, the loss of a loved one causes anyone to experience emotional pain, distress, and a temporary impairment in functioning. **Impairment** refers to a limited ability to engage in activities of daily living (i.e., they cannot maintain personal hygiene, prepare meals, or pay bills) or participate in social events, work, or school. Impairment can also interfere with the ability to perform important life roles such as a caregiver, parent, or student.[17]

Deviance refers to behavior that violates social norms or cultural expectations because one's culture determines what is "normal." When a person is described as "deviant," it means they are not following the stated and unstated rules of their society (referred to as **social norms**).[18]

Nurses complete and document initial and ongoing assessments of dysfunction, distress, and behavior associated with an individual's diagnosed mental health disorder. The World Health Organization Disability Assessment Scale (WHODAS) is a tool recommended in the *DSM-5* to assess impairments resulting from mental illness.[19] The **WHODAS** is a generic assessment instrument that provides a standardized method for measuring health and disability across cultures.[20] The WHODAS assesses functioning in six domains: cognition, mobility, self-care, getting along, life activities, and participation.[21]

View the WHODAS 2.0 web page.

The Global Assessment of Functioning (GAF) was historically used to rate the seriousness of a mental illness and measure how symptoms affect an individual's day-to-day life on a scale of 0 to 100. It is an overall (global) measure of how clients are doing and rates psychological, social, and occupational functioning on the continuum from mental well-being to serious mental illness. The higher the score, the better the daily functioning. The GAF was omitted from the *DSM-5* because it had questionable validity and reliability, but some government agencies and insurance companies continue to include it in paperwork to assess client functioning.[22]

---

16 *Culture and Psychology* by Worthy, Lavigne, and Romero is licensed under CC BY-NC-SA 4.0

17 *Culture and Psychology* by Worthy, Lavigne, and Romero is licensed under CC BY-NC-SA 4.0

18 *Culture and Psychology* by Worthy, Lavigne, and Romero is licensed under CC BY-NC-SA 4.0

19 Office of Federal Contract Compliance Programs. (2009, January 1). *ADA Amendments Act of 2008 frequently asked questions.* U.S. Department of Labor. https://www.dol.gov/agencies/ofccp/faqs/americans-with-disabilities-act-amendments

20 World Health Organization. (2012). *Measuring health and disability: Manual for WHO disability assessment schedule (WHODAS 2.0).* [Manual]. https://www.who.int/publications/i/item/measuring-health-and-disability-manual-for-who-disability-assessment-schedule-(-whodas-2.0)

21 National Academies of Sciences, Engineering, and Medicine. (2016). *Measuring specific mental illness diagnoses with functional impairment: Work-shop summary.* J. C. Rivard and K. Marton, Rapporteurs. Committee on National Statistics and Board on Behavioral, Cognitive, and Sensory Sciences, Division of Behavioral and Social Sciences and Education. Board on Health Sciences Policy, Institute of Medicine. The National Academies Press. http://elibrary.pcu.edu.ph:9000/digi/NA02/2016/21920.pdf

22 Smith, M. (2021, February 6). *What is the global assessment of functioning (GAF) scale?* WebMD. https://www.webmd.com/mental-health/gaf-scale-facts

My Notes

Recovery

Mental illness is treatable. Research shows that people with mental illness can get better, and many recover completely.[23] The majority of individuals with mental illness continue to function in their daily lives. **Recovery** refers to a process of change through which individuals improve their health and wellness, live a self-directed life, and strive to reach their full potential.[24] Dimensions that support a life in recovery include the following:

- **Health:** Overcoming or managing one's disease(s), as well as living in a physically and emotionally healthy way
- **Home:** Having a stable and safe place to live
- **Purpose:** Participating in meaningful daily activities, such as a job, school, volunteerism, family caretaking, or creative endeavors, and the independence, income, and resources to participate in society
- **Community:** Enjoying relationships and social networks that provide support, friendship, love, and hope

Early Signs of Mental Health Problems

Mental health problems are common. We all experience problems and stressors from daily living at the milder end of the mental health continuum, and at some point in our lives, we are likely to experience emotional problems or concerns. Mental illness, though less common, is nevertheless a frequent occurrence, and it is estimated that approximately one in five Americans will personally experience a mental illness in their lifetime.[25,26]

Nurses in all care settings must recognize signs and symptoms of diagnosed and undiagnosed emotional and mental health problems in clients. Each mental health disorder has specific signs and symptoms, but common signs of mental health problems in adults and adolescents are as follows[27]:

- Excessive worrying or fear
- Excessive sad or low feelings
- Confused thinking or problems concentrating and learning
- Extreme mood changes, including uncontrollable "highs" or feelings of euphoria
- Prolonged or strong feelings of irritability or anger
- Avoidance of friends and social activities

---

23 Centers for Disease Control and Prevention. (2021, July 20). *Mental health.* https://www.cdc.gov/mentalhealth/index.htm

24 Center for Substance Abuse Treatment (US). (2014). *Trauma-informed care in behavioral health services.* https://www.ncbi.nlm.nih.gov/books/NBK207201/

25 William, S. (2021, January 18). The continuum between temperament and mental illness as dynamical phases and transitions. *Frontiers in Psychiatry, 11,* 1617. https://doi.org/10.3389/fpsyt.2020.614982

26 National Alliance on Mental Illness (NAMI). (2022, June). *Mental health by the numbers.* https://www.nami.org/mhstats#:~:text=21%25%20of%20U.S.%20adults%20experienced,represents%201%20in%2020%20adults

27 National Alliance on Mental Illness. (n.d.). *Warning signs and symptoms.* https://nami.org/About-Mental-Illness/Warning-Signs-and-Symptoms

My Notes

- Difficulty understanding or relating to other people
- Changes in sleeping habits or feeling tired and low energy
- Changes in eating habits, such as increased hunger or lack of appetite
- Changes in sex drive
- Disturbances in perceiving reality referred to as hallucinations (i.e., when a person senses things that don't exist in reality)
- Inability to perceive changes in one's own feelings, behavior, or personality (i.e., lack of insight)
- Misuse of substances like alcohol, drugs, or prescription medications
- Multiple physical ailments without obvious causes (such as headaches, stomachaches, or vague and ongoing "aches and pains")
- Thoughts of suicide
- Inability to carry out daily activities or handle daily problems and stress
- Intense fear of weight gain or being overly concerned with appearance

Mental health disorders can also be present in young children. Because children are still learning how to identify and talk about thoughts and emotions, their most obvious symptoms are behavioral or complaints of physical symptoms. Behavioral symptoms in children can include the following[28]:

- Changes in school performance
- Excessive worry or anxiety, for example fighting to avoid going to bed or school
- Hyperactive behavior
- Frequent nightmares
- Frequent disobedience or aggression
- Frequent temper tantrums

View the following YouTube video about warning signs of mental health problems[29]: 10 Common Warning Signs of a Mental Health Condition.

Cultural Impact

Cultural values and beliefs impact how a person views certain ideas or behaviors. In the case of mental health, it can impact whether or not the individual seeks help, the type of help sought, and the support available. Every individual has different cultural beliefs and faces a unique journey to recovery. In general, historically marginalized

28 National Alliance on Mental Illness. (n.d.). *Warning signs and symptoms.* https://nami.org/About-Mental-Illness/Warning-Signs-and-Symptoms

29 NAMI. (2015, February 2). *10 common warning signs of a mental health condition* [Video]. YouTube. All rights reserved. https://youtu.be/zt4sOjWwV3M

My Notes

communities in the United States are less likely to access mental health treatment, or they wait until symptoms are severe before seeking assistance.[30]

Four ways that culture can impact mental well-being are the following[31]:

- **Cultural stigma.** Every culture has a different perspective on mental health, and most cultures have a stigma surrounding mental health. Mental health challenges may be considered a weakness and something to hide, which can make it harder for those struggling to talk openly and ask for help.
- **Describing symptoms.** Culture can influence how people describe or feel about their symptoms. It can affect whether someone chooses to recognize and talk openly about physical symptoms, emotional symptoms, or both. For example, members of the Amish community are typically stoic and endure physical and emotional pain without complaining.
- **Community support.** Cultural factors can determine how much support someone gets from their family and community when it comes to mental health. Because of existing stigma, it can be challenging for individuals to find mental health treatment and support.
- **Resources.** When looking for mental health treatment, it can be difficult to find resources and treatment options that take into account a specific culture's concerns and needs.

Nurses can help clients by understanding the role culture plays in their mental health. If potential signs of undiagnosed or poorly managed mental health disorders are present, nurses should make appropriate referrals for further assessment and follow-up.

Read more about cultural diversity and providing culturally responsive care in the "Diverse Patients" chapter of Open RN *Nursing Fundamentals.*

Causes of Mental Illness

Mental health researchers have developed several theories to explain the causes of mental health disorders, but they have not reached consensus. One factor in which they all agree is that an individual is not at fault for the condition, and they cannot simply turn symptoms on or off at will. There are likely several factors that combine to trigger a mental health disorder, including environmental, biological, and genetic factors.[32]

30 Mental Health First Aid USA. (2019, July 11). *Four ways culture impacts mental health.* National Council for Mental Wellbeing. https://www.mentalhealthfirstaid.org/2019/07/four-ways-culture-impacts-mental-health/

31 Mental Health First Aid USA. (2019, July 11). *Four ways culture impacts mental health.* National Council for Mental Wellbeing. https://www.mentalhealthfirstaid.org/2019/07/four-ways-culture-impacts-mental-health/

32 University of Michigan Human Resources. (n.d.). *Section 1: What you need to know about mental health problems and substance misuse.* https://hr.umich.edu/benefits-wellness/health-well-being/mhealthy/faculty-staff-well-being/mental-emotional-health/mental-emotional-health-classes-training-events/online-tutorial-supervisors/section-1-what-you-need-know-about-mental-health-problems-substance-misuse

My Notes

Environmental Factors

Individuals are affected by broad social and cultural factors, as well as by unique factors in their personal environments. Social factors such as racism, discrimination, poverty, and violence (often referred to as "social determinants of health") can contribute to mental illness.

> Read more about addressing social determinants of health in the "Advocacy" chapter of Open RN *Nursing Management and Professional Concepts.*

Additionally, it is estimated that 61% of adults have experienced early **adverse childhood experiences (ACEs)** such as abuse, neglect, or growing up in a household with violence, mental illness, substance misuse, incarceration, or divorce. Chronic stress from ACEs can change brain development and affect how the body responds to stress. ACEs are linked to chronic health problems, mental illness, and substance misuse in adulthood.[33,34] See Figure 1.2[35] for an image of adverse childhood experiences.

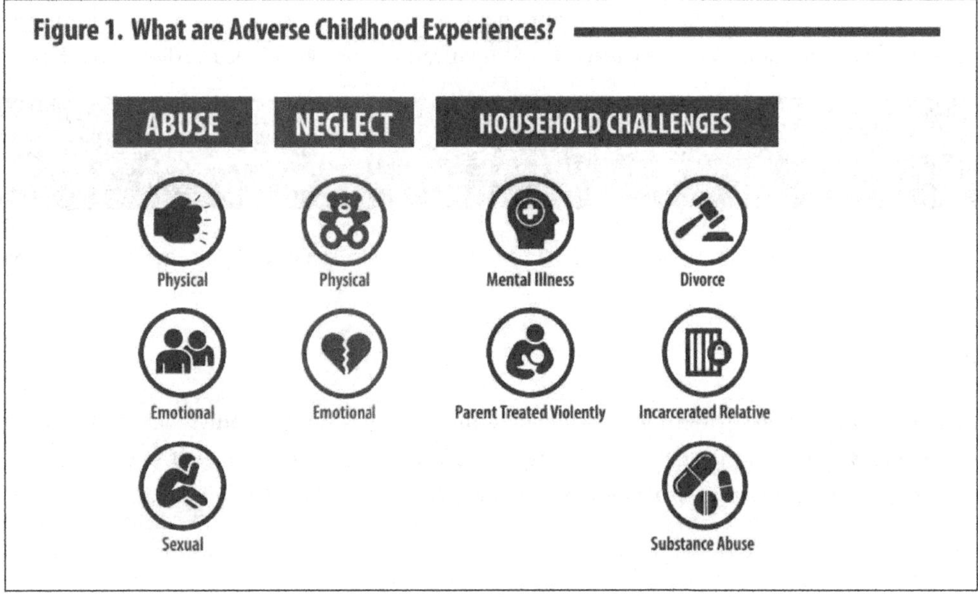

Figure 1.2 Adverse Childhood Experiences (ACEs)

Individual trauma resulting from an event, series of events, or set of circumstances that is experienced as physically or emotionally harmful can have lasting adverse effects on the individual's functioning and mental, physical, social,

---

33 University of Michigan Human Resources. (n.d.). *Section 1: What you need to know about mental health problems and substance misuse.* https://hr.umich.edu/benefits-wellness/health-well-being/mhealthy/faculty-staff-well-being/mental-emotional-health/mental-emotional-health-classes-training-events/online-tutorial-supervisors/section-1-what-you-need-know-about-mental-health-problems-substance-misuse

34 National Human Trafficking Training and Technical Assistance Center. (n.d.) *The original ACE study.* https://nhttac.acf.hhs.gov/soar/eguide/stop/adverse_childhood_experiences

35 "ACEs.png" by unknown author for Centers for Disease Control and Prevention is licensed in the Public Domain. Access for free at https://www.cdc.gov/injury/pdfs/priority/ACEs-Strategic-Plan_Final_508.pdf

My Notes

emotional, or spiritual well-being.[36] Read more about ACEs and addressing individual trauma in the "Introduction to Trauma-Informed Care" section of this chapter.

Take the Adverse Childhood Experiences Questionnaire for Adults to better understand how previous experiences can affect one's well-being.

Current stressors such as relationship difficulties, the loss of a job, the birth of a child, a move, or prolonged problems at work can also be important contributory environmental factors.[37]

Read more about stress in the "Stress, Coping, and Crisis Intervention" chapter.

Biological Factors

Scientists believe the brain can have an imbalance of neurotransmitters, such as dopamine, acetylcholine, gamma-aminobutyric acid (GABA), norepinephrine, glutamate, and serotonin, resulting in changes in behavior, mood, and thought. While causes of fluctuations in brain chemicals aren't fully understood, contributing factors can include physical illness, hormonal changes, reactions to medication, substance misuse, diet, and stress.[38]

Read more about neurotransmitters and the central nervous system in the "Psychotropic Medications" chapter.

Some studies also suggest that depressive and bipolar disorders are accompanied by immune system dysregulation and inflammation.[39]

Genetics

There appears to be a hereditary pattern to some mental illnesses. For example, individuals with major depressive disorder often have parents or other close relatives with the same illness. Research continues to investigate genes involved in specific disorders so that treatment can be effectively targeted to the individual.[40]

---

36 U.S. Department of Health & Human Services. (2020, January 24). *Strategic goal 3: Strengthen the economic and social well-being of Americans across the lifespan.* https://www.hhs.gov/about/strategic-plan/strategic-goal-3/index.html

37 University of Michigan Human Resources. (n.d.). *Section 1: What you need to know about mental health problems and substance misuse.* https://hr.umich.edu/benefits-wellness/health-well-being/mhealthy/faculty-staff-well-being/mental-emotional-health/mental-emotional-health-classes-training-events/online-tutorial-supervisors/section-1-what-you-need-know-about-mental-health-problems-substance-misuse

38 University of Michigan Human Resources. (n.d.). *Section 1: What you need to know about mental health problems and substance misuse.* https://hr.umich.edu/benefits-wellness/health-well-being/mhealthy/faculty-staff-well-being/mental-emotional-health/mental-emotional-health-classes-training-events/online-tutorial-supervisors/section-1-what-you-need-know-about-mental-health-problems-substance-misuse

39 Kraybill, O. (2019, May 31). Inflammation and mental health symptoms. *Psychology Today.* https://www.psychologytoday.com/us/blog/expressive-trauma-integration/201905/inflammation-and-mental-health-symptoms

40 University of Michigan Human Resources. (n.d.). *Section 1: What you need to know about mental health problems and substance misuse.* https://hr.umich.edu/benefits-wellness/health-well-being/mhealthy/faculty-staff-well-being/mental-emotional-health/mental-emotional-health-classes-training-events/online-tutorial-supervisors/section-1-what-you-need-know-about-mental-health-problems-substance-misuse

My Notes

View the following YouTube video on causes of mental illness[41]: Understanding the Biology of Mental Illness.

WHO Guidelines for Mental Health Care

It is vital for nurses to protect and promote the mental well-being of all individuals and address the needs of individuals with diagnosed mental disorders.[42] The World Health Organization (WHO) published the *Mental Health Intervention Guide* for nurses and primary health care providers that provides evidence-based guidance and tools for assessing and managing priority mental health and substance use disorders using clinical decision-making protocols. Essential principles for providing mental health care include promoting respect and dignity for the individuals seeking care; using effective communication skills to ensure care is provided in a nonjudgmental, nonstigmatizing, and supportive manner; and conducting comprehensive assessments.[43]

Promoting Respect and Dignity

Individuals with mental health and substance use conditions should be treated with respect and dignity in a culturally appropriate manner. Health care professionals should promote the preferences of people with mental health and substance use disorders and support them, their family members, and their loved ones in an inclusive and equitable manner. These are some tips discussed in the WHO *Mental Health Intervention Guide*[44]:

Do:

- Treat people with mental health and substance use conditions with respect and dignity.
- Protect confidentiality.
- Ensure privacy.
- Provide access to information and explain the proposed treatment risks and benefits in writing when possible.
- Make sure the person provides consent to treatment.
- Promote autonomy and independent living in the community.
- Provide access to decision-making options.

Don't:

- Discriminate against people with mental health and substance use conditions.
- Ignore individual preferences.

---

41 Alabama Department of Health. (2011, July 29). *Understanding the biology of mental illness* [Video]. YouTube. All rights reserved. https://youtu.be/LLUoG9Se77w

42 World Health Organization. (2018, March 30). *Mental health: Strengthening our response.* https://www.who.int/news-room/fact-sheets/detail/mental-health-strengthening-our-response

43 *mhGAP Intervention Guide - Version 2.0* by World Health Organization is licensed under CC BY-NC-SA 3.0

44 *mhGAP Intervention Guide - Version 2.0* by World Health Organization is licensed under CC BY-NC-SA 3.0

My Notes

- Make decisions for or on behalf of individuals.
- Use overly technical language when explaining proposed treatment.

Using Effective Communication Skills

Using effective communication skills promotes quality mental health care. Tips for effective communication from the WHO *Mental Health Intervention Guide* include the following[45]:

Create an Environment That Facilitates Open Communication.

- Meet the person in a private space, if possible.
- Be welcoming and conduct introductions in a culturally appropriate manner.
- Use culturally appropriate eye contact, body language, and facial expressions that facilitate trust.
- Explain to adults that information discussed during the visit will be kept confidential. (Special considerations regarding "conditional confidentiality" and mandatory reporting for minors are discussed in the "Childhood and Adolescence Disorders" chapter.)
- If caregivers are present, suggest speaking with the client alone (except for young children) and obtain consent from the client to share clinical information.
- When interviewing a young person, consider having another person present who identifies with the same gender to maintain feelings of a psychologically safe environment.

Involve the Person.

- Include the person (and with their consent, their caregivers and family members) in all aspects of assessment and management as much as possible. This includes children, adolescents, adults, and older adults.

Start by Listening.

- Actively listen. Be empathic and sensitive. (Read more about active listening in the "Therapeutic Communication and the Nurse-Client Relationship" chapter.)
- Allow the person to speak without interruption.
- Be patient and ask for clarification of unclear information.
- For children, use language that they can understand. For example, ask about their interests (toys, friends, school, etc.).
- For adolescents, convey that you understand their feelings and situation.

Be Friendly, Respectful, and Nonjudgmental.

- Always be respectful.
- Be nonjudgmental about an individual's behaviors and appearances.
- Remain calm and professional.

---

45 *mhGAP Intervention Guide - Version 2.0* by World Health Organization is licensed under CC BY-NC-SA 3.0

Use Good Verbal Communication Skills.

- Use simple language. Be clear and concise. Avoid medical terminology only understood by health care professionals.
- Use open-ended questions and other therapeutic communication techniques. (Read more about specific techniques in the "Therapeutic Communication and the Nurse-Client Relationship" chapter.) For example:
    - Use open-ended questions: "Tell me more about what happened?"
    - Summarize: "So, your brother pushed you off your bike and then laughed when you fell and started crying?"
    - Clarify: "To clarify, were you at home or a neighbor's house when this happened?"
- Summarize and repeat key points at the end of the conversation.
- Allow the person to ask questions about the information provided. For example, "What questions do you have about what we have discussed today?"

Respond With Sensitivity When People Disclose Traumatic Experiences (E.G., Sexual Assault, Violence, or Self-Harm).

- Thank the person for sharing this sensitive information.
- Show extra sensitivity when discussing difficult topics.
- Remind the person that what they tell you will only be shared with the immediate treatment team to provide the best possible care.
- Acknowledge that it may have been difficult for the person to disclose the information.

Therapeutic Relationship

In all nursing care, the therapeutic relationship with the client is essential. This is especially so in psychiatric care, where the therapeutic relationship is considered to be the foundation of client care and healing.[46] Although nurse generalists are not expected to perform advanced psychiatric interventions, all nurses are expected to engage in compassionate, supportive relationships with their patients and use therapeutic communication as part of the "art of nursing."[47]

The nurse-client relationship establishes trust and rapport with a specific purpose. It facilitates therapeutic communication and engages the client in decision-making regarding their plan of care. Read more about therapeutic communication and the nurse-client relationship in the "Therapeutic Communication and the Nurse-Client Relationship" chapter.

---

46 Ross, C. A., & Goldner, E. M. (2009). Stigma, negative attitudes and discrimination towards mental illness within the nursing profession: A review of the literature. *Journal of Psychiatric and Mental Health Nursing, 16*(6), 558-567. https://doi.org/10.1111/j.1365-2850.2009.01399.x

47 Centers for Disease Control & Prevention. (2021, July 22). *Coping with stress.* https://www.cdc.gov/mentalhealth/stress-coping/cope-with-stress/index.html

My Notes

Conducting Comprehensive Assessments

Clients undergo comprehensive assessments related to their disorder, including mental status examination, psychosocial assessment, physical examination, and review of laboratory results. Specific nursing assessments are further discussed in the "Application of the Nursing Process in Mental Health Care" chapter, as well in each "Disorder" chapter. Persons with severe mental health and substance use disorders are two to three times more likely to die of preventable disease like infections and cardiovascular disorders, so it is also important for nurses to advocate for the medical treatment of existing physical disorders.[48]

View the WHO's Mental Health Gap Intervention Guide.

48 *mhGAP Intervention Guide - Version 2.0* by World Health Organization is licensed under CC BY-NC-SA 3.0

1.3 INTRODUCTION TO TRAUMA-INFORMED CARE

My Notes

Many individuals experience trauma during their lifetimes that can have a lasting impact on their mental health. **Trauma** results from an event, series of events, or set of circumstances that are experienced by an individual as physically or emotionally harmful and can have lasting adverse effects on the individual's functioning and physical, social, emotional, or spiritual well-being. Events may be human-made, such as war, terrorism, sexual abuse, violence, or medical trauma, or they can be the products of nature (e.g., flooding, hurricanes, and tornadoes). Nurses must keep in mind to not interject their own experiences or perspectives because something minor to them may be major to the client.

It's not just the event itself that determines if it is traumatic, but the individual's experience of the event. Two people may be exposed to the same event or series of events but experience and interpret these events in vastly different ways. Various biopsychosocial and cultural factors influence an individual's immediate response and long-term reactions to trauma. For most individuals, regardless of the severity of the trauma, the effects of trauma are met with **resilience**, defined as the ability to rise above circumstances or meet challenges with fortitude. Resilience includes the process of using available resources to negotiate hardship and/or the consequences of adverse events.[1]

Trauma can affect people of any culture, age, gender, or sexual orientation. Individuals may also experience trauma even if the event didn't happen to them. A traumatic experience can be a single event, a series of events, or adverse childhood experiences (ACEs). Review information about ACEs in the "Mental Health and Mental Illness" section of this chapter. There has been an increased focus on the ways in which trauma, psychological distress, quality of life, health, mental illness, and substance misuse are linked. For example, the terrorist attacks of September 11, 2001, the wars in Iraq and Afghanistan, disastrous hurricanes, and the COVID pandemic have moved traumatic experiences to the forefront of national consciousness. Trauma can affect individuals, families, groups, communities, specific cultures, and generations. It can overwhelm an individual's ability to cope; stimulate the "fight, flight, or freeze" stress reaction; and produce a sense of fear, vulnerability, and helplessness.[2]

Read more information about the stress reaction in the "Stress, Coping, and Crisis Intervention" chapter.

For some people, reactions to a traumatic event are temporary, whereas other people have prolonged reactions to trauma with enduring mental health consequences, such as post-traumatic stress disorder, anxiety disorder, substance use disorder, mood disorder, or psychotic disorder. Others may exhibit culturally mediated physical symptoms referred to as **somatization**, in which psychological stress is expressed through physical concerns such as chronic headaches, pain, and stomachaches. Traumatic experiences can significantly impact how an individual functions in daily life and how they seek medical care.[3]

Individuals may not recognize the significant effects of trauma or may avoid the topic altogether. Likewise, nurses may not ask questions that elicit a client's history of trauma. They may feel unprepared to address trauma-related

---

1 Center for Substance Abuse Treatment (US). (2014). *Trauma-informed care in behavioral health services.* https://www.ncbi.nlm.nih.gov/books/NBK207201/

2 Center for Substance Abuse Treatment (US). (2014). *Trauma-informed care in behavioral health services.* https://www.ncbi.nlm.nih.gov/books/NBK207201/

3 Center for Substance Abuse Treatment (US). (2014). *Trauma-informed care in behavioral health services.* https://www.ncbi.nlm.nih.gov/books/NBK207201/

My Notes

issues proactively or struggle to effectively address traumatic experiences within the constraints of their agency's policies.[4]

By recognizing that traumatic experiences are closely tied to mental health, nurses can provide trauma-informed care and promote resilience. **Trauma-informed care (TIC)** is a strengths-based framework that acknowledges the prevalence and impact of traumatic experiences in clinical practice. TIC emphasizes physical, psychological, and emotional safety for both survivors and health professionals and creates opportunities for survivors to rebuild a sense of control and empowerment (i.e., resilience).[5] TIC acknowledges that clients can be retraumatized by unexamined agency policies and practices and stresses the importance of providing patient-centered care rather than applying general treatment approaches.[6]

TIC enhances therapeutic communication between the client and the nurse. It decreases risks associated with misunderstanding clients' reactions or underestimating the need for referrals for trauma-specific treatment. TIC encourages patient-centered care by involving the client in setting goals and planning care that optimizes therapeutic outcomes and minimizes adverse effects. Clients are more likely to feel empowered, invested, and satisfied when they receive TIC.[7]

Implementing TIC requires specific training, but it begins with the first contact a person has with an agency. It requires all staff members (e.g., receptionists, direct patient-care staff, nurses, supervisors, and administrators) to recognize that an individual's traumatic experiences can greatly influence their receptivity and engagement with health services. It can affect their interactions with staff, as well as their responsiveness to care plans and interventions.[8]

View the following YouTube video on trauma-informed approach to health care[9]: Dr. Pickens Explains Trauma-Informed Approach.

Read more details about trauma-informed care (TIC) in the "Trauma, Abuse, and Violence" chapter.

4 Center for Substance Abuse Treatment (US). (2014). *Trauma-informed care in behavioral health services.* https://www.ncbi.nlm.nih.gov/books/NBK207201/

5 Center for Substance Abuse Treatment (US). (2014). *Trauma-informed care in behavioral health services.* https://www.ncbi.nlm.nih.gov/books/NBK207201/

6 Center for Substance Abuse Treatment (US). (2014). *Trauma-informed care in behavioral health services.* https://www.ncbi.nlm.nih.gov/books/NBK207201/

7 Center for Substance Abuse Treatment (US). (2014). *Trauma-informed care in behavioral health services.* https://www.ncbi.nlm.nih.gov/books/NBK207201/

8 Center for Substance Abuse Treatment (US). (2014). *Trauma-informed care in behavioral health services.* https://www.ncbi.nlm.nih.gov/books/NBK207201/

9 Washington State Health Care Authority. (2019, June 24). *Dr. Pickens explains trauma-informed approach* [Video]. YouTube. All rights reserved. https://youtu.be/6syEFO4OSFU

My Notes

1.4 STIGMA

Despite a recent focus on mental health in the United States, there are still many harmful attitudes and misunderstandings surrounding mental illnesses that can cause people to ignore their mental health and make it more difficult for them to reach out for help.[1,2] **Stigma** has been defined as a cluster of negative attitudes and beliefs that motivates the general public to fear, reject, avoid, and discriminate against people with mental health disorders.[3]

It estimated that nearly two thirds of people with diagnosable mental health disorders do not seek treatment due to the stigma of mental illness. The *U.S. Surgeon General's Report* in 1999 was a milestone report that sought to dispel the stigma of mental illness and its impact on those seeking care.[4] The National Alliance on Mental Illness (NAMI) seeks to improve the lives of those with mental illness and reduce stigma through education, support, and advocacy. NAMI encourages people to share their stories to discredit stereotypes, break the silence, and document discrimination.[5]

Take a quiz in the following box to separate facts from myths about mental illness.

Take the CDC's Mental Health Quiz.

However, stigma and negative attitudes toward mental illness can still be found among nurses. A review of nursing literature by Ross and Golder explored negative attitudes and discrimination towards mental illness in the nursing profession. Several studies from a variety of countries indicated that health care professionals can be classified in three categories in relation to stigma, including "stigmatizers," "the stigmatized," and "de-stigmatizers." "Stigmatizers" refer to nurses in medical settings with stereotypical attitudes towards clients with mental illnesses, psychiatric-mental health nurses, and/or psychiatry. Nurses classified as "the stigmatized" have mental health disorders or perceive stigma regarding their roles as psychiatric-mental health nurses. "De-stigmatizers" actively work to reduce stigma surrounding mental health disorders. The authors found that many nurses share commonly held stereotypical beliefs portrayed in the media. For example, clients with mental health disorders have been portrayed in the media as dangerous, unpredictable, violent, or bizarre, and these portrayals can cause fearful attitudes. Nurses in the studies were also concerned about inadvertently saying or doing "the wrong thing" or "setting off" uncontrollable behavior. Many nurses in general medical settings felt they lacked the skills to confidently and competently manage behavioral symptoms of clients with mental health disorders. The authors of the review

---

1 Centers for Disease Control and Prevention. (2021, July 20). *Mental health.* https://www.cdc.gov/mentalhealth/index.htm

2 Corrigan, P. W., & Watson, A. C. (2002). Understanding the impact of stigma on people with mental illness. *World Psychiatry: Official Journal of the World Psychiatric Association (WPA), 1*(1), 16-20. https://www.ncbi.nlm.nih.gov/pmc/articles/PMC1489832/

3 *School Materials for a Mental Health Friendly Classroom: Training Package* by SAMHSA is available in the Public Domain

4 Hegner, R. E. (2000). Dispelling the myths and stigma of mental illness: The surgeon general's report on mental health. *Issue Brief,* 754. https://www.ncbi.nlm.nih.gov/books/NBK559750/

5 Abderholden, S. (2019, March 7). *It's not stigma, it's discrimination* [Blog]. National Alliance on Mental Illness. https://www.nami.org/Blogs/NAMI-Blog/March-2019/It-s-Not-Stigma-It-s-Discrimination

My Notes

reported that nursing literature supports additional mental health education for entry-level nurses and practicing nurses to enhance their knowledge base on mental health.[6]

Nurses can reduce stigma and advocate for a client's needs and dignity by establishing a therapeutic nurse-client relationship. A therapeutic nurse-client relationship is essential in all settings, but it is especially important in mental health care where the therapeutic relationship is considered the foundation of client care and healing. Although nurse generalists are not expected to perform advanced psychiatric-mental health nursing interventions, all nurses are expected to engage in compassionate, supportive relationships with their clients.[7] In fact, in *Nursing: Scope and Standards of Practice (2021)*, the American Nurses Association states, "The nursing profession, rooted in caring relationships, demands that nurses reflect unconditional positive regard for every patient."[8]

Read more about establishing a therapeutic nurse-client relationship in the "Therapeutic Communication and the Nurse-Client Relationship" chapter.

The first step in resolving stigma is to become aware of one's personal beliefs. Take the survey in the following box to become more aware of your own attitudes and biases toward mental health care.

Take the Personal Attitudes Survey (page 8) from the Canadian Mental Health Association.

6 Ross, C. A., & Goldner, E. M. (2009). Stigma, negative attitudes and discrimination towards mental illness within the nursing profession: A review of the literature. *Journal of Psychiatric and Mental Health Nursing, 16*(6), 558-567. https://doi.org/10.1111/j.1365-2850.2009.01399.x

7 Ross, C. A., & Goldner, E. M. (2009). Stigma, negative attitudes and discrimination towards mental illness within the nursing profession: A review of the literature. *Journal of Psychiatric and Mental Health Nursing, 16*(6), 558-567. https://doi.org/10.1111/j.1365-2850.2009.01399.x

8 American Nurses Association. (2021). *Nursing: Scope and standards of practice* (4th ed.). American Nurses Association.

1.5 BOUNDARIES

My Notes

Boundaries are limits we set as individuals that define our levels of comfort when interacting with others. Personal boundaries include limits in physical, sexual, intellectual, emotional, sexual, and financial areas of our lives.

Boundaries promote psychological safety in relationships at work, home, and with partners by protecting one's well-being and limiting the stress response. For example, if you come away from a meeting or conversation with someone feeling depleted, anxious, or tense, consider if your boundaries were crossed. A lack of healthy personal boundaries can lead to emotional and physical fatigue.[1]

Five major types of personal boundaries include the following[2]:

- **Physical:** Physical boundaries refer to one's personal space, privacy, and body. For example, some people are comfortable with public displays of affection (hugs, kisses, and hand-holding), while others prefer not to be touched in public.
- **Sexual:** Sexual boundaries refer to one's comfort level with intimacy and attention of a sexual nature. This can include sexual comments and touch, not just sexual acts.
- **Intellectual:** Intellectual boundaries refer to one's thoughts and beliefs. Intellectual boundaries are not respected when someone dismisses another person's ideas and opinions.
- **Emotional:** Emotional boundaries refer to a person's feelings. For example, an individual might not feel comfortable sharing feelings with another person and prefer to share information gradually over time.
- **Financial:** Financial boundaries refer to how one prefers to spend or save money.

When caring for clients with mental health disorders, it is common to notice problems with setting appropriate boundaries. For example, a client experiencing bipolar disorder may exhibit a lack of financial and sexual boundaries. When they are experiencing a manic episode, they may spend thousands of dollars on a credit card over a weekend or have sexual relations with someone they just met. Another example of boundary issues is an individual with a depressive disorder who is treated poorly by their partner but does not leave or assert boundaries because they don't feel that they deserve to be treated any better.

Nurses must establish professional boundaries with all clients while also maintaining a respectful and caring relationship. Due to their professional role, nurses have authority and access to sensitive information that can make clients feel vulnerable. *A Nurses Guide to Professional Boundaries* by the National Council of State Boards of Nursing (NCSBN) states that it is the nurse's responsibility to use clinical judgment to determine and maintain professional boundaries. Nurses should limit self-disclosure of personal information and avoid situations where they have a personal or business relationship with a client. The difference between a caring nurse-client relationship and an over-involved relationship can be difficult to discern, especially in small communities or in community health nursing where roles may overlap. In these circumstances, it is important for the nurse to openly

1 Pattemore, C. (2021, June 2). *10 ways to build and preserve better boundaries.* PsychCentral. https://psychcentral.com/lib/10-way-to-build-and-preserve-better-boundaries#types

2 Pattemore, C. (2021, June 2). *10 ways to build and preserve better boundaries.* PsychCentral. https://psychcentral.com/lib/10-way-to-build-and-preserve-better-boundaries#types

My Notes

acknowledge their dual relationship and emphasize when they are performing in a professional capacity. Signs of inappropriate boundaries include the following[3]:

- Self-disclosing intimate or personal issues with a client
- Engaging in behaviors that could be interpreted as flirting
- Keeping secrets with a client
- Believing you are the only one who truly understands or can help the client
- Spending more time than is necessary with a particular client
- Speaking poorly about colleagues or your employment setting with the client and/or their family
- Showing favoritism to a particular client
- Meeting a client in settings outside of work
- Contacting a client and/or their family members using social media

Establishing professional boundaries with clients diagnosed with mental health disorders is essential due to the vulnerability of the client population, as well as the behavioral manifestations of some disorders. For safety purposes, nurses and nursing students should keep their last name, home address, personal telephone number, and social media handles private.

 View the NCSBN video: "Professional Boundaries in Nursing."

 Read A Nurse's Guide to Professional Boundaries PDF from the National Council of State Boards of Nursing (NCSBN).

3 National Council of State Boards of Nursing. (2018). *A nurse's guide to professional boundaries*. https://www.ncsbn.org/ProfessionalBoundaries_Complete.pdf

1.6 ESTABLISHING SAFETY

My Notes

Suicidal thoughts are a common symptom of mental health disorders and typically resolve with effective treatment. However, despite a recent increased focus on mental health care, there has been no documented decrease of suicide rates in the United States, and suicide remains the tenth leading cause of death in the country.[1]

Warning Signs of Suicide

Everyone can help prevent suicide by recognizing warning signs of suicide and intervening appropriately. Warning signs of suicide include client statements or nurse observations of the following[2]:

- Feeling like a burden
- Being isolated
- Increasing levels of anxiety
- Feeling trapped
- Being in unbearable pain
- Increasing substance use
- Looking for a way to access lethal means
- Increasing anger or rage
- Exhibiting extreme mood swings
- Expressing hopelessness
- Sleeping too little or too much
- Talking or posting about wanting to die
- Making plans for suicide

See Figure 1.3[3] for five action steps for anyone to take to prevent suicide in someone experiencing suicidal thoughts or ideations. Nurses can educate others to take the following steps if they believe someone may be in danger of suicide[4]:

- Call 911 if danger for self-harm seems imminent.
- Ask the person if they are thinking about killing themselves. Although asking this question can feel invasive, it is common for individuals with mental health problems to share their thoughts and plans regarding suicide. Asking them about suicide will not "put the idea into their head" or

---

1 The Joint Commission. (2021). *2021 Behavioral health care and human services: National patient safety goals.* https://www.jointcommission.org/-/media/tjc/documents/standards/national-patient-safety-goals/2021/simplified-2021-bhc-npsg-goals-final-11420.pdf

2 Centers for Disease Control and Prevention. (2021, July 20). *Mental health.* https://www.cdc.gov/mentalhealth/index.htm

3 "5actionsteps_t.jpg" by unknown author for National Institute of Mental Health is licensed in the Public Domain. Access for free at https://www.nimh.nih.gov/health/topics/suicide-prevention

4 Substance Abuse and Mental Health Services Administration. (2021, November 29). *Help prevent suicide.* https://www.samhsa.gov/suicide

My Notes

make it more likely that they will attempt suicide. In fact, by responding appropriately, you can help save their life by asking this question.

- Listen without judging and show you care.
- Stay with the person or make sure the person is in a private, secure place with another caring person until you can get further help.
- Remove any objects that could be used in a suicide attempt.
- Call or text 988 to reach the new nationwide Suicide and Crisis Line for a direct connection with compassionate, accessible care and support for anyone experiencing mental health-related distress.

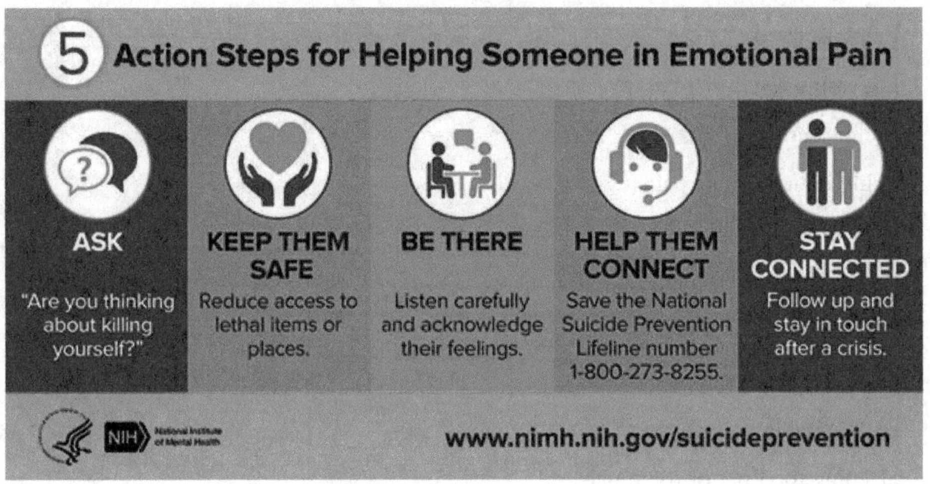

Figure 1.3 Preventing Suicide

Establishing a Safe Care Environment for Clients

In addition to encouraging these general action steps to prevent suicide, nurses can further prevent suicide by establishing a safe care environment. Establishing a safe care environment is a priority nursing intervention.

Reducing the risk for suicide is one of the National Patient Safety Goals for Behavioral Health Care established by The Joint Commission. New requirements were established in 2020 that apply to patients in psychiatric hospitals, patients being evaluated or treated for behavioral health conditions as their primary reason for care in general hospital units or critical access hospitals, and all patients who express **suicidal ideation** during their course of care.[5] These requirements include performing an environmental risk assessment, screening for suicidal ideation, assessing suicide risk, documenting risk of suicide, following evidence-based written policies and procedures, providing information on follow-up care on discharge, and monitoring effectiveness of these actions in preventing suicides. These requirements are discussed in further detail in the following subsections.[6]

---

5 The Joint Commission. (2021). *2021 Behavioral health care and human services: National patient safety goals.* https://www.jointcommission.org/-/media/tjc/documents/standards/national-patient-safety-goals/2021/simplified-2021-bhc-npsg-goals-final-11420.pdf

6 The Joint Commission. (2019, November 20). *R3 report | Requirement, rationale, reference.* https://www.jointcommission.org/-/media/tjc/documents/standards/r3-reports/r3_18_suicide_prevention_hap_bhc_cah_11_4_19_final1.pdf

My Notes

Read more about suicide prevention at Joint Commission's Suicide Prevention web page.

Perform Environmental Risk Assessment

An **environmental risk assessment** identifies physical environment features that could be used by clients to attempt suicide. Nurses implement actions to safeguard individuals identified at a high risk of suicide from environmental risks, such as continuous monitoring, routinely removing objects from rooms that could be used for self-harm, assessing objects brought into a facility by clients and visitors, and using safe transportation procedures when moving clients to other parts of the hospital.

In psychiatric hospitals and on psychiatric units within general hospitals, additional measures are taken to prevent suicide by hanging by removing anchor points, door hinges, and hooks. The Veteran's Health Administration showed that the use of a Mental Health Environment of Care Checklist to facilitate a thorough, systematic environmental assessment reduced the rate of suicide from 4.2 per 100,000 admissions to 0.74 per 100,000 admissions.[7]

Read more about the VA Mental Health at the Mental Health Environment of Care Checklist (MHEOCC) web page.[8]

Screen for Suicidal Ideation With a Validated Tool

Clients being evaluated or treated for mental health conditions often have suicidal ideation (i.e., thoughts of killing themselves). Additionally, clients being treated for medical conditions often have coexisting mental health disorders or psychosocial issues that can cause suicidal ideation. Therefore, all patients aged 12 and older admitted for acute health care should be screened for suicidal ideation with a validated tool. An example of a validated screening tool is the Patient Safety Screener.[9,10] View more information about the Patient Safety Screener tool in the following boxes.

Visit the Suicide Prevention Resource Center's web page to read more about the The Patient Safety Screener: A Brief Tool to Detect Suicide Risk.[11]

7 The Joint Commission. (2019, November 20). *R3 report | Requirement, rationale, reference.* https://www.jointcommission.org/-/media/tjc/documents/standards/r3-reports/r3_18_suicide_prevention_hap_bhc_cah_11_4_19_final1.pdf

8 U.S. Department of Veterans Affair. (2021, April 1). *VHA national center for patient safety.* https://www.patientsafety.va.gov/professionals/onthejob/mentalhealth.asp

9 The Joint Commission. (2019, November 20). *R3 report | Requirement, rationale, reference.* https://www.jointcommission.org/-/media/tjc/documents/standards/r3-reports/r3_18_suicide_prevention_hap_bhc_cah_11_4_19_final1.pdf

10 Suicide Prevention Resource Center. (n.d.). *The patient safety screener: A brief tool to detect suicide risk.* https://sprc.org/micro-learning/patientsafetyscreener

11 Suicide Prevention Resource Center. (n.d.). *The patient safety screener: A brief tool to detect suicide risk.* https://sprc.org/micro-learning/patientsafetyscreener

My Notes

View the following YouTube video on administering the Patient Safety Screener[12]: The Patient Safety Screener 3.

Assess Suicide Risk

An evidence-based **suicide risk assessment** should be completed on patients who have screened positive for suicidal ideation. Patients with suicidal ideation vary widely in their risk for a suicide attempt depending upon whether they have a plan, intent, or past history of attempts. An in-depth assessment of patients who screen positive for suicide risk must be completed to determine how to appropriately keep them safe from harm. Assessment for suicide risk includes asking about their suicidal ideation (i.e., thoughts of suicide), if they have a plan for committing suicide, their intent on completing the plan, previous suicidal or self-harm behaviors, risk factors, and protective factors.[13] When assessing for a suicide plan, notice if the plan is specific and the method they plan to use. The risk of acting on suicide thoughts increases with a specific plan. The risk also increases if the plan includes use of a lethal method that is accessible to the client.

An example of an evidence-based suicide risk assessment tool that anyone can use with anyone, anywhere is the Columbia Protocol, also known as the Columbia-Suicide Severity Rating Scale (C-SSRS). Read more about the C-SSRS in the following box. The C-SSRS uses a series of simple, plain-language questions that anyone can ask. The answers help identify if a person is at risk for suicide, assess the severity and immediacy of that risk, and gauge the level of support that the person needs. Examples of questions include the following[14]:

- Have you had thoughts of killing yourself?
- Have you thought about how you might do this?
- Have you done anything, started to do anything, or prepared to do anything to end your life?

Columbia Suicide Severity Rating Scale (C-SSRS)[15]

Read more about using the C-SSRS at Columbia Lighthouse Project website.

View a video: Saving Lives Worldwide – A Call to Action – The Columbia Lighthouse Project.[16]

---

12 SPRC. (2018, April 26). *The Patient Safety Screener 3* [Video]. YouTube. All rights reserved. https://youtu.be/4GmGiRBMnYc

13 The Joint Commission. (2019, November 20). *R3 report | Requirement, rationale, reference.* https://www.jointcommission.org/-/media/tjc/documents/standards/r3-reports/r3_18_suicide_prevention_hap_bhc_cah_11_4_19_final1.pdf

14 The Columbia Lighthouse Project. (n.d.). *Identify risk. Prevent suicide.* https://cssrs.columbia.edu/

15 The Columbia Lighthouse Project. (n.d.). *Identify risk. Prevent suicide.* https://cssrs.columbia.edu/

16 The Columbia Lighthouse Project. (2016, October 19). *Saving lives worldwide - A call to action - The Columbia Lighthouse Project* [Video]. YouTube. All rights reserved. https://youtu.be/csPPsstf2og

My Notes

Develop a Safety Plan

If a client is assessed as high risk for suicide, a safety plan should be created in collaboration with the client. A **safety plan** is a prioritized written list of coping strategies and sources of support that clients can use before or during a suicidal crisis. The plan should be brief, in the client's own words, and easy to read. After the plan is developed, the nurse should problem solve with the client to identify barriers or obstacles to using the plan. It should be discussed where the client will keep the safety plan and how it will be located during a crisis.[17,18]

Read the Safety Planning Guide PDF by the Western Interstate Commission for Higher Education.[19]

Document Level of Risk for Suicide

After suicide screening and suicide risk are assessed, it should be documented and communicated with the treatment team, along with the plan to keep the client safe. It is vital for all health care team members caring for the client to be aware of their level of risk and plans to reduce that risk as they provide care.[20] Nurses complete documentation regarding the level of a client's suicide risk and associated interventions every shift or more frequently as needed, depending upon the client status.

Follow Written Policies and Procedures

Nurses must strictly follow agency policies and procedures addressing the care of individuals who are identified at risk for suicide to keep them safe. For example, in some suicide cases reported to The Joint Commission, the root cause was a failure of staff to adhere to agency policies, such as a period of time when one-to-one monitoring was in place for a client identified as high risk for suicide.[21]

Provide Information for Follow-Up Care on Discharge

Nurses should provide written information at discharge regarding follow-up care to clients identified at risk for suicide and share it with their family members and loved ones as appropriate. Studies have shown that a patient's risk for suicide is high after discharge from psychiatric inpatient or emergency department settings. Developing a safety plan with the patient and providing the number of crisis call centers can decrease suicidal behavior after the patient leaves the care of the organization.[22]

---

17 Western Interstate Commission for Higher Education. (2008). *Safety planning guide* [Handout]. https://www.sprc.org/sites/default/files/SafetyPlanningGuide%20Quick%20Guide%20for%20Clinicians.pdf

18 Schuster, H., Jones, N., & Qadri, S. F. (2021). Safety planning: Why it is essential on the day of discharge from in-patient psychiatric hospitalization in reducing future risks of suicide. *Cureus, 13*(12), e20648. https://doi.org/10.7759/cureus.20648

19 Western Interstate Commission for Higher Education. (2008). *Safety planning guide* [Handout]. https://www.sprc.org/sites/default/files/SafetyPlanningGuide%20Quick%20Guide%20for%20Clinicians.pdf

20 The Joint Commission. (2019, November 20). *R3 report | Requirement, rationale, reference.* https://www.jointcommission.org/-/media/tjc/documents/standards/r3-reports/r3_18_suicide_prevention_hap_bhc_cah_11_4_19_final1.pdf

21 The Joint Commission. (2019, November 20). *R3 report | Requirement, rationale, reference.* https://www.jointcommission.org/-/media/tjc/documents/standards/r3-reports/r3_18_suicide_prevention_hap_bhc_cah_11_4_19_final1.pdf

22 The Joint Commission. (2019, November 20). *R3 report | Requirement, rationale, reference.* https://www.jointcommission.org/-/media/tjc/documents/standards/r3-reports/r3_18_suicide_prevention_hap_bhc_cah_11_4_19_final1.pdf

My Notes

Monitor Effectiveness of Suicide Prevention Interventions

The effectiveness of policies and protocols regarding suicide prevention should be evaluated on a periodic basis as part of overall quality improvement initiatives of the agency.[23] Research demonstrates implementation of the Zero Suicide Model results in lower suicidal behaviors.

Zero Suicide Toolkit[24]

Read the American Psychiatric Association *Psych News Alert*, "'Zero Suicide' Practices at Mental Health Clinics Reduce Suicide Among Patients."

Visit the Zero Suicide Toolkit web page.

View a video: Preventing Suicide: Information for Health Care Workers.[25]

One or more interactive elements has been excluded from this version of the text. You can view them online here: https://wtcs.pressbooks.pub/nursingmhcc/?p=73#oembed-1

Establishing a Safe Care Environment for Nurses and Other Health Care Team Members

The American Nurses Association states, "No staff nurse should have to deal with violence in the workplace, whether from staff, patients, or visitors."[26] **Workplace violence** is the act or threat of violence, ranging from verbal abuse to physical assaults directed toward persons at work or on duty. The impact of workplace violence can range from psychological issues to physical injury or even death. Violence can occur in any workplace and among any type of worker, but the risk for nonfatal violence resulting in days away from work is greatest for health care workers.[27] Research indicates the rate of physical assaults on nurses is 13.2 per 100 nurses per year, and 25% of psychiatric nurses experienced disabling injuries from client assault. Many experts believe these figures represent

23 The Joint Commission. (2019, November 20). *R3 report | Requirement, rationale, reference.* https://www.jointcommission.org/-/media/tjc/documents/standards/r3-reports/r3_18_suicide_prevention_hap_bhc_cah_11_4_19_final1.pdf

24 Zero Suicide. (n.d.). *Zero suicide toolkit.* https://zerosuicide.edc.org/toolkit/zero-suicide-toolkitsm

25 World Health Organization (WHO). (2019, October 8). *Preventing suicide: Information for health workers* [Video]. YouTube. Licensed in the Public Domain. https://youtu.be/Fy7n8SfwS_A

26 American Nurses Association. (n.d.). *Safety on the job.* https://www.nursingworld.org/practice-policy/work-environment/health-safety/safety-on-the-job/

27 Centers for Disease Control and Prevention. (2021, August 11). *Occupational violence.* https://www.cdc.gov/niosh/topics/violence/default.html

My Notes

only the tip of the iceberg and that most incidents of violence go unreported.[28] See Figure 1.4[29] for an illustration of safety first.

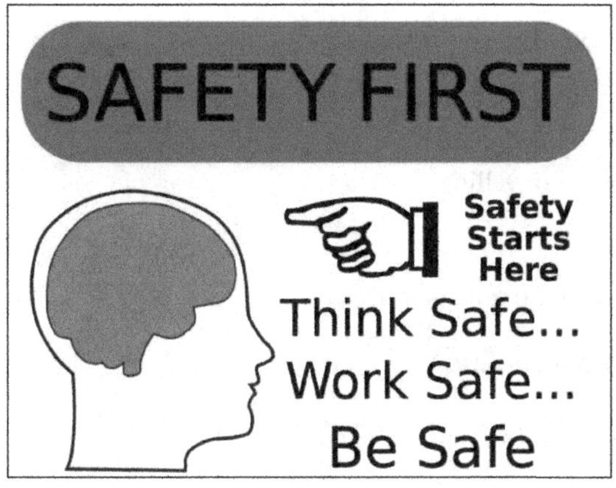

Figure 1.4 Safety First

Safety strategies for nurses and nursing students providing client care include the following[30]:

Dress for Safety

- Tuck away long hair so that it can't be grabbed
- Avoid earrings or necklaces that can be pulled
- Avoid overly tight clothing that can restrict movement or overly loose clothing or scarves that can be caught
- Use breakaway safety lanyards for glasses, keys, or name tags
- Do not wear your stethoscope around your neck

Be Aware of Your Work Environment

- When in a room with a client or visitor who is demonstrating warning signs of escalation, position yourself between the door and the client so you can exit quickly if needed
- Note exits and emergency phone numbers, especially if you float to other areas
- Recognize that confusion, background noises, and crowding can increase clients' stress levels
- Be aware that mealtimes, shift changes, and transporting patients are times of increased disruptive behaviors

---

28 Centers for Disease Control and Prevention. (2021, August 11). *Occupational violence: Workplace violence prevention for nurses*. https://www.cdc.gov/niosh/topics/violence/training_nurses.html

29 "Safety-First--Arvin61r58.png" by unknown author at freesvg.org is licensed under CC0 1.0. Access for free at https://freesvg.org/safety-first

30 Centers for Disease Control and Prevention. (2021, August 11). *Occupational violence: Workplace violence prevention for nurses*. https://www.cdc.gov/niosh/topics/violence/training_nurses.html

My Notes

Be Attuned to Patient Behaviors

- Most violent behavior is preceded by warning signs, including verbal cues and nonverbal cues. The greater the number of cues, the greater the risk for violence. Be aware of these verbal and nonverbal cues indicating a client's potential escalation to violence:

Verbal Cues

- Speaking loudly or yelling
- Swearing
- Using a threatening tone of voice

Nonverbal and Behavioral Cues

- Evidence of confusion or disorientation
- Irritability or easily angered
- Boisterous behavior (i.e., overly loud, shouting, slamming doors)
- Disheveled physical appearance (i.e., neglected hygiene)
- Holding arms tightly across chest
- Clenching fists
- Heavy breathing
- Pacing or agitated restlessness
- Looking terrified (signifying fear and high anxiety)
- Staring with a fixed look
- Holding oneself in an aggressive or threatening posture
- Throwing objects
- Exhibiting sudden changes in behavior or signs of being under the influence of a substance

Use Violence Risk Assessment Tools

- Use risk assessment tools to evaluate individuals for potential violence, enabling all health care providers to share a common frame of reference and understanding. This minimizes the possibility that communications regarding a person's potential for violence will be misinterpreted. These tools can be used as an initial assessment upon admission to determine potential risk for violence and repeated daily to assist in predicting imminent violent behavior within the next 24 hours. See sample risk assessment tools in the box at the end of this section.

Be Attuned to Your Own Responses

- Be aware of your own feelings, responses, and sensitivities and pay attention to your instincts. For example, your "fight or flight" response can be an early warning sign of impending danger to get help or get out.
- Be aware of how you express yourself and how others respond to you. Those who know you well may respond differently than do strangers. Effective therapeutic communication skills are an essential tool in preventing violence.

My Notes

- Use self-awareness and acknowledge if you have a personal history of abuse, trauma, or adverse childhood experiences (ACEs) that can affect how you respond to situations.
- If coworkers are engaging in abusive behaviors, consider if you are exhibiting similar behaviors.
- Be aware that fatigue can diminish your alertness and your ability to respond appropriately to a challenging situation.

Check Your Cultural Biases

- A key aspect of self-awareness is recognizing how our own particular cultural heritage, values, and belief systems affect how we respond to our clients and coworkers and how they, in turn, respond to us.

Sample Violence Risk Assessment Tools from the CDC:

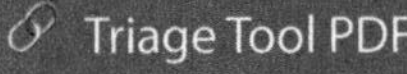
Triage Tool PDF

Indicator for Violent Behavior PDF

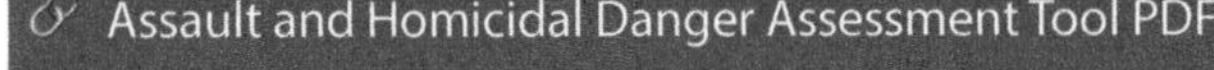
Assault and Homicidal Danger Assessment Tool PDF

If travelling to a home setting as a home health nurse, additional safety strategies are as follows[31]:

- Review agency files to confirm that a background check was done on a patient regarding any history of violence or crime, drug or alcohol abuse, and mental health diagnoses. Also, check to see if a patient's family member has a record of violence or arrest.
- If entering a situation assessed as potentially dangerous, you should be accompanied by a team member who has training in de-escalation and crisis intervention.
- Always carry a charged cell phone.
- Make sure someone always knows where you are.
- Have a code word to use with your office or coworkers to let them know you're in trouble if you can't call the police.

The CDC offers a free, online course called Workplace Violence Prevention for Nurses to better understand the scope and nature of violence in the workplace. Access the free CDC course on workplace violence with nurse videos at the Workplace Violence Prevention for Nurses web page.

31 Centers for Disease Control and Prevention. (2021, August 11). *Occupational violence: Workplace violence prevention for nurses.* https://www.cdc.gov/niosh/topics/violence/training_nurses.html

My Notes

1.7 PSYCHIATRIC-MENTAL HEALTH NURSING

What is Psychiatric-Mental Health Nursing?

Registered nurses (RNs) in a variety of settings provide care for clients with medical illnesses who may also be experiencing concurrent mental health disorders. Nurses who specialize in psychiatric-mental health nursing promote clients' well-being through prevention strategies and patient education, while also using the nursing process to provide care for clients with mental health and substance use disorders.[1] According to the American Psychiatric Nurses Association, psychiatric-mental health nurse specialists perform the following activities[2]:

- Partner with individuals to achieve their recovery goals
- Provide health promotion and maintenance
- Conduct intake screening, evaluation, and triage
- Provide case management
- Teach self-care activities
- Administer and monitor psychobiological treatment regimens
- Practice crisis intervention and stabilization
- Engage in psychiatric rehabilitation and intervention
- Educate patients, families, and communities
- Coordinate care
- Work within interdisciplinary teams

Within the specialty of psychiatric-mental health nursing, there is an opportunity to become board certified. Eligibility requirements include a bachelor's degree, two years of full-time work, 30 hours of continuing education, and passing a certification exam. The nurse earns the credential of PMH-BC (Psychiatric-Mental Health-Board Certified) or RN-BC.

Psychiatric-mental health advanced practice registered nurses (PMH-APRN) and nurse practitioners (PMHNP-BC) are registered nurses with a Master of Science in Nursing (MSN) or Doctor of Nursing Practice (DNP) degree in psychiatric nursing. PMH-APRNs perform the following activities:

- Provide individual, group, couples, and/or family psychotherapy
- Prescribe medication for acute and chronic illnesses
- Conduct comprehensive assessments
- Provide clinical supervision
- Diagnose, treat, and manage chronic or acute illness
- Provide integrative therapy interventions
- Order, perform, and interpret lab tests and other diagnostic studies

---

1 American Psychiatric Nurses Association. (n.d.). *About psychiatric-mental health nursing*. https://www.apna.org/about-psychiatric-nursing/

2 American Psychiatric Nurses Association. (n.d.). *About psychiatric-mental health nursing*. https://www.apna.org/about-psychiatric-nursing/

My Notes

- Provide preventative care, including screening
- Develop policies for programs and systems
- Make referrals for health problems outside their scope of practice
- Perform procedures

Standards of Psychiatric-Mental Health Nursing

The American Psychiatric Nurses Association establishes standards of practice in psychiatric-mental health nursing that are built on the ANA Scope and Standards of Practice (2021). These standards are published in the *Psychiatric-Mental Health Nursing: Scope and Standards of Practice* document.[3] The standards are very similar to the ANA Scope and Standards of Practice, with additional activities included in the *Intervention* standard of care. These interventions will be further discussed in the "Implementation" section of the "Application of the Nursing Process in Mental Health Care" chapter.

Read the About Psychiatric-Mental Health Nursing web page to learn more about the American Psychiatric Nursing Association.

There are specific legal and ethical considerations that apply to caring for clients with mental illness. See the "Legal and Ethical Considerations in Mental Health Care" chapter for further information.

Treatment Settings

There are many settings where psychiatric-mental health nurses collaboratively provide services to clients with mental health disorders, ranging from outpatient settings to inpatient care to state mental hospitals.

Outpatient Services

Clients often initially visit their primary care provider when concerned about their mental health. If a client has a more severe disorder, they are typically referred to specialized psychiatric care providers such as psychiatrists, psychiatric-mental health advanced practice registered nurses/nurse practitioners, psychologists, social workers, counselors, or other licensed therapists.

There are many different types of mental health services offered in the community:

- Patient-centered medical homes that are comprehensive, coordinated, patient-centered models of primary care.[4]
- Community mental health centers that offer free, low-cost, or sliding scale care for those who lack funding for mental health care.
- Country programs, such as Comprehensive Community Services (CSC) or Community Support Programs (CSP).
- Psychiatric mental health care in correctional facilities.

---

3 American Nurses Association, American Psychiatric Nurses Association, and International Society of Psychiatric-Mental Health Nurses. (2014). *Psychiatric-Mental Health Nursing: Scope and Standards of Practice* (2nd ed.). Nursebooks.org

4 AHRQ. (n.d.). *Defining the PCMH.* https://pcmh.ahrq.gov/page/defining-pcmh

My Notes

- Psychiatric home care that provides community-based treatment for clients who are homebound.
- Certified peer specialists.
- Telepsychiatry that provides therapy and prescription services through videoconferencing.[5]

Inpatient Care Settings

Clients with acute mental health symptoms, or those who are at-risk for hurting themselves or others, may be hospitalized. They are often initially seen in the emergency department for emergency psychiatric care. Clients may seek voluntary admission, or in some situations, may be involuntarily admitted after referral for emergency evaluation by law enforcement, schools, friends, or family members. Read more about involuntary admissions in the "Patient Rights" section of the "Legal and Ethical Considerations in Mental Health Care" chapter.

Acute-care psychiatric units in general hospitals are typically locked units on a separate floor of the hospital with the purpose of maintaining environmental safety for its clients. State-operated psychiatric hospitals serve clients who have chronic serious mental illness. They also provide court-related care for criminal cases where the client was found "not guilty by reason of insanity." This judgment means the client was deemed to be so mentally ill when they committed a crime that they cannot be held responsible for the act, but instead require treatment.[6]

Terminology Used in Psychiatric-Mental Health Nursing

Specific terminology is used in psychiatry and mental health nursing to document and describe signs, symptoms, and behaviors related to mental health disorders. Using specific mental health terminology when documenting and communicating with interprofessional health care team members is vital to ensure continuity of care. See the definitions of common terms in the "Assessment" section of the "Application of the Nursing Process in Mental Health Care" chapter, as well as in chapters related to specific mental health disorders.

---

5 Halter, M. J. (2022). *Varcarolis' foundations of psychiatric-mental health nursing* (9th ed.). Saunders.

6 Halter, M. J. (2022). *Varcarolis' foundations of psychiatric-mental health nursing* (9th ed.). Saunders.

1.8 LEARNING ACTIVITIES

My Notes

Interactive Activities

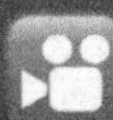

An interactive H5P element has been excluded from this version of the text. You can view it online here: https://wtcs.pressbooks.pub/nursingmhcc/?p=86#h5p-2

An interactive H5P element has been excluded from this version of the text. You can view it online here: https://wtcs.pressbooks.pub/nursingmhcc/?p=86#h5p-1

An interactive H5P element has been excluded from this version of the text. You can view it online here: https://wtcs.pressbooks.pub/nursingmhcc/?p=86#h5p-3

My Notes

GLOSSARY

Adverse childhood experiences (ACEs): Traumatic circumstances experienced during childhood such as abuse, neglect, or growing up in a household with violence, mental illness, substance use, incarceration, or divorce.

Boundaries: Limits that we set as individuals that define our levels of comfort when interacting with others. Personal boundaries include limits in physical, sexual, intellectual, emotional, sexual, and financial areas of our lives.

Deviance: Behavior that violates social norms or cultural expectations because one's culture determines what is "normal."

Distress: Psychological and/or physical pain.

Dysfunction: Disturbances in a person's thinking, emotional regulation, or behavior that reflects significant dysfunction in psychological, biological, or developmental processes underlying mental functioning.

Environmental risk assessment: Identification of physical environment features that could be used to attempt suicide in clients identified as at a high risk for suicide.

Health: A state of complete physical, mental, and social well-being and not merely the absence of disease or infirmity.

Impairment: A limited ability to engage in activities of daily living (i.e., they cannot maintain personal hygiene, prepare meals, or pay bills) or participate in social events, work, or school.

Major life activities: Activities of daily living such as caring for oneself, performing manual tasks, seeing, hearing, eating, sleeping, walking, standing, lifting, bending, speaking, breathing, learning, reading, concentrating, thinking, communicating, and working.[1]

Mental health: A state of well-being in which an individual realizes their own abilities, copes with the normal stresses of life, works productively, and contributes to their community.[2]

Mental health continuum: A continuum of mental health, ranging from well-being to emotional problems to mental illness.

Mental illness: A health condition involving changes in emotion, thinking, or behavior (or a combination of these) associated with emotional distress and problems functioning in social, work, or family activities.[3]

Recovery: A process of change through which individuals improve their health and wellness, live a self-directed life, and strive to reach their full potential.[4]

Resilience: The ability to rise above circumstances or meet challenges with fortitude.[5]

---

1 Office of Federal Contract Compliance Programs. (2009, January 1). *ADA Amendments Act of 2008 frequently asked questions. U.S. Department of Labor.* https://www.dol.gov/agencies/ofccp/faqs/americans-with-disabilities-act-amendments

2 World Health Organization. (2018, March 30). *Mental health: Strengthening our response.* https://www.who.int/news-room/fact-sheets/detail/mental-health-strengthening-our-response

3 American Psychiatric Association. (n.d.). *What is mental illness?* https://www.psychiatry.org/patients-families/what-is-mental-illness

4 Center for Substance Abuse Treatment (US). (2014). *Trauma-informed care in behavioral health services.* https://www.ncbi.nlm.nih.gov/books/NBK207201/

5 Center for Substance Abuse Treatment (US). (2014). *Trauma-informed care in behavioral health services.* https://www.ncbi.nlm.nih.gov/books/NBK207201/

My Notes

Safety plan: A prioritized written list of coping strategies and sources of support that clients can use before or during a suicidal crisis. The plan should be brief, in the client's own words, and easy to read. After the plan is developed, the nurse should problem solve with the client to identify barriers or obstacles to using the plan. It should be discussed where the client will keep the safety plan and how it will be located during a crisis.

Serious mental illness: Mental illness that causes disabling functional impairment that substantially interferes with one or more major life activities. Examples of serious mental illnesses that commonly interfere with major life activities include major depressive disorder, schizophrenia, and bipolar disorder.[6]

Social norms: Stated and unstated rules of an individual's society.

Stigma: A cluster of negative attitudes and beliefs that motivates the general public to fear, reject, avoid, and discriminate against people with mental health disorders.

Suicidal ideation: Thoughts of killing oneself.

Suicide risk assessment: Identifying the risk of a client dying by suicide by assessing suicidal ideation, plan, intent, suicidal or self-harm behaviors, risk factors, and protective factors.

Trauma: An event, series of events, or set of circumstances that is experienced by an individual as physically or emotionally harmful and can have lasting adverse effects on the individual's functioning and physical, social, emotional, or spiritual well-being.

Trauma-informed care (TIC): A strengths-based framework that acknowledges the prevalence and impact of traumatic experiences in clinical practice. TIC emphasizes physical, psychological, and emotional safety for both survivors and health professionals and creates opportunities for survivors to rebuild a sense of control and empowerment referred to as resilience.[7]

Well-being: The "healthy" range of the mental health continuum where individuals are experiencing a state of good mental and emotional health.

Workplace violence: The act or threat of violence, ranging from verbal abuse to physical assaults, directed toward persons at work or on duty.

World Health Organization Disability Assessment Scale (WHODAS): A generic assessment instrument that provides a standardized method for measuring health and disability across cultures.

6 American Psychiatric Association. (n.d.). *What is mental illness?* https://www.psychiatry.org/patients-families/what-is-mental-illness

7 Center for Substance Abuse Treatment (US). (2014). *Trauma-informed care in behavioral health services.* https://www.ncbi.nlm.nih.gov/books/NBK207201/

Chapter 2

Therapeutic Communication and the Nurse-Client Relationship

2.1 INTRODUCTION

My Notes

Learning Objectives

- Review basic concepts of client-centered communication
- Outline effective therapeutic communication techniques
- Describe barriers to effective therapeutic communication
- Explore guidelines for effective communication during teletherapy

Nurses engage in compassionate, supportive, professional relationships with their clients as part of the "art of nursing."[1] This chapter will review the nurse-client relationship, therapeutic communication, and motivational interviewing. It will also introduce teletherapy and telehealth.

1 American Nurses Association. (2021). *Nursing: Scope and standards of practice* (4th ed.). American Nurses Association.

My Notes

2.2 BASIC CONCEPTS OF COMMUNICATION

Communication Standard of Professional Performance

The Standard of Professional Performance for *Communication* established by the American Nurses Association (ANA) is defined as, "The registered nurse communicates effectively in all areas of professional practice."[1] See the following box for the competencies associated with the *Communication* standard.

ANA's Communication Competencies

The registered nurse:

- Assesses one's own communication skills and effectiveness.
- Demonstrates cultural humility, professionalism, and respect when communicating.
- Assesses communication ability, health literacy, resources, and preferences of health care consumers to inform the interprofessional team and others.
- Uses language translation resources to ensure effective communication.
- Incorporates appropriate alternative strategies to communicate effectively with health care consumers who have visual, speech, language, or communication difficulties.
- Uses communication styles and methods that demonstrate caring, respect, active listening, authenticity, and trust.
- Conveys accurate information to health care consumers, families, community stakeholders, and members of the interprofessional team.
- Advocates for the health care consumer and their preferences and choices when care processes and decisions do not appear to be in the best interest of the health care consumer.
- Maintains communication with interprofessional team members and others to facilitate safe transitions and continuity in care delivery.
- Confirms with the recipient if the communication was heard and if the recipient understands the message.
- Contributes the nursing perspective in interactions and discussions with the interprofessional team and other stakeholders.
- Promotes safety in the care or practice environment by disclosing and reporting concerns related to potential or actual hazards or deviations from the standard of care.
- Demonstrates continuous improvement of communication skills.

1 American Nurses Association. (2021). *Nursing: Scope and standards of practice* (4th ed.). American Nurses Association.

Review basic communication concepts for nurses in the "Communication" chapter in Open RN *Nursing Fundamentals.*

Nurse-Client Relationship

Establishment of the therapeutic nurse-client relationship is vital in nursing care. Nurses engage in compassionate, supportive, professional relationships with their clients as part of the "art of nursing."[2] This is especially true in psychiatric care, where the therapeutic relationship is considered to be the foundation of client care and healing.[3] The **nurse-client relationship** establishes trust and rapport with a specific purpose; it facilitates therapeutic communication and engages the client in decision-making regarding their plan of care.

Therapeutic nurse-client relationships vary in depth, length, and focus. Brief therapeutic encounters might last only a few minutes and focus on the client's immediate needs, current feelings, or behaviors. For example, in the emergency department setting, a nurse may therapeutically communicate with a client in crisis who recently experienced a situational trauma. During longer periods of time, such as inpatient care, nurses work with clients in setting short-term goals and outcomes that are documented in the nursing care plan and evaluated regularly. In long-term care settings, such as residential facilities, the therapeutic nurse-client relationship may last several months and include frequent interactions focusing on behavior modification.

Read more about crisis and crisis intervention in the "Stress, Coping, and Crisis Intervention" chapter.

Phases of Development of a Therapeutic Relationship

The nurse-client relationship goes through three phases. A well-known nurse theorist named Hildegard Peplau described these three phases as orientation, working, and termination.[4]

Orientation Phase

During the brief orientation phase, clients may realize they need assistance as they adjust to their current status. Simultaneously, nurses introduce themselves and begin to obtain essential information about clients as individuals with unique needs, values, beliefs, and priorities. During this brief phase, trust is established, and rapport begins to develop between the client and the nurse. Nurses ensure privacy when talking with the client and providing care and respect the client's values, beliefs, and personal boundaries.

A common framework used for introductions during patient care is AIDET, a mnemonic for Acknowledge, Introduce, Duration, Explanation, and Thank You.

- **Acknowledge:** Greet the patient by the name documented in their medical record. Make eye contact, smile, and acknowledge any family or friends in the room. Ask the patient their preferred

---

2 American Nurses Association. (2021). *Nursing: Scope and standards of practice* (4th ed.). American Nurses Association.

3 Ross, C. A., & Goldner, E. M. (2009). Stigma, negative attitudes and discrimination towards mental illness within the nursing profession: A review of the literature. *Journal of Psychiatric and Mental Health Nursing, 16*(6), 558-567. https://doi.org/10.1111/j.1365-2850.2009.01399.x

4 Hagerty, T. A., Samuels, W., Norcini-Pala, A., & Gigliotti, E. (2018). Peplau's Theory of Interpersonal Relations: An alternate factor structure for patient experience data? *Nursing Science Quarterly, 30*(2), 160-167. https://dx.doi.org/10.1177%2F0894318417693286

My Notes

way of being addressed (for example, "Mr. Doe," "Jonathon," or "Johnny") and their preferred pronouns (e.g., he/him, she/her, or they/them).

- **Introduce:** Introduce yourself by your name and role. For example, "I'm John Doe, and I am a nursing student working with your nurse to take care of you today."
- **Duration:** Estimate a timeline for how long it will take to complete the task you are doing. For example, "I am here to perform an admission assessment. This should take about 15 minutes."
- **Explanation:** Explain step by step what to expect next and answer questions. For example, "I will be putting this blood pressure cuff on your arm and inflating it. It will feel as if it is squeezing your arm for a few moments."
- **Thank You:** At the end of the encounter, thank the patient and ask if anything is needed before you leave. In an acute or long-term care setting, ensure the call light is within reach and the patient knows how to use it. If family members are present, thank them for being there to support the patient as appropriate. For example, "Thank you for taking time to talk with me today. Is there anything I can get for you before I leave the room? Here is the call light (Place within reach). Press the red button if you would like to call the nurse."

Working Phase

The majority of a nurse's time with a client is in the working phase. During this phase, nurses use active listening and begin by asking the reason the client is seeking care to determine what is important to them. They use assessment findings to develop a nursing plan of care and plan patient education. If a care plan has already been established on admission, nurses use this time to implement interventions targeted to meet short-term outcomes and long-term goals. During the working phase, clients begin to accept nurses as health educators, counselors, and care providers. Nurses use therapeutic communication techniques to facilitate clients' awareness of their thoughts and feelings and mutually develop goals and an individualized plan of care. Nurses provide reflective and nonjudgmental feedback to clients to help them clarify their thoughts, goals, and coping strategies.[5] Therapeutic communication techniques used during this phase, including motivational interviewing, are discussed later in this chapter.

Termination Phase

The final phase of a nurse-client relationship is the termination phase. This phase typically occurs at the end of a shift or on discharge from care. If the previous working phase has been successful, the client's needs have been successfully met by collaboration among the client, nurses, and interprofessional health care team members. The nurse should be aware the client may try to return to the working phase to avoid termination of the relationship. During the termination phase, the nurse can encourage the client to reflect on progress they have made and review post-discharge goals.

The nurse also makes community referrals for follow-up and continuation of support in meeting goals.

---

5 Hagerty, T. A., Samuels, W., Norcini-Pala, A., & Gigliotti, E. (2018). Peplau's Theory of Interpersonal Relations: An alternate factor structure for patient experience data? *Nursing Science Quarterly, 30*(2), 160-167. https://dx.doi.org/10.1177%2F0894318417693286

My Notes

2.3 THERAPEUTIC COMMUNICATION

Therapeutic communication has roots going back to Florence Nightingale, who insisted on the importance of building trusting relationships with patients. She taught that therapeutic healing resulted from nurses' presence with patients.[1] Since then, several professional nursing associations have highlighted therapeutic communication as one of the most vital elements in nursing. **Therapeutic communication** is a type of professional communication defined as the purposeful, interpersonal, information-transmitting process that leads to client understanding and participation.[2] Read an example of a nursing student using therapeutic communication in the following box.

Example of Nurse Using Therapeutic Listening

Ms. Z. is a nursing student (as simulated in Figure 2.1[3]) who enjoys interacting with patients. When she goes to patients' rooms, she greets them and introduces herself and her role in a calm tone. She kindly asks patients about their problems and notices their reactions. She provides information and answers their questions. Patients perceive that she wants to help them. She treats patients professionally by respecting boundaries and listening to them in a nonjudgmental manner. She addresses communication barriers and respects patients' cultural beliefs. She notices patients' health literacy and ensures they understand her messages and patient education. As a result, patients trust her and feel as if she cares about them, so they feel comfortable sharing their health care needs with her.[4]

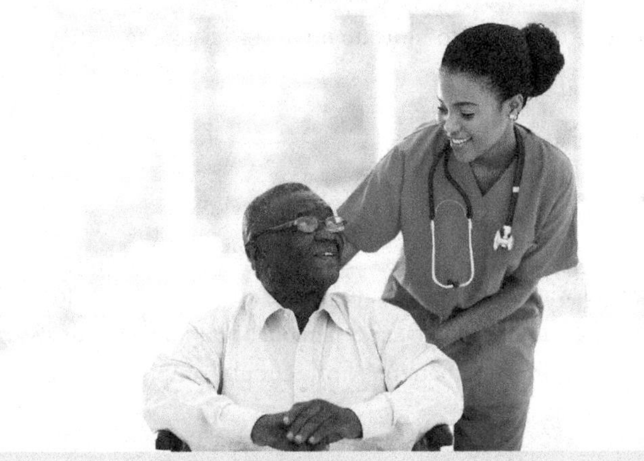

Figure 2.1 Nursing Student Using Therapeutic Communication

Therapeutic communication is different from social interaction. Social interaction does not have a goal or purpose and includes casual sharing of information, whereas therapeutic communication has a goal or purpose for the

1 Karimi, H., & Masoudi Alavi, N. (2015). Florence Nightingale: The mother of nursing. *Nursing and Midwifery Studies, 4*(2), e29475. https://doi.org/10.17795/nmsjournal29475

2 Abdolrahimi, M., Ghiyasvandian, S., Zakerimoghadam, M., & Ebadi, A. (2017). Therapeutic communication in nursing students: A Walker & Avant concept analysis. *Electronic Physician, 9*(8), 4968–4977. https://doi.org/10.19082/4968

3 "beautiful african nurse taking care of senior patient in wheelchair" by agilemktg1 is in the Public Domain.

4 Abdolrahimi, M., Ghiyasvandian, S., Zakerimoghadam, M., & Ebadi, A. (2017). Therapeutic communication in nursing students: A Walker & Avant concept analysis. *Electronic Physician, 9*(8), 4968–4977. https://doi.org/10.19082/4968

My Notes

conversation. An example of a nursing goal before using therapeutic communication is, "The client will share feelings or concerns about their treatment plan by the end of the conversation."

Therapeutic communication includes active listening, professional touch, and a variety of therapeutic communication techniques.

Active Listening

Listening is an important part of communication. There are three main types of listening, including competitive, passive, and active listening. Competitive listening occurs when we are mostly focused on sharing our own point of view instead of listening to someone else. Passive listening occurs when we are not interested in listening to the other person, and we assume we understand what the person is communicating correctly without verifying their message. During **active listening**, we communicate both verbally and nonverbally that we are interested in what the other person is saying while also actively verifying our understanding with them. For example, an active listening technique is to restate what the person said and then verify our understanding is correct. This feedback process is the major difference between passive listening and active listening.[5]

Nonverbal communication is an important component of active listening. **SOLER** is a mnemonic for establishing good nonverbal communication with clients. SOLER stands for the following[6]:

- **S:** **S**itting and squarely facing the client
- **O:** Using **o**pen posture (i.e., avoid crossing arms)
- **L:** **L**eaning towards the client to indicate interest in listening
- **E:** Maintaining good **e**ye contact
- **R:** Maintaining a **r**elaxed posture

Touch

Professional touch is a powerful way to communicate caring and empathy if done respectfully while also being aware of the client's preferences, cultural beliefs, and personal boundaries. Nurses use professional touch when assessing, expressing concern, or comforting patients. For example, simply holding a patient's hand during a painful procedure can effectively provide comfort.

For individuals with a history of trauma, touch can be negatively perceived, so it is important to ask permission before touching. Inform the person before engaging in medical procedures requiring touch such as, "I need to hold down your arm so I can draw blood."

Nurses should avoid using touch with individuals who are becoming agitated or experiencing a manic or psychotic episode because it can cause escalation. It is also helpful to maintain a larger interpersonal distance when interacting with an individual who is experiencing paranoia or psychosis.

---

5 This work is a derivative of *Human Relations* by LibreTexts and is licensed under CC BY-NC-SA 4.0

6 Stickley, T. (2011). From SOLER to SURETY for effective non-verbal communication. *Nurse Education in Practice, 11*(6), 395–398. https://doi.org/10.1016/j.nepr.2011.03.021

Therapeutic Communication Techniques

My Notes

There are a variety of therapeutic techniques that nurses use to engage clients in verbalizing emotions, establishing goals, and discussing coping strategies. See Table 2.3a for definitions of various therapeutic communication techniques discussed in the *American Nurse*, the official journal of the American Nurses Association.

Table 2.3a Therapeutic Communication Techniques[7]

Therapeutic Techniques	Definition	Examples
Acceptance	Acceptance acknowledges a client's emotions or message and affirms they have been heard. Acceptance isn't necessarily the same thing as agreement; it can be enough to simply make eye contact and say, "I hear what you are saying." Clients who feel their nurses are listening to them and taking them seriously are more likely to be receptive to care.	Client: "I hate taking all this medicine. It makes me feel numb." Nurse (making eye contact): "Yes, I understand."
Clarification	Clarification asks the client to further define what they are communicating. Similar to active listening, asking for clarification when a client says something confusing or ambiguous is important. It helps nurses ensure they understand what is actually being said and can help clients process their ideas more thoroughly.	Client: "I feel useless to everyone and everything." Nurse: "I'm not sure I understand what you mean by useless. Can you give an example of a time you felt useless?"
Focusing	Focusing on a specific statement made by a client that seems particularly important prompts them to discuss it further. Clients don't always have an objective perspective on their situation or past experiences, but as impartial observers, nurses can more easily pick out important topics on which to focus.	Client: "I grew up with five brothers and sisters. We didn't have much money, so my mom was always working and never home. We had to fend for ourselves, and there was never any food in the house." Nurse: "It sounds as if you experienced some stressful conditions growing up."
Exploring	Exploring gathers more information about what the client is communicating.	Client: "I had to lie when I found out a dark secret about my sister." Nurse: "If you feel comfortable doing so, tell me more about the situation and your sister's dark secret."

7 American Nurse. (n.d.). *Therapeutic communication techniques*. https://www.myamericannurse.com/therapeutic-communication-techniques/

My Notes

Therapeutic Techniques	Definition	Examples
Giving Recognition	Giving recognition acknowledges and validates the client's positive health behaviors. Recognition acknowledges a patient's behavior and highlights it without giving an overt compliment. A compliment can sometimes be taken as condescending, especially when it concerns a routine task like making the bed.	Nurse: "I noticed you took all of your medications."
Open-Ended Questions/ Offering General Leads	Using open questions or offering general leads provides keywords to "open" the discussion while also seeking more information. Therapeutic communication is most effective when clients direct the flow of conversation and decide what to talk about. Giving patients a broad opening such as "What's on your mind today?" or "What would you like to talk about?" is a good way to encourage clients to discuss what's on their mind.	Client: "I'm unsure of what to do next." Nurse: "Tell me more about your concerns."
Paraphrasing	Paraphrasing rephrases the client's words and key ideas to clarify their message and encourage additional communication.	Client: "I've been way too busy today." Nurse: "Participating in the support groups today has kept you busy."
Presenting Reality	Presenting reality restructures the client's distorted thoughts with valid information.	Client: "I can't go in that room; there are spiders on the walls." Nurse: "I see no evidence of spiders on the walls."
Restating	Restating uses different word choices for the same content stated by the client to encourage elaboration.	Client: "The nurses hate me here." Nurse: "You feel as though the nurses dislike you?"
Reflecting	Reflecting asks clients what they think they should do, encourages them to be accountable for their own actions, and helps them come up with solutions.	Client: "Do you think I should do this new treatment or not?" Nurse: "What do you think the pros and cons are for the new treatment plan?"
Providing Silence	Providing silence allows quiet time for self-reflection by the client.	The nurse does not verbally respond after a client makes a statement, although they may nod or use other nonverbal communication to demonstrate active listening and validation of the client's message.

My Notes

Therapeutic Techniques	Definition	Examples
Making Observations	Observations about the appearance, demeanor, or behavior of patients can help draw attention to areas that might pose a problem for them.	Nurse: "You look tired today." Client: "I haven't been getting much sleep lately because of so many racing thoughts in my head at night."
Offering Self/ Providing Presence	Offering self provides support by being present. Inpatient care can be lonely and stressful at times. When nurses provide presence and spend time with their clients, it shows clients they value them and are willing to give them time and attention.	Offering to simply sit with clients for a few minutes is a powerful way to create a caring connection.
Encouraging Descriptions of Perceptions	Asking about perceptions in an encouraging, nonjudgmental way is important for clients experiencing sensory issues or hallucinations. It gives clients a prompt to explain what they're perceiving without casting their perceptions in a negative light. It is also important to establish safety by ensuring the hallucinations are not encouraging the client to harm themselves or others.	The client looks distracted and frightened as if they see or hear something. Nurse: "It looks as though you might be hearing something. What do you hear now?" or "It looks as if you might be seeing something. What does it look like to you?"
Encouraging Comparisons	Encouraging comparisons helps clients reflect on previous situations in which they have coped effectively. In this manner, nurses can help clients discover solutions to their problems.	Nurse: "It must have been difficult when you went through a divorce. How did you cope with that?" Client: "I walked my dog outside a lot." Nurse: "It sounds as though walking your dog outside helps you cope with stress and feel better?"
Offering Hope	Offering hope encourages a client to persevere and be resilient.	Nurse: "I remember you shared with me how well you coped with difficult situations in the past."
Offering Humor	Humor can lighten the mood and contribute to feelings of togetherness, closeness, and friendliness. However, it is vital for the nurse to tailor humor to the client's sense of humor.	Nurse: "Knock, knock." Client: "Who's there?" Nurse: "Orange." Client: "Orange who?" Nurse: "Orange you glad to see me?" (Laughs with the client)

My Notes

Therapeutic Techniques	Definition	Examples
Confronting	Confronting presents reality or challenges a client's assumptions. Nurses should only apply this technique during the working phase after they have established trust. Confrontation, when used correctly, can help clients break destructive routines or understand the state of their current situation.	Client: "I haven't drunk much this year." Nurse: "Yesterday you told me that every weekend you go out and drink so much you don't know where you are when you wake up."
Summarizing	Summarizing demonstrates active listening to clients and allows the nurse to verify information. Ending a discussion with a phrase such as "Does that sound correct?" gives clients explicit permission to make corrections if they're necessary.	Client: "I don't like to take my medications because they make me tired, and I gain a lot of weight." Nurse: "You haven't been taking your medications this month because of the side effects of fatigue and weight gain. Is that correct?"

Nontherapeutic Responses

Nurses must be aware of potential barriers to communication and avoid nontherapeutic responses. Nonverbal communication such as looking at one's watch, crossing arms across one's chest, or not actively listening may be perceived as barriers to communication. Nontherapeutic verbal responses often block the client's communication of feelings or ideas. See Table 2.3b for a description of nontherapeutic responses to avoid.

Table 2.3b Nontherapeutic Responses[8,9]

Nontherapeutic Response	Description	Examples
Asking Personal Questions	Asking personal questions that are not relevant to the situation is not professional or appropriate. Don't ask questions just to satisfy your curiosity.	Nontherapeutic: "Why have you and Mary never gotten married?" Therapeutic: "How would you describe your relationship with Mary?"
Giving Personal Opinions	Giving personal opinions takes away the decision-making from the client. Effective problem-solving must be accomplished by the client and not provided by the nurse.	Nontherapeutic: "If I were you, I would put your father in a nursing home to reduce your stress." Therapeutic: "Let's explore options for your father's care."

8 Abdolrahimi, M., Ghiyasvandian, S., Zakerimoghadam, M., & Ebadi, A. (2017). Therapeutic communication in nursing students: A Walker & Avant concept analysis. *Electronic Physician, 9*(8), 4968–4977. https://doi.org/10.19082/4968

9 *StatPearls* by Sharma & Gupta is licensed under CC BY 4.0

My Notes

Nontherapeutic Response	Description	Examples
Changing the Subject	Changing the subject when someone is trying to communicate with you demonstrates lack of empathy and blocks further communication. It communicates that you don't care about what they are sharing.	Nontherapeutic: "Let's not talk about your insurance problems; it's time for your walk now." Therapeutic: "After your walk, let's look into what is going on with your insurance company."
Stating Generalizations and Stereotypes	Generalizations and stereotypes can threaten nurse-patient relationships.	Nontherapeutic: "Older adults are always confused." Therapeutic: "Tell me more about your concerns about your father's confusion."
Providing False Reassurances	When a client is seriously ill or distressed, the nurse may be tempted to offer false hope with statements that everything will be alright. These comments can discourage further expressions of a client's feelings.	Nontherapeutic: "You'll be fine; don't worry." Therapeutic: "It must be difficult not to know what will happen next. What can I do to help?"
Showing Sympathy	Sympathy focuses on the nurse's feelings rather than the client. It demonstrates pity rather than trying to help the client cope with the situation.	Nontherapeutic: "I'm so sorry about your amputation; I can't imagine losing my leg due to a car crash." Therapeutic: "The loss of your leg is a major change. How do you think this will affect your life?"
Asking "Why" Questions	A nurse may be tempted to ask the client to explain "why" they believe, feel, or act in a certain way. However, clients and family members can interpret "why" questions as accusations and become defensive. It is best to rephrase a question to avoid using the word "why."	Nontherapeutic: "Why are you so upset?" Therapeutic: "You seem upset. Tell me more about that."

My Notes

Nontherapeutic Response	Description	Examples
Approving or Disapproving	Nurses should not impose their own attitudes, values, beliefs, and moral standards on others while in the professional nursing role. Judgmental messages contain terms such as "should," "shouldn't," "ought to," "good," "bad," "right," or "wrong." Agreeing or disagreeing sends the subtle message that a nurse has the right to make value judgments about the client's decisions. Approving implies that the behavior being praised is the only acceptable one, and disapproving implies that the client must meet the nurse's expectations or standards. Instead, the nurse should assist the client to explore their own values, beliefs, goals, and decisions.	Nontherapeutic: "You shouldn't consider elective surgery; there are too many risks involved." Therapeutic: "You are considering having elective surgery. Tell me more about the pros and cons of surgery."
Giving Defensive Responses	When clients or family members express criticism, nurses should listen to the message. Listening does not imply agreement. To discover reasons for the client's anger or dissatisfaction, the nurse should listen without criticizing, avoid being defensive or accusatory, and attempt to defuse anger.	Client: "Everyone is lying to me!" Nontherapeutic: "No one here would intentionally lie to you." Therapeutic: "You believe people have been dishonest with you. Tell me more about what happened." (After obtaining additional information, the nurse may elect to follow the chain of command at the agency and report the client's concerns for follow-up.)
Providing Passive or Aggressive Responses	Passive responses serve to avoid conflict or sidestep issues, whereas aggressive responses provoke confrontation. Nurses should use assertive communication.	Nontherapeutic: "It's your fault you are feeling ill because you didn't take your medicine." Therapeutic: "Taking your medicine every day can prevent these symptoms from returning."
Arguing	Arguing against client perceptions denies that they are real and valid. They imply that the other person is lying, misinformed, or uneducated. The skillful nurse can provide information or present reality in a way that avoids argument.	Nontherapeutic: "How can you say you didn't sleep last night when I heard you snoring!" Therapeutic: "You don't feel rested this morning? Let's talk about ways to improve the quality of your rest."

See the following box for a summary of tips for using therapeutic communication and avoiding common barriers to therapeutic communication.

My Notes

Tips for Effective Therapeutic Communication

- Establish a goal for the conversation.
- Be self-aware of one's nonverbal messages.
- Observe the client's nonverbal behaviors and actions as 'cues' for assessments and planning interventions.
- Avoid self-disclosure of personal information and use professional boundaries. (Review boundary setting in the "Boundaries" section of Chapter 1.)
- Be patient-centered and actively listen to what the client is expressing (e.g., provide empathy, not sympathy; show respect; gain the client's trust; and accept the person as who they are as an individual).
- Be sensitive to the values, cultural beliefs, attitudes, practices, and problem-solving strategies of the client.
- Effectively use therapeutic communication techniques.
- Recognize themes in a conversation (e.g., Is there a theme emerging of poor self-esteem, guilt, shame, loneliness, helplessness, hopelessness, or suicidal thoughts?).

Common Barriers to Therapeutic Communication

- Using a tone of voice that is distant, condescending, or disapproving.
- Using medical jargon or too many technical terms.
- Asking yes/no questions instead of open-ended questions.
- Continually asking "why," causing the client to become defensive or feel challenged by your questions.
- Using too many probing questions, causing the client to feel you are interrogating them, resulting in defensiveness or refusal to talk with the nurse.
- Lacking awareness of one's biases, fears, feelings, or insecurities.
- Causing sensory overload in the client with a high emotional level of the content.
- Giving advice.
- Blurring the nurse-client relationship boundaries (e.g., assuming control of the conversation, disclosing personal information, practicing outside one's scope of practice).

My Notes

Recognizing and Addressing Escalation

When communicating therapeutically with a client, it is important to recognize if the client is escalating with increased agitation and becoming a danger to themselves, staff, or other patients. When escalation occurs, providing safety becomes the nurse's top priority, and the focus is no longer on therapeutic communication. Read more information in the "Crisis and Crisis Intervention" section of the "Stress, Coping, and Crisis Intervention" chapter.

Cultural Considerations

Recall the discussion from Chapter 1 on how cultural values and beliefs can impact a client's mental health in many ways. Every culture has a different perspective on mental health. For many cultures, there is stigma surrounding mental health. Mental health challenges may be considered a weakness and something to hide, which can make it harder for those struggling to talk openly and ask for help. Culture can also influence how people describe and feel about their symptoms. It can affect whether someone chooses to recognize and talk openly about physical symptoms, emotional symptoms, or both. Cultural factors can determine how much support someone gets from their family and community when it comes to mental health.[10]

Nurses can help clients understand the role culture plays in their mental health by encouraging therapeutic communication about their symptoms and treatment. For example, a nurse should ask, "What do you think is wrong? How would you treat your symptoms?"

> Read more about providing culturally responsive care in the "Diverse Clients" chapter of Open RN *Nursing Fundamentals.*

10 Mental Health First Aid USA. (2019, July 11). *Four ways culture impacts mental health.* National Council for Mental Wellbeing. https://www.mentalhealthfirstaid.org/2019/07/four-ways-culture-impacts-mental-health/

2.4 MOTIVATIONAL INTERVIEWING

My Notes

Patient education and health promotion are core nursing interventions. **Motivational interviewing (MI)** is a communication skill used to elicit and emphasize a client's personal motivation for modifying behavior to promote health. MI has been effectively used for several health issues such as smoking cessation, diabetes, substance use disorders, and adherence to a treatment plan.[1]

The spirit of motivational interviewing is a collaborative partnership between nurses and clients, focused on patient-centered care, autonomy, and personal responsibility. It is a technique that explores a client's motivation, confidence, and roadblocks to change. During motivational interviewing, nurses pose questions, actively listen to client responses, and focus on where the client is now with a current health behavior and where they want to be in the future.[2]

Motivational interviewing uses these principles[3]:

- **Express empathy.** Use reflective listening to convey acceptance and a nonjudgmental attitude. Rephrase client comments to convey active listening and let clients know they are being heard.
- **Highlight discrepancies.** Help clients become aware of the gap between their current behaviors and their values and goals. Present objective information that highlights the consequences of continuing their current behaviors to motivate them to change their behavior.
- **Adjust to resistance.** Adjust to a client's resistance and do not argue. The client may demonstrate resistance by avoiding eye contact, becoming defensive, interrupting you, or seeming distracted by looking at their watch or cell phone. Arguing can place the client on the defensive and in a position of arguing against the change. Focus on validating the client's feelings.
- **Understand motivations.** Uncover a client's personal reasons for making behavioral changes and build on them.
- **Support self-efficacy.** Encourage the client's optimistic belief in the prospect of change and encourage them to commit to positive behavioral changes. Ask clients to elaborate on past successes to build self-confidence and support self-efficacy.
- **Resist the reflex to provide advice.** Avoid imposing your own perspective and advice.

When implementing motivational interviewing, it is important to assess the client's readiness for change. Motivational interviewing is especially useful for clients in the contemplation stage who are feeling ambivalent about making change. Recall these five stages of behavioral change[4]:

1 Rubak, S., Sandbaek, A., Lauritzen, T., & Christensen, B. (2005). Motivational interviewing: A systematic review and meta-analysis. *The British Journal of General Practice: The Journal of the Royal College of General Practitioners, 55*(513), 305–312. https://www.ncbi.nlm.nih.gov/pmc/articles/PMC1463134/

2 Droppa, M., & Lee, H. (2014). Motivational interviewing: A journey to improve health. *Nursing, 44*(3), 40–46. https://doi.org/10.1097/01.NURSE.0000443312.58360.82

3 Droppa, M., & Lee, H. (2014). Motivational interviewing: A journey to improve health. *Nursing, 44*(3), 40–46. https://doi.org/10.1097/01.NURSE.0000443312.58360.82

4 Droppa, M., & Lee, H. (2014). Motivational interviewing: A journey to improve health. *Nursing, 44*(3), 40–46. https://doi.org/10.1097/01.NURSE.0000443312.58360.82

My Notes

- **Precontemplation:** Not considering change.
- **Contemplation:** Ambivalent about making change.
- **Preparation:** Taking steps toward implementing change.
- **Action:** Actively involved in the change process.
- **Maintenance:** Sustaining the target behavior.

Identify clients who are ambivalent about making a behavioral change or following a treatment plan by listening for the phrase, "Yes, but." The "but" holds the key for opening the conversation about ambivalence. For example, a client may state, "I want to take my medication, but I hate gaining weight." The content in the sentence after the "but" reveals the client's personal roadblock to making a change and should be taken into consideration when planning outcomes and interventions.[5]

See the following box for an example of a nurse using motivational interviewing with a client.

Example of Motivational Interviewing

Mr. L. had been in treatment for bipolar I disorder with medication management and supportive therapy for many years. He had a history of alcohol dependence but was in full recovery. Mr. L. was admitted to the intensive care unit with a toxic lithium level. He had been seen in the emergency room the preceding evening and was noted to have a very high blood alcohol level. The next day the nurse asked the client about his alcohol use using motivational interviewing.

Client: I am so sick of everyone always blaming everything on my drinking!

Nurse (Using reflective listening): You seem pretty angry about the perception that you were hospitalized because you had been drinking.

Client: You better believe it! I am a man! I can have a few drinks if I want to!

Nurse: (Expressing empathy and acceptance): You want to be respected even when you are drinking.

Client: I have had some trouble in the past with drinking, but that is not now. I can quit if I want to! Compared to what I used to drink, this is nothing.

Nurse (Rolling with resistance): So you see yourself as having had drinking problems in the past, but the drinking you've done recently is not harmful for you.

Client: Well, I guess I did end up in the hospital.

Nurse (Using open-ended questioning): Tell me more about what happened.

Client: I was pretty angry after an argument with my girlfriend, and I decided to buy a bottle of whiskey.

Nurse (Exploring): And then?

5 Droppa, M., & Lee, H. (2014). Motivational interviewing: A journey to improve health. *Nursing, 44*(3), 40–46. https://doi.org/10.1097/01.NURSE.0000443312.58360.82

My Notes

Client: Well, I meant to have a couple of shots, but I ended up drinking the whole fifth. I really don't remember what happened next. They said I nearly died.

Nurse (Summarizing): So after many years of not drinking, you decided to have a couple of drinks after the argument with your girlfriend, but unintentionally drank enough to have a blackout and nearly die.

Client: I guess that does sound like a problem . . . but I don't want anyone else telling me whether or not I can drink!

Nurse (Emphasizing autonomy): Tell me how the choice to drink or not continues to support or oppose your health goals.

View the following supplementary YouTube videos about motivational interviewing:

Introduction to Motivational Interviewing[6]

Motivational Interviewing – Good Example – Alan Lyme[7]

Complete Western Region Public Health Training Center's Motivational Interviewing course and receive a certificate of completion.

6 Matulich, B. (2013, May 30). *Introduction to motivational interviewing* [Video]. YouTube. All rights reserved. https://youtu.be/s3MCJZ7OGRk

7 TheRETAchannel. (2013, July 18). *Motivational interviewing - Good example - Alan Lyme* [Video]. YouTube. All rights reserved. https://youtu.be/67I6g1I7Zao

My Notes

2.5 TELETHERAPY AND TELEHEALTH

Telehealth is the use of digital technologies to deliver medical care, health education, and public health services by remotely connecting multiple users in separate locations. Nurses must be aware of potential barriers affecting client use of telehealth (such as lack of Internet access or lack of support for individuals learning new technologies), as well as state and federal policies regarding telehealth and their nursing license across state lines.

Read more about telehealth licensing requirements and interstate compacts at the Telehealth.hss.gov web page.

Teletherapy is mental health counseling over the phone or online with videoconferencing. COVID-19 has led to reduced access to medical and mental health care, so delivering behavioral health care via telehealth is one way to address this issue. When using teletherapy, nurses should treat clients as if they are sitting across from them and focus on eye contact and empathetic expressions to build a connection, just like during a face-to-face encounter.[1]

Group therapy can be accomplished via telehealth. Connecting clients through telehealth creates a group dynamic that can build community, reduce feelings of isolation, and offer new perspectives. Group therapy via telehealth can create a sense of belonging and build a trusted support system.

Here are a few guidelines for group therapy telehealth sessions[2]:

- **Prescreen group members:** Group members may have various needs, experiences, or personalities. It is helpful to screen each potential client to ensure every member can benefit from group therapy and that their needs match the goals of the group.
- **Require completion of online consent forms:** Group telehealth sessions involve multiple people and are conducted outside of a controlled setting like an office. Client consent forms should be required and available online. The consent forms should outline any associated risks, benefits, and limits to confidentiality.
- **Develop group guidelines:** Make clear ground rules covering what is acceptable and what is not acceptable. Some common ground rules include requiring all participants to have their camera on, attend from a room where they can be alone during the session, and use the digital "raise hand" feature (or raise their hand) when they want to speak. Prohibiting recording of the session is a common ground rule to protect confidentiality. Address logistical topics like how many missed sessions are allowed and how to contact the group leader(s).
- **Select your settings and technology:** Choose the telehealth video platform that best suits your needs for encryption and privacy, user controls, and more. Go through all of the settings ahead of time to select the options that provide the highest level of privacy. Think about what will help you and the group communicate effectively such as screen sharing options or a virtual whiteboard.
- **Be engaging:** When you are on screen instead of in person, it is even more important to be conscious of the group dynamic and take steps to keep group members interested, energized, and engaged. Start with introductions and greetings using first names only for privacy. Make

---

1 TELEHEALTH.HHS.GOV. (2021, July 2). *Individual teletherapy.* Health Resources & Services Administration. https://telehealth.hhs.gov/providers/telehealth-for-behavioral-health/individual-teletherapy/

2 TELEHEALTH.HHS.GOV. (2021, July 2). *Individual teletherapy.* Health Resources & Services Administration. https://telehealth.hhs.gov/providers/telehealth-for-behavioral-health/individual-teletherapy/

My Notes

eye contact with group members by looking into the camera and use body language and hand gestures to help express your ideas. Build in moments for clients to interact and contribute to the conversation, such as breakout rooms or paired discussions.

My Notes

2.6 LEARNING ACTIVITIES

Interactive Activities

An interactive H5P element has been excluded from this version of the text. You can view it online here: https://wtcs.pressbooks.pub/nursingmhcc/?p=194#h5p-4

An interactive H5P element has been excluded from this version of the text. You can view it online here: https://wtcs.pressbooks.pub/nursingmhcc/?p=194#h5p-6

An interactive H5P element has been excluded from this version of the text. You can view it online here: https://wtcs.pressbooks.pub/nursingmhcc/?p=194#h5p-9

An interactive H5P element has been excluded from this version of the text. You can view it online here: https://wtcs.pressbooks.pub/nursingmhcc/?p=194#h5p-10

II GLOSSARY

My Notes

Active listening: Communicating both verbally and nonverbally that we are interested in what the other person is saying while also actively verifying our understanding with them.

Motivational interviewing (MI): A communication skill used to elicit and emphasize a client's personal motivation for modifying behavior to promote health.

Nurse-client relationship: A relationship that establishes trust and rapport with a specific purpose of facilitating therapeutic communication and engaging the client in decision-making regarding their plan of care.

SOLER: A mnemonic for effective nonverbal communication that stands for the following[1]:

- S: Sit and squarely face the client
- O: Open posture
- L: Lean towards the client to indicate interest in listening
- E: Eye contact
- R: Relax

Telehealth: The use of digital technologies to deliver medical care, health education, and public health services by remotely connecting multiple users in separate locations.

Teletherapy: Mental health counseling over the phone or online with videoconferencing tools.

Therapeutic communication: A type of professional communication defined as the purposeful, interpersonal, information-transmitting process that leads to client understanding and participation.[2]

---

1 Stickley, T. (2011). From SOLER to SURETY for effective non-verbal communication. *Nurse Education in Practice, 11*(6), 395–398. https://doi.org/10.1016/j.nepr.2011.03.021

2 Abdolrahimi, M., Ghiyasvandian, S., Zakerimoghadam, M., & Ebadi, A. (2017). Therapeutic communication in nursing students: A Walker & Avant concept analysis. *Electronic Physician, 9(*8), 4968–4977. https://doi.org/10.19082/4968

Chapter 3

Stress, Coping, and Crisis Intervention

3.1 INTRODUCTION

My Notes

Learning Objectives

- Recognize nonverbal cues for physical and/or psychological stressors
- Provide patient education on stress management techniques
- Promote adaptive coping strategies
- Recognize the use of defense mechanisms
- Recognize a client in crisis
- Describe crisis intervention

Nurses support the emotional, mental, and social well-being of all clients experiencing stressful events and those with acute and chronic mental illnesses.[1] This chapter will review stressors, stress management, coping strategies, defense mechanisms, and crisis intervention.

1 NCSBN. (n.d.). *Test plans*. https://www.ncsbn.org/testplans.htm

My Notes

3.2 STRESS

Everyone experiences stress during their lives. High levels of stress can cause symptoms like headaches, back pain, and gastrointestinal symptoms. Chronic stress contributes to the development of chronic illnesses, as well as acute physical illnesses due to decreased effectiveness of the immune system. It is important for nurses to recognize signs and symptoms of stress in themselves and others, as well as encourage effective stress management strategies. We will begin this section by reviewing the stress response and signs and symptoms of stress and then discuss stress management techniques.

Stress Response

Stressors are any internal or external event, force, or condition that results in physical or emotional stress.[1] The body's sympathetic nervous system (SNS) responds to actual or perceived stressors with the "fight, flight, or freeze" stress response. Several reactions occur during the **stress response** that help the individual to achieve the purpose of either fighting or running. The respiratory, cardiovascular, and musculoskeletal systems are activated to breathe rapidly, stimulate the heart to pump more blood, dilate the blood vessels, and increase blood pressure to deliver more oxygenated blood to the muscles. The liver creates more glucose for energy for the muscles to use to fight or run. Pupils dilate to see the threat (or the escape route) more clearly. Sweating prevents the body from overheating from excess muscle contraction. Because the digestive system is not needed during this time of threat, the body shunts oxygen-rich blood to the skeletal muscles. To coordinate all these targeted responses, hormones, including epinephrine, norepinephrine, and glucocorticoids (including cortisol, often referred to as the "stress hormone"), are released by the endocrine system via the hypothalamic-pituitary-adrenal axis (HPA) and dispersed to the many SNS neuroreceptors on target organs simultaneously.[2] After the response to the stressful stimuli has resolved, the body returns to the pre-emergency state facilitated by the parasympathetic nervous system (PNS) that has opposing effects to the SNS. See Figure 3.1[3] for an image comparing the effects of stimulating the SNS and PNS.

1 American Psychological Association. (n.d.). Stressor. *APA Dictionary of Psychology*. https://dictionary.apa.org

2 This work is a derivative of *Anatomy and Physiology* by OpenStax licensed under CC BY 4.0. Access for free at https://openstax.org/books/anatomy-and-physiology/pages/1-introduction

3 Untitled image by Meredith Pomietlo for Chippewa Valley Technical College is licensed under CC BY 4.0

My Notes

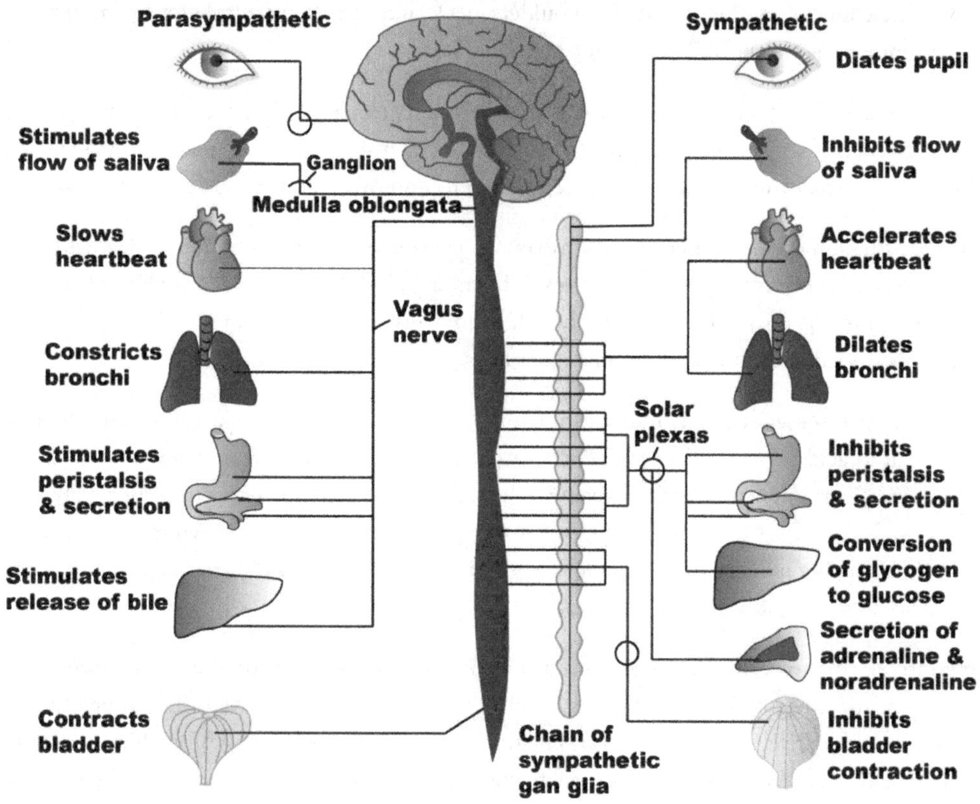

Figure 3.1 SNS and PNS Simulation

Effects of Chronic Stress

The "fight or flight or freeze" stress response equips our bodies to quickly respond to life-threatening stressors. However, exposure to long-term stress can cause serious effects on the cardiovascular, musculoskeletal, endocrine, gastrointestinal, and reproductive systems.[4] Consistent and ongoing increases in heart rate and blood pressure and elevated levels of stress hormones contribute to inflammation in arteries and can increase the risk for hypertension, heart attack, or stroke.[5]

During sudden onset stress, muscles contract and then relax when the stress passes. However, during chronic stress, muscles in the body are often in a constant state of vigilance that may trigger other reactions of the body and even promote stress-related disorders. For example, tension-type headaches and migraine headaches are associated

4 Shaw, W., Labott-Smith, S., Burg, M. M., Hostinar, C., Alen, N., van Tilburg, M. A. L., Berntson, G. G., Tovian, S. M., & Spirito, M. (2018, November 1). *Stress effects on the body.* American Psychological Association. https://www.apa.org/topics/stress/body

5 Shaw, W., Labott-Smith, S., Burg, M. M., Hostinar, C., Alen, N., van Tilburg, M. A. L., Berntson, G. G., Tovian, S. M., & Spirito, M. (2018, November 1). *Stress effects on the body.* American Psychological Association. https://www.apa.org/topics/stress/body

My Notes

with chronic muscle tension in the area of the shoulders, neck, and head. Musculoskeletal pain in the lower back and upper extremities has also been linked to job stress.[6]

Relaxation techniques and other stress-relieving activities have been shown to effectively reduce muscle tension, decrease the incidence of stress-related disorders, and increase a sense of well-being. For individuals with chronic pain conditions, stress-relieving activities have been shown to improve mood and daily function.[7]

During an acute stressful event, an increase in cortisol can provide the energy required to deal with prolonged or extreme challenges. However, chronic stress can result in an impaired immune system that has been linked to the development of numerous physical and mental health conditions, including chronic fatigue, metabolic disorders (e.g., diabetes, obesity), depression, and immune disorders.[8]

When chronically stressed, individuals may eat much more or much less than usual. Increased food, alcohol, or tobacco can result in acid reflux. Stress can induce muscle spasms in the bowel and can affect how quickly food moves through the gastrointestinal system, causing either diarrhea or constipation. Stress especially affects people with chronic bowel disorders, such as inflammatory bowel disease or irritable bowel syndrome. This may be due to the nerves in the gut being more sensitive, changes in gut microbiota, changes in how quickly food moves through the gut, and/or changes in gut immune responses.[9]

Excess amounts of cortisol can affect the normal biochemical functioning of the male reproductive system. Chronic stress can affect testosterone production, resulting in a decline in sex drive or libido, erectile dysfunction, or impotence. It can negatively impact sperm production and maturation, causing difficulties in couples who are trying to conceive. Researchers have found that men who experienced two or more stressful life events in the past year had a lower percentage of sperm motility and a lower percentage of sperm of normal morphology (size and shape) compared with men who did not experience any stressful life events.[10]

In the female reproductive system, stress affects menstruation and may be associated with absent or irregular menstrual cycles, more painful periods, and changes in the length of cycles. It may make premenstrual symptoms worse or more difficult to cope with, such as cramping, fluid retention, bloating, negative mood, and mood swings. Chronic stress may also reduce sexual desire. Stress can negatively impact a woman's ability to conceive, the health

---

6 Shaw, W., Labott-Smith, S., Burg, M. M., Hostinar, C., Alen, N., van Tilburg, M. A. L., Berntson, G. G., Tovian, S. M., & Spirito, M. (2018, November 1). *Stress effects on the body.* American Psychological Association. https://www.apa.org/topics/stress/body

7 Shaw, W., Labott-Smith, S., Burg, M. M., Hostinar, C., Alen, N., van Tilburg, M. A. L., Berntson, G. G., Tovian, S. M., & Spirito, M. (2018, November 1). *Stress effects on the body.* American Psychological Association. https://www.apa.org/topics/stress/body

8 Shaw, W., Labott-Smith, S., Burg, M. M., Hostinar, C., Alen, N., van Tilburg, M. A. L., Berntson, G. G., Tovian, S. M., & Spirito, M. (2018, November 1). *Stress effects on the body.* American Psychological Association. https://www.apa.org/topics/stress/body

9 Shaw, W., Labott-Smith, S., Burg, M. M., Hostinar, C., Alen, N., van Tilburg, M. A. L., Berntson, G. G., Tovian, S. M., & Spirito, M. (2018, November 1). *Stress effects on the body.* American Psychological Association. https://www.apa.org/topics/stress/body

10 Shaw, W., Labott-Smith, S., Burg, M. M., Hostinar, C., Alen, N., van Tilburg, M. A. L., Berntson, G. G., Tovian, S. M., & Spirito, M. (2018, November 1). *Stress effects on the body.* American Psychological Association. https://www.apa.org/topics/stress/body

My Notes

of her pregnancy, and her postpartum adjustment. Maternal stress can negatively impact fetal development, disrupt bonding with the baby following delivery, and increase the risk of postpartum depression.[11]

Adverse Childhood Experiences

Adults with adverse childhood experiences or exposure to adverse life events often experience ongoing chronic stress with an array of physical, mental, and social health problems throughout adulthood. Some of the most common health risks include physical and mental illness, substance use disorder, and a high level of engagement in risky sexual behavior.[12]

As previously discussed in Chapter 1, **adverse childhood experiences (ACEs)** include sexual abuse, physical abuse, emotional abuse, physical neglect, emotional neglect, parental loss, or parental separation before the child is 18 years old. Individuals who have experienced four or more ACEs are at a significantly higher risk of developing mental, physical, and social problems in adulthood. Research has established that early life stress is a predictor of smoking, alcohol consumption, and drug dependence. Adults who experienced ACEs related to maladaptive family functioning (parental mental illness, substance use disorder, criminality, family violence, physical and sexual abuse, and neglect) are at higher risk for developing mood, substance abuse, and anxiety disorders. ACEs are also associated with an increased risk of the development of malignancy, cardiovascular disease, metabolic syndrome, and other chronic debilitating conditions.[13]

Signs and Symptoms of Stress

Nurses are often the first to notice signs and symptoms of stress and can help make their clients aware of these symptoms. Common signs and symptoms of chronic stress are as follows[14,15]:

- Irritability
- Fatigue
- Headaches
- Difficulty concentrating
- Rapid, disorganized thoughts
- Difficulty sleeping
- Digestive problems

---

11 Shaw, W., Labott-Smith, S., Burg, M. M., Hostinar, C., Alen, N., van Tilburg, M. A. L., Berntson, G. G., Tovian, S. M., & Spirito, M. (2018, November 1). *Stress effects on the body.* American Psychological Association. https://www.apa.org/topics/stress/body

12 Amnie, A. G. (2018). Emerging themes in coping with lifetime stress and implication for stress management education. *SAGE Open Medicine, 6.* https://doi.org/10.1177%2F2050312118782545

13 Amnie, A. G. (2018). Emerging themes in coping with lifetime stress and implication for stress management education. *SAGE Open Medicine, 6.* https://doi.org/10.1177%2F2050312118782545

14 Shaw, W., Labott-Smith, S., Burg, M. M., Hostinar, C., Alen, N., van Tilburg, M. A. L., Berntson, G. G., Tovian, S. M., & Spirito, M. (2018, November 1). *Stress effects on the body.* American Psychological Association. https://www.apa.org/topics/stress/body

15 Kelly, J. F., & Coons, H. L. (2019, October 25). *Stress won't go away? Maybe you are suffering from chronic stress.* American Psychological Association. https://www.apa.org/topics/stress/chronic

My Notes

- Changes in appetite
- Feeling helpless
- A perceived loss of control
- Low self-esteem
- Loss of sexual desire
- Nervousness
- Frequent infections or illnesses
- Vocalized suicidal thoughts

Stress Management

Recognizing signs and symptoms of stress allows individuals to implement stress management strategies. Nurses can educate clients about effective strategies for reducing the stress response. Effective strategies include the following[16,17]:

- Set personal and professional boundaries
- Maintain a healthy social support network
- Select healthy food choices
- Engage in regular physical exercise
- Get an adequate amount of sleep each night
- Set realistic and fair expectations

Setting limits is essential for effectively managing stress. Individuals should list all of the projects and commitments making them feel overwhelmed, identify essential tasks, and cut back on nonessential tasks. For work-related projects, responsibilities can be discussed with supervisors to obtain input on priorities. Encourage individuals to refrain from accepting any more commitments until they feel their stress is under control.[18]

Maintaining a healthy social support network with friends and family can provide emotional support.[19] Caring relationships and healthy social connections are essential for achieving resilience.

---

16 Shaw, W., Labott-Smith, S., Burg, M. M., Hostinar, C., Alen, N., van Tilburg, M. A. L., Berntson, G. G., Tovian, S. M., & Spirito, M. (2018, November 1). *Stress effects on the body.* American Psychological Association. https://www.apa.org/topics/stress/body

17 Kelly, J. F., & Coons, H. L. (2019, October 25). *Stress won't go away? Maybe you are suffering from chronic stress.* American Psychological Association. https://www.apa.org/topics/stress/chronic

18 Kelly, J. F., & Coons, H. L. (2019, October 25). *Stress won't go away? Maybe you are suffering from chronic stress.* American Psychological Association. https://www.apa.org/topics/stress/chronic

19 Kelly, J. F., & Coons, H. L. (2019, October 25). *Stress won't go away? Maybe you are suffering from chronic stress.* American Psychological Association. https://www.apa.org/topics/stress/chronic

My Notes

Physical activity increases the body's production of endorphins that boost the mood and reduce stress. Nurses can educate clients that a brisk walk or other aerobic activity can increase energy and concentration levels and lessen feelings of anxiety.[20]

People who are chronically stressed often suffer from lack of adequate sleep and, in some cases, stress-induced insomnia. Nurses can educate individuals how to take steps to increase the quality of sleep. Experts recommend going to bed at a regular time each night, striving for at least 7-8 hours of sleep, and, if possible, eliminating distractions, such as television, cell phones, and computers from the bedroom. Begin winding down an hour or two before bedtime and engage in calming activities such as listening to relaxing music, reading an enjoyable book, taking a soothing bath, or practicing relaxation techniques like meditation. Avoid eating a heavy meal or engaging in intense exercise immediately before bedtime. If a person tends to lie in bed worrying, encourage them to write down their concerns and work on quieting their thoughts.[21]

Nurses can encourage clients to set realistic expectations, look at situations more positively, see problems as opportunities, and refute negative thoughts to stay positive and minimize stress. Setting realistic expectations and positively reframing the way one looks at stressful situations can make life seem more manageable. Clients should be encouraged to keep challenges in perspective and do what they can reasonably do to move forward.[22]

Mindfulness is a form of meditation that uses breathing and thought techniques to create an awareness of one's body and surroundings. Research suggests that mindfulness can have a positive impact on stress, anxiety, and depression.[23] Additionally, guided imagery may be helpful for enhancing relaxation. The use of guided imagery provides a narration that the mind can focus in on during the activity. For example, as the nurse encourages a client to use mindfulness and relaxation breathing, they may say, "As you breathe in, imagine waves rolling gently in. As you breathe out, imagine the waves rolling gently back out to sea."

WHO Stress Management Guide

In addition to the stress management techniques discussed in the previous section, the World Health Organization (WHO) shares additional techniques in a guide titled *Doing What Matters in Times of Stress*. This guide is comprised of five categories. Each category includes techniques and skills that, based on evidence and field testing, can reduce overall stress levels even if only used for a few minutes each day. These categories include 1) Grounding, 2) Unhooking, 3) Acting on our values, 4) Being kind, and 5) Making room.[24]

Nurses can educate clients that powerful thoughts and feelings are a natural part of stress, but problems can occur if we get "hooked" by them. For example, one minute you might be enjoying a meal with family, and the next moment you get "hooked" by angry thoughts and feelings. Stress can make someone feel as if they are being pulled

---

20 Kelly, J. F., & Coons, H. L. (2019, October 25). *Stress won't go away? Maybe you are suffering from chronic stress.* American Psychological Association. https://www.apa.org/topics/stress/chronic

21 Kelly, J. F., & Coons, H. L. (2019, October 25). *Stress won't go away? Maybe you are suffering from chronic stress.* American Psychological Association. https://www.apa.org/topics/stress/chronic

22 Kelly, J. F., & Coons, H. L. (2019, October 25). *Stress won't go away? Maybe you are suffering from chronic stress.* American Psychological Association. https://www.apa.org/topics/stress/chronic

23 Kandola, A. (2018, October 12). *What are the health effects of chronic stress? MedicalNewsToday.* https://www.medicalnewstoday.com/articles/323324#treatment

24 This work is a derivative of *Doing What Matters in Times of Stress: An Illustrated Guide* by World Health Organization and is licensed under CC BY-NC-SA 3.0 IGO

My Notes

away from the values of the person they want to be, such as being calm, caring, attentive, committed, persistent, and courageous.[25]

There are many kinds of difficult thoughts and feelings that can "hook us," such as, "This is too hard," "I give up," "I am never going to get this," "They shouldn't have done that," or memories about difficult events that have occurred in our lives. When we get "hooked," our behavior changes. We may do things that make our lives worse, like getting into more disagreements, withdrawing from others, or spending too much time lying in bed. These are called "away moves" because they move us away from our values. Sometimes emotions become so strong they feel like emotional storms. However, we can "unhook" ourselves by focusing and engaging in what we are doing, referred to as "grounding."[26]

Grounding

"Grounding" is a helpful tool when feeling distracted or having trouble focusing on a task and/or the present moment. The first step of grounding is to notice how you are feeling and what you are thinking. Next, slow down and connect with your body by focusing on your breathing. Exhale completely and wait three seconds, and then inhale as slowly as possible. Slowly stretch your arms and legs and push your feet against the floor. The next step is to focus on the world around you. Notice where you are and what you are doing. Use your five senses. What are five things you can see? What are four things you can hear? What can you smell? Tap your leg or squeeze your thumb and count to ten. Touch your knees or another object within reach. What does it feel like? Grounding helps us engage in life, refocus on the present moment, and realign with our values.[27]

Unhooking

At times we may have unwanted, intrusive, negative thoughts that negatively affect us. "Unhooking" is a tool to manage and decrease the impact of these unwanted thoughts. First, NOTICE that a thought or feeling has hooked you, and then NAME it. Naming it begins by silently saying, "Here is a thought," or "Here is a feeling." By adding "I notice," it unhooks us even more. For example, "I notice there is a knot in my stomach." The next step is to REFOCUS on what you are doing, fully engage in that activity, and pay full attention to whoever is with you and whatever you are doing. For example, if you are having dinner with family and notice feelings of anger, note "I am having feelings of anger," but choose to refocus and engage with family.[28]

Acting on Our Values

The third category of skills is called "Acting on Our Values." This means, despite challenges and struggles we are experiencing, we will act in line with what is important to us and our beliefs. Even when facing difficult situations, we can still make the conscious choice to act in line with our values. The more we focus on our own actions, the more we can influence our immediate world and the people and situations we encounter every day. We must continually ask ourselves, "Are my actions moving me toward or away from my values?" Remember that even the

---

25 This work is a derivative of *Doing What Matters in Times of Stress: An Illustrated Guide* by World Health Organization and is licensed under CC BY-NC-SA 3.0 IGO

26 This work is a derivative of *Doing What Matters in Times of Stress: An Illustrated Guide* by World Health Organization and is licensed under CC BY-NC-SA 3.0 IGO

27 This work is a derivative of *Doing What Matters in Times of Stress: An Illustrated Guide* by World Health Organization and is licensed under CC BY-NC-SA 3.0 IGO

28 This work is a derivative of *Doing What Matters in Times of Stress: An Illustrated Guide* by World Health Organization and is licensed under CC BY-NC-SA 3.0 IGO

My Notes

smallest actions have impact, just as a giant tree grows from a small seed. Even in the most stressful of times, we can take small actions to live by our values and maintain or create a more satisfying and fulfilling life. These values should also include self-compassion and care. By caring for oneself, we ultimately have more energy and motivation to then help others.[29]

Being Kind

"Being Kind" is a fourth tool for reducing stress. Kindness can make a significant difference to our mental health by being kind to others, as well as to ourselves.

Making Room

"Making Room" is a fifth tool for reducing stress. Sometimes trying to push away painful thoughts and feelings does not work very well. In these situations, it is helpful to notice and name the feeling, and then "make room" for it. "Making room" means allowing the painful feeling or thought to come and go like the weather. Nurses can educate clients that as they breathe, they should imagine their breath flowing into and around their pain and making room for it. Instead of fighting with the thought or feeling, they should allow it to move through them, just like the weather moves through the sky. If clients are not fighting with the painful thought or feeling, they will have more time and energy to engage with the world around them and do things that are important to them.[30]

Read Doing What Matters in Times of Stress by the World Health Organization (WHO).

View a video: Doing What Matters in Times of Stress: An Illustrated Guide.[31]

One or more interactive elements has been excluded from this version of the text. You can view them online here: https://wtcs.pressbooks.pub/nursingmhcc/?p=135#oembed-1

29 This work is a derivative of *Doing What Matters in Times of Stress: An Illustrated Guide* by World Health Organization and is licensed under CC BY-C-SA 3.0 IGO

30 This work is a derivative of *Doing What Matters in Times of Stress: An Illustrated Guide* by World Health Organization and is licensed under CC BY-NC-SA 3.0 IGO

31 World Health Organization (WHO). (2020, November 4). *Doing what matters in times of stress: An illustrated guide* [Video]. YouTube. Licensed in the Public Domain. https://youtu.be/E3Cts45FNrk

My Notes

Stress Related to the COVID-19 Pandemic and World Events

The COVID-19 pandemic had a major effect on many people's lives. Many health care professionals faced challenges that were stressful, overwhelming, and caused strong emotions.[32] See Figure 3.2[33] for a message from the World Health Organization regarding stress and health care workers.

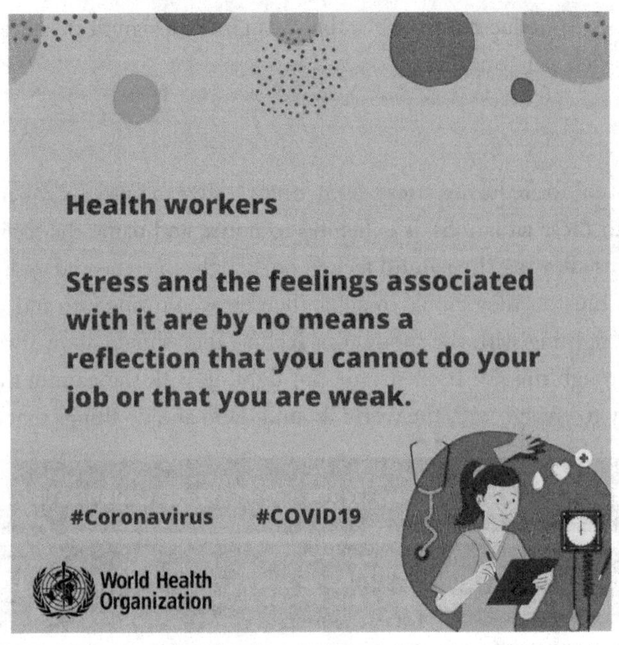

Figure 3.2 Stress and Healthcare Workers

Learning to cope with stress in a healthy way can increase feelings of resiliency for health care professionals. Here are ways to help manage stress resulting from world events[34]:

- Take breaks from watching, reading, or listening to news stories and social media. It's good to be informed but consider limiting news to just a couple times a day and disconnecting from phones, TVs, and computer screens for a while.
    - It can be important to do a self check-in before reading any news. "Do I have the emotional energy to handle a difficult headline if I see one?"

---

32 Centers for Disease Control and Prevention. (2021, December 2). *Healthcare personnel and first responders: How to cope with stress and build resilience during the COVID-19 pandemic.* https://www.cdc.gov/coronavirus/2019-ncov/hcp/mental-health-healthcare.html

33 "89118597-2933268333403014-548082632068431872-n.jpg" by unknown author for World Health Organization (WHO) is licensed in the Public Domain. Access for free at https://www.who.int/campaigns/connecting-the-world-to-combat-coronavirus/healthyathome/healthyathome---mental-health?gclid=Cj0KCQiA0MD_BRCTARIsADXoopa7YZldaIqCtKlGrxDV8YcUBtpVSD2HaOtT9NsdT8ajyCXbnPot-bsaAvlQEALw_wcB

34 Centers for Disease Control and Prevention. (2021, December 2). *Healthcare personnel and first responders: How to cope with stress and build resilience during the COVID-19 pandemic.* https://www.cdc.gov/coronavirus/2019-ncov/hcp/mental-health-healthcare.html

My Notes

- Take care of your body.
  - Take deep breaths, stretch, or meditate
  - Try to eat healthy, well-balanced meals
  - Exercise regularly
  - Get plenty of sleep
  - Avoid excessive alcohol, tobacco, and substance use
  - Continue routine preventive measures (such as vaccinations, cancer screenings, etc.) as recommended by your health care provider
- Make time to unwind. Plan activities you enjoy.
- Purposefully connect with others. It is especially important to stay connected with your friends and family. Helping others cope through phone calls or video chats can help you and your loved ones feel less lonely or isolated. Connect with your community or faith-based organizations.
- Use the techniques described in the WHO stress management guide.[35]

Strategies for Self-Care

By becoming self-aware regarding signs of stress, you can implement self-care strategies to prevent compassion fatigue and burnout. Use the following "A's" to assist in building resilience, connection, and compassion[36]:

- **Attention:** Become aware of your physical, psychological, social, and spiritual health. What are you grateful for? What are your areas of improvement? This protects you from drifting through life on autopilot.
- **Acknowledgement:** Honestly look at all you have witnessed as a health care professional. What insight have you experienced? Acknowledging the pain of loss you have witnessed protects you from invalidating the experiences.
- **Affection:** Choose to look at yourself with kindness and warmth. Affection and self-compassion prevent you from becoming bitter and "being too hard" on yourself.
- **Acceptance:** Choose to be at peace and welcome all aspects of yourself. By accepting both your talents and imperfections, you can protect yourself from impatience, victim mentality, and blame.

Many individuals have had to cope with grief and loss during the COVID pandemic. Read more about coping with grief and loss during COVID at the CDC's Mental Health Grief and Loss web page.

35 This work is a derivative of *Doing What Matters in Times of Stress: An Illustrated Guide* by World Health Organization and is licensed under CC BY-NC-SA 3.0 IGO

36 This work is a derivative of *Nursing Care at the End of Life* by Lowey and is licensed under CC BY-NC-SA 4.0

My Notes

3.3 COPING

The health consequences of chronic stress depend on an individual's coping styles and their resilience to real or perceived stress. **Coping** refers to cognitive and behavioral efforts made to master, tolerate, or reduce external and internal demands and conflicts.[1]

Coping strategies are actions, a series of actions, or thought processes used in meeting a stressful or unpleasant situation or in modifying one's reaction to such a situation. Coping strategies are classified as adaptive or maladaptive. **Adaptive coping strategies** include problem-focused coping and emotion-focused coping. **Problem-focused coping** typically focuses on seeking treatment such as counseling or cognitive behavioral therapy. **Emotion-focused coping** includes strategies such as mindfulness, meditation, and yoga; using humor and jokes; seeking spiritual or religious pursuits; engaging in physical activity or breathing exercises; and seeking social support.

Maladaptive coping responses include avoidance of the stressful condition, withdrawal from a stressful environment, disengagement from stressful relationships, and misuse of drugs and/or alcohol.[2] Nurses can educate individuals and their family members about adaptive, emotion-focused coping strategies and make referrals to interprofessional team members for problem-focused coping and treatment options for individuals experiencing maladaptive coping responses to stress.

Emotion-Focused Coping Strategies

Nurses can educate clients about many emotion-focused coping strategies, such as meditating, practicing yoga, journaling, praying, spending time in nature, nurturing supportive relationships, and practicing mindfulness.

Meditation

Meditation can induce feelings of calm and clearheadedness and improve concentration and attention. Research has shown that meditation increases the brain's gray matter density, which can reduce sensitivity to pain, enhance the immune system, help regulate difficult emotions, and relieve stress. Meditation has been proven helpful for people with depression and anxiety, cancer, fibromyalgia, chronic pain, rheumatoid arthritis, type 2 diabetes, chronic fatigue syndrome, and cardiovascular disease.[3] See Figure 3.3[4] for an image of an individual participating in meditation.

---

1 Amnie, A. G. (2018). Emerging themes in coping with lifetime stress and implication for stress management education. *SAGE Open Medicine, 6*. https://doi.org/10.1177%2F2050312118782545

2 Amnie, A. G. (2018). Emerging themes in coping with lifetime stress and implication for stress management education. *SAGE Open Medicine, 6*. https://doi.org/10.1177%2F2050312118782545

3 Delagran, L. (n.d.). *What is spirituality?* University of Minnesota. https://www.takingcharge.csh.umn.edu/what-spirituality

4 "yoga-class-a-cross-legged-palms-up-meditation-position-850x831.jpg" by Amanda Mills, USCDCP on Pixnio is licensed under CC0

My Notes

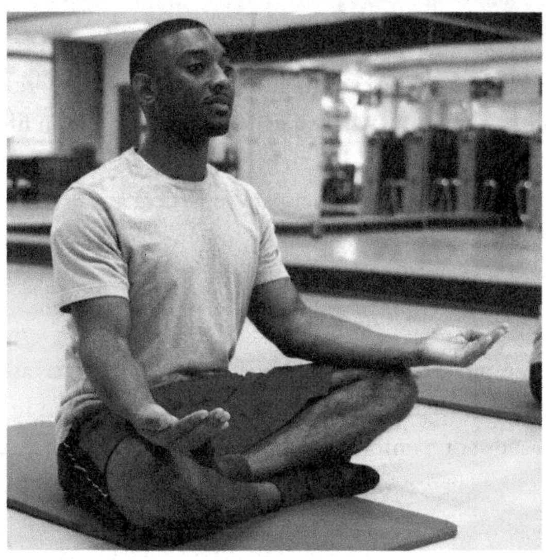

Figure 3.3 Meditation

Yoga

Yoga is a centuries-old spiritual practice that creates a sense of union within the practitioner through physical postures, ethical behaviors, and breath expansion. The systematic practice of yoga has been found to reduce inflammation and stress, decrease depression and anxiety, lower blood pressure, and increase feelings of well-being.[5] See Figure 3.4[6] for an image of an individual participating in yoga.

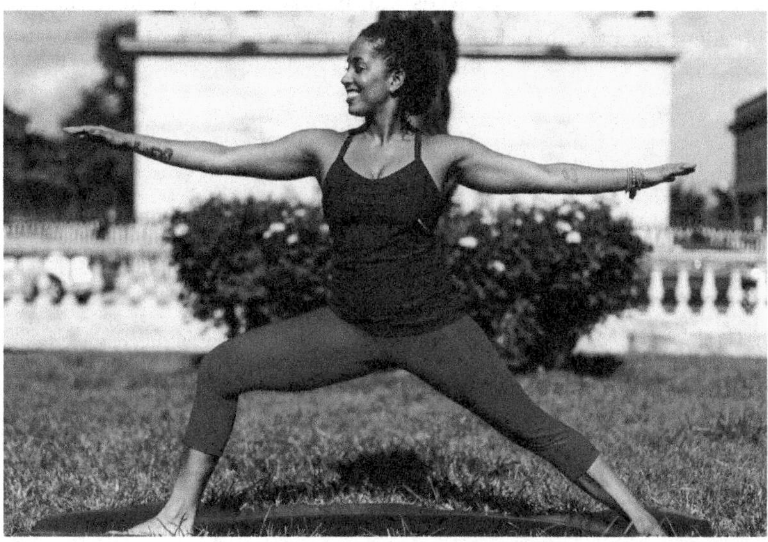

Figure 3.4 Yoga

5 Delagran, L. (n.d.). *What is spirituality?* University of Minnesota. https://www.takingcharge.csh.umn.edu/what-spirituality

6 "9707554768.jpg" by Dave Rosenblum is licensed under CC BY 2.0

My Notes

Journaling

Journaling can help a person become more aware of their inner life and feel more connected to experiences. Studies show that writing during difficult times may help a person find meaning in life's challenges and become more resilient in the face of obstacles. When journaling, it can be helpful to focus on three basic questions: What experiences give me energy? What experiences drain my energy? Were there any experiences today where I felt alive and experienced "flow"? Allow yourself to write freely, without stopping to edit or worry about spelling and grammar.[7]

Prayer

Prayer can elicit the relaxation response, along with feelings of hope, gratitude, and compassion, all of which have a positive effect on overall well-being. There are several types of prayer rooted in the belief that there is a higher power. This belief can provide a sense of comfort and support in difficult times. A recent study found that adults who were clinically depressed who believed their prayers were heard by a concerned presence responded much better to treatment than those who did not believe.[8]

Individuals can be encouraged to find a spiritual community, such as a church, synagogue, temple, mosque, meditation center, or other local group that meets to discuss spiritual issues. The benefits of social support are well-documented, and having a spiritual community to turn to for fellowship can provide a sense of belonging and support.[9]

Spending Time in Nature

Spending time in nature is cited by many individuals as a spiritual practice that contributes to their mental health.[10] Spirituality is defined as a dynamic and intrinsic aspect of humanity through which persons seek ultimate meaning, purpose, and transcendence and experience relationship to self, family, others, community, society, nature, and the significant or sacred.[11] Spiritual needs and spirituality are often mistakenly equated with religion, but spirituality is a broader concept. Other elements of spirituality include meaning, love, belonging, forgiveness, and connectedness.[12]

---

7 Delagran, L. (n.d.). *What is spirituality?* University of Minnesota. https://www.takingcharge.csh.umn.edu/what-spirituality

8 Delagran, L. (n.d.). *What is spirituality?* University of Minnesota. https://www.takingcharge.csh.umn.edu/what-spirituality

9 Delagran, L. (n.d.). *What is spirituality?* University of Minnesota. https://www.takingcharge.csh.umn.edu/what-spirituality

10 Yamada, A., Lukoff, D., Lim, C. S. F., & Mancuso, L. L. (2020). Integrating spirituality and mental health: Perspectives of adults receiving public mental health services in California. *Psychology of Religion and Spirituality, 12*(3), 276–287. https://doi.org/10.1037/rel0000260

11 Puchalski, C. M., Vitillo, R., Hull, S. K., & Reller, N. (2014). Improving the spiritual dimension of whole person care: Reaching national and international consensus. *Journal of Palliative Medicine, 17*(6), 642–656. https://doi.org/10.1089/jpm.2014.9427

12 Rudolfsson, G., Berggren, I., & da Silva, A. B. (2014). Experiences of spirituality and spiritual values in the context of nursing - An integrative review. *The Open Nursing Journal, 8*, 64–70. https://dx.doi.org/10.2174%2F1874434601408010064

Supportive Relationships

Individuals should be encouraged to nurture supportive relationships with family, significant others, and friends. Relationships aren't static – they are living, dynamic aspects of our lives that require attention and care. To benefit from strong connections with others, individuals should take charge of their relationships and devote time and energy to support them. It can be helpful to create rituals together. With busy schedules and the presence of online social media that offer the façade of real contact, it's very easy to drift from friends. Research has found that people who deliberately make time for gatherings enjoy stronger relationships and more positive energy. An easy way to do this is to create a standing ritual that you can share and that doesn't create more stress, such as talking on the telephone on Fridays or sharing a walk during lunch breaks.[13]

Mindfulness

Mindfulness has been defined as, "Awareness that arises through paying attention, on purpose, in the present moment, and nonjudgmentally." Mindfulness has also been described as, "Non-elaborative, nonjudgmental, present-centered awareness in which each thought, feeling, or sensation that arises is acknowledged and accepted as it is." Mindfulness helps us be present in our lives and gives us some control over our reactions and repetitive thought patterns. It helps us pause, get a clearer picture of a situation, and respond more skillfully. Compare your default state to mindfulness when studying for an exam in a difficult course or preparing for a clinical experience. What do you do? Do you tell yourself, "I am not good at this" or "I am going to look stupid"? Does this distract you from paying attention to studying or preparing? How might it be different if you had an open attitude with no concern or judgment about your performance? What if you directly experienced the process as it unfolded, including the challenges, anxieties, insights, and accomplishments, while acknowledging each thought or feeling and accepting it without needing to figure it out or explore it further? If practiced regularly, mindfulness helps a person start to see the habitual patterns that lead to automatic negative reactions that create stress. By observing these thoughts and emotions instead of reacting to them, a person can develop a broader perspective and can choose a more effective response.[14]

> Try free mindfulness activities at the Free Mindfulness Project.

Coping With Loss and Grief

In addition to assisting individuals to recognize and cope with their stress and anxiety, nurses can also use this knowledge regarding coping strategies to support clients and their family members as they cope with life changes, grief, and loss that can cause emotional problems and feelings of distress.

> Review concepts and nursing care related to coping with grief and loss in the "Grief and Loss" chapter of Open RN *Nursing Fundamentals*.

---

13 Delagran, L. (n.d.). *What is spirituality?* University of Minnesota. https://www.takingcharge.csh.umn.edu/what-spirituality

14 Delagran, L. (n.d.). *What is spirituality?* University of Minnesota. https://www.takingcharge.csh.umn.edu/what-spirituality

My Notes

3.4 DEFENSE MECHANISMS

When providing clients with stress management techniques and effective coping strategies, nurses must be aware of common defense mechanisms. **Defense mechanisms** are reaction patterns used by individuals to protect themselves from anxiety that arises from stress and conflict.[1] Excessive use of defense mechanisms is associated with specific mental health disorders. With the exception of suppression, all other defense mechanisms are unconscious and out of the awareness of the individual. See Table 3.4 for a description of common defense mechanisms.

Table 3.4 Common Defense Mechanisms

Defense Mechanisms	Definitions	Examples
Conversion	Anxiety caused by repressed impulses and feelings are converted into a physical symptoms.[2]	An individual scheduled to see their therapist to discuss a past sexual assault experiences a severe headache and cancels the appointment.
Denial	Unpleasant thoughts, feelings, wishes, or events are ignored or excluded from conscious awareness to protect themselves from overwhelming worry or anxiety.[3,4]	A client recently diagnosed with cancer states there was an error in diagnosis and they don't have cancer. Other examples include denial of a financial problem, an addiction, or a partner's infidelity.
Dissociation	A feeling of being disconnected from a stressful or traumatic event – or feeling that the event is not really happening – to block out mental trauma and protect the mind from too much stress.[5]	A person experiencing physical abuse may feel as if they are floating above their bodies observing the situation.
Displacement	Unconscious transfer of one's emotions or reaction from an original object to a less-threatening target to discharge tension.[6]	An individual who is angry with their partner kicks the family dog. An angry child breaks a toy or yells at a sibling instead of attacking their father. A frustrated employee criticizes their spouse instead of their boss.[7]

1 American Psychological Association. (n.d.). Stressor. *APA Dictionary of Psychology*. https://dictionary.apa.org

2 American Psychological Association. (n.d.). Stressor. *APA Dictionary of Psychology*. https://dictionary.apa.org

3 American Psychological Association. (n.d.). Stressor. *APA Dictionary of Psychology*. https://dictionary.apa.org

4 Sissons, C. (2020, July 31). Defense mechanisms in psychology: What are they? *MedicalNewsToday*. https://www.medicalnewstoday.com/articles/defense-mechanisms

5 Sissons, C. (2020, July 31). Defense mechanisms in psychology: What are they? *MedicalNewsToday*. https://www.medicalnewstoday.com/articles/defense-mechanisms

6 American Psychological Association. (n.d.). Stressor. *APA Dictionary of Psychology*. https://dictionary.apa.org

7 American Psychological Association. (n.d.). Stressor. *APA Dictionary of Psychology*. https://dictionary.apa.org

My Notes

Defense Mechanisms	Definitions	Examples
Introjection	Unconsciously incorporating the attitudes, values, and qualities of another person's personality.[8]	A client talks and acts like one of the nurses they admire.
Projection	A process when one attributes their individual positive or negative characteristics, affects, and impulses to another person or group.[9]	A person conflicted over expressing anger changes "I hate him" to "He hates me."[10]
Rationalization	Logical reasons are given to justify unacceptable behavior to defend against feelings of guilt, maintain self-respect, and protect oneself from criticism.[11]	A client who is overextended on several credit cards rationalizes it is okay to buy more clothes to be in style when spending money that was set aside to pay for the monthly rent and utilities. A student caught cheating on a test rationalizes, "Everybody cheats."
Reaction Formation	Unacceptable or threatening impulses are denied and consciously replaced with an opposite, acceptable impulse.[12]	A client who hates their mother writes in their journal that their mom is a wonderful mother.
Regression	A return to a prior, lower state of cognitive, emotional, or behavioral functioning when threatened with overwhelming external problems or internal conflicts.[13]	A child who was toilet trained reverts to wetting their pants after their parents' divorce.
Repression	Painful experiences and unacceptable impulses are unconsciously excluded from consciousness as a protection against anxiety.[14]	A victim of incest indicates they have always hated their brother (the molester) but cannot remember why.
Splitting	Objects provoking anxiety and ambivalence are viewed as either all good or all bad.[15]	A client tells the nurse they are the most wonderful person in the world, but after the nurse enforces the unit rules with them, the client tells the nurse they are the worst person they have ever met.

8 American Psychological Association. (n.d.). Stressor. *APA Dictionary of Psychology*. https://dictionary.apa.org

9 American Psychological Association. (n.d.). Stressor. *APA Dictionary of Psychology*. https://dictionary.apa.org

10 American Psychological Association. (n.d.). Stressor. *APA Dictionary of Psychology*. https://dictionary.apa.org

11 American Psychological Association. (n.d.). Stressor. *APA Dictionary of Psychology*. https://dictionary.apa.org

12 American Psychological Association. (n.d.). Stressor. *APA Dictionary of Psychology*. https://dictionary.apa.org

13 American Psychological Association. (n.d.). Stressor. *APA Dictionary of Psychology*. https://dictionary.apa.org

14 American Psychological Association. (n.d.). Stressor. *APA Dictionary of Psychology*. https://dictionary.apa.org

15 American Psychological Association. (n.d.). Stressor. *APA Dictionary of Psychology*. https://dictionary.apa.org

My Notes

Defense Mechanisms	Definitions	Examples
Suppression	A conscious effort to keep disturbing thoughts and experiences out of mind or to control and inhibit the expression of unacceptable impulses and feelings. Suppression is similar to repression, but it is a conscious process.[16,17]	An individual has an impulse to tell their boss what they think about them and their unacceptable behavior, but the impulse is suppressed because of the need to keep the job.
Sublimation	Unacceptable sexual or aggressive drives are unconsciously channeled into socially acceptable modes of expression that indirectly provide some satisfaction for the original drives and protect individuals from anxiety induced by the original drive.[18]	An individual with an exhibitionistic impulse channels this impulse into creating dance choreography. A person with a voyeuristic urge completes scientific research and observes research subjects. An individual with an aggressive drive joins the football team.[19]
Symbolization	The substitution of a symbol for a repressed impulse, affect, or idea.[20]	A client unconsciously wears red clothing due a repressed impulse to physically harm someone.

16 American Psychological Association. (n.d.). Stressor. *APA Dictionary of Psychology*. https://dictionary.apa.org

17 Sissons, C. (2020, July 31). Defense mechanisms in psychology: What are they? *MedicalNewsToday*. https://www.medicalnewstoday.com/articles/defense-mechanisms

18 American Psychological Association. (n.d.). Stressor. *APA Dictionary of Psychology*. https://dictionary.apa.org

19 American Psychological Association. (n.d.). Stressor. *APA Dictionary of Psychology*. https://dictionary.apa.org

20 American Psychological Association. (n.d.). Stressor. *APA Dictionary of Psychology*. https://dictionary.apa.org

3.5 CRISIS AND CRISIS INTERVENTION

My Notes

If you were asked to describe someone in crisis, what would come to your mind? Many of us might draw on traditional images of someone anxiously wringing their hands, pacing the halls, having a verbal outburst, or acting erratically. Health care professionals should be aware that crisis can be reflected in these types of behaviors, but it can also be demonstrated in various verbal and nonverbal signs. There are many potential causes of crisis, and there are four phases an individual progresses through to crisis. Nurses and other health care professionals are often the frontline care providers when an individual faces a crisis, so it is important to recognize signs of crisis, know what to assess, intervene appropriately, and evaluate crisis resolution.

Definition of Crisis

A **crisis** can be broadly defined as the inability to cope or adapt to a stressor. Historically, the first examination of crisis and development of formal crisis intervention models occurred among psychologists in the 1960s and 1970s. Although definitions of crisis have evolved, there are central tenets related to an individual's stress management.

Consider the historical context of crisis as first formally defined in the literature by Gerald Caplan. Crisis was defined as a situation that produces psychological disequilibrium in an individual and constitutes an important problem in which they can't escape or solve with their customary problem-solving resources.[1] This definition emphasized the imbalance created by situation stressors.

Albert Roberts updated the concept of crisis management in more recent years to include a reflection on the level of an individual's dysfunction. He defined crisis as an acute disruption of psychological homeostasis in which one's usual coping mechanisms fail with evidence of distress and functional impairment.[2] A person's subjective reaction to a stressful life experience compromises their ability (or inability) to cope or function.

Causes of Crisis

A crisis can emerge for individuals due to a variety of events. It is also important to note that events may be managed differently by different individuals. For example, a stressful stimulus occurring for Patient A may not induce the same crisis response as it does for Patient B. Therefore, nurses must remain vigilant and carefully monitor each patient for signs of emerging crisis.

A crisis commonly occurs when individuals experience some sort of significant life event. These events may be unanticipated, but that is not always the case. An example of anticipated life events that may cause a crisis include the birth of a baby. For example, the birth (although expected) can result in a crisis for some individuals as they struggle to cope with and adapt to this major life change. Predictable, routine schedules from before the child was born are often completely upended. Priorities shift to an unyielding focus on the needs of the new baby. Although many individuals welcome this change and cope effectively with the associated life changes, it can induce crises in those who are unprepared for such a change.

Crisis situations are more commonly associated with unexpected life events. Individuals who experience a newly diagnosed critical or life-altering illness are at risk for experiencing a crisis. For example, a client experiencing a life-threatening myocardial infarction or receiving a new diagnosis of cancer may experience a crisis. Additionally,

---

1 Caplan, G. (1964). *Principles of preventive psychiatry*. Basic Books.

2 Roberts, A. R. (2005). Bridging the past and present to the future of crisis intervention and crisis management. In A. R. Roberts (Ed.), *Crisis intervention handbook: Assessment, treatment, and research* (3rd ed.). Oxford University Press. pp. 3-34.

My Notes

the crisis may be experienced by family and loved ones of the patient as well. Nurses should be aware that crisis intervention and the need for additional support may occur in these types of situations and often extend beyond the needs of the individual patient.

Other events that may result in crisis development include stressors such as the loss of a job, loss of one's home, divorce, or death of a loved one. It is important to be aware that clustering of multiple events can also cause stress to build sequentially so that individuals can no longer successfully manage and adapt, resulting in crisis.

Categories of Crises

Due to a variety of stimuli that can cause the emergence of a crisis, crises can be categorized to help nurses and health care providers understand the crisis experience and the resources that may be most beneficial for assisting the client and their family members. Crises can be characterized into one of three categories: maturational, situational, or social crisis. Table 3.5a explains characteristics of the different categories of crises and provides examples of stressors associated with that category.

Table 3.5a Categories of Crises

Category	Characteristics	Examples
Maturational (also known as Developmental crisis)	■ The result of normal processes of growth and development. ■ Commonly occurs at specific developmental periods of life. ■ It is predictable in nature and normally occurs as a part of life. ■ An individual is vulnerable based on their equilibrium.	■ Birth ■ Adolescence ■ Marriage ■ Death
Situational	■ An unexpected personal stressful event occurs with little advance warning. ■ It is less predictable in nature. ■ The event threatens an individual's equilibrium.	■ Accident ■ Illness or serious injury of self or family member ■ Loss of a job ■ Bankruptcy ■ Relocation/geographical move ■ Divorce
Social (also known as Adventitious crisis)	■ An event that is uncommon or unanticipated. ■ The event often involves multiple losses or extensive losses. ■ It can occur due to a major natural or man-made event. ■ It is unpredictable in nature. ■ The event poses a severe threat to an individual's equilibrium.	■ Flood ■ Fire ■ Tornado ■ Hurricane ■ Earthquake ■ War ■ Riot ■ Violent crime

My Notes

Phases of Crisis

The process of crisis development can be described as four distinct phases. The phases progress from initial exposure to the stressor, to tension escalation, to an eventual breaking point. These phases reflect a sequential progression in which resource utilization and intervention are critical for assisting a client in crisis. Table 3.5b describes the various phases of crisis, their defining characteristics, and associated signs and symptoms that individuals may experience as they progress through each phase.

Table 3.5b Crisis Phases[3,4]

Crisis Phase	Defining Characteristics	Signs and Symptoms
Phase 1: **Normal Stress & Anxiety**	Exposure to a precipitating stressor. Stressors may be considered minor annoyances and inconveniences of everyday life.	Anxiety levels or the stress response begin to elevate. Individuals try using previously successful problem-solving techniques to attempt resolution of the stressor. Individuals are rational and in control of their behavior and emotions.
Phase 2: **Rising Anxiety Level**	Problem-solving techniques do not relieve the stressor. Use of past coping strategies are not successful.	Anxiety levels increase and individuals experience increased discomfort. Feelings of helplessness, confusion, and disorganized thinking may occur. Individuals may complain of "feeling lost" in how to proceed. Individuals may experience elevated heart rate and respiration rate. Their voice pitch may be higher with a more rapid speech pattern. Nervous habits such as finger or foot tapping may occur.
Phase 3: **Severe Level of Stress and Anxiety**	Individuals use all possible internal and external resources. Problems are explored from different perspectives, and new problem-solving techniques are attempted.	Equilibrium may be restored if new problem-solving approaches are successful. Individuals experience decreased anxiety if resolution occurs. If new problem-solving techniques are not successful, the level of anxiety worsens, and functioning is impaired as the stressor continues to impact the individual. Capacity to reason becomes significantly diminished, and behaviors become more disruptive. Communication processes may include yelling and swearing. Individuals may become very argumentative or use threats. Individuals may pace; clench their fists; perspire heavily; or demonstrate rapid, shallow, panting breaths.

3 Caplan, G. (1964). *Principles of preventive psychiatry*. Basic Books.

4 Centers for Disease Control and Prevention. (2018, May 25). *The National Institute for Occupational Health and Safety*. https://www.cdc.gov/niosh/

My Notes

Crisis Phase	Defining Characteristics	Signs and Symptoms
Phase 4: **Crisis**	If resolution is not achieved, tension escalates to a critical breaking point.	Individuals experience unbearable anxiety, increased feelings of panic, and disordered thinking processes. There is an urgent need to end emotional discomfort. Many cognitive functions are impaired as the crisis event becomes thought consuming. Emotions are labile, and some patients may experience psychotic thinking. *It is important to note that some individuals at this level of crisis may be a danger to themselves and others.

Crisis Assessment

Nurses must be aware of the potential impact of stressors for their clients and the ways in which they may manifest in a crisis. The first step in assessing for crisis occurs with the basic establishment of a therapeutic nurse-patient relationship. Understanding who your patient is, what is occurring in their life, what resources are available to them, and their individual beliefs, supports, and general demeanor can help a nurse determine if a patient is at risk for ineffective coping and possible progression to crisis. Crisis symptoms can manifest in various ways. Nurses should carefully monitor for signs of the progression through the phases of crisis such as the following:

- Escalating anxiety
- Denial
- Confusion or disordered thinking
- Anger and hostility
- Helplessness and withdrawal
- Inefficiency
- Hopelessness and depression
- Steps toward resolution and reorganization

When a nurse identifies these signs in a patient or their family members, it is important to carefully explore the symptoms exhibited and the potential stressors. Collecting information regarding the severity of the stress response, the individual's or family's resources, and the crisis phase can help guide the nurse and health care team toward appropriate intervention.

Crisis Interventions

Crisis intervention is an important role for the nurse and health care team to assist patients and families toward crisis resolution. Resources are employed, and interventions are implemented to therapeutically assist the individual in whatever phase of crisis they are experiencing. Depending on the stage of the crisis, various strategies and resources are used.

The goals of crisis intervention are the following:

- Identify, assess, and intervene
- Return the individual to a prior level of functioning as quickly as possible
- Lessen negative impact on future mental health

During the crisis intervention process, new skills and coping strategies are acquired, resulting in change. A crisis state is time-limited, usually lasting several days but no longer than four to six weeks.

Various factors can influence an individual's ability to resolve a crisis and return to equilibrium, such as realistic perception of an event, adequate situational support, and adequate coping strategies to respond to a problem. Nurses can implement strategies to reinforce these factors.

Strategies for Crisis Phase 1 and 2

Table 3.5c describes strategies and techniques for early phases of a crisis that can help guide the individual toward crisis resolution.

Table 3.5c Phase 1 & 2 Early Crisis Intervention Strategies[5]

Verbal	**Strategies**	**Examples**
Therapeutic use of words holds significant power to defuse the stress response.	Encourage the person to express their thoughts and concerns.	"I understand how hard this must be for you."
Be attuned to the individual's tone of voice and body language.	Use a shared problem-solving approach. Avoid being defensive.	"I understand your feelings of frustration. How can we correct this problem?"
Be attuned to word choice.	Use empathetic inquiry.	"You seem to be upset. Tell me more about what is bothering you."
Nonverbal	**Strategies**	**Example**
Be aware of your nonverbal messages and be in control of your body positions.	Be calm and act calm. Invite the client to sit to help them calm down and demonstrate you are calm.	Maintain nonthreatening eye contact, smile, and keep hands open and visible.
	Listen.	Nod your head to demonstrate that you are engaged with the individual.
	Respect personal space.	Maintain distance and avoid touching an individual who is upset.
	Approach the patient from an angle or from the side.	Avoid directly approaching an individual, as it can feel confrontational.
	Avoid threatening gestures.	Avoid finger pointing or crossing arms.
	Demonstrate respect.	Mirror the individual's nonverbal messaging. Avoid laughing or joking.

5 Centers for Disease Control and Prevention. (2018, May 25). *The National Institute for Occupational Health and Safety.* https://www.cdc.gov/niosh/

My Notes

Strategies for Crisis Phase 3

If an individual continues to progress in severity to higher levels of crisis, the previously identified verbal and nonverbal interventions for Phase 1 and Phase 2 may be received with a variability of success. For example, for a receptive individual who is still in relative control of their emotions, the verbal and nonverbal interventions may still be well-received. However, if an individual has progressed to Phase 3 with emotional lability, the nurse must recognize this escalation and take additional measures to protect oneself. If an individual demonstrates loss of problem-solving ability or the loss of control, the nurse must take measures to ensure safety for themselves and others in all interactions with the patient. This can be accomplished by calling security or other staff to assist when engaging with the patient. It is important to always note the location of exits in the patient's room and ensure the patient is never between the nurse and the exit. Rapid response devices may be worn, and nurses should feel comfortable using them if a situation begins to escalate.

Verbal cues can still hold significant power even in a late phase of crisis. The nurse should provide direct cues to an escalating patient such as, "Mr. Andrews, please sit down and take a few deep breaths. I understand you are angry. You need to gain control of your emotions, or I will have to call security for assistance." This strategy is an example of limit-setting that can be helpful for de-escalating the situation and defusing tension. Setting limits is important for providing behavioral guidance to a patient who is escalating, but it is very different from making threats. Limit-setting describes the desired behavior whereas making threats is nontherapeutic. See additional examples contrasting limit-setting and making threats in the following box.[6]

Examples of Limit-Setting Versus Making Threats[7]

- **Threat:** "If you don't stop, I'm going to call security!"
- **Limit-Setting:** "Please sit down. I will have to call for assistance if you can't control your emotions."
- **Threat:** "If you keep pushing the call button over and over like that, I won't help you."
- **Limit-Setting:** "Ms. Ferris, I will come as soon as I am able when you need assistance, but please give me a chance to get to your room."
- **Threat:** "That type of behavior won't be tolerated!"
- **Limit-Setting:** "Mr. Barron, please stop yelling and screaming at me. I am here to help you."

Strategies for Crisis Phase 4

A person who is experiencing an elevated phase of crisis is not likely to be in control of their emotions, cognitive processes, or behavior. It is important to give them space so they don't feel trapped. Many times these individuals

6 Centers for Disease Control and Prevention. (2018, May 25). *The National Institute for Occupational Health and Safety.* https://www.cdc.gov/niosh/

7 Centers for Disease Control and Prevention. (2018, May 25). *The National Institute for Occupational Health and Safety.* https://www.cdc.gov/niosh/

My Notes

are not responsive to verbal intervention and are solely focused on their own fear, anger, frustration, or despair. Don't try to argue or reason with them. Individuals in Phase 4 of crisis often experience physical manifestations such as rapid heart rate, rapid breathing, and pacing.

If you can't successfully de-escalate an individual who is becoming increasingly more agitated, seek assistance. If you don't believe there is an immediate danger, call a psychiatrist, psychiatric-mental health nurse specialist, therapist, case manager, social worker, or family physician who is familiar with the person's history. The professional can assess the situation and provide guidance, such as scheduling an appointment or admitting the person to the hospital. If you can't reach someone and the situation continues to escalate, consider calling your county mental health crisis unit, crisis response team, or other similar contacts. If the situation is life-threatening or if serious property damage is occurring, call 911 and ask for immediate assistance. When you call 911, tell them someone is experiencing a mental health crisis and explain the nature of the emergency, your relationship to the person in crisis, and whether there are weapons involved. Ask the 911 operator to send someone trained to work with people with mental illnesses such as a Crisis Intervention Training (CIT) officer.[8]

A nurse who assesses a patient in this phase should observe the patient's behaviors and take measures to ensure the patient and others remain safe. A person who is out of control may require physical or chemical restraints to be safe. Nurses must be aware of organizational policies and procedures, as well as documentation required for implementing restraints, if the patient's or others' safety is in jeopardy.

Review guidelines for safe implementation of restraints in the "Restraints" section of Open RN *Nursing Fundamentals*.

Crisis Resources

Depending on the type of stressors and the severity of the crisis experienced, there are a variety of resources that can be offered to patients and their loved ones. Nurses should be aware of community and organizational resources that are available in their practice settings. Support groups, hotlines, shelters, counseling services, and other community resources like the Red Cross may be helpful. Read more about potential national and local resources in the following box.

Mental Health Crisis Resources

NAMI: National Alliance on Mental

Health ADRC of Central Wisconsin

Wisconsin County Crisis Lines

Wisconsin Suicide & Crisis Hotlines

8 Brister, T. (2018). *Navigating a mental health crisis: A NAMI resource guide for those experiencing a mental health emergency.* National Alliance on Mental Illness. https://www.nami.org/Support-Education/Publications-Reports/Guides/Navigating-a-Mental-Health-Crisis/Navigating-A-Mental-Health-Crisis?utm_source=website&utm_medium=cta&utm_campaign=crisisguide

My Notes

Mental Health Crisis

When an individual is diagnosed with a mental health disorder, the potential for crisis is always present. Risk of suicide is always a priority concern for people with mental health conditions in crisis. Any talk of suicide should always be taken seriously. Most people who attempt suicide have given some warning. If someone has attempted suicide before, the risk is even greater.

Read more about assessing suicide risk in the "Establishing Safety" section of Chapter 1. Encouraging someone who is having suicidal thoughts to get help is a safety priority.

Common signs that a mental health crisis is developing are as follows:

- Inability to perform daily tasks like bathing, brushing teeth, brushing hair, or changing clothes
- Rapid mood swings, increased energy level, inability to stay still, pacing, suddenly depressed or withdrawn, or suddenly happy or calm after period of depression
- Increased agitation with verbal threats; violent, out-of-control behavior or destruction of property
- Abusive behavior to self and others, including substance misuse or self-harm (cutting)
- Isolation from school, work, family, or friends
- Loss of touch with reality (psychosis) – unable to recognize family or friends, confused, doesn't understand what people are saying, hearing voices, or seeing things that aren't there
- Paranoia

Clients with mental illness and their loved ones need information for what to do if they are experiencing a crisis. *Navigating a Mental Health Crisis: A NAMI Resource Guide for Those Experiencing a Mental Health Emergency* provides important, potentially life-saving information for people experiencing mental health crises and their loved ones. It outlines what can contribute to a crisis, warning signs that a crisis is emerging, strategies to help de-escalate a crisis, and available resources.

Read NAMI's Navigating a Mental Health Crisis: A NAMI Resource Guide for Those Experiencing a Mental Health Emergency.

3.6 APPLYING THE NURSING PROCESS TO STRESS AND COPING

My Notes

This section will review the nursing process as it applies to stress and coping.

Assessments Related to Stress and Coping

Here are several nursing assessments used to determine an individual's response to stress and their strategies for stress management and coping:

- Recognize nonverbal cues of physical or psychological stress
- Assess for environmental stressors affecting client care
- Assess for signs of abuse or neglect
- Assess client's ability to cope with life changes
- Assess family dynamics
- Assess the potential for violence
- Assess client's support systems and available resources
- Assess client's ability to adapt to temporary/permanent role changes
- Assess client's reaction to a diagnosis of acute or chronic mental illness (e.g., rationalization, hopefulness, anger)
- Assess constructive use of defense mechanisms by a client
- Assess if the client has successfully adapted to situational role changes (e.g., accept dependency on others)
- Assess client's ability to cope with end-of-life interventions
- Recognize the need for psychosocial support to the family/caregiver
- Assess clients for maladaptive coping such as substance abuse
- Identify a client in crisis

Diagnoses Related to Stress and Coping

Nursing diagnoses related to stress and coping are *Stress Overload* and *Ineffective Coping*. See Table 3.6 to compare the definitions and defining characteristics for these nursing diagnoses.

Table 3.6 Stress and Coping Nursing Diagnoses

Nursing Diagnosis	Definition	Selected Defining Characteristics
Stress Overload	Excessive amounts and types of demands that require action.	■ Excessive stress ■ Impaired decision-making ■ Impaired functioning ■ Increase in anger ■ Increased impatience

My Notes

Nursing Diagnosis	Definition	Selected Defining Characteristics
Ineffective Coping	A pattern of invalid appraisal of stressors, with cognitive and/or behavioral efforts, that fails to manage demands related to well-being.	■ Alteration in concentration ■ Alteration in sleep pattern ■ Change in communication pattern ■ Fatigue ■ Inability to ask for help ■ Inability to deal with a situation ■ Ineffective coping strategies ■ Insufficient social support ■ Substance misuse

Outcomes Identification

An outcome is a measurable behavior demonstrated by the patient responsive to nursing interventions. Outcomes should be identified before nursing interventions are planned. Outcome identification includes setting short- and long-term goals and then creating specific expected outcome statements for each nursing diagnosis. Goals are broad, general statements, and outcomes are specific and measurable. Expected outcomes are statements of measurable action for the patient within a specific time frame that are responsive to nursing interventions.

Expected outcome statements should contain five components easily remembered using the "SMART" mnemonic:

- Specific
- Measurable
- Attainable/Action oriented
- Relevant/Realistic
- Time frame

An example of a SMART outcome related to *Stress Overload* is, "The client will identify two stressors that can be modified or eliminated by the end of the week."

An example of a SMART outcome related to *Ineffective Coping* is, "The client will identify three preferred coping strategies to implement by the end of the week."

Read more information about establishing SMART outcome statements in the "Outcome Identification" section of Chapter 4.

Planning Interventions Related to Stress and Coping

Common nursing interventions that are implemented to facilitate effective coping in their clients include the following[1]:

1 NCSBN. (n.d.). *Test plans.* https://www.ncsbn.org/testplans.htm

My Notes

- Implement measures to reduce environmental stressors
- Teach clients about stress management techniques and coping strategies
- Provide caring interventions for a client experiencing grief or loss, as well as resources to adjust to loss/bereavement
- Identify the client in crisis and tailor crisis intervention strategies to assist them to cope
- Guide the client to resources for recovery from crisis (i.e., social supports)

Implementation

When implementing nursing interventions to enhance client coping, it is important to recognize signs of a crisis and maintain safety for the client, oneself, and others. Review signs of a client in crisis and crisis intervention strategies in the "Crisis and Crisis Intervention" section of this chapter.

Evaluation

After implementing individualized interventions for a client, it is vital to evaluate their effectiveness. Review the specific SMART outcomes and deadlines that have been established for a client and determine if interventions were effective in meeting these outcomes or if the care plan requires modification.

My Notes

3.7 LEARNING ACTIVITIES

Interactive Activities

An interactive H5P element has been excluded from this version of the text. You can view it online here: https://wtcs.pressbooks.pub/nursingmhcc/?p=165#h5p-26

An interactive H5P element has been excluded from this version of the text. You can view it online here: https://wtcs.pressbooks.pub/nursingmhcc/?p=165#h5p-12

An interactive H5P element has been excluded from this version of the text. You can view it online here: https://wtcs.pressbooks.pub/nursingmhcc/?p=165#h5p-13

III GLOSSARY

My Notes

Adaptive coping strategies: Coping strategies, including problem-focused coping and emotion-focused coping.

Adverse childhood experiences: Potentially traumatic events that occur in childhood such as sexual abuse, physical abuse, emotional abuse, physical neglect, emotional neglect, parental loss, or parental separation before the child is 18 years old.

Coping: Cognitive and behavioral efforts made to master, tolerate, or reduce external and internal demands and conflicts.[1]

Coping strategies: An action, series of actions, or a thought process used in meeting a stressful or unpleasant situation or in modifying one's reaction to such a situation.[2]

Crisis: The inability to cope or adapt to a stressor.

Defense mechanisms: Unconscious reaction patterns used by individuals to protect themselves from anxiety that arises from stress and conflict.[3]

Emotion-focused coping: Adaptive coping strategies such as practicing mindfulness, meditation, and yoga; using humor and jokes; seeking spiritual or religious pursuits; engaging in physical activity or breathing exercises; and seeking social support.

Maladaptive coping responses: Ineffective responses to stressors such as avoidance of the stressful condition, withdrawal from a stressful environment, disengagement from stressful relationships, and misuse of drugs and/or alcohol.

Problem-focused coping: Adaptive coping strategies that typically focus on seeking treatment such as counseling or cognitive behavioral therapy.

Stress response: The body's physiological response to a real or perceived stressor. For example, the respiratory, cardiovascular, and musculoskeletal systems are activated to breathe rapidly, stimulate the heart to pump more blood, dilate the blood vessels, and increase blood pressure to deliver more oxygenated blood to the muscles.

Stressors: Any internal or external event, force, or condition that results in physical or emotional stress.

1 Amnie, A. G. (2018). Emerging themes in coping with lifetime stress and implication for stress management education. *SAGE Open Medicine, 6*. https://doi.org/10.1177%2F2050312118782545

2 American Psychological Association. (n.d.). Stressor. *APA Dictionary of Psychology*. https://dictionary.apa.org

3 American Psychological Association. (n.d.). Stressor. *APA Dictionary of Psychology*. https://dictionary.apa.org

Chapter 4

Application of the Nursing Process to Mental Health Care

4.1 INTRODUCTION

My Notes

Learning Objectives

- Apply the nursing process to mental health care
- Describe nursing assessments when providing mental health care
- Incorporate respectful and equitable practice
- Consider developmental levels when providing care
- Identify common nursing diagnoses/problems related to mental health conditions
- Promote a therapeutic environment
- Apply the subcategories of the *Implementation* standard of care to mental health care
- Create effective nursing care plans for clients with various mental health disorders
- Compare NCLEX Next Generation terminology to the nursing process

Psychiatric-mental health nursing is, "The nursing practice specialty committed to promoting mental health through the assessment, diagnosis, and treatment of behavioral problems, mental disorders, and comorbid conditions across the life span. Psychiatric-mental health nursing intervention is an art and a science, employing a purposeful use of self and a wide range of nursing, psychosocial, and neurobiological evidence to produce effective outcomes."[1]

In 2014 the American Psychiatric Nurses Association (APNA) and the International Society of Psychiatric-Mental Health Nurses (ISPN) published the *Psychiatric-Mental Health Nursing: Scope and Standards of Practice* resource in alignment with the second edition of the ANA's *Nursing: Scope and Standard of Practice Nursing*. The *Psychiatric-Mental Health Nursing: Scope and Standards of Practice* resource guides psychiatric-mental health nurses in the application of their professional skills and responsibilities and should be reviewed in conjunction with state Board of Nursing policies and practices that govern the practice of nursing.[2] The Standards of Practice for Psychiatric-Mental Health Nursing mirror the ANA Standards of Professional Nursing Practice of *Assessment, Diagnosis, Outcome Identification, Planning, Implementation*, and *Evaluation*, but also have additional competencies for Psychiatric-Mental Health Registered Nurse Specialists (PMH-RNs) and Advanced Practice Registered Nurse Specialists (PMH-APRNs) and additional components for the *Implementation* standard of care.

This chapter will review how nurse generalists apply the nursing process and the ANA Standards of Professional Nursing Practice to clients experiencing a mental health condition. Assessments, nursing diagnoses, expected outcomes, and interventions pertaining to mental health will be reviewed while incorporating life span and cultural considerations. For specific assessments, nursing diagnoses, expected outcomes, and interventions related to specific mental health conditions, see each corresponding "disorder" chapter.

---

1 American Nurses Association, American Psychiatric Nurses Association, and International Society of Psychiatric-Mental Health Nurses. (2014). *Psychiatric-Mental Health Nursing: Scope and Standards of Practice* (2nd ed.). Nursebooks.org

2 American Nurses Association, American Psychiatric Nurses Association, and International Society of Psychiatric-Mental Health Nurses. (2014). *Psychiatric-Mental Health Nursing: Scope and Standards of Practice* (2nd ed.). Nursebooks.org

My Notes

4.2 APPLYING THE NURSING PROCESS

The nursing process is a critical thinking model based on a systematic approach to patient-centered care. Nurses use the **nursing process** to perform clinical reasoning and make clinical judgments when providing patient care. The nursing process is based on the Standards of Professional Nursing Practice established by the American Nurses Association (ANA). These standards are authoritative statements of the actions and behaviors that all registered nurses, regardless of role, population, specialty, and setting, are expected to perform competently.[1]

The mnemonic **ADOPIE** is an easy way to remember the six ANA standards regarding the nursing process. Each letter refers to one of the six components of the nursing process: *Assessment, Diagnosis, Outcomes Identification, Planning, Implementation*, and *Evaluation*. The nursing process is a continuous, cyclic process that is constantly adapting to the patient's current health status. See Figure 4.1[2] for an illustration of the nursing process.

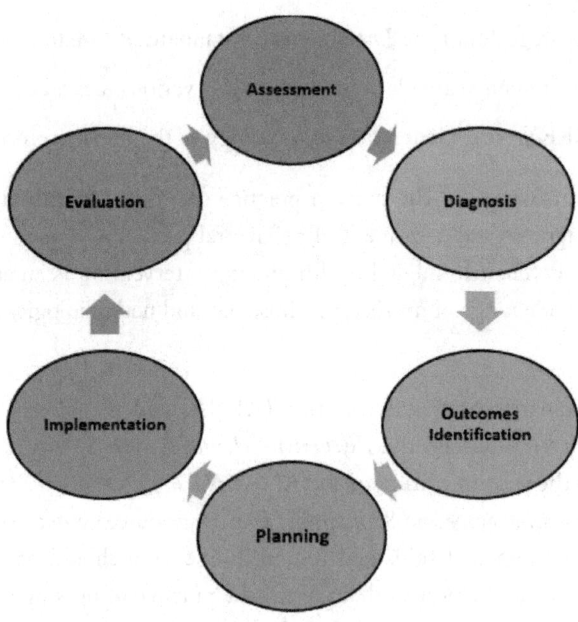

Figure 4.1 The Nursing Process

Review using the nursing process in the "Nursing Process" chapter in Open RN *Nursing Fundamentals*.

---

1 American Nurses Association. (2021). *Nursing: Scope and standards of practice* (4th ed.). American Nurses Association.

2 "The Nursing Process" by Kim Ernstmeyer at Chippewa Valley Technical College is licensed under CC BY 4.0

4.3 ASSESSMENT

My Notes

The *Assessment* Standard of Practice established by the American Nurses Association (ANA) states, "The registered nurse collects pertinent data to the health care and information relative to the health care consumer's health or the situation."[1] Review the competencies for the *Assessment* Standard of Practice for registered nurses in the following box.

ANA's Assessment Competencies[2]

The registered nurse:

- Creates the safest environment possible for conducting assessments.
- Collects pertinent data related to health and quality of life in a systematic, ongoing manner, with compassion and respect for the wholeness, the inherent dignity, worth, and unique attributes of every person, including, but not limited to, demographics, environmental and occupational exposures, social determinants of health, health disparities, physical, functional, psychosocial, emotional, cognitive, spiritual/transpersonal, sexual, sociocultural, age-related, environmental, and lifestyle/economic assessments.
- Utilizes a health and wellness model of assessment that incorporates integrative approaches to data collection and honors the whole person.
- Recognizes the health care consumer or designated person as the decision-maker regarding their own health.
- Explores the health care consumer's culture, values, preferences, expressed and unexpressed needs, and knowledge of the heath care situation.
- Assesses the impact of family dynamics on the health care consumer's health and wellness.
- Identifies enhancements and barriers to effective communication based on personal, cognitive, physiological, psychosocial, literacy, financial, and cultural considerations.
- Engages the health care consumer, family, significant others, and interprofessional team members in holistic, culturally sensitive data collection.
- Integrates knowledge from current local, regional, national, and global health initiatives and environmental factors into the assessment process.
    - State and local departments of health
    - *World Health Organization*
    - *World Health Organization health topics*

1 American Nurses Association. (2021). *Nursing: Scope and standards of practice* (4th ed.). American Nurses Association.

2 American Nurses Association. (2021). *Nursing: Scope and standards of practice* (4th ed.). American Nurses Association.

My Notes

- *Healthy People*
- *Centers for Disease Control and Prevention*

- Prioritizes data collection based on the health care consumer's immediate condition, the anticipated needs of the health care consumer or situation, or both.
- Uses evidence-based assessment techniques and available data and information to identify patterns and variances in the consumer's health.
- Remains knowledgeable about constantly changing technologies that impact the assessment process (e.g., telehealth, artificial intelligence).
- Analyzes assessment data to identify patterns, trends, and situations that impact the person's health and wellness.
- Validates the analysis with the health care consumer.
- Documents data accurately and makes accessible to the interprofessional team in a timely manner.
- Communicates changes in a person's condition to the interprofessional team.
- Applies the provisions of the ANA Code of Ethics, legal guidelines, and policies to the collection, maintenance, use, and dissemination of data and information.
- Recognizes the impact of one's own personal attitudes, values, beliefs, and biases on the assessment process.

Review the components of a nursing assessment in the "Nursing Process" chapter of Open RN *Nursing Fundamentals*.

Nursing assessments related to mental health disorders differ from physiological assessments with a greater focus on collecting subjective data. For example, prior to administering a cardiac medication to a client with a heart condition, a nurse will assess objective data such as blood pressure and an apical heart rate to determine the effectiveness of the medication treatment. However, prior to administering an antidepressant, a nurse uses therapeutic communication to ask questions and gather subjective data about how the patient is feeling to determine the effectiveness of the medication. The nurse will also observe client behaviors, speech, mood, and thought processes as part of the assessment.

As a nurse, you cannot directly measure a neurotransmitter to determine the effects of the medication, but you can ask questions to determine how your patient is feeling emotionally and perceiving the world, which are influenced by neurotransmitter levels. An example of a nurse using therapeutic communication to perform subjective assessment is, "Tell me more about how you are feeling today." The nurse may also use general survey techniques such as simply observing the patient to assess for cues of behavior. Examples of objective data collected by a general survey could be assessing the patient's mood, hygiene, appearance, or movement.

Recall the mental health continuum introduced in the "Foundational Mental Health Concepts" chapter (see Figure 4.2[3]). Nurses in any setting holistically assess their clients' physical, emotional, and mental health, as well as any impairments impacting their functioning. They must recognize subtle cues of undiagnosed or poorly managed physical and mental disorders and follow up appropriately with other members of the interprofessional health care team.

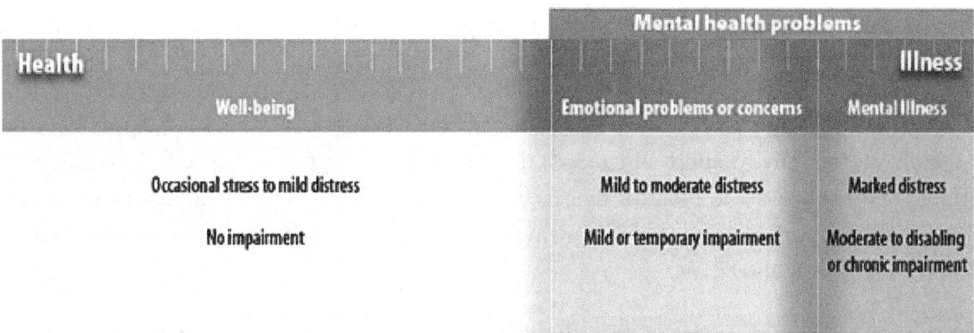

Figure 4.2 Mental Health Continuum (Used with permission.)

When assessing a client's mental health, the nurse incorporates a variety of assessments, in addition to the traditional physical examination. Assessments may include the following:

- Performing a mental status examination
- Completing a psychosocial assessment
- Reviewing the client's use of psychotropic medications (drugs that treat psychiatric symptoms) and/or other medications that can cause psychiatric symptoms as side effects
- Screening for suicidal ideation, exposure to trauma or violence, and substance misuse
- Incorporating a spiritual assessment while assessing the client's coping status
- Incorporating life span, developmental, and cultural considerations
- Reviewing specific laboratory results related to the client's use of psychotropic and other medications

Mental Status Examination

Registered nurses must use effective clinical interviewing skills while performing a mental status assessment and developing a therapeutic nurse-client relationship.[4] Read more about establishing a therapeutic nurse-client rela-

---

3 "continuum.jpg" by University of Michigan is used with permission. Access the original at https://hr.umich.edu/benefits-wellness/health-well-being/mhealthy/faculty-staff-well-being/mental-emotional-health/mental-emotional-health-classes-training-events/online-tutorial-supervisors/section-1-what-you-need-know-about-mental-health-problems-substance-misuse

4 American Nurses Association, American Psychiatric Nurses Association, and International Society of Psychiatric-Mental Health Nurses. (2014). *Psychiatric-Mental Health Nursing: Scope and Standards of Practice* (2nd ed.). Nursebooks.org

My Notes

tionship in the "Therapeutic Communication and the Nurse-Client Relationship" chapter. Assessing a client with a suspected or previously diagnosed mental health disorder focuses on both verbal and nonverbal assessments. New assessment findings are compared to the baseline admission findings to determine if the client's condition is improving, worsening, or remaining the same.

When conducting a focused assessment on a client's mental health, the mental status examination is a priority component of the overall assessment. A successful nurse develops a style in which the bulk of the mental status examination is performed through unstructured observations made during the routine physical examination, also referred to as the "general survey." When the nurse recognizes cues of possible mental health disorders, such as aberrant behavior or difficulties in day-to-day functioning, then a focused mental status examination should be completed.

A **mental status examination** assesses a client's level of consciousness and orientation, appearance and general behavior, speech, motor activity, affect and mood, thought and perception, attitude and insight, and cognitive abilities. The examiner should also monitor their personal reaction to a client when performing a mental status examination. The structured components of a mental status examination are outlined in Table 4.3 and further described in the following subsections.

Read about the components of a general survey in the "General Survey Assessment" chapter of Open RN *Nursing Skills*.

Table 4.3 Mental Status Examination[5]

Assessment	Expected Findings/Optimal Level of Functioning	Unexpected Findings/Impaired Functioning
Signs of Distress	■ Calm and comfortable with no signs of distress	■ Unresponsive ■ Difficulty breathing ■ Chest pain ■ New onset of confusion ■ Moaning ■ Grimacing
Level of Consciousness and Orientation	■ Alert ■ Oriented to person, place, and time ■ Aware of the situation	■ Unable to provide name, location, or day ■ Clouded consciousness ■ Delirium ■ Obtundation ■ Stupor ■ Coma

5 Martin, D. C. (1990). The mental status examination. In Walker, H. K., Hall, W. D., Hurst, J. W., (Eds.), *Clinical methods: The history, physical, and laboratory examinations*. (3rd ed.). Butterworths. https://www.ncbi.nlm.nih.gov/books/NBK320/

My Notes

Assessment	Expected Findings/Optimal Level of Functioning	Unexpected Findings/Impaired Functioning
Appearance and General Behavior	■ Appears stated age ■ Well-groomed ■ Dressed appropriately for the weather and situation ■ Erect posture ■ Good oral hygiene ■ Culturally appropriate eye contact ■ Socializes with others ■ No threatening behaviors	■ Appears older than stated age ■ Unkempt ■ Not dressed appropriately for the weather and/or situation ■ Slumped posture ■ Poor eye contact ■ Does not socialize with others ■ Demonstrates threatening behavior
Speech	■ Exhibiting spontaneous speech ■ Even speech rate, rhythm, and tone ■ Responds to verbal questions ■ Speech is clear and understandable ■ Follows instructions appropriately for developmental level	■ Does not respond to verbal questions ■ Does not follow instructions appropriately for development level ■ Speech is unclear ■ Rapid or pressured speech ■ Halting speech
Motor Activity	■ Good balance ■ Moves extremities equally bilaterally ■ Smooth gait	■ Poor balance ■ Uneven gait ■ Slow movements ■ Lack of spontaneous movement ■ Motor restlessness (**akathisia**) ■ Repetitive movements ■ Tremors ■ Pacing ■ Uncontrolled, involuntary movement (**dyskinesia**)
Affect and Mood	■ Displays wide range of emotions that are appropriate to situation ■ Congruent with mood ■ Bright ■ Hopeful with goals ■ Positive self-worth	■ Inappropriate or incongruent with the situation ■ Subdued ■ Tearful ■ Labile ■ Blunted ■ Flat ■ Dysphoric ■ Euphoric

My Notes

Assessment	Expected Findings/Optimal Level of Functioning	Unexpected Findings/Impaired Functioning
Thought and Perception	■ Realistic ■ Logical ■ Goal-directed ■ Organized ■ Ability to focus or concentrate ■ Absence of suicidal ideation ■ Absence of homicidal ideation ■ Absence of violence ideation	■ Inability to focus or concentrate ■ Irrational fear ■ Exaggerated response ■ Delusions ■ Hallucinations ■ Illusions ■ Obsessions ■ Racing thoughts ■ Flight of ideas ■ Loose associations ■ Clang associations ■ Suicidal ideation ■ Homicidal ideation
Attitude and Insight	■ Looks toward improvement and/or recovery ■ Demonstrates understanding of the situation	■ Exhibits hostility, anger, helplessness, pessimism, overdramatization, self-centeredness, or passivity ■ Demonstrates little or no understanding of the situation
Cognitive Abilities	■ Focused attention ■ Good immediate recall, short-term memory, and long-term storage	■ Distractibility ■ Poor immediate recall ■ Poor short-term memory ■ Poor long-term memory
Examiner's Reaction to Client	■ Noticing and managing examiner's internal responses to the client such as frustration, boredom, sadness, anxiousness, or countertransference	■ Lack of awareness of examiner's internal responses to the client such as frustration, boredom, sadness, anxiousness, countertransference

Signs of Distress

If a client is exhibiting signs of distress during an examination, the nurse must quickly obtain focused assessment data and obtain additional assistance based on the level of emergency care required and agency policy. For example, if a client is found unresponsive, a "code" is typically called during inpatient care, or 911 is called in an outpatient setting as the nurse begins cardiopulmonary resuscitation (CPR). If a client is demonstrating difficulty breathing, new onset confusion, or other signs of a deteriorating condition, the rapid response team may be called, or other emergency assistance may be obtained per agency policy. Keep in mind that the emergency administration of naloxone may be required in cases of a suspected opioid overdose.

My Notes

Level of Consciousness and Orientation

A normal level of consciousness is when the client is alert (i.e., the ability to respond to stimuli at the same level as most people) and oriented to person, place, and time. **Clouded consciousness** refers to a state of reduced awareness to stimuli. **Delirium** is an acute onset of an abnormal mental state, often with fluctuating levels of consciousness, disorientation, irritability, and hallucinations. Delirium is often associated with infection, metabolic disorders, or toxins in the central nervous system. **Obtundation** refers to a moderate reduction in the client's level of awareness so that mild to moderate stimuli do not awaken the client. When arousal does occur, the patient is slow to respond. **Stupor** refers to unresponsiveness unless a vigorous stimulus is applied, such as a sternal rub. The client quickly drifts back into a deep sleep-like state on cessation of the stimulation. **Coma** refers to unarousable unresponsiveness, where vigorous noxious stimuli may not elicit reflex motor responses. For example, a client in a coma may not pull their foot away from a painful prick of their toe with a needle. When documenting reduced levels of consciousness, note the type of stimulus required to arouse the patient and the degree to which the patient can respond when aroused.[6]

Appearance and General Behavior

This component refers to an overall impression of the client, including their physical appearance regarding their age, grooming, dressing, posture, eye contact, ability to socialize with others, and general behaviors. There are several terms used to describe a client's appearance and behavior. For example, the appearance of one's age can be altered due to chronic illness and pain. Providers may document that a client "appears their stated age" or "appears older than their stated age." Clients may be described as well-groomed (i.e., exhibit good hygiene) or **disheveled** (i.e., their hair, clothes, or hygiene appears untidy, disordered, unkempt, or messy). Their dress may be described as "appropriate" or "inappropriate" according to the weather and situation. A client's posture may be described as "erect" or "slumped." Clients may be described as having "good eye contact" (i.e., they maintain a direct gaze into the examiner's eyes) or "poor eye contact" (i.e., they avoid direct eye contact).[7] Life span and cultural considerations must always be kept in mind when assessing a client's appearance and general behavior. For example, some cultures consider direct eye contact disrespectful.

Speech

Evaluating speech as the client answers open-ended questions provides useful information. A client demonstrates normal speech when responding to verbal questions appropriately with an even rate, rhythm, and tone. Their speech is clear and understandable, and the client follows instructions appropriately.

Characteristics of speech can be described as normal, rapid, slow (i.e., delayed rhythm of conversation), loud, or soft. Stuttering and aphasia may occur.

Examples of speech difficulties include lack of appropriate responses to verbal questions, rapid and/or pressured speech of a client experiencing mania or amphetamine intoxication, or halting speech of a client experiencing word-finding difficulties due to a previous stroke.[8]

---

6 Martin, D. C. (1990). The mental status examination. In Walker, H. K., Hall, W. D., Hurst, J. W., (Eds.), *Clinical methods: The history, physical, and laboratory examinations.* (3rd ed.). Butterworths. https://www.ncbi.nlm.nih.gov/books/NBK320/

7 Martin, D. C. (1990). The mental status examination. In Walker, H. K., Hall, W. D., Hurst, J. W., (Eds.), *Clinical methods: The history, physical, and laboratory examinations.* (3rd ed.). Butterworths. https://www.ncbi.nlm.nih.gov/books/NBK320/

8 Martin, D. C. (1990). The mental status examination. In Walker, H. K., Hall, W. D., Hurst, J. W., (Eds.), *Clinical methods: The history, physical, and laboratory examinations.* (3rd ed.). Butterworths. https://www.ncbi.nlm.nih.gov/books/NBK320/

My Notes

Other terms used to describe speech include **circumstantial** (i.e., speaking with many unnecessary or tedious details without getting to the point of the conversation) and **poverty of content** (i.e., a conversation in which the client talks without stating anything related to the question, or their speech in general is vague and meaningless).

Motor Activity

Overall motor activity should be noted, including any tics or unusual mannerisms. Normal motor activity refers to the client having good balance, moving all extremities equally bilaterally, and walking with a smooth gait. Slow movements or lack of spontaneity in movement can occur due to depression or dementia. **Dyskinesia** (uncontrolled, involuntary movement) and **akathisia** (i.e., motor restlessness) may occur if the client is experiencing extrapyramidal syndrome related to psychotropic medication use.[9]

Terminology used to describe motor activity includes **psychomotor agitation** (i.e., a condition of purposeless, non goal-directed activity) and **psychomotor retardation** (i.e., a condition of extremely slow physical movements, slumped posture, or slow speech patterns).

Affect and Mood

Affect refers to the client's expression of emotion, and mood refers to the predominant emotion expressed by an individual.[10] Sustained emotions influence a person's behavior, personality, and perceptions. **Mood** can be described using various terms such as neutral, elevated, or **labile** (i.e., a rapid change in emotional responses, mood, or affect that are inappropriate for the moment or the situation). It can also be described as anxious, angry, sad, irritable, **dysphoric** (i.e., exhibiting depression), or **euphoric** (i.e., a pathologically elevated sense of well-being). People may express feelings of emptiness, impaired self-esteem, indecisiveness, or crying spells.[11]

Normal affect and mood are described as **euthymic** (i.e., displays a wide range of emotion that is appropriate for the situation). Abnormal findings related to affect include inappropriateness for the situation (e.g., laughing at the recent death of a loved one) or incongruent. **Congruence** refers to the consistency of verbal and nonverbal communication. Affect may also be described as subdued, tearful, labile, **blunted** (i.e., diminished range and intensity), or **flat** (no emotional expression).

Other terminology related to documenting a client's mood includes **alexithymia** (i.e., the inability to describe emotions with how one is feeling), **anhedonia** (i.e, the lack of experiencing pleasure in activities normally found enjoyable), and **apathy** (i.e., a lack of feelings, emotions, interests, or concerns).

Thoughts and Perceptions

The manner in which a client perceives and responds to stimuli is a critical psychiatric assessment. The inability to process information accurately is a component of the definition of psychotic thinking. For example, does the client

---

9 Martin, D. C. (1990). The mental status examination. In Walker, H. K., Hall, W. D., Hurst, J. W., (Eds.), *Clinical methods: The history, physical, and laboratory examinations.* (3rd ed.). Butterworths. https://www.ncbi.nlm.nih.gov/books/NBK320/

10 Martin, D. C. (1990). The mental status examination. In Walker, H. K., Hall, W. D., Hurst, J. W., (Eds.), *Clinical methods: The history, physical, and laboratory examinations.* (3rd ed.). Butterworths. https://www.ncbi.nlm.nih.gov/books/NBK320/

11 Martin, D. C. (1990). The mental status examination. In Walker, H. K., Hall, W. D., Hurst, J. W., (Eds.), *Clinical methods: The history, physical, and laboratory examinations.* (3rd ed.). Butterworths. https://www.ncbi.nlm.nih.gov/books/NBK320/

My Notes

harbor realistic concerns or are their concerns elevated to the level of irrational fear? Is the client responding in an exaggerated fashion to actual events? Is there no discernible basis in reality for the patient's beliefs or behavior?[12]

Clients with mental health disorders may experience intrusive thoughts, delusions, and/or obsessions. **Delusions** are a fixed, false belief not held by cultural peers and persisting in the face of objective contradictory evidence. For example, a client may have the delusion that the CIA is listening to their conversations via satellites. **Grandiose delusions** refer to a state of false attribution to the self of great ability, knowledge, importance or worth, identity, prestige, power, or accomplishment.[13] Clients may withdraw into an inner fantasy world that's not equivalent to reality, where they have inflated importance, powers, or a specialness that is opposite of what their actual life is like.[14] **Paranoia** is a condition characterized by delusions of persecution.[15] Clients often experience extreme suspiciousness or mistrust or express fear. For example, a resident of a long-term care facility may have delusions that the staff is trying to poison them.

Obsessions are persistent thoughts, ideas, images, or impulses that are experienced as intrusive or inappropriate and result in anxiety, distress, or discomfort. Common obsessions include repeated thoughts about contamination, a need to have things in a particular order or sequence, repeated doubts, aggressive impulses, and sexual imagery. Obsessions are distinguished from excessive worries about everyday occurrences because they are not concerned with real-life problems.[16] **Rumination** is obsessional thinking involving excessive, repetitive thoughts that interfere with other forms of mental activity.[17]

Clients may also experience altered perceptions such as hallucinations and illusions. **Hallucinations** are false sensory perceptions not associated with real external stimuli and can include any of the five senses (auditory, visual, gustatory, olfactory, and tactile). For example, a client may see spiders climbing on the wall or hear voices telling them to do things. These are referred to as "visual hallucinations" or "auditory hallucinations."

Illusions are misperceptions of real stimuli. For example, a client may misperceive tree branches blowing in the wind at night to be the arms of monsters trying to grab them.

It is important for nurses to remember that delusions, hallucinations, and illusions feel very real to clients and cause internal emotional reactions, even when a caregiver reassures them they are not based in reality. Because clients often conceal these experiences, it is helpful to ask leading questions, such as, "Have you ever seen or heard things that other people could not see or hear? Have you ever seen or heard things that later turned out not to be there?"[18]

Other terms used to document clients' thought processes include racing thoughts, flight of ideas, loose associations, and clang associations. **Racing thoughts** are fast moving and often repetitive thought patterns that can be

---

12 Martin, D. C. (1990). The mental status examination. In Walker, H. K., Hall, W. D., Hurst, J. W., (Eds.), *Clinical methods: The history, physical, and laboratory examinations.* (3rd ed.). Butterworths. https://www.ncbi.nlm.nih.gov/books/NBK320/

13 American Psychological Association. (n.d.). *APA Dictionary of Psychology.* https://dictionary.apa.org/

14 Raypole, C. (2019, November 20). *10 signs of covert narcissism.* Healthline. https://www.healthline.com/health/covert-narcissist#fantasies

15 American Psychological Association. (n.d.). *APA Dictionary of Psychology.* https://dictionary.apa.org/

16 American Psychological Association. (n.d.). *APA Dictionary of Psychology.* https://dictionary.apa.org/

17 American Psychological Association. (n.d.). *APA Dictionary of Psychology.* https://dictionary.apa.org/

18 Martin, D. C. (1990). The mental status examination. In Walker, H. K., Hall, W. D., Hurst, J. W., (Eds.), *Clinical methods: The history, physical, and laboratory examinations.* (3rd ed.). Butterworths. https://www.ncbi.nlm.nih.gov/books/NBK320/

My Notes

overwhelming. They may focus on a single topic, or they may represent multiple different lines of thought. For example, a client may have racing thoughts about a financial issue or an embarrassing moment.

Flight of ideas indicates the client frequently shifts from one topic to another with rapid speech, making it seem fragmented. The examiner may feel the client is rambling and changing topics faster than they can keep track, and they probably can't get a word in edgewise.[19] An example of client exhibiting a flight of ideas is, "My father sent me here. He drove me in a car. The car is yellow in color. Yellow color looks good on me."[20]

Loose associations refers to jumping from one idea to an unrelated idea in the same sentence. For example, the client might state, "I like to dance, and my feet are wet."[21] The term **word salad** refers to severely disorganized and virtually incomprehensible speech or writing, marked by severe loosening of associations.[22]

Clang associations refers to stringing words together that rhyme without logical association and do not convey rational meaning. For example, a client exhibiting clang associations may state, "Here she comes with a cat catch a rat match."

Clients with altered perceptions, especially when experiencing hallucinations and delusions, may have violent thoughts regarding themselves or others. If a client is having auditory hallucinations, it is vital for the nurse to determine if the voices are encouraging the client to hurt themselves or others. **Homicidal ideation** refers to threats or acts of life-threatening harm toward another person. **Suicidal ideation** is used to describe an individual who has been thinking about suicide but does not necessarily have an intention to act on that idea. **Suicide attempt** is a term used to describe an individual who harms themselves with intent to end their life but does not die as a result of their actions. **Suicide plan** refers to an individual who has a plan for suicide, has the means to injure oneself, and has the intent to die.

Of all portions of the mental status examination, the evaluation of thought disorders is the most difficult and requires a thorough assessment.[23] Psychiatric-mental health nurse specialists receive additional training in assessing thought disorders. These types of thought disorders are associated with mental illnesses like bipolar disorder and schizophrenia and may precede an episode of psychosis, so it is important to obtain further assistance if you notice a client is newly exhibiting these types of behaviors.[24]

Read more information about how to help individuals experiencing hallucinations and delusions in the "Applying the Nursing Process to Schizophrenia" section of the "Psychosis and Schizophrenia" chapter.

---

19 Martin, D. C. (1990). The mental status examination. In Walker, H. K., Hall, W. D., Hurst, J. W., (Eds.), *Clinical methods: The history, physical, and laboratory examinations.* (3rd ed.). Butterworths. https://www.ncbi.nlm.nih.gov/books/NBK320/

20 PsychologGenie. (n.d.). *The true meaning of flight of ideas explained with examples.* https://psychologenie.com/flight-of-ideas-meaning-examples

21 American Psychological Association. (n.d.). *APA Dictionary of Psychology.* https://dictionary.apa.org/

22 American Psychological Association. (n.d.). *APA Dictionary of Psychology.* https://dictionary.apa.org/

23 Martin, D. C. (1990). The mental status examination. In Walker, H. K., Hall, W. D., Hurst, J. W., (Eds.), *Clinical methods: The history, physical, and laboratory examinations.* (3rd ed.). Butterworths. https://www.ncbi.nlm.nih.gov/books/NBK320/

24 Joy, R. (2020, January 20). *Clang association: When a mental health condition disrupts speech.* Healthline. https://www.healthline.com/health/clang-association#whats-it-sound-like

My Notes

Attitude and Insight

The client's attitude is the emotional tone displayed toward the examiner, other individuals, or their illness. It may convey a sense of hostility, anger, helplessness, pessimism, overdramatization, self-centeredness, or passivity. It is important to determine the client's attitude toward emotional problems or diagnosed mental health disorders. Does the client look forward to improvement and recovery or are they resigned to suffer?[25]

Insight is the client's ability to identify the existence of a problem and to have an understanding of its nature.

Nurses must also be aware of transference. **Transference** occurs when the client projects (i.e., transfers) their feelings onto the nurse. For example, a client is feeling angry at a family member related to a previous disagreement and displaces the anger onto the nurse during the interview.

Cognitive Abilities

Cognition is the mental action or process of acquiring knowledge and understanding through thought, experience, and the senses. It includes thinking, knowing, remembering, judging, and problem-solving. When performing focused assessments on cognition, the examiner assesses attention and memory.[26] A term related to assessing attention is **distractibility**, referring to the client's attention being easily drawn to unimportant or irrelevant external stimuli.

Memory disturbance is a common complaint and is often a presenting symptom in the elderly. Memory can be grouped into three categories: immediate recall, short-term memory, and long-term storage. Short-term memory is the most clinically pertinent, and the most important to be tested. Short-term retention requires that the patient process and store information so that they can move on to a second intellectual task and then call up the remembrance after completion of the second task. For example, short-term memory may be tested by having the patient repeat the names of four unrelated objects and then asking the patient to recall the information in 3 to 5 minutes after performing a second, unrelated mental task.[27]

Examiner's Reaction to the Client

Assessing a client sometimes results in the nurse developing subtle and easily overlooked feelings toward the client. For example, it can be difficult to repeatedly address a client's negative state. Examiners may experience feelings of frustration, which can be taken by patients to mean there's something wrong with them. In such cases, nurses should examine their reactions to the client and be alert to feelings of distraction, boredom, or frustration. They should also be aware that clients perceive a nurse's feelings through their nonverbal communication, such as facial expressions, posture, tone of voice, and lack of eye contact.[28]

Nurses should also be aware of countertransference. **Countertransference** refers to a tendency for the examiner to displace (transfer) their own feelings onto the client and then these feelings may influence the client. For example,

---

25 Martin, D. C. (1990). The mental status examination. In Walker, H. K., Hall, W. D., Hurst, J. W., (Eds.), *Clinical methods: The history, physical, and laboratory examinations.* (3rd ed.). Butterworths. https://www.ncbi.nlm.nih.gov/books/NBK320/

26 Martin, D. C. (1990). The mental status examination. In Walker, H. K., Hall, W. D., Hurst, J. W., (Eds.), *Clinical methods: The history, physical, and laboratory examinations.* (3rd ed.). Butterworths. https://www.ncbi.nlm.nih.gov/books/NBK320/

27 Martin, D. C. (1990). The mental status examination. In Walker, H. K., Hall, W. D., Hurst, J. W., (Eds.), *Clinical methods: The history, physical, and laboratory examinations.* (3rd ed.). Butterworths. https://www.ncbi.nlm.nih.gov/books/NBK320/

28 DeAngelis, T. (2019). Better relationships with patients lead to better outcomes. *Monitor on Psychology, 50*(10), 38. https://www.apa.org/monitor/2019/11/ce-corner-relationships

My Notes

a nurse finds themself providing advice about how to raise children to a client. Upon self-reflection, they realize it is a countertransference reaction related to their previous parenting experience.[29]

Review a brief mental status examination PDF form from TherapistAid.

Psychosocial Assessment

A **psychosocial assessment** (also referred to as a health history) is a component of the nursing assessment process that obtains additional subjective data to detect risks and identify treatment opportunities and resources. Agencies have specific forms used for psychosocial assessments/health histories that typically consist of several components[30,31]:

- Cultural assessment
- Reason for seeking health care (i.e., "chief complaint")
- Thoughts of self-harm or suicide
- Current and past medical history
- Current medications
- History of previously diagnosed mental health disorders
- Previous hospitalizations
- Educational background
- Occupational background
- Family dynamics
- History of exposure to psychological trauma, violence, and domestic abuse
- Substance use (tobacco, alcohol, recreational drugs, misused prescription drugs)
- Family history of mental illness
- Coping mechanisms
- Functional ability/Activities of daily living
- Spiritual assessment

Review specific questions used during a psychosocial assessment/health history in the "Health History" chapter in Open RN *Nursing Skills*.

29 DeAngelis, T. (2019). Better relationships with patients lead to better outcomes. *Monitor on Psychology, 50*(10), 38. https://www.apa.org/monitor/2019/11/ce-corner-relationships

30 GW School of Medicine & Health Sciences. (n.d.). *Clinical FICA tool.* https://smhs.gwu.edu/spirituality-health/program/transforming-practice-health-settings/clinical-fica-tool

31 Glasner, J., Baltag, V., & Ambresin, A. E. (2021). Previsit multidomain psychosocial screening tools for adolescents and young adults: A system review. *Journal of Adolescent Health, 68*, 449-459. https://www.jahonline.org/article/S1054-139X(20)30600-5/pdf

Cultural Formulation Interview Questions

My Notes

While performing a psychosocial assessment, it is important to begin by performing a cultural assessment. We all bring our own cultural beliefs, values, and expectations to the clinical encounter, which influences how we approach specific aspects of care. The American Psychiatric Association developed evidence-based Cultural Formulation Interview (CFI) questions as a way to incorporate cultural assessment into the care of all clients that enhances clinical understanding and decision-making.[32] The CFI questions are used to clarify key aspects of the presenting clinical problem from the point of view of the individual and other members of the individual's social network (e.g., family, friends, or others involved in the current problem). This includes the problem's meaning, potential sources of help, and expectations for health care services.

CFI questions used with all clients include the following[33]:

1. What brings you here today?
2. What troubles you most about this problem?
3. Why do you think this is happening to you? What do you think is the cause of this problem?
4. Are there any kinds of support that make this problem better, such as support from family, friends, or others?
5. Are there any kinds of stresses that make this problem worse, such as difficulties with money or family problems?
6. Sometimes aspects of people's background or identity can make their problem better or worse, such as the communities they belong to, the languages they speak, where they or their family are from, their race or ethnic background, their gender or sexual orientation, or their faith or religion. Are there any aspects of your background or identity that make a difference to this problem?
7. Sometimes people have various ways of dealing with problems. What have you done on your own to cope with this problem?
8. Often, people look for help from many different sources, including different kinds of doctors, helpers, or healers. In the past, what kinds of treatment, help, advice, or healing have you sought for this problem?
9. Has anything prevented you from getting the help you need?
10. What kinds of help do you think would be most useful to you at this time for this problem?
11. Are there other kinds of help that your family, friends, or other people have suggested that would be helpful for you now?
12. Sometimes health care professionals and patients misunderstand each other because they come from different backgrounds or have different expectations. Have you been concerned about misaligned care expectations and is there anything that we can do to provide you with the care you need?

---

32 DeSilva, R., Aggarwall, N. K., & Lewis-Fernandez, R. (2015). The DSM-5 cultural formulation interview and the evolution of cultural assessment in psychiatry. *Psychiatric Times, 32*(6). https://www.psychiatrictimes.com/view/dsm-5-cultural-formulation-interview-and-evolution-cultural-assessment-psychiatry

33 American Psychiatric Association. (2013). Cultural formulation. In *Diagnostic and Statistical Manual of Mental Disorders* (5th ed.). American Psychiatric Association. pp. 749-759.

My Notes

Findings from the cultural formulation interview are used to individualize a client's plan of care to their preferences, values, beliefs, and goals.

Reason for Seeking Health Care

It is helpful to begin the psychosocial assessment by obtaining the reason why the patient is seeking health care in their own words. During a visit to a clinic or emergency department or on admission to a health care agency, the patient's primary reasons for seeking care are referred to as the **chief complaint**. Assessing a client's chief complaint recognizes that clients are complex beings, with potentially multiple coexisting health needs, but there is often a pressing issue that requires most immediate care. Questions used to evaluate a client's chief complaint are as follows:

- What brought you in today?
- How long has this been going on?
- How is this affecting you?

After identifying the reason the patient is seeking health care, additional focused questions are used to obtain detailed information about priority concerns, such as pain or other symptoms causing discomfort. The mnemonic PQRSTU is used to ask the patient questions in an organized fashion. See Table 4.3b for examples of questions used to assess a client's report of pain.

Table 4.3b Sample PQRSTU Questions

PQRSTU	Sample Questions
Provocation/ Palliation	What makes your pain worse? What makes your pain feel better?
Quality	What does the pain feel like? Note: You can provide suggestions for pain characteristics such as "aching," "stabbing," or "burning."
Region	Where exactly do you feel the pain? Does it move around or radiate elsewhere?
Severity	How would you rate your pain on a scale of 0 to 10, with "0" being no pain and "10" being the worst pain you've ever experienced?
Timing/ Treatment	When did the pain start? What were you doing when the pain started? Is the pain constant or does it come and go? If the pain is intermittent, when does it occur? How long does the pain last? Have you taken anything to help relieve the pain?
Understanding	What do you think is causing the pain?

Thoughts of Suicide

As discussed in Chapter 1, all clients aged 12 and older presenting for acute care should be screened for suicidal ideation. Clients being evaluated or treated for mental health conditions often have suicidal ideation, and up to

10 percent of emergency department clients presenting with medical issues have a hidden risk for suicide, such as recent suicidal ideation or previous suicide attempts.[34] Universal screening allows for the detection of suicide risk and implementation of early interventions before a person attempts suicide.

It is important to introduce suicide screening in a way that helps the patient understand its purpose and normalize questions that might otherwise seem intrusive. A nurse might introduce the topic in the following way: "Now I'm going to ask you some questions that we ask everyone treated here, no matter what problem they are here for. It is part of the hospital's policy, and it helps us to make sure we are not missing anything important."[35]

The Patient Safety Screener (PSS-3) is an example of a brief screening tool to detect suicide risk in all patients presenting to acute care settings.[36] See Figure 4.3[37] for an image of the PSS-3.

The PSS-3 consists of assessing for three items: depression, active suicidal ideation, and lifetime suicide attempt. Each of these items taps a different aspect of suicide risk[38]:

- Depression is a common precipitant of suicidal ideation and behavior and is the most common diagnosis among those who die by suicide.
- Suicidal ideation (i.e., thoughts about killing oneself) is a precondition for suicidal behavior.
- A previous suicide attempt is one of the most consistent risk factors for suicide.

---

34 Suicide Prevention Resource Center. (n.d.). *The patient safety screener: A brief tool to detect suicide risk.* https://sprc.org/micro-learning/patientsafetyscreener

35 Suicide Prevention Resource Center. (n.d.). *The patient safety screener: A brief tool to detect suicide risk.* https://sprc.org/micro-learning/patientsafetyscreener

36 Suicide Prevention Resource Center. (n.d.). *The patient safety screener: A brief tool to detect suicide risk.* https://sprc.org/micro-learning/patientsafetyscreener

37 "Patient Safety Screener (PSS-3) Pocket Card" by University of Massachusetts Medical School (UMass Medical) is used on the basis of Fair Use.

38 Suicide Prevention Resource Center. (n.d.). *The patient safety screener: A brief tool to detect suicide risk.* https://sprc.org/micro-learning/patientsafetyscreener

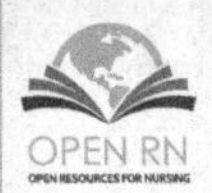

My Notes

Use this pocket card as a job aid or training tool when implementing universal suicide screening in acute care settings.

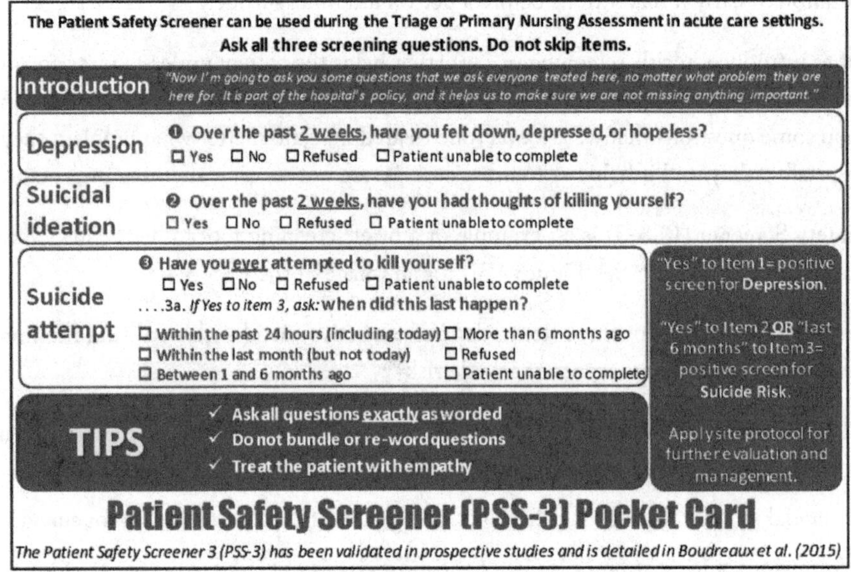

The Patient Safety Screener can be used during the Triage or Primary Nursing Assessment in acute care settings.
Ask all three screening questions. Do not skip items.

Introduction *"Now I'm going to ask you some questions that we ask everyone treated here, no matter what problem they are here for. It is part of the hospital's policy, and it helps us to make sure we are not missing anything important."*

Depression
❶ Over the past 2 weeks, have you felt down, depressed, or hopeless?
☐ Yes ☐ No ☐ Refused ☐ Patient unable to complete

Suicidal ideation
❷ Over the past 2 weeks, have you had thoughts of killing yourself?
☐ Yes ☐ No ☐ Refused ☐ Patient unable to complete

Suicide attempt
❸ Have you ever attempted to kill yourself?
☐ Yes ☐ No ☐ Refused ☐ Patient unable to complete
....3a. *If Yes to item 3, ask:* when did this last happen?
☐ Within the past 24 hours (including today) ☐ More than 6 months ago
☐ Within the last month (but not today) ☐ Refused
☐ Between 1 and 6 months ago ☐ Patient unable to complete

"Yes" to Item 1= positive screen for **Depression**.

"Yes" to Item 2 OR "last 6 months" to Item 3= positive screen for **Suicide Risk**.

Apply site protocol for further evaluation and management.

TIPS
✓ Ask all questions exactly as worded
✓ Do not bundle or re-word questions
✓ Treat the patient with empathy

Patient Safety Screener (PSS-3) Pocket Card

The Patient Safety Screener 3 (PSS-3) has been validated in prospective studies and is detailed in Boudreaux et al. (2015)

Figure 4.3 Patient Safety Screener for Suicide Risk. Used under Fair Use.

Self-Injury

Non-suicidal self-injury (NSSI) refers to intentional self-inflicted destruction of body tissue without suicidal intention and for purposes not socially sanctioned. Common forms of NSSI include behaviors such as cutting, burning, scratching, and self-hitting. It is considered a maladaptive coping strategy without the desire to die. NSSI is a common finding among adolescents and young adults in psychiatric inpatient settings.[39]

Family Dynamics

Family dynamics are included in a psychosocial assessment, especially for children, adolescents, and older adults. **Family dynamics** refers to the patterns of interactions among relatives, their roles and relationships, and the various factors that shape their interactions. Because family members rely on each other for emotional, physical, and economic support, they are primary sources of relationship security or stress. Family dynamics and the quality of family relationships can have either a positive or negative impact on an individual's health. For example, secure and supportive family relationships can provide love, advice, and care, whereas stressful family relationships can be burdened with arguments and constant critical feedback.[40]

Unhealthy family dynamics can cause children to experience trauma and stress as they grow up. This type of exposure, known as adverse childhood experiences (ACEs), is linked to an increased risk of developing physical and mental health problems such as heart, lung, and liver disease; depression; and anxiety. Unhealthy family dynamics also correlate with an increased risk of substance use and addiction among adolescents.[41]

---

39 Cipriano, A., Cella, S., & Cotrufo, P. (2017). Nonsuicidal self-injury: A systematic review. *Frontiers in Psychology*, 8. https://www.frontiersin.org/articles/10.3389/fpsyg.2017.01946/full

40 This work is a derivative of *StatPearls* by Jabbari & Rouster and is licensed under CC BY 4.0

41 This work is a derivative of *StatPearls* by Jabbari & Rouster and is licensed under CC BY 4.0

Review information about adverse childhood experiences (ACEs) in the "Mental Health and Mental Illness" section of Chapter 1.

Effectively assessing and addressing a client's family dynamic and its role in health and disease require an interprofessional team of health professionals, including nurses, physicians, social workers, and therapists. Nurses are in a unique position to observe and document interaction patterns, assess family relationships, and tend to family concerns in the clinical setting because they are in frequent contact with family members.[42]

Spiritual Assessment

Spiritual assessment is included in a psychosocial assessment. It is common for people in the process of recovery from mental health disorders and substance use to search for spiritual support.[43] **Spirituality** includes a sense of connection to something larger than oneself and typically involves a search for meaning and purpose in life. Basic questions used to assess spirituality include the following:

- Who or what provides you with strength or hope?
- How do you express your spirituality?
- What spiritual needs can we advocate for you during this health care experience?

Over the past decade, research has demonstrated the importance of spirituality in health care.[44,45] Spiritual distress is very common for clients experiencing serious illness, injury, or the dying process, and nurses are on the front lines as they assist these individuals to cope with these life events. Addressing a patient's spirituality and advocating spiritual care have been shown to improve patients' health and quality of life, including how they experience pain, cope with stress and suffering associated with serious illness, and approach end of life.[46,47]

---

42 This work is a derivative of *StatPearls* by Jabbari & Rouster and is licensed under CC BY 4.0

43 Neto, G. L., Rodrigues, L., Rozendo da Silva, D. A., Turato, E. R., & Campos, C. J. G. (2018). Spirituality review on mental health and psychiatric nursing. *Revista Brasileira de Enfermagem, 71* (Suppl 5), 2323-2333. https://doi.org/10.1590/0034-7167-2016-0429

44 Pilger, C., Molzahn, A. E., de Oliveira, M. P., & Kusumota, L. (2016). The relationship of the spiritual and religious dimensions with quality of life and health of patients with chronic kidney disease: An integrative literature review. *Nephrology Nursing Journal: Journal of the American Nephrology Nurses' Association, 43*(5), 411–426. https://pubmed.ncbi.nlm.nih.gov/30550069/

45 Puchalski, C., Jafari, N., Buller, H., Haythorn, T., Jacobs, C., & Ferrell, B. (2020). Interprofessional spiritual care education curriculum: A milestone toward the provision of spiritual care. *Journal of Palliative Medicine, 23*(6), 777–784. https://doi.org/10.1089/jpm.2019.0375

46 Pilger, C., Molzahn, A. E., de Oliveira, M. P., & Kusumota, L. (2016). The relationship of the spiritual and religious dimensions with quality of life and health of patients with chronic kidney disease: An integrative literature review. *Nephrology Nursing Journal: Journal of the American Nephrology Nurses' Association, 43*(5), 411–426. https://pubmed.ncbi.nlm.nih.gov/30550069/

47 Puchalski, C., Jafari, N., Buller, H., Haythorn, T., Jacobs, C., & Ferrell, B. (2020). Interprofessional spiritual care education curriculum: A milestone toward the provision of spiritual care. *Journal of Palliative Medicine, 23*(6), 777–784. https://doi.org/10.1089/jpm.2019.0375

My Notes

The FICA Spiritual History Tool© is a common tool used to gather information about a patient's spiritual history and preferences.[48] FICA© is a mnemonic for Faith, Importance, Community, and Address in Care. Read more about the FICA© tool in the following box.

The FICA© Spiritual History Tool[49]

F – Faith and Belief: Determine if the patient identifies with a particular belief system or spirituality.

I – Importance: Ask, "Is this belief important to you? Does it influence how you think about health and illness? Does it influence your health care decisions?"

C – Community: Determine if the client belongs to a spiritual community (e.g., a church, temple, mosque, or other group). If not, ask, "Would it be helpful to you to find a spiritual community?"

A – Address in Care: Evaluate what should be addressed during the client's care. Ask, "What should be included in your treatment plan? Are there spiritual practices you want to develop? Would you like to see a chaplain, spiritual director, or pastoral counselor while you are here?"

Based on the assessment findings, nurses may refer clients to agency chaplains or to the client's religious leaders for spiritual support to enhance coping.

 Read more about spiritual assessment and providing spiritual care in the "Spirituality" chapter of Open RN *Nursing Fundamentals*.

Screening Tools

Screening tools are evidence-based methods to assess specific information related to mental health disorders. These tools may be used on admission to the hospital or treatment facility, as well as at different times throughout the client's stay. Findings may be used to compare client progress during the hospital stay or from a previous admission. The registered nurse often conducts these screening tools as part of the interprofessional health care treatment team. Read more about specific screening tools in each "disorder" chapter.

Laboratory and Diagnostic Testing

Nurses review laboratory and diagnostic testing results as part of the assessment process.

Nurses monitor electrolytes and medication levels as they evaluate the need for medication adjustment. For example, serum sodium levels may be out of range due to conditions such as polydipsia, and poor nutritional or hydration status related to mental health disorders may require additional interventions by the nurse. Specific laboratory and diagnostic tests will be discussed in each "disorder" chapter, as well as in the "Psychotropic Medications" chapter.

48 GW School of Medicine & Health Sciences. (n.d.). *Clinical FICA tool.* https://smhs.gwu.edu/spirituality-health/program/transforming-practice-health-settings/clinical-fica-tool

49 GW School of Medicine & Health Sciences. (n.d.). *Clinical FICA tool.* https://smhs.gwu.edu/spirituality-health/program/transforming-practice-health-settings/clinical-fica-tool

Life Span Considerations

Life span considerations influence nursing assessments, care planning, and interventions. Mental health disorders occur across the life span, from the very young to the very old, and developmental stages must be considered when identifying impairments. Assessments and interventions must be individualized to the age and developmental level of the client. **Development** encompasses physical, social, and cognitive changes that occur continuously throughout one's life. See Figure 4.4[50] for an image of the human life cycle.

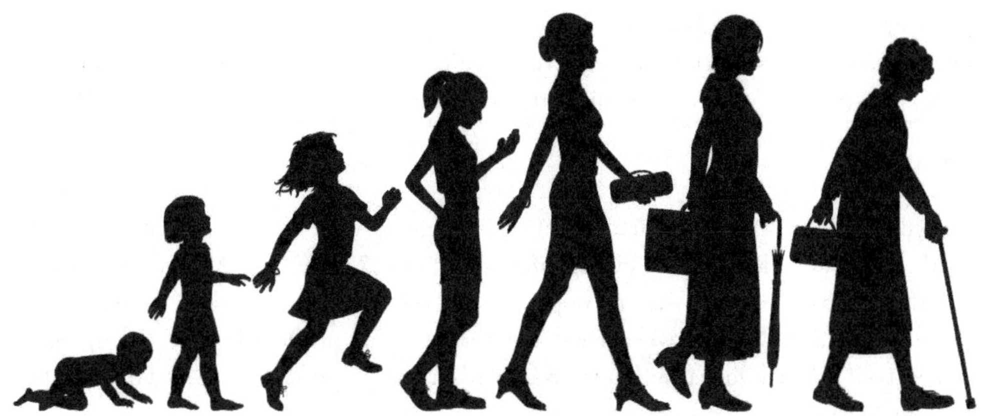

Figure 4.4 Human Life Cycle

There are multiple factors that affect human development with expected milestones along the way. Cognitive development encompasses several different skills that develop at different rates. Each human has their own individual experience that influences development of intelligence and reasoning as they interact with one another. With these unique experiences, everyone has a memory of feelings and events that is exclusive to them.[51]

There are many theories regarding how infants and children grow and develop into happy, healthy adults. Three major theories that have historically impacted nursing care are Freud's Psychosexual Theory of Development, Erikson's Psychosocial Stages of Development, and Piaget's Cognitive Theory of Development.

Freud's Psychosexual Theory of Development

Sigmund Freud (1856–1939) believed that personality develops during early childhood, and childhood experiences shape our personalities and behavior as adults. Freud believed that each individual must pass through a series of stages during childhood, and if we lack proper nurturance and parenting during a stage, we may become stuck, or fixated, in that stage. According to Freud, children's pleasure-seeking urges are focused on different areas of the body, called erogenous zones, at each of the five stages of development: oral, anal, phallic, latency, and genital.[52]

---

50 "shutterstock_149010437.jpg" by Robert Adrian Hillman is used under license from Shutterstock.com

51 Vallotton, C. D., & Fischer, K. W. (2008). Cognitive development. *Encyclopedia of Infant and Early Childhood Development.* Academic Press. pp. 286-298. https://doi.org/10.1016/B978-012370877-9.00038-4

52 This work is a derivative of *Psychology 2e* by OpenStax and is licensed under CC BY 4.0. Access for free at https://openstax.org/books/psychology-2e/pages/1-introduction

My Notes

While most of Freud's ideas are not supported by research and modern psychologists dispute Freud's psychosexual stages as a legitimate explanation for how one's personality develops, Freud's original theory supported that one's personality is shaped, in some part, by childhood experiences.[53]

Erikson's Psychosocial Stages of Development

Erik Erikson (1902–1994) took Freud's theory and modified it as psychosocial theory. Erikson's psychosocial development theory emphasizes the social nature of our development rather than its sexual nature. It describes eight sequential stages of individual human development influenced by biological, psychological, and social factors throughout the life span that contribute to an individual's personality. Erikson's stages of development are trust versus mistrust, autonomy versus shame, initiative versus guilt, industry versus inferiority, identity versus identity confusion, intimacy versus isolation, generativity versus stagnation, and integrity versus despair.[54,55]

Trust Vs. Mistrust

The first stage that develops is trust (or mistrust) that basic needs, such as nourishment and affection, will be met. Trust is the basis of our development during infancy (birth to 12 months). Infants are dependent upon their caregivers for their needs. Caregivers who are responsive and sensitive to their infant's needs help their baby to develop a sense of trust, and the infant will perceive the world as a safe, predictable place. Unresponsive caregivers who do not meet their baby's needs can engender feelings of anxiety, fear, and mistrust, and the infant will perceive the world as unpredictable.[56]

Autonomy Vs. Shame

Toddlers begin to explore their world and learn that they can control their actions and act on the environment to get results. They begin to show clear preferences for certain elements of the environment, such as food, toys, and clothing. A toddler's main task is to resolve the issue of autonomy versus shame and doubt by working to establish independence. For example, we might observe a budding sense of autonomy in a two-year-old child who wishes to choose their own clothes and dress themselves. Although the outfits might not be appropriate for the situation, the input in basic decisions has an effect on the toddler's sense of independence. If denied the opportunity to act on their environment, they may begin to doubt their abilities, which could lead to low self-esteem and feelings of shame.[57]

Initiative Vs. Guilt

After children reach the preschool stage (ages 3–6 years), they are capable of initiating activities and asserting control over their world through social interactions and play. By learning to plan and achieve goals while interacting

---

53 This work is a derivative of *Psychology 2e* by OpenStax and is licensed under CC BY 4.0. Access for free at https://openstax.org/books/psychology-2e/pages/1-introduction

54 This work is a derivative of *StatPearls* by Orenstein & Lewis and is licensed under CC BY 4.0

55 This work is a derivative of *Psychology 2e* by OpenStax and is licensed under CC BY 4.0. Access for free at https://openstax.org/books/psychology-2e/pages/1-introduction

56 This work is a derivative of *Psychology 2e* by OpenStax and is licensed under CC BY 4.0. Access for free at https://openstax.org/books/psychology-2e/pages/1-introduction

57 This work is a derivative of *Psychology 2e* by OpenStax and is licensed under CC BY 4.0. Access for free at https://openstax.org/books/psychology-2e/pages/1-introduction

My Notes

with others, preschool children can master a feeling of initiative and develop self-confidence and a sense of purpose. Those who are unsuccessful at this stage may develop feelings of guilt.[58]

Industry Vs. Inferiority

During the elementary school stage (ages 7–11), children begin to compare themselves to their peers to see how they measure up. They either develop a sense of pride and accomplishment in their schoolwork, sports, social activities, and family life, or they may feel inferior and inadequate if they feel they don't measure up to their peers.[59]

Identity Vs. Identity Confusion

In adolescence (ages 12–18), children develop a sense of self. Adolescents struggle with questions such as, "Who am I?" and "What do I want to do with my life?" Along the way, adolescents try on many different selves to see which ones fit. Adolescents who are successful at this stage have a strong sense of identity and are able to remain true to their beliefs and values in the face of problems and other people's perspectives. Teens who do not make a conscious search for identity, or those who are pressured to conform to their parents' ideas for the future, may have a weak sense of self and experience role confusion as they are unsure of their identity and confused about the future.[60]

Intimacy Vs. Isolation

People in early adulthood (i.e., 20s through early 40s) are ready to share their lives and become intimate with others after they have developed a sense of self. Adults who do not develop a positive self-concept in adolescence may experience feelings of loneliness and emotional isolation.[61]

Generativity Vs. Stagnation

When people reach their 40s, they enter a time period known as middle adulthood that extends to the mid-60s. The developmental task of middle adulthood is generativity versus stagnation. Generativity involves finding your life's work and contributing to the development of others through activities such as volunteering, mentoring, and raising children. Adults who do not master this developmental task may experience stagnation with little connection to others and little interest in productivity and self-improvement.[62]

Integrity Vs. Despair

The mid-60s to the end of life is a period of development known as late adulthood. People in late adulthood reflect on their lives and feel either a sense of satisfaction or a sense of failure. People who feel proud of their accomplishments feel a sense of integrity and often look back on their lives with few regrets. However, people who are not

---

58 This work is a derivative of *Psychology 2e* by OpenStax and is licensed under CC BY 4.0. Access for free at https://openstax.org/books/psychology-2e/pages/1-introduction

59 This work is a derivative of *Psychology 2e* by OpenStax and is licensed under CC BY 4.0. Access for free at https://openstax.org/books/psychology-2e/pages/1-introduction

60 This work is a derivative of *Psychology 2e* by OpenStax and is licensed under CC BY 4.0. Access for free at https://openstax.org/books/psychology-2e/pages/1-introduction

61 This work is a derivative of *Psychology 2e* by OpenStax and is licensed under CC BY 4.0. Access for free at https://openstax.org/books/psychology-2e/pages/1-introduction

62 This work is a derivative of *Psychology 2e* by OpenStax and is licensed under CC BY 4.0. Access for free at https://openstax.org/books/psychology-2e/pages/1-introduction

My Notes

successful at this stage may feel as if their life has been wasted. They focus on what "would have," "should have," or "could have" been. They face the end of their lives with feelings of bitterness, depression, and despair.[63]

Piaget's Cognitive Theory of Development

Jean Piaget (1896–1980) studied childhood development by focusing on children's cognitive growth. He believed that thinking is a central aspect of development and that children are naturally inquisitive but do not think and reason like adults. Children explore the world as they attempt to make sense of their experiences. His theory explains that humans move from one stage to another as they seek cognitive equilibrium and mental balance. There are four stages in Piaget's theory of development that occur in children from all cultures[64,65]:

- **Sensorimotor period.** The first stage extends from birth to approximately two years and is a period of rapid cognitive growth. During this period, infants develop an understanding of the world by coordinating sensory experiences (seeing, hearing) with motor actions (reaching, touching). The main development during the sensorimotor stage is the understanding that objects exist, and events occur in the world independently of one's own actions. Infants develop an understanding of what they want and what they must do to have their needs met. They begin to understand language used by those around them to make needs met.
- **Preoperational period.** The second stage begins in the toddler years. This continues through early school-age years. This is the time frame when children learn to think in images and symbols. Play is an important part of cognitive development during this period.
- **Concrete Operations period.** Older school-age children (age 7 years to 11 years) learn to think in terms of processes and can understand that there is more than one perspective when discussing a concept. This stage is considered a major turning point in the child's cognitive development because it marks the beginning of logical or operational thought.
- **Formal Operations period.** Children enter this stage around age 12 as they become self-conscious and egocentric. Adolescents gain the ability to think in an abstract manner by manipulating ideas in their head. Moving toward adulthood, this further develops into the ability to critically reason.

Cognitive Impairment

Cognitive impairment is a term used to describe impairment in mental processes that drive how an individual understands and acts in the world, affecting the acquisition of information and knowledge. Cognitive impairments can range from mild impairments, such as impairments in cognitive operations, to profound intellectual impairments causing minimal independent functioning. Components of cognitive functioning include attention, decision-making, general knowledge, judgment, language, memory, perception, planning, and reasoning.[66]

---

63 This work is a derivative of *Psychology 2e* by OpenStax and is licensed under CC BY 4.0. Access for free at https://openstax.org/books/psychology-2e/pages/1-introduction

64 Vallotton, C. D., & Fischer, K. W. (2008). Cognitive development. *Encyclopedia of Infant and Early Childhood Development.* Academic Press. pp. 286-298. https://doi.org/10.1016/B978-012370877-9.00038-4

65 McLeod, S. (2020, December 7). *Piaget's theory and stages of development.* SimplyPsychology. https://www.simplypsychology.org/piaget.html

66 Schofield, D. W. (2018, December 26). *Cognitive deficits.* Medscape. https://emedicine.medscape.com/article/917629-overview

My Notes

Review information about cognitive impairments associated with dementia and Alzheimer's disease in the "Cognitive Impairments" chapter of Open RN *Nursing Fundamentals*.

Intellectual disability (formerly referred to as mental retardation) is a diagnostic term that describes intellectual and adaptive functioning deficits identified during the developmental period. In the United States, the developmental period refers to the span of time prior to the age of 18 years. Children with intellectual disabilities may demonstrate a delay in developmental milestones (e.g., sitting, speaking, walking) or demonstrate mild cognitive impairments that may not be identified until school-age. Intellectual disability is typically nonprogressive and lifelong. It is diagnosed by multidisciplinary clinical assessments and standardized testing and is treated with a multidisciplinary treatment plan that maximizes quality of life.[67]

Resilience

When assessing an individual's developmental level, it is important to consider possible effects of adverse childhood events (ACEs) on their development. Science tells us that some children develop **resilience**, the ability to overcome serious hardship or traumatic experiences, while others do not. One way to understand the development of resilience is to visualize a seesaw. Protective experiences and coping skills on one side counterbalance significant adversity on the other. Resilience is evident when a child's health and development tip toward positive outcomes – even when a heavy load of factors is stacked on the negative outcome side.[68]

The most common factor for children who develop resilience is at least one stable and committed relationship with a supportive parent, caregiver, or other adult. These relationships provide the personalized responsiveness and protection that buffer children from developmental disruption. They also build their ability to plan, monitor, and regulate behavior that enables children to respond adaptively to adversity and thrive. This combination of supportive relationships, adaptive skill-building, and positive experiences is the foundation of resilience.[69]

The capabilities that underlie resilience can be strengthened at any age. It is never too late to build resilience. Age-appropriate, health-promoting activities can significantly improve the chances that an individual will recover from stress-inducing experiences. For example, regular physical exercise, stress management activities, and programs that actively promote self-regulation skills can improve the abilities of children and adults to cope with adversity in their lives.[70]

Read more about promoting resilience across the life span at Harvard's Center on the Developing Child Resilience web page.

---

67 Schofield, D. W. (2018, December 26). *Cognitive deficits.* Medscape. https://emedicine.medscape.com/article/917629-overview

68 Center on the Developing Child. (n.d.). *Resilience.* Harvard University. https://developingchild.harvard.edu/science/key-concepts/resilience/

69 Center on the Developing Child. (n.d.). *Resilience.* Harvard University. https://developingchild.harvard.edu/science/key-concepts/resilience/

70 Center on the Developing Child. (n.d.). *Resilience.* Harvard University. https://developingchild.harvard.edu/science/key-concepts/resilience/

My Notes

Cultural Considerations

Cultures and communities exhibit and explain symptoms of mental illness and manifest stress in various ways. Nurses should be aware of relevant contextual information stemming from a patient's culture, race, ethnicity, religion, or geographical origin. For example, uncontrollable crying and headaches are symptoms of panic attacks in some cultures, whereas difficulty breathing may be the primary symptom in another culture. Understanding such distinctions will help nurses effectively treat them.[71]

At the center of patient-centered care is practicing with cultural humility and inclusiveness. In the 2021 edition of *Nursing: Scope and Standards of Practice*, the American Nurses Association (ANA) established a Standard of Professional Performance called *Respectful and Equitable Practice*. This standard is defined as, "The registered nurse practices with cultural humility and inclusiveness." **Cultural humility** is "a humble and respectful attitude toward individuals of other cultures that pushes one to challenge their own cultural biases, realize they cannot know everything about other cultures, and approach learning about other cultures as a life-long goal and process."[72] **Inclusiveness** is defined as "the practice of providing equal access to opportunities and resources for people who might otherwise be excluded or marginalized, such as those having physical or mental disabilities or belonging to other minority groups."[73] Read the ANA competencies for the *Respectful and Equitable Practice* standard in the following box.

ANA's Respectful and Equitable Practice Competencies[74]

The registered nurse:

- Demonstrates respect, equity, and empathy in actions and interactions with all health care consumers.
- Respects consumer decisions without bias.
- Participates in life-long learning to understand cultural preferences, worldviews, choices, and decision-making processes of diverse consumers.
- Reflects upon personal and cultural values, beliefs, biases, and heritage.
- Applies knowledge of differences in health beliefs, practices, and communication patterns without assigning values to the differences.
- Addresses the effects and impact of discrimination and oppression on practice within and among diverse groups.
- Uses appropriate skills and tools for the culture, literacy, and language of the individuals and population served.

71 American Psychiatric Association. (n.d.). *DSM-5 fact sheets.* https://www.psychiatry.org/psychiatrists/practice/dsm/educational-resources/dsm-5-fact-sheets

72 American Nurses Association. (2021). *Nursing: Scope and standards of practice* (4th ed.). American Nurses Association.

73 Oxford Learner's Dictionaries. (n.d.). *Inclusion*. Oxford University Press. https://www.oxfordlearnersdictionaries.com/us/definition/english/inclusion

74 American Nurses Association. (2021). *Nursing: Scope and standards of practice* (4th ed.). American Nurses Association.

My Notes

- Communicates with appropriate language and behaviors, including the use of qualified health care interpreters and translators in accordance with consumer needs and preferences.
- Serves as a role model and educator for the cultural humility and the recognition and appreciation of diversity and inclusivity.
- Identifies the cultural-specific meaning of interactions, terms, and content.
- Advocates for policies that promote health and prevent harm among diverse health care consumers and groups.
- Promotes equity in all aspects of health and health care.
- Advances organizational policies, programs, services, and practices that reflect respect, equity, and values for diversity and inclusion.

Read more about cultural humility and advocating for the values, beliefs, and preferences of diverse clients in the "Diverse Clients" chapter of Open RN *Nursing Fundamentals*.

My Notes

4.4 DIAGNOSIS

The *Diagnosis* Standard of Practice by the American Nurses Association states, "The registered nurse analyzes assessment data to determine actual or potential diagnoses, problems, and issues."[1] Review the competencies for the *Diagnosis* Standard of Practice for registered nurses in the following box.

ANA's Diagnosis Competencies[2]

The registered nurse:

- Identifies actual or potential risks to the health care consumer's health and safety or barriers to health, which may include, but are not limited to, interpersonal, systematic, cultural, socioeconomic, or environmental circumstances.
- Uses assessment data, standardized classification systems, technology, and clinical decision support tools to articulate actual or potential diagnoses, problems, and issues.
- Identifies the health care consumer's strengths and abilities, including, but not limited to, support systems, health literacy, and engagement in self-care.
- Verifies the diagnoses, problems, and issues with the health care consumer and interprofessional colleagues.
- Prioritizes diagnoses, problems, and issues based on mutually established goals to meet the needs of the health care consumer across the health-illness continuum and the care continuum.
- Documents diagnoses, problems, strengths, and issues in a manner that facilitates the development of the expected outcomes and collaborative plan.

Review how to analyze assessment data, make hypotheses, and create nursing diagnoses statements in the "Diagnosis" section of the "Nursing Process" chapter in Open RN *Nursing Fundamentals*.

Nursing Diagnoses

A nursing diagnosis is "a clinical judgment concerning a human response to health conditions/life processes, or a vulnerability to that response, by an individual, family, group, or community."[3] Nursing diagnoses are customized to each patient and drive the development of the nursing care plan. The nurse should refer to an evidence-based care planning resource and review the definitions and defining characteristics of the hypothesized nursing diagnoses.

1 American Nurses Association. (2021). *Nursing: Scope and standards of practice* (4th ed.). American Nurses Association.

2 American Nurses Association. (2021). *Nursing: Scope and standards of practice* (4th ed.). American Nurses Association.

3 Herdman, T. H., & Kamitsuru, S. (Eds.). (2018). *Nursing diagnoses: Definitions and classification, 2018-2020.* Thieme Publishers New York.

My Notes

Recall that nursing diagnoses are different from medical diagnoses and mental health diagnoses. Medical diagnoses focus on medical problems that have been identified by the physician, physician's assistant, or advanced nurse practitioner. Mental health diagnoses are established by mental health experts, such as psychiatrists, psychologists, and advanced practice psychiatric-mental health nurses, using the *Diagnostic and Statistical Manual of Mental Disorders (DSM-5)*. See Figure 4.5[4] for an illustration of several mental health diagnoses.

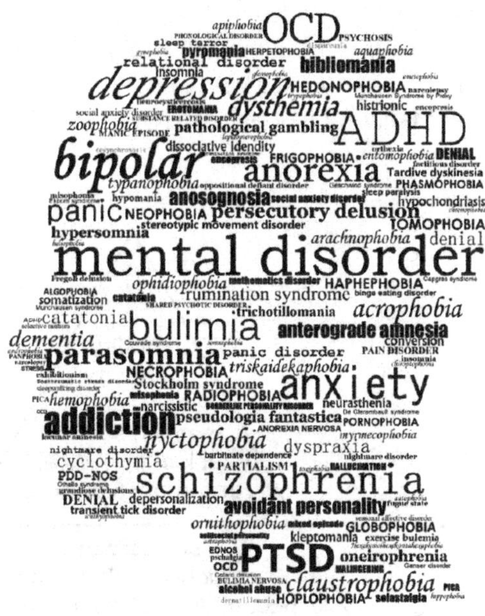

Figure 4.5 Mental Health Diagnoses

Nursing diagnoses focus on the human response to health conditions and life processes and are established by registered nurses. Patients with the same mental health diagnosis will often respond differently and thus have different nursing diagnoses. For example, two clients may have the same diagnosis of Major Depressive Disorder. However, one client may demonstrate a high risk for suicide whereas another patient may experience impaired nutrition due to lack of appetite. The nurse must consider these different responses when creating an individualized nursing care plan.

Prioritization

After identifying nursing diagnoses, the next step is prioritizing specific needs of the patient. Prioritization is the process of identifying the most significant problems and the most important interventions to implement based on a client's current status.

It is essential that life-threatening concerns and crises are quickly identified and addressed immediately. Depending on the severity of a problem, the steps of the nursing process may be performed in a matter of seconds for life-threatening concerns. Nurses must recognize cues signaling a change in patient condition, apply evidence-based practices in a crisis, and communicate effectively with interprofessional team members. Most client care situations fall somewhere between a crisis and routine care.

4 "Mental_Disorder_Silhouette.png" by Paget Michael Creelman is licensed under CC BY-SA 4.0

My Notes

Maslow's Hierarchy of Needs is commonly used to prioritize the most urgent patient needs. It is based on the theory that people are motivated by five levels of needs: physiological, safety, love, esteem, and self-actualization. The bottom levels of the pyramid represent the priority physiological needs intertwined with safety, whereas the upper levels focus on belonging, esteem, and self-actualization. Physiological needs must be met before focusing on higher level needs.[5] For example, priorities for a client experiencing mania are the need for food, fluid, and sleep, as well as controlling the agitation and impulsivity to ensure safety. These needs would need to be met before focusing on strategies to improve relationships with family and friends, build respect and acceptance for self and others, and engage in activities promoting personal growth. It is important to note that although safety is not described as a top priority in this theory, nurses must always prioritize safety needs in addition to physiological needs. See Figure 4.6[6] for an image of Maslow's Hierarchy of Needs.

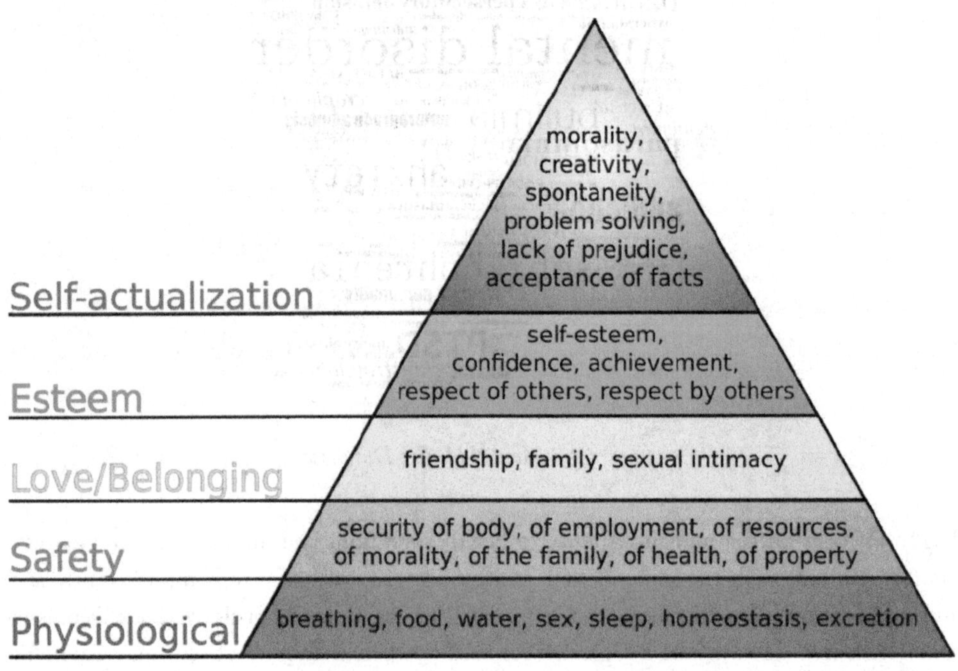

Figure 4.6 Maslow's Hierarchy of Needs

Common Nursing Diagnosis for Mental Health Conditions

Commonly used nursing diagnoses related to caring for clients with mental health conditions are included in Table 4.4. As always, when providing client care, refer to a current, evidence-based nursing care planning resource.

5 Maslow, A. H. (1943). A theory of human motivation. *Psychological Review*, 50(4), 370–396. https://doi.org/10.1037/h0054346

6 "Maslow's hierarchy of needs.svg" by J. Finkelstein is licensed under CC BY-SA 3.0

My Notes

Table 4.4 Common Nursing Diagnoses Related to Mental Health[7]		
Nursing Diagnosis	**Definition**	**Selected Defining Characteristics**
Risk for Suicide	Susceptible to self-inflicted, life-threatening injury.	■ Reports desire to die ■ Threats of killing self ■ Hopelessness ■ Social isolation ■ Giving away possessions ■ Substance misuse ■ Chronic pain ■ Sudden change in mood
Ineffective Coping	A pattern of impaired appraisal of stressors with cognitive and/or behavioral efforts that fails to manage demands related to well-being.	■ Alteration in concentration ■ Alteration in sleep pattern ■ Change in communication pattern ■ Inability to meet basic needs ■ Ineffective coping strategies ■ Insufficient goal-directed behavior ■ Risk-taking behavior ■ Substance misuse
Readiness for Enhanced Coping	A pattern of effective appraisal of stressors with cognitive and behavioral efforts to manage demands related to well-being, which can be strengthened.	■ Expresses desire to enhance: • Knowledge of stress management strategies • Social support • Use of problem and emotion-oriented strategies • Use of spiritual resources
Self-Neglect	A collection of culturally framed behaviors involving one or more self-care activities in which there is a failure to maintain a socially accepted standard of health and well-being.	■ Insufficient personal hygiene ■ Insufficient environmental hygiene ■ Nonadherence to health activity

7 McLeod, S. (2020, December 7). *Piaget's theory and stages of development*. SimplyPsychology. https://www.simplypsychology.org/piaget.html

My Notes

Nursing Diagnosis	Definition	Selected Defining Characteristics
Fatigue	An overwhelming sustained sense of exhaustion and decreased capacity for physical and mental work at the usual level.	■ Alteration in concentration ■ Alteration in libido ■ Apathy ■ Impaired ability to maintain usual routines ■ Ineffective role performance ■ Nonrestorative sleep patterns
Imbalanced Nutrition: Less than Body Requirements	Intake of nutrients insufficient to meet metabolic needs.	■ Food intake less than recommended daily allowance ■ Insufficient interest in food ■ Body weight 20% or more below ideal weight range ■ Read more in the "Nutrition" chapter in Open RN *Nursing Fundamentals*
Constipation	Decrease in normal frequency of defecation accompanied by difficult or incomplete passage of stool and/or passage of excessively dry, hard stool.	■ Read more in the "Constipation" section of the "Elimination" chapter in Open RN *Nursing Fundamentals* ■ Related factors: depression, emotional disturbance, medication side effects, imbalanced nutrition, and poor intake
Sleep Deprivation	Prolonged periods of time without sustained natural, periodic suspension of relative consciousness that provides rest.	■ Anxiety ■ Agitation ■ Irritability ■ Restlessness ■ Alteration in concentration ■ Fatigue ■ Transient paranoia ■ Read more in the "Sleep and Rest" chapter of Open RN *Nursing Fundamentals*
Social Isolation	Aloneness experienced by the individual and perceived as imposed by others and as a negative or threatening state.	■ Absence of support system ■ Flat or sad affect ■ Feeling different from others ■ Values incongruent with social norms

My Notes

Nursing Diagnosis	Definition	Selected Defining Characteristics
Chronic Low Self-Esteem	Negative evaluation and/or feelings about one's own capabilities, lasting at least three months.	■ Repeatedly unsuccessful in life events ■ Underestimates ability to deal with situation ■ Exaggerates negative feedback about self ■ Excessive seeking of reassurance ■ Nonassertive behavior
Hopelessness	Subjective state in which an individual sees limited or no alternatives or personal choices available and is unable to mobilize energy on own behalf.	■ Decrease in: • Appetite • Affect • Verbalization • Initiative ■ Shrugging in response to speaker
Spiritual Distress	A state of suffering related to the impaired ability to experience meaning in life through connections with self, others, the world, or a superior being.	■ Ineffective coping strategies ■ Perceived insufficient meaning in life ■ Separation from support system ■ Anger ■ Hopelessness
Readiness for Enhanced Knowledge	A pattern of cognitive information related to a specific topic or its acquisition, which can be strengthened.	■ Expresses desire to enhance learning

Sample Case A

During an interview with a 32-year-old client diagnosed with Major Depressive Disorder, Mr. J. exhibited signs of a sad affect and hopelessness. He expressed desire to die and reported difficulty sleeping and a lack of appetite with weight loss. He reports he has not showered in over a week, and his clothes have a strong body odor. The nurse analyzed this data and created four nursing diagnoses using a nurse care plan reference[8]:

- *Hopelessness* related to social isolation
- *Risk for Suicide* as manifested by reported desire to die

8 Ackley, B., Ladwig, G., Makic, M. B., Martinez-Kratz, M., & Zanotti, M. (2020). *Nursing diagnosis handbook: An evidence-based guide to planning care* (12th ed.). Elsevier.

My Notes

- *Imbalanced Nutrition: Less than Body Requirements* related to insufficient dietary intake
- *Self-Neglect* related to insufficient personal hygiene

The nurse established the top priority nursing diagnosis of *Risk for Suicide* and immediately screened for suicidal ideation and a plan using the Patient Safety Screener.

My Notes

4.5 OUTCOMES IDENTIFICATION

The *Outcomes Identification* Standard of Practice by the American Nurses Association states, "The registered nurse identifies expected outcomes for a plan individualized to the health care consumer or the situation."[1] Review the competencies for the *Outcomes Identification* Standard of Practice for registered nurses in the following box.

ANA's Outcomes Identification Competencies[2]

The registered nurse:

- Engages with the health care consumer, interprofessional team, and others to identify expected outcomes.
- Collaborates with the health care consumer to define expected outcomes integrating the health care consumer's culture, values, and ethical considerations.
- Formulates expected outcomes derived from assessments and diagnoses.
- Integrates evidence and best practices to identify expected outcomes.
- Develops expected outcomes that facilitate coordination of care.
- Identifies a time frame for the attainment of expected outcomes.
- Documents expected outcomes as measurable goals.
- Identifies the actual outcomes in relation to expected outcomes, safety, and quality standards.
- Modifies expected outcomes based on the evaluation of the status of the health care consumer and situation.

An **outcome** is a "measurable behavior demonstrated by the patient who is responsive to nursing interventions."[3] After nursing interventions are implemented, the nurse evaluates if the outcomes were met in the time frame indicated for that patient.

Outcome identification includes setting short-term and long-term goals and then creating specific expected outcome statements for each nursing diagnosis. Outcome statements are always patient-centered. They should be developed collaboratively with the client and individualized to meet the client's unique needs, values, and cultural beliefs. They should start with the phrase *"The client will . . . "* Outcome statements should be directed at resolving the defining characteristics for that nursing diagnosis. Additionally, the outcome must be something the patient is willing to cooperate in achieving.

1 American Nurses Association. (2021). *Nursing: Scope and standards of practice* (4th ed.). American Nurses Association.

2 American Nurses Association. (2021). *Nursing: Scope and standards of practice* (4th ed.). American Nurses Association.

3 Herdman, T. H., & Kamitsuru, S. (Eds.). (2018). *Nursing diagnoses: Definitions and classification, 2018-2020.* Thieme Publishers New York.

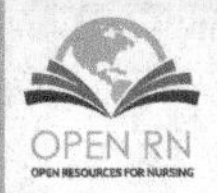

My Notes

Read more about how to use the "Motivational Interviewing" technique in setting individualized goals and expected outcomes with a client in the "Therapeutic Communication and Nurse-Client Relationship" chapter.

Outcome statements should contain five components easily remembered using the "SMART" mnemonic:

- **S**pecific
- **M**easurable
- **A**ttainable/Action-oriented
- **R**elevant/Realistic
- **T**ime frame

See Figure 4.7[4] for an image of the SMART components of outcome statements.

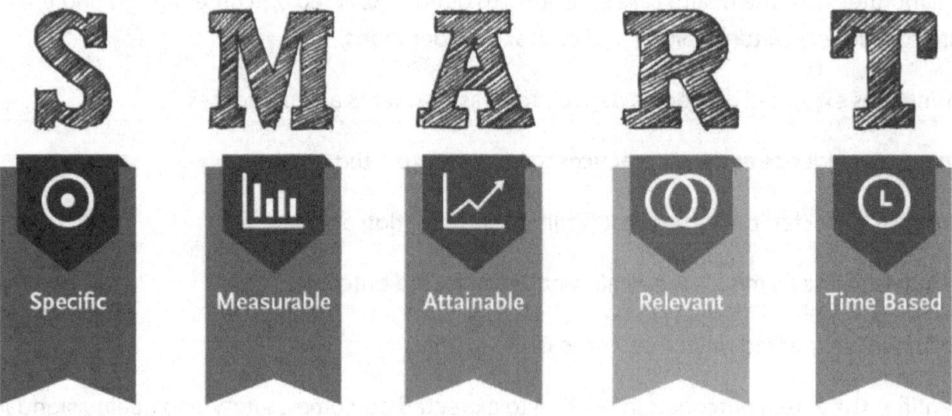

Figure 4.7 SMART Components

Review how to create "SMART" expected outcomes in the "Nursing Process" chapter of Open RN *Nursing Fundamentals*.

Unfolding Case A

Recall Sample Case A in the "Diagnosis" section regarding the 32-year-old male diagnosed with Major Depressive Disorder. The nurse created these four nursing diagnoses:

- *Hopelessness* related to social isolation
- *Risk for Suicide* as manifested by reported desire to die
- *Imbalanced Nutrition: Less than Body Requirements* related to insufficient dietary intake
- *Self-Neglect* related to insufficient personal hygiene

4 "SMART-goals.png" by Dungdm93 is licensed under CC BY-SA 4.0

My Notes

The nurse established the top priority nursing diagnosis of *Risk for Suicide* and immediately screened for suicidal ideation and a plan using the Patient Safety Screener.

The nurse then identified the following SMART expected outcome for the nursing diagnosis *Risk for Suicide* related to reported desire to die: *The client will remain free from self-harm self during the hospitalization stay.*

My Notes

4.6 PLANNING

The *Planning* Standard of Practice by the American Nurses Association states, "The registered nurse develops a collaborative plan encompassing strategies to achieve expected outcomes."[1]

Review the competencies for the *Planning* Standard of Practice for registered nurses in the following box.

ANA's Planning Competencies[2]

The registered nurse:

- Develops an individualized, holistic, evidence-based plan in partnership with the health care consumer, family, significant others, and interprofessional team.
- Designs innovative nursing practices that can be incorporated into the plan.
- Prioritizes elements of the plan based on the assessment of the health care consumer's level of safety needs to include risks, benefits, and alternatives.
- Establishes the plan priorities with the health care consumer, family, significant others, and interprofessional team.
- Advocates for compassionate, responsible, and appropriate use of interventions to minimize unwarranted or unwanted treatment, health care consumer suffering, or both.
- Includes strategies designed to address each of the identified diagnoses, health challenges, issues, or opportunities. These strategies may include, but are not limited to, maintaining health and wellness; promotion of comfort; promotion of wholeness, growth, and development; promotion and restoration of health and wellness; prevention of illness, injury, disease, complications, and trauma; facilitation of healing; alleviation of suffering; supportive care; and mitigation of environmental or occupational risks.
- Incorporates an implementation pathway that describes an overall timeline, steps, and milestones.
- Provides for the coordination and continuity of care.
- Identifies cost and economic implications of the plan.
- Develops a plan that reflects compliance with current statutes, rules, regulations, and standards.
- Modifies the plan according to the ongoing assessment of the health care consumer's response and other outcome indicators.

1 American Nurses Association. (2021). *Nursing: Scope and standards of practice* (4th ed.). American Nurses Association.

2 American Nurses Association. (2021). *Nursing: Scope and standards of practice* (4th ed.). American Nurses Association.

My Notes

- Documents the plan using standardized language or recognized terminology.
- Actively contributes at all levels in the development and continuous improvement of systems that support the planning process.

As always, consult a current, evidence-based nursing care planning resource when planning nursing interventions individualized to each client's needs. You might be asking yourself, "How do I know what evidence-based nursing interventions to include in the nursing care plan regarding mental health care?" There are several sources that can be used to select nursing interventions. Many agencies have care planning tools and references included in the electronic health record that are easily documented in the patient chart. Additionally, the Substance Abuse and Mental Health Services Administration (SAMHSA) maintains an evidence-based resource center.[3]

Access the Evidence-Based Resource Center maintained by the Substance Abuse and Mental Services Administration (SAMHSA).

See sample planned nursing interventions for a client who has been diagnosed with *Risk for Suicide* in Table 4.6.

Table 4.6 Sample Nursing Interventions for Risk for Suicide

Nursing Intervention The nurse will…	**Rationale**
Use an evidence-based process to conduct a suicide risk assessment.	Patients with suicidal ideation vary widely in their risk for a suicide attempt depending on whether they have a plan, intent, and past history of attempts. In-depth assessment of patients who screen positive for suicide risk must be completed to determine how to appropriately treat them.[4]
Document and communicate the client's overall level of risk for suicide with the treatment team and the plan for mitigating their risk for suicide.	All interprofessional health care team members who might come in contact with a client at risk for suicide must be aware of the level of risk and the mitigation plans to reduce that risk. This information should be explicitly documented in the patient's record.[5]

3 Substance Abuse and Mental Health Services Administration. (n.d.). *Evidence-based practices resource center.* https://www.samhsa.gov/resource-search/ebp

4 DeAngelis, T. (2019). Better relationships with patients lead to better outcomes. *Monitor on Psychology, 50*(10), 38. https://www.apa.org/monitor/2019/11/ce-corner-relationships

5 DeAngelis, T. (2019). Better relationships with patients lead to better outcomes. *Monitor on Psychology, 50*(10), 38. https://www.apa.org/monitor/2019/11/ce-corner-relationships

My Notes

Nursing Intervention The nurse will…	Rationale
Perform an environmental risk assessment and remove features that could be used to attempt suicide.	The Veteran's Health Administration showed that use of a Mental Health Environment of Care Checklist to facilitate a thorough, systematic environmental assessment reduced the rate of suicide from 4.2 per 100,000 admissions to 0.74 per 100,000 admissions.[6]
Administer prescribed treatment and collaboratively manage psychiatric symptoms that may be contributing to the client's suicidal ideation or behavior.	Symptoms of the disorder may require treatment with antidepressant, antipsychotic, or antianxiety medications. A systematic review has shown a significant effect for cognitive behavioral therapy in reducing suicidal behavior.[7]
Express desire to help the client and validate the client's experience of psychological pain while maintaining a safe environment for the client.	The nurse must reconcile their goal of preventing suicide with recognition of the client's goal to alleviate their psychological pain.[8]
Develop a positive therapeutic relationship with the client; do not make promises that may not be kept.	Nurses connect suicidal clients with humanity by guiding the client, encouraging effective coping strategies, and helping them connect appropriately with others.[9]
Determine the client's need for supervision and assign a room near the nursing station as necessary.	Close assignment increases ease of observation and availability for a rapid response in the event of a suicide attempt.[10]
Search the newly hospitalized client and the client's personal belongings for weapons or potential weapons and hoarded medications during the admission process and remove dangerous items.	Clients with suicidal ideation may bring the means with them. This action is necessary to maintain a hazard-free environment and client safety.[11]
Limit access to windows and exits unless locked and shatterproof, as appropriate. Ensure exits are secure.	Suicidal behavior may include attempts to jump out of windows or escape to find other means of suicide.[12]

6 DeAngelis, T. (2019). Better relationships with patients lead to better outcomes. *Monitor on Psychology, 50*(10), 38. https://www.apa.org/monitor/2019/11/ce-corner-relationships

7 Ackley, B., Ladwig, G., Makic, M. B., Martinez-Kratz, M., & Zanotti, M. (2020). *Nursing diagnosis handbook: An evidence-based guide to planning care* (12th ed.). Elsevier.

8 Ackley, B., Ladwig, G., Makic, M. B., Martinez-Kratz, M., & Zanotti, M. (2020). *Nursing diagnosis handbook: An evidence-based guide to planning care* (12th ed.). Elsevier.

9 Ackley, B., Ladwig, G., Makic, M. B., Martinez-Kratz, M., & Zanotti, M. (2020). *Nursing diagnosis handbook: An evidence-based guide to planning care* (12th ed.). Elsevier.

10 Ackley, B., Ladwig, G., Makic, M. B., Martinez-Kratz, M., & Zanotti, M. (2020). *Nursing diagnosis handbook: An evidence-based guide to planning care* (12th ed.). Elsevier.

11 Ackley, B., Ladwig, G., Makic, M. B., Martinez-Kratz, M., & Zanotti, M. (2020). *Nursing diagnosis handbook: An evidence-based guide to planning care* (12th ed.). Elsevier.

12 Ackley, B., Ladwig, G., Makic, M. B., Martinez-Kratz, M., & Zanotti, M. (2020). *Nursing diagnosis handbook: An evidence-based guide to planning care* (12th ed.). Elsevier.

My Notes

Nursing Intervention The nurse will…	**Rationale**
Place the client in the least restrictive, safe, and monitored environment that allows for the necessary level of observation. Assess suicidal risk at least daily and more frequently as warranted.	Close observation of the client is necessary for safety as long as the intent remains high. Suicide risk should be assessed at frequent intervals to adjust suicide precautions and ensure restrictions continue to be appropriate.[13]
Consider strategies to decrease isolation and opportunity to act on harmful thoughts (e.g., use of a sitter).	Clients have reported feeling safe and having their hope restored in response to close observation.[14]
Create a safety plan that includes a no-suicide contract. Contract verbally or in writing with the client for no self-harm and recontract at appropriate intervals.	Discussing thoughts of suicide and self-harm with a trusted person can provide relief for the client. A safety plan gets the subject out in the open and places some of the responsibility for safety with the client. However, research has suggested that self-harm is not prevented by contracts, and ongoing assessment of suicide risk is necessary.[15]
Explain suicide precautions and relevant safety issues to the client and family (purpose, duration, behavioral expectations, and behavioral consequences).	Suicide precautions may be viewed as restrictive. Clients have reported the loss of privacy as distressing.[16] Explaining the reasoning for safety precautions helps the client understand why they are being used even though they may feel restrictive and distressing. When clients and family members understand the reasoning for the precautions, they are more likely to comply.
Verify the client has taken medications as ordered (e.g., conduct mouth checks after medication administration).	The client may attempt to hoard medications for a later suicide attempt.[17]

13 Ackley, B., Ladwig, G., Makic, M. B., Martinez-Kratz, M., & Zanotti, M. (2020). *Nursing diagnosis handbook: An evidence-based guide to planning care* (12th ed.). Elsevier.

14 Ackley, B., Ladwig, G., Makic, M. B., Martinez-Kratz, M., & Zanotti, M. (2020). *Nursing diagnosis handbook: An evidence-based guide to planning care* (12th ed.). Elsevier.

15 Ackley, B., Ladwig, G., Makic, M. B., Martinez-Kratz, M., & Zanotti, M. (2020). *Nursing diagnosis handbook: An evidence-based guide to planning care* (12th ed.). Elsevier.

16 Ackley, B., Ladwig, G., Makic, M. B., Martinez-Kratz, M., & Zanotti, M. (2020). *Nursing diagnosis handbook: An evidence-based guide to planning care* (12th ed.). Elsevier.

17 Ackley, B., Ladwig, G., Makic, M. B., Martinez-Kratz, M., & Zanotti, M. (2020). *Nursing diagnosis handbook: An evidence-based guide to planning care* (12th ed.). Elsevier.

My Notes

Nursing Intervention The nurse will…	Rationale
Maintain increased surveillance of the client whenever the use of an antidepressant has been initiated or the dose increased.	Antidepressant medications take anywhere from 2 to 6 weeks to achieve full efficacy. During that period, the client's energy level may increase although the depression has not yet lifted, which increases the potential for suicide.[18]
Involve the client in treatment planning and self-care management of psychiatric disorders.	Self-care management promotes feelings of self-efficacy. The more clients participate in their own care, the less powerless and hopeless they feel.[19]
Assist the client in identifying a network of supportive persons and resources (e.g., family, clergy, care providers).	Social support and positive events were found to have a protective effect against suicidal ideation.[20]
Document client behavior in detail to support involuntary admission if actively suicidal.	Read more about involuntary admissions in the "Patient Rights" section of the "Legal and Ethical Considerations in Mental Health Care" chapter. Involuntary inpatient admissions serve to keep the client safe from harm. Involuntary outpatient commitment is also available in many states and can improve treatment, reduce the likelihood of hospital readmission, and reduce episodes of violent behavior in persons with severe psychiatric illnesses.[21]
Involve the family in discharge planning (e.g., illness/medication teaching, recognition of increasing suicidal risk, client's plan for dealing with recurring suicidal thoughts, and community resources).	Family members must learn how to respond to cues early, support the treatment regimen, and encourage the client to initiate an emergency plan.[22] When family members are aware of cues, treatments, and emergency plans, clients are less likely to act on thoughts of suicide or self-harm.

18 Ackley, B., Ladwig, G., Makic, M. B., Martinez-Kratz, M., & Zanotti, M. (2020). *Nursing diagnosis handbook: An evidence-based guide to planning care* (12th ed.). Elsevier.

19 Ackley, B., Ladwig, G., Makic, M. B., Martinez-Kratz, M., & Zanotti, M. (2020). *Nursing diagnosis handbook: An evidence-based guide to planning care* (12th ed.). Elsevier.

20 Ackley, B., Ladwig, G., Makic, M. B., Martinez-Kratz, M., & Zanotti, M. (2020). *Nursing diagnosis handbook: An evidence-based guide to planning care* (12th ed.). Elsevier.

21 Ackley, B., Ladwig, G., Makic, M. B., Martinez-Kratz, M., & Zanotti, M. (2020). *Nursing diagnosis handbook: An evidence-based guide to planning care* (12th ed.). Elsevier.

22 Ackley, B., Ladwig, G., Makic, M. B., Martinez-Kratz, M., & Zanotti, M. (2020). *Nursing diagnosis handbook: An evidence-based guide to planning care* (12th ed.). Elsevier.

My Notes

Nursing Intervention The nurse will…	**Rationale**
Before discharge from the hospital, ensure the client has a safety plan to use after discharge, including a supply of prescribed medications and a plan for outpatient follow-up. Ensure they understand the plan or have a caregiver able and willing to follow the plan, as well as the ability to access outpatient treatment.	Clients may have difficulty concentrating on the plan for follow-up. They may need assistance from others to ensure prescriptions are filled, appointments are attended, and transportation is available to appointments.[23]
In the event of a client's suicide, refer the family to a support group for survivors of suicide.	Psychoeducational support group participants found relief in sharing their bereavement with others.[24]

Review the "Establishing Safety" section for clients at risk for suicide in Chapter 1.

23 Ackley, B., Ladwig, G., Makic, M. B., Martinez-Kratz, M., & Zanotti, M. (2020). *Nursing diagnosis handbook: An evidence-based guide to planning care* (12th ed.). Elsevier.

24 Ackley, B., Ladwig, G., Makic, M. B., Martinez-Kratz, M., & Zanotti, M. (2020). *Nursing diagnosis handbook: An evidence-based guide to planning care* (12th ed.). Elsevier.

My Notes

4.7 IMPLEMENTATION

The *Implementation* Standard of Practice by the American Nurses Association (ANA) states, "The registered nurse implements the identified plan."[1] Review the competencies for the *Implementation* Standard of Practice for registered nurses in the following box.

ANA's Implementation Competencies[2]

The registered nurse:

- Demonstrates caring behaviors to develop therapeutic relationships.
- Provides care that focuses on the health care consumer.
- Advocates for the needs of diverse populations across the life span.
- Uses critical thinking and technology solutions to implement the nursing process to collect, measure, record, retrieve, trend, and analyze data and information to enhance health care consumer outcomes and nursing practice.
- Partners with the health care consumer to implement the plan in a safe, effective, efficient, timely, and equitable manner.
- Engages interprofessional team partners with implementation of the plan through collaboration and communication across the continuum of care.
- Uses evidence-based interventions and strategies to achieve mutually identified goals and outcomes specific to the problem or needs.
- Delegates according to the health, safety, and welfare of the health care consumer.
- Delegates after considering the circumstance, person, task, direction or communication, supervision, and evaluation.
- Considers the state's Nurse Practice Act regulations, institution, and regulatory entities while maintaining accountability for the care.
- Documents implementation and any modifications, including changes or omissions, of the identified nursing care plan.

In addition to these competencies, the American Nurses Association established two additional subcategories for the *Implementation* standard: *Coordination of Care* and *Health Teaching and Health Promotion*. In addition to these basic subcategories, the American Psychiatric established additional subcategories for registered nurses working in psychiatric/mental health settings: *Pharmacological, Biological, and Integrative Therapies; Milieu Therapy;* and

1 American Nurses Association. (2021). *Nursing: Scope and standards of practice* (4th ed.). American Nurses Association.

2 American Nurses Association. (2021). *Nursing: Scope and standards of practice* (4th ed.). American Nurses Association.

My Notes

Therapeutic Relationship and Counseling. Each of these additional subcategories of *Implementation* is discussed in the following subsections.

Coordination of Care

Review the competencies for the *Coordination of Care* Standard of Care in the following box.

ANA's Coordination of Care Competencies[3]

The registered nurse:

- Collaborates with the health care consumer and the interprofessional team to help manage health care based on mutually agreed-upon outcomes.
- Organizes the components of the plan with input from the health care consumer and other stakeholders.
- Manages the health care consumer's care to reach mutually agreed-upon outcomes.
- Engages health care consumers in self-care to achieve preferred goals for quality of life.
- Assists the health care consumer to identify options for care and navigate the health care system and its services.
- Communicates with the health care consumer, interprofessional team, and community-based resources to effect safe transitions in continuity of care.
- Advocates for the delivery of dignified and person-centered care by the interprofessional team.
- Documents the coordination of care.

Health Teaching and Health Promotion

Review the competencies for *Health Teaching and Health Promotion* in the following box.

ANA's Health Teaching and Health Promotion Competencies[4]

The registered nurse:

- Provides opportunities for the health care consumer to identify needed health promotion, disease prevention, and self-management topics such as:
    - Healthy lifestyles

---

3 American Nurses Association. (2021). *Nursing: Scope and standards of practice* (4th ed.). American Nurses Association.

4 American Nurses Association. (2021). *Nursing: Scope and standards of practice* (4th ed.). American Nurses Association.

My Notes

- Self-care and risk management
- Coping, adaptability, and resiliency

- Uses health promotion and health teaching methods in collaboration with the health care consumer's values, beliefs, health practices, developmental level, learning needs, readiness and ability to learn, language preference, spirituality, culture, and socioeconomic status.
- Uses feedback from the health care consumer and other assessments to determine the effectiveness of the employed strategies.
- Uses technologies to communicate health promotion and disease prevention information to the health care consumer.
- Provides health care consumers with information and education about intended effects and potential adverse effects of the plan of care.
- Engages consumer alliance and advocacy groups in health teaching and health promotion activities for health care consumers.
- Provides anticipatory guidance to health care consumers to promote health and prevent or reduce risk

Pharmacological, Biological, and Integrative Therapies

Biological therapies are "any form of treatment for mental disorders that attempts to alter physiological functioning, including drug therapies, electroconvulsive therapy, and psychosurgery."[5] **Integrative therapies** are defined by the American Psychiatric Association (APA) as "psychotherapy that selects theoretical models or techniques from various therapeutic schools to suit the client's particular problems."[6] **Psychotherapy interventions** include "all generally accepted and evidence-based methods of brief or long-term therapy, including individual therapy, group therapy, marital or couple therapy, and family therapy. These interventions use a range of therapy models, including, but not limited to, psychodynamic, cognitive, behavioral, and supportive interpersonal therapies to promote insight, produce behavioral change, maintain function, and promote recovery."[7] Review the competencies for this Standard of Care in the following box.

5 American Psychological Association. (n.d.). *APA Dictionary of Psychology.* https://dictionary.apa.org/

6 American Psychological Association. (n.d.). *APA Dictionary of Psychology.* https://dictionary.apa.org/

7 American Nurses Association, American Psychiatric Nurses Association, and International Society of Psychiatric-Mental Health Nurses. (2014). *Psychiatric-Mental Health Nursing: Scope and Standards of Practice* (2nd ed.). Nursebooks.org

My Notes

APNA's Pharmacological, Biological, and Integrative Therapies Competencies[8]

"The psychiatric-mental health registered nurse (PMH-RN) incorporates knowledge of pharmacological, biological, and complementary interventions with applied clinical skills to restore the health care consumer's health and prevent future disability."[9]

The PMH-RN:

- Applies current research findings to guide nursing actions related to pharmacology, other biological therapies, and integrative therapies.
- Assesses the health care consumer's response to biological interventions based on current knowledge of pharmacological agent's intended actions, interactive effects, potential untoward effects, and therapeutic doses.
- Includes health teaching for medication management to support health care consumers in managing their own medications and adhering to a prescribed regimen.
- Provides health teaching about mechanism of action, intended effects, potential adverse effects of the proposed prescription, ways to cope with transitional side effects, and other treatment options, including the selection of a no-treatment option.
- Directs interventions toward alleviating untoward effects of biological interventions.
- Communicates observations about the health care consumer's response to biological interventions to other health clinicians.

Milieu Therapy

A **therapeutic milieu** is defined by the American Psychiatric Nursing Association as, "A safe, welcoming, supportive, and functional physical treatment environment." **Milieu therapy** includes nursing interventions used to assist health care consumers to make positive change and promote recovery in a therapeutic milieu. Nursing interventions include providing empathy, assisting in problem-solving, acting as a role model, demonstrating leadership, confronting discrepancies, encouraging self-efficacy, decreasing stimuli when necessary, and manipulating the environment so that the above interventions can be effective."[10] Review the APNA competencies for this Standard of Care in the following box.

8 American Nurses Association, American Psychiatric Nurses Association, and International Society of Psychiatric-Mental Health Nurses. (2014). *Psychiatric-Mental Health Nursing: Scope and Standards of Practice* (2nd ed.). Nursebooks.org

9 American Nurses Association, American Psychiatric Nurses Association, and International Society of Psychiatric-Mental Health Nurses. (2014). *Psychiatric-Mental Health Nursing: Scope and Standards of Practice* (2nd ed.). Nursebooks.org

10 American Nurses Association, American Psychiatric Nurses Association, and International Society of Psychiatric-Mental Health Nurses. (2014). *Psychiatric-Mental Health Nursing: Scope and Standards of Practice* (2nd ed.). Nursebooks.org

My Notes

APNA's Milieu Therapy Competencies[11]

"The psychiatric-mental health registered nurse (PMH-RN) provides, structures, and maintains a safe, therapeutic, recovery-oriented environment in collaboration with health care consumers, families, and other health care clinicians."[12]

The PMH-RN:

- Orients the health care consumer and family to the care environment, including the physical environment, the roles of the different health care providers, self-involvement in the treatment and care delivery processes, schedules of events pertinent to their care and treatment, and expectations regarding safe and therapeutic behaviors.
- Orients health care consumers to their rights and responsibilities particular to the treatment or care environment.
- Establishes a welcome, trauma-sensitive environment using therapeutic interventions, including, but not limited to, sensory or relaxation rooms.
- Conducts ongoing assessments of the health care consumer in relation to the environment to guide nursing interventions in maintaining a safe environment.
- Selects specific activities (both individual and group) that meet the health care consumer's physical and mental health needs for meaningful participation in the milieu and promotion of personal growth.
- Advocates that the health care consumer is treated in the least restrictive environment necessary to maintain the safety of the individual and others.
- Informs the health care consumer in a culturally sensitive manner about the need for limits related to safety and the conditions necessary to remove the restrictions.
- Provides support and validation to health care consumers when discussing their illness experience and seeks to prevent complications of illness.

Therapeutic Relationship and Counseling

The American Nurses Association states, "Nursing integrates the art and science of caring . . . It facilitates healing and alleviates suffering through compassionate presence . . . The act of caring is the first step in the power to heal."[13] Jean Watson's Human Caring Science Theory emphasizes the therapeutic relationship between the patient and nurse and highlights the role of the nurse in defining the patient as a unique human being to be

11 American Nurses Association, American Psychiatric Nurses Association, and International Society of Psychiatric-Mental Health Nurses. (2014). *Psychiatric-Mental Health Nursing: Scope and Standards of Practice* (2nd ed.). Nursebooks.org

12 American Nurses Association, American Psychiatric Nurses Association, and International Society of Psychiatric-Mental Health Nurses. (2014). *Psychiatric-Mental Health Nursing: Scope and Standards of Practice* (2nd ed.). Nursebooks.org

13 American Nurses Association. (2021). *Nursing: Scope and standards of practice* (4th ed.). American Nurses Association.

valued, respected, nurtured, understood, and assisted.[14] In a caring, therapeutic relationship, the nurse implements interventions to promote interpersonal connection, such as listening attentively, making eye contact, using verbal reassurances, and using professional touch with permission.[15] Nurses use several therapeutic techniques during a nurse-client relationship. Read more information in the "Therapeutic Communication and the Nurse-Client Relationship" chapter.

Read the APNA competencies regarding therapeutic relationship and counseling in the following box.

APNA's Therapeutic Relationship and Counseling Competencies[16]

"The psychiatric-mental health registered nurse (PMH-RN) uses the therapeutic relationship and counseling interventions to assist health care consumers in their individual recovery journeys by improving and regaining their previous coping abilities, fostering mental health, and preventing mental disorder and disability."[17]

The PMH-RN:

- Uses therapeutic relationship and counseling techniques to promote the health care consumer's stabilization of symptoms and personal recovery goals.
- Uses the therapeutic relationship and counseling techniques, both in the individual and group setting, to reinforce healthy behaviors and interaction patterns and helps the health care consumer discover individualized health care behaviors to replace unhealthy ones.
- Documents counseling interventions, including, but not limited to, communication and interviewing techniques, problem-solving activities, crisis intervention, stress management, supportive skill building and educational groups, relaxation techniques, assertiveness training, and conflict resolution.

Read more information about stress management, relaxation techniques, and crisis intervention in the "Stress, Coping, and Crisis Management" chapter.

Categories of Interventions

Nurses implement several interventions related to each subcategory of the *Implementation* Standard of Care for clients in mental health settings. See Table 4.7 for common nursing interventions in mental health settings for each subcategory.

---

14 American Nurses Association. (2021). *Nursing: Scope and standards of practice* (4th ed.). American Nurses Association.

15 American Nurses Association. (2021). *Nursing: Scope and standards of practice* (4th ed.). American Nurses Association.

16 American Nurses Association, American Psychiatric Nurses Association, and International Society of Psychiatric-Mental Health Nurses. (2014). *Psychiatric-Mental Health Nursing: Scope and Standards of Practice* (2nd ed.). Nursebooks.org

17 American Nurses Association, American Psychiatric Nurses Association, and International Society of Psychiatric-Mental Health Nurses. (2014). *Psychiatric-Mental Health Nursing: Scope and Standards of Practice* (2nd ed.). Nursebooks.org

My Notes

Table 4.7 Categories of Nursing Mental Health Interventions	
Subcategories: Implementation Standard of Care	**Sample Nursing Interventions**
Coordination of Care	■ Refer to community support groups for optimal recovery. ■ Advocate for dignified care with the interprofessional team. ■ Communicate client trends with interprofessional team members such as cheeking (i.e., not swallowing medications), increased agitation, or propensity toward violence.
Health Teaching and Health Promotion	■ Deliver health teaching to clients about self-care and stress management techniques. ■ Promote health by teaching about adaptive coping strategies such as journaling and daily exercise.
Pharmacological, Biological, and Integrative Therapies	■ Provide health teaching about medications' mechanisms of action, intended effects, potential adverse effects, and ways to cope with transitional side effects.
Milieu Therapy	■ Encourage client participation within the therapeutic milieu by attending support groups and exercise groups. ■ Perform intentional rounding at varying times between every 15-60 minutes and document. Varying rounding times helps prevent suicide attempts. ■ Advocate for the least restrictive environment necessary to maintain the safety of the individual and others. ■ Perform environmental safety scans and eliminate any devices or objects that can cause injury. Remove strings, cords, and drawstrings.
Therapeutic Relationship and Counseling	■ Observe for, document, and communicate changes in behavior. ■ Demonstrate caring behaviors. ■ Utilize therapeutic communication techniques.

Implementing Interventions

Implementation of interventions requires the RN to use critical thinking and clinical judgment. After the initial plan of care is developed, continual reassessment of the patient is necessary to detect any changes in the patient's condition requiring modification of the plan. The need for continual patient reassessment underscores the dynamic nature of the nursing process and is crucial to providing safe care.

During the *Implementation* phase of the nursing process, the nurse prioritizes planned interventions, assesses patient safety while implementing interventions, delegates interventions as appropriate, and documents interventions performed.

Prioritizing implementation of interventions follows a similar method as to prioritizing nursing diagnoses. Maslow's Hierarchy of Needs and the ABCs of airway, breathing, and circulation are used to establish top priority interventions. When possible, least restrictive interventions are preferred.

My Notes

Read more about methods for prioritization under the "Diagnosis" section of this chapter.

It is essential to consider patient safety when implementing interventions. At times, patients may experience a change in condition that makes a planned nursing intervention or provider prescription no longer safe to implement. For example, an established nursing care plan for a patient states, "The nurse will ambulate the patient 100 feet three times daily." However, during assessment this morning, the patient reports feeling dizzy today, and their blood pressure is 90/60. Using critical thinking and clinical judgment, the nurse decides to not implement the planned intervention of ambulating the patient and notifies the provider of suspected side effects of the client's antidepressant medication. This decision, supporting assessment findings, and notification of the provider should be documented in the patient's chart and also communicated during the shift handoff report.

Read more about delegating interventions in the "Delegation and Supervision" chapter of Open RN *Nursing Management and Professional Concepts.*

My Notes

4.8 EVALUATION

The *Evaluation* Standard of Practice by the American Nurses Association states, "The registered nurse evaluates progress toward attainment of goals and outcomes."[1] Review the competencies for the *Evaluation* Standard of Practice for registered nurses in the following box.

ANA's Evaluation Competencies[2]

The registered nurse:

- Uses applicable standards and defined criteria (e.g., Quality and Safety Education for Nurses [QSEN], Quadruple Aim, Institute for Healthcare Improvement [IHI]).
- Conducts a systematic, ongoing, and criterion-based evaluation of the goals and outcomes in relation to the structure, processes, and timelines prescribed in the plan.
- Collaborates with the health care consumer, stakeholders, interprofessional team, and others involved in the care or situation in the evaluation process.
- Determines, in partnership with the health care consumer and other stakeholders, the person-centeredness, effectiveness, efficiency, safety, timeliness, and equitability of the strategies in relation to the responses to the plan and attainment of outcomes.
- Uses ongoing assessment data, other data and information resources and benchmarks, research, and meta-analyses for the analytic activities to revise the diagnoses, outcomes, plan, implementation, and evaluation strategies as needed.
- Documents the results of the evaluation.
- Reports evaluation data in a timely fashion.
- Shares evaluation data and conclusions with the health care consumer and other stakeholders to promote clarity and transparency in accordance with state, federal, organizational, and professional requirements.

Evaluation focuses on the effectiveness of the nursing interventions by reviewing the expected outcomes to determine if they were met by the time frames indicated. Evaluation includes analysis of data from assessments, screening tools, laboratory results, and pharmacologic interventions, as well as the effectiveness of nursing interventions related to thought process and content. During the *Evaluation* phase, nurses use critical thinking to analyze reassessment data and determine if a patient's expected outcomes have been met, partially met, or not met by the time frames established. If outcomes are not met or only partially met by the time frame indicated, the care plan should be revised. If revision is necessary, the nurse should consider which step of the nursing process requires modification. Have additional assessment data been obtained, or have assessment data changed? Has a

1 American Nurses Association. (2021). *Nursing: Scope and standards of practice* (4th ed.). American Nurses Association.

2 American Nurses Association. (2021). *Nursing: Scope and standards of practice* (4th ed.). American Nurses Association.

My Notes

different nursing diagnosis become a priority? Were the identified goals or expected outcomes unrealistic? Were any interventions not effective?

Reassessment should occur every time the nurse interacts with a patient, discusses the care plan with others on the interprofessional team, or reviews updated laboratory or diagnostic test results. Nursing care plans should be updated as higher priority goals emerge. The results of the evaluation must be documented in the patient's medical record.

Ideally, when the planned interventions are implemented, the patient will respond positively, and the expected outcomes are achieved. However, when interventions do not assist in progressing the patient toward the expected outcomes, the nursing care plan must be revised to more effectively address the needs of the patient. These questions can be used as a guide when revising the nursing care plan:

- Did anything unanticipated occur?
- Has the patient's condition changed?
- Have the patient's goals and priorities shifted?
- Were the expected outcomes and their time frames realistic?
- Are the nursing diagnoses accurate for this patient at this time?
- Are the planned interventions appropriately focused on supporting outcome attainment?
- What barriers were experienced as interventions were implemented?
- Do ongoing assessment data indicate the need to revise diagnoses, outcome criteria, planned interventions, or implementation strategies?
- Are different interventions required?

My Notes

4.9 NCLEX NEXT GENERATION TERMINOLOGY

The National Council Licensure Examination for Registered Nurses (NCLEX- RN) is the exam that all nursing graduates must successfully pass to obtain their nursing license and become a registered nurse. The purpose of the NCLEX is to evaluate if a nursing graduate (i.e., candidate) is competent to provide safe, competent, entry-level nursing care. The NCLEX-RN is developed by the National Council of State Board of Nursing (NCSBN), an independent, nonprofit organization composed of the 50 state boards of nursing and other regulatory agencies.[1]

A new edition of NCLEX will be released in 2023 that includes "Next Generation" questions. (If you take the NCLEX before the new edition is released, you may be asked to voluntarily participate in a special research section that tests the accuracy of these new types of questions without your performance counting toward your final score.) The Next Generation NCLEX (Next Gen) uses evolving case studies and other types of test questions based on the new NCSBN Clinical Judgment Measurement Model (NCJMM). The NCJMM assesses how well the candidate can think critically and use clinical judgment when providing safe nursing care.[2]

Five new Next Generation test item types are called extended multiple response, extended drag and drop, cloze (drop-down), extended hot spot (highlighting), and matrix-grid[3]:

- **Extended Multiple Response:** Extended Multiple Response items allow candidates to select one or more answer options at a time. This item type is similar to the current NCLEX multiple response item but has more options and uses partial credit scoring.
- **Extended Drag and Drop:** Extended Drag and Drop items allow candidates to move or place response options into answer spaces. This item type is like the current NCLEX ordered response items but not all of the response options may be required to answer the item. In some items, there may be more response options than answer spaces.
- **Cloze (Drop – Down):** Cloze (Drop – Down) items allow candidates to select one option from a drop-down list. There can be more than one drop-down list in a cloze item. These drop-down lists can be used as words or phrases within a sentence or within tables and charts.
- **Enhanced Hot Spot (Highlighting):** Enhanced Hot Spot items allow candidates to select their answer by highlighting predefined words or phrases. Candidates can select and deselect the highlighted parts by clicking on the words or phrases. These types of items allow an individual to read a portion of a client medical record (e.g., a nursing note, medical history, lab values, medication record, etc.), and then select the words or phrases that answer the item.
- **Matrix/Grid:** Matrix/Grid items allow the candidate to select one or more answer options for each row and/or column. This item type can be useful in measuring multiple aspects of the clinical scenario with a single item.

1 NCSBN. https://www.ncsbn.org/nclex.htm

2 NCSBN. https://www.ncsbn.org/nclex.htm

3 NCSBN. https://www.ncsbn.org/nclex.htm

My Notes

View the following YouTube video[4] from NCSBN on Next Generation test items: The Right Decisions Come from the Right Questions.

The NCJMM complements the nursing process but uses different terminology in exam questions while assessing the candidate's clinical judgment. This terminology includes recognize cues, analyze cues, prioritize hypotheses, generate solutions, take actions, and evaluate outcomes. See Table 4.9 for a comparison of these terms and actions to the nursing process.[5,6,7]

Table 4.9 Comparison of the NCSBN Clinical Judgment Measurement Model to the Nursing Process

NCSBN Clinical Judgment Skill	Description	Corresponding Step of the Nursing Process
Recognize Cues	*What data is clinically significant?* Determining what client findings are significant, most important, and of immediate concern to the nurse (i.e., identifying "relevant cues").	Assessment
Analyze Cues	*What does the data mean?* Analyzing data to determine if it is "expected" or "unexpected" or "normal" or "abnormal" for this client at this time according to their age, development, and clinical status. Making a clinical judgment concerning the client's "human response to health conditions/life processes, or a vulnerability for that response," also referred to as "forming a hypothesis."	Diagnosis (Analysis of Data)
Prioritize Hypotheses	*What hypotheses should receive priority attention?* Ranking client conditions and problems according to urgency, complexity, and time.	Planning
Generate Solutions	*What should be done?* Planning individualized interventions that meet the desired outcomes for the client; may include gathering additional assessment data.	Planning

4 NCSBN. (2019, December 17). *The right decisions come from the right questions* [Video]. YouTube. All rights reserved. https://youtu.be/ZBXfkINlRF0

5 NCSBN. (n.d.). *NCSBN Clinical Judgment Measurement Model.* https://www.ncsbn.org/14798.htm

6 Ignatavicius, V., & Silvestri, L. (2022). *Preparing for the Next-Generation NCLEX (NGN): A "how-to" step-by-step faculty resource manual.* Elsevier. https://evolve.elsevier.com/education/wp-content/uploads/sites/2/NGN_FacultyGuide_Final.pdf

7 American Nurses Association. (2021). *Nursing: Scope and standards of practice* (4th ed.). American Nurses Association.

My Notes

NCSBN Clinical Judgment Skill	Description	Corresponding Step of the Nursing Process
Take Action	*What will I do now?* Implementing interventions that are safe and most appropriate for the client's current priority conditions and problems.	Implementation
Evaluate Outcomes	*Did the interventions work?* Comparing actual client outcomes with desired client outcomes to determine effectiveness of care and making appropriate revisions to the nursing care plan.	Evaluation

It is important to note that NANDA Nursing Diagnoses are not specifically assessed on the NCLEX. However, the ability of a candidate to cluster client data, make hypotheses, prioritize hypotheses, and plan nursing interventions is based on a nursing knowledge base of potential human responses to health problems and life processes (otherwise known as nursing diagnoses).

Learning activities are incorporated throughout the chapters of this book to assist students in learning how to respond to NCLEX Next Generation-style test questions.

4.10 SPOTLIGHT APPLICATION

My Notes

Let's review how the nursing process can be applied to Sample Case A introduced in the "Diagnosis" section of this chapter regarding caring for a suicidal client.

Assessment

During an interview with a 32-year-old male client diagnosed with Major Depressive Disorder, the client exhibited signs of a sad affect and hopelessness. He expressed desire to die and reported difficulty sleeping and a lack of appetite. He reports he has not showered in over a week, and his clothes have a strong body odor.

Diagnosis

The nurse analyzed this data and created four nursing diagnoses:

- *Hopelessness* related to social isolation
- *Risk for Suicide* as manifested by the reported desire to die
- *Imbalanced Nutrition: Less than Body Requirements* related to insufficient dietary intake
- *Self-Neglect* related to insufficient personal hygiene

The nurse established the top priority nursing diagnosis of *Risk for Suicide* and immediately screened for suicidal ideation and a plan using the Columbia Suicide Severity Rating Scale (C-SSRS).

Outcomes Identification

The nurse identified the following SMART expected outcomes:

- The client will verbalize feelings by the end of the shift.
- The client will remain free from injury during the hospitalization stay.
- The client will progressively gain at least one pound per week toward his ideal body weight (180 pounds).
- The client will participate in daily bathing.

Planning and Implementation

The nurse implemented planned nursing interventions for *Risk for Suicide* as previously discussed in Table 4.6.

Evaluation

Day 1: Outcomes partially met. By the end of the shift, the client verbalized feelings related to hopelessness and did not harm himself. He did not agree to participate in taking a bath and only ate 25% of his meal tray. Interventions will be re-attempted on Day 2 and reassessed for effectiveness.

Sample Documentation

0900: 32-year-old male client diagnosed with Major Depressive Disorder admitted for active suicidal ideation with a plan to do so with a gun. He has the means to accomplish this plan at home. He has expressed the desire

My Notes

to die and reports difficulty sleeping and a lack of appetite for the past two weeks. He reports he has not showered in over a week, and his clothes have a strong body odor. Client was placed in a room near the nursing station and assigned a 1:1 sitter. His personal belongings were removed and placed in a secure area. An environmental scan was completed, and all hazards were removed from the room. He agreed to complete a no-harm contract. Dr. Delgado was notified at 0930. She assessed the client at 0945, and new orders for medications were received and administered.— Zerimiah Alimi, Nursing Student

4.11 LEARNING ACTIVITIES

My Notes

Interactive Activities

An interactive H5P element has been excluded from this version of the text. You can view it online here: https://wtcs.pressbooks.pub/nursingmhcc/?p=296#h5p-16

An interactive H5P element has been excluded from this version of the text. You can view it online here: https://wtcs.pressbooks.pub/nursingmhcc/?p=296#h5p-61

My Notes

IV GLOSSARY

ADOPIE: A mnemonic for the components of the nursing process: Assessment, Diagnosis, Outcomes Identification, Planning, Implementation, and Evaluation.

Affect: A client's expression of emotion.

Akathisia: Motor restlessness.

Alexithymia: The inability to describe emotions with how one is feeling.

Anhedonia: The lack of experiencing pleasure in activities normally found enjoyable.

Apathy: A lack of feelings, emotions, interests, or concerns.

Biological therapies: Any form of treatment for mental health disorders that attempts to alter physiological functioning, including drug therapies, electroconvulsive therapy, and psychosurgery."[1]

Blunted: A diminished range and intensity of affect or mood.

Chief complaint: The patient's primary reasons for seeking care.

Circumstantial: Speaking with many unnecessary or tedious details without getting to the point of the conversation.

Clang associations: Stringing words together that rhyme without logical association and do not convey rational meaning. For example, a client exhibiting clang associations may state, "Here she comes with a cat catch a rat match."

Clouded consciousness: A state of reduced awareness to stimuli.

Cognition: The mental action or process of acquiring knowledge and understanding through thought, experience, and the senses. It includes thinking, knowing, remembering, judging, and problem-solving.

Cognitive impairment: Impaired mental processes that drive how an individual understands and acts in the world, affecting the acquisition of information and knowledge. Components of cognitive functioning include attention, decision-making, general knowledge, judgment, language, memory, perception, planning, and reasoning.[2]

Coma: A state of unarousable unresponsiveness, where vigorous noxious stimuli may not elicit reflex motor responses.

Congruence: Consistency of verbal and nonverbal communication.

Countertransference: A tendency for the examiner to displace (transfer) their own feelings onto the client, and these feelings may influence the client.

Cultural humility: A humble and respectful attitude toward individuals of other cultures that pushes one to challenge their own cultural biases, realize they cannot know everything about other cultures, and approach learning about other cultures as a life-long goal and process.[3]

Delirium: An onset of an abnormal mental state, often with fluctuating levels of consciousness, disorientation, irritability, and hallucinations. Delirium is often associated with infection, metabolic disorders, or toxins in the central nervous system.

Delusions: A fixed, false belief not held by cultural peers and persisting in the face of objective contradictory evidence. For example, a client may have the delusion that the CIA is listening to their conversations via satellites.

---

1 American Psychological Association. (n.d.). *APA Dictionary of Psychology.* https://dictionary.apa.org/

2 Schofield, D. W. (2018, December 26). *Cognitive deficits.* Medscape. https://emedicine.medscape.com/article/917629-overview

3 American Nurses Association. (2021). *Nursing: Scope and standards of practice* (4th ed.). American Nurses Association.

My Notes

Development: Physical, social, and cognitive changes that occur continuously throughout one's life.

Diagnostic and Statistical Manual of Mental Disorders (DSM-5): The manual used to make mental health diagnoses established by mental health experts.

Disheveled: A client's hair, clothes, or hygiene appears untidy, disordered, unkempt, or messy.

Distractibility: A state when the client's attention is easily drawn to unimportant or irrelevant external stimuli.

Dyskinesia: Uncontrolled, involuntary movements.

Dysphoric: A client's mood or affect exhibiting persistent sadness or depression.

Euphoric: A pathologically elevated sense of well-being.

Euthymic: Normal affect and mood with a wide range of emotion appropriate for the situation.

Family dynamics: Patterns of interactions among relatives, their roles and relationships, and the various factors that shape their interactions. Because family members rely on each other for emotional, physical, and economic support, they are primary sources of relationship security or stress. Family dynamics and the quality of family relationships can have either a positive or negative impact on an individual's health.

Flat: No emotional expression.

Flight of ideas: A state where the client frequently shifts from one topic to another with rapid speech, making it seem fragmented. The examiner may feel the client is rambling and changing topics faster than they can keep track, and they probably can't get a word in edgewise.[4] An example of client exhibiting a flight of ideas is, "My father sent me here. He drove me in a car. The car is yellow in color. Yellow color looks good on me."[5]

Grandiose delusions: A state of false attribution to the self of great ability, knowledge, importance or worth, identity, prestige, power, accomplishment.[6] Clients may withdraw into an inner fantasy world that's not equivalent to reality, where they have inflated importance, powers, or a specialness that is opposite of what their actual life is like.

Hallucinations: False sensory perceptions not associated with real external stimuli that can include any of the five senses (auditory, visual, gustatory, olfactory and tactile). For example, a client may see spiders climbing on the wall or hear voices telling them to do things. These are referred to as "visual hallucinations" or "auditory hallucinations."

Homicidal ideation: Threats or acts of life-threatening harm towards another person.

Illusions: Misperceptions of real stimuli. For example, a client may misperceive tree branches blowing in the wind at night to be the arms of monsters trying to grab them.

Inclusiveness: The practice of providing equal access to opportunities and resources for people who might otherwise be excluded or marginalized, such as those having physical or mental disabilities or belonging to other minority groups.[7]

---

4 Martin, D. C. (1990). The mental status examination. In Walker, H. K., Hall, W. D., Hurst, J. W., (Eds.), *Clinical methods: The history, physical, and laboratory examinations.* (3rd ed.). Butterworths. https://www.ncbi.nlm.nih.gov/books/NBK320/

5 PsychologGenie. (n.d.). *The true meaning of flight of ideas explained with examples.* https://psychologenie.com/flight-of-ideas-meaning-examples

6 American Psychological Association. (n.d.). *APA Dictionary of Psychology.* https://dictionary.apa.org/

7 Oxford Learner's Dictionaries. (n.d.). *Inclusion.* Oxford University Press. https://www.oxfordlearnersdictionaries.com/us/definition/english/inclusion

My Notes

Insight: The client demonstrates awareness of their situation.

Integrative therapies: Psychotherapy that selects theoretical models or techniques from various therapeutic schools to suit the client's particular problems.[8]

Intellectual disability: A diagnostic term that describes intellectual and adaptive functioning deficits identified during the developmental period prior to the age 18.

Labile: Rapid changes in emotional responses, mood, or affect that are inappropriate for the moment or the situation.

Loose associations: Jumping from one idea to an unrelated idea in the same sentence. For example, the client might state, "I like to dance; my feet are wet."[9] The term "word salad" refers to severely disorganized and virtually incomprehensible speech or writing, marked by severe loosening of associations.[10]

Maslow's Hierarchy of Needs: A theory commonly used to prioritize the most urgent patient needs.

Mental status examination: An assessment of a client's level of consciousness and orientation, appearance and general behavior, speech, motor activity, affect and mood, thought and perception, attitude and insight, and cognitive abilities.

Milieu therapy: Nursing interventions used to assist health care consumers to make positive change and promote recovery by creating a therapeutic milieu. Milieu therapy includes interventions such as providing empathy, assisting in problem-solving, acting as a role model, demonstrating leadership, confronting discrepancies, encouraging self-efficacy, decreasing stimuli when necessary, and manipulating the environment so that the above interventions can be effective.[11]

Mood: The predominant emotion expressed by an individual.[12]

Non-suicidal self-injury (NSSI): Intentional self-inflicted destruction of body tissue without suicidal intention and for purposes not socially sanctioned. Common forms of NSSI include behaviors such as cutting, burning, scratching, and self-hitting.

Nursing diagnosis: A clinical judgment concerning a human response to health conditions/life processes or a vulnerability for that response, by an individual, family, group, or community.

Nursing process: A critical thinking model based on a systematic approach to patient-centered care. Nurses use the nursing process to perform clinical reasoning and make clinical judgments when providing patient care.

8 American Psychological Association. (n.d.). *APA Dictionary of Psychology.* https://dictionary.apa.org/

9 American Psychological Association. (n.d.). *APA Dictionary of Psychology.* https://dictionary.apa.org/

10 American Psychological Association. (n.d.). *APA Dictionary of Psychology.* https://dictionary.apa.org/

11 American Nurses Association, American Psychiatric Nurses Association, and International Society of Psychiatric-Mental Health Nurses. (2014). *Psychiatric-Mental Health Nursing: Scope and Standards of Practice* (2nd ed.) Nursebooks.org.

12 Martin, D. C. (1990). The mental status examination. In Walker, H. K., Hall, W. D., Hurst, J. W., (Eds.), C*linical methods: The history, physical, and laboratory examinations.* (3rd ed.). Butterworths. https://www.ncbi.nlm.nih.gov/books/NBK320/

My Notes

Obsessions: Persistent thoughts, ideas, images, or impulses that are experienced as intrusive or inappropriate and result in anxiety, distress, or discomfort. Common obsessions include repeated thoughts about contamination, a need to have things in a particular order or sequence, repeated doubts, aggressive impulses, and sexual imagery. Obsessions are distinguished from excessive worries about everyday occurrences because they are not concerned with real-life problems.[13]

Obtundation: A moderate reduction in the client's level of awareness so that mild to moderate stimuli do not awaken the client. When arousal does occur, the patient is slow to respond.

Outcome: A measurable behavior demonstrated by the patient who is responsive to nursing interventions.

Paranoia: A condition characterized by delusions of persecution.[14] Clients often experience extreme suspiciousness, mistrust, or expression of fear. For example, a resident of a long-term care facility may have delusions that the staff is trying to poison him.

Poverty of content: A conversation in which the client talks without stating anything related to the question, or their speech in general is vague and meaningless.

Prioritization: The process of identifying the most significant problems and the most important interventions to implement based on a client's current status.

Psychiatric-mental health nursing: The nursing practice specialty committed to promoting mental health through the assessment, diagnosis, and treatment of behavioral problems, mental disorders, and comorbid conditions across the life span. Psychiatric-mental health nursing intervention is an art and a science, employing a purposeful use of self and a wide range of nursing, psychosocial, and neurobiological evidence to produce effective outcomes.[15]

Psychomotor agitation: A condition of purposeless, non-goal-directed activity.

Psychomotor retardation: A condition of extremely slow physical movements, slumped posture, or slow speech patterns.

Psychosocial assessment: A component of the nursing assessment process that obtains additional subjective data to detect risks and identify treatment opportunities and resources.

Psychotherapy interventions: Generally accepted and evidence-based methods of brief or long-term therapy, including individual therapy, group therapy, marital or couple therapy, and family therapy. These interventions use a range of therapy models including, but not limited to, psychodynamic, cognitive, behavioral, and supportive interpersonal therapies to promote insight, produce behavioral change, maintain function, and promote recovery.[16]

Racing thoughts: Fast-moving and often repetitive thought patterns that can be overwhelming. They may focus on a single topic, or they may represent multiple different lines of thought. For example, a client may have racing thoughts about a financial issue or an embarrassing moment.

Resilience: The ability to overcome serious hardship or traumatic experiences.

---

13 American Psychological Association. (n.d.). *APA Dictionary of Psychology*. https://dictionary.apa.org/

14 American Psychological Association. (n.d.). *APA Dictionary of Psychology*. https://dictionary.apa.org/

15 American Nurses Association, American Psychiatric Nurses Association, and International Society of Psychiatric-Mental Health Nurses. (2014). *Psychiatric-Mental Health Nursing: Scope and Standards of Practice* (2nd ed.). Nursebooks.org

16 American Nurses Association, American Psychiatric Nurses Association, and International Society of Psychiatric-Mental Health Nurses. (2014). *Psychiatric-Mental Health Nursing: Scope and Standards of Practice* (2nd ed.). Nursebooks.org

My Notes

Rumination: Obsessional thinking involving excessive, repetitive thoughts that interfere with other forms of mental activity.[17]

Safety plan: A prioritized written list of coping strategies and sources of support that clients can use before or during a suicidal crisis. The plan should be brief, in the client's own words, and easy to read. After the plan is developed, the nurse should problem solve with the client to identify barriers or obstacles to using the plan. It should be discussed where the client will keep the safety plan and how it will be located during a crisis.

SMART outcomes: Outcome statements should contain five components easily remembered using the "SMART" mnemonic: Specific, Measurable, Attainable/Action-oriented, Relevant/Realistic, with a Time frame.

Spirituality: A sense of connection to something larger than oneself that typically involves a search for meaning and purpose in life.

Stupor: A state of unresponsiveness unless a vigorous stimulus is applied, such as a sternal rub. The client quickly drifts back into a deep sleep-like state on cessation of the stimulation.

Suicide attempt: An action in which there is intent to end one's life but the individual does not die as a result of their actions.

Suicidal ideation: When an individual has been thinking about suicide but does not necessarily have an intention to act on that idea.

Suicide plan: An individual who has a plan for suicide, has the means to injury oneself, and has the intent to die.

Therapeutic milieu: A safe, welcoming, supportive, and functional physical treatment environment.

Transference: When the client projects (i.e., transfers) their feelings to the nurse. For example, a client is feeling angry at a family member related to a previous disagreement and displaces the anger to the nurse during the interview.

17 American Psychological Association. (n.d.). *APA Dictionary of Psychology*. https://dictionary.apa.org/

Chapter 5

Legal and Ethical Considerations in Mental Health Care

5.1 INTRODUCTION

My Notes

Learning Objectives

- Explore the nurse's role and legal and ethical responsibilities when providing care to clients with mental health disorders
- Describe standards of care for nurses
- Discuss the elements of a malpractice lawsuit
- Explain patient rights based on the Patient Self-Determination Act

The *Code of Ethics for Nurses With Interpretive Statements* states, "The nurse promotes, advocates for, and protects the rights, health, and safety of the patient."[1] This chapter describes nurses' legal and ethical responsibilities while protecting the safety and rights of clients receiving mental health care.

1 American Nurses Association. (2015). *Code of ethics for nurses with interpretive statements.* American Nurses Association. https://www.nursingworld.org/practice-policy/nursing-excellence/ethics/code-of-ethics-for-nurses/coe-view-only/

My Notes

5.2 ETHICAL PRINCIPLES

The American Nurses Association (ANA) designates *Ethics* as the first Standard of Professional Performance in *Nursing: Scope and Standards of Practice*, stating, "The registered nurse integrates ethics in all aspects of practice."[1] See the following box for competencies associated with the ANA's *Ethics* Standard of Professional Performance.

ANA's Ethics Competencies[2]

The registered nurse:

- Uses the *Code of Ethics for Nurses With Interpretive Statements* as a moral foundation to guide nursing practice and decision-making.
- Demonstrates that every person is worthy of nursing care through the provision of respectful, person-centered, compassionate care, regardless of personal history or characteristics (Beneficence).
- Advocates for health care consumer perspectives, preferences, and rights to informed decision-making and self-determination (Respect for autonomy).
- Demonstrates a primary commitment to the recipients of nursing and health care services in all settings and situations (Fidelity).
- Maintains therapeutic relationships and professional boundaries.
- Safeguards sensitive information within ethical, legal, and regulatory parameters (Nonmaleficence).
- Identifies ethics resources within the practice setting to assist and collaborate in addressing ethical issues.
- Integrates principles of social justice in all aspects of nursing practice (Justice).
- Refines ethical competence through continued professional education and personal self-development activities.
- Depicts one's professional nursing identity through demonstrated values and ethics, knowledge, leadership, and professional comportment.
- Engages in self-care and self-reflection practices to support and preserve personal health, well-being, and integrity.
- Contributes to the establishment and maintenance of an ethical environment that is conducive to safe, quality health care.

---

1 American Nurses Association. (2021). *Nursing: Scope and standards of practice* (4th ed.). American Nurses Association.

2 American Nurses Association. (2015). *Code of ethics for nurses with interpretive statements.* American Nurses Association. https://www.nursingworld.org/practice-policy/nursing-excellence/ethics/code-of-ethics-for-nurses/coe-view-only/

My Notes

- Collaborates with other health professionals and the public to protect human rights, promote health diplomacy, enhance cultural sensitivity and congruence, and reduce health disparities.
- Represents the nursing perspective in clinic, institutional, community, or professional association ethics discussions.

American Nurses Association Code of Ethics

The American Nurses Association *Code of Ethics for Nurses With Interpretive Statements* is an ethical standard that guides nursing practice and ethical decision-making. It states, "Individuals who become nurses are expected to adhere to the ideals and moral norms of the profession and also to embrace them as a part of what it means to be a nurse. The ethical tradition of nursing is self-reflective, enduring, and distinctive. A code of ethics makes explicit the primary goals, values, and obligations of the profession."[3]

The *Code of Ethics for Nurses* contains nine provisions. Each provision contains several clarifying or "interpretive" statements. Read a summary of the nine provisions in the following box.

Nine Provisions of the ANA's Code of Ethics for Nurses[4]

Provision 1: The nurse practices with compassion and respect for the inherent dignity, worth, and unique attributes of every person.

Provision 2: The nurse's primary commitment is to the patient, whether an individual, family, group, community, or population.

Provision 3: The nurse promotes, advocates for, and protects the rights, health, and safety of the patient.

Provision 4: The nurse has authority, accountability, and responsibility for nursing practice; makes decisions; and takes action consistent with the obligation to promote health and to provide optimal care.

Provision 5: The nurse owes the same duties to self as to others, including the responsibility to promote health and safety, preserve wholeness of character and integrity, maintain competence, and continue personal and professional growth.

Provision 6: The nurse, through individual and collective effort, establishes, maintains, and improves the ethical environment of the work setting and conditions of employment that are conducive to safe, quality health care.

3 American Nurses Association. (2015). *Code of ethics for nurses with interpretive statements.* American Nurses Association. https://www.nursingworld.org/practice-policy/nursing-excellence/ethics/code-of-ethics-for-nurses/coe-view-only/

4 American Nurses Association. (2015). *Code of ethics for nurses with interpretive statements.* American Nurses Association. https://www.nursingworld.org/practice-policy/nursing-excellence/ethics/code-of-ethics-for-nurses/coe-view-only/

My Notes

Provision 7: The nurse, in all roles and settings, advances the profession through research and scholarly inquiry, professional standards development, and the generation of both nursing and health policy.

Provision 8: The nurse collaborates with other health professionals and the public to protect human rights, promote health diplomacy, and reduce health disparities.

Provision 9: The profession of nursing, collectively through its professional organizations, must articulate nursing values, maintain the integrity of the profession, and integrate principles of social justice into nursing and health policy.

Read the free, online, full version of the Code of Ethics for Nurses With Interpretive Statements.

Ethical Principles

Ethical principles are used to define right from wrong action. Although there are many ethical principles that guide nursing practice, foundational ethical principles include respect for autonomy (self-determination), beneficence (do good), nonmaleficence (do no harm), justice (fairness), fidelity (keep promises), and veracity (tell the truth).

Autonomy

The ethical principle of autonomy recognizes each individual's right to self-determination and decision-making based on their unique values, beliefs, and preferences. The American Nurses Association (ANA) defines **autonomy** as, "the capacity to determine one's own actions through independent choice, including demonstration of competence."[5] The nurse's primary ethical obligation is client autonomy.[6] Based on autonomy, clients have the right to refuse nursing care and medical treatment.

Beneficence

Beneficence is defined by the ANA as, "the bioethical principle of benefiting others by preventing harm, removing harmful conditions, or affirmatively acting to benefit another or others, often going beyond what is required by law."[7] When caring for clients with mental health disorders, nurses implement beneficence when advocating for evidence-based treatment for clients' mental health.

5 American Nurses Association. (2021). *Nursing: Scope and standards of practice* (4th ed.). American Nurses Association.

6 American Nurses Association. (2015). *Code of ethics for nurses with interpretive statements.* American Nurses Association. https://www.nursingworld.org/practice-policy/nursing-excellence/ethics/code-of-ethics-for-nurses/coe-view-only/

7 American Nurses Association. (2015). *Code of ethics for nurses with interpretive statements.* American Nurses Association. https://www.nursingworld.org/practice-policy/nursing-excellence/ethics/code-of-ethics-for-nurses/coe-view-only/

Nonmaleficence

My Notes

Nonmaleficence is defined by the ANA as, "the bioethical principle that specifies a duty to do no harm and balances avoidable harm with benefits of good achieved."[8] A classic example of doing no harm in nursing practice is reflected by nurses checking medication rights three times before administering medications. In this manner, medication errors can be avoided, and the duty to do no harm is met. An example of nurses implementing nonmaleficence in mental health care is ensuring that clients are not harmed by adverse effects of psychotropic medications (such as lithium toxicity or tardive dyskinesia).

Justice

Justice is defined by the ANA as, "a moral obligation to act on the basis of equality and equity and a standard linked to fairness for all in society."[9] The principle of justice requires health care to be provided in a fair and equitable way. Nurses provide quality care for all individuals with the same level of fairness despite their personalities or characteristics, such as financial status, cultural beliefs, religion, gender, or sexual orientation. Nurses have a social contract to "provide compassionate care that addresses the individual's needs for protection, advocacy, empowerment, optimization of health, prevention of illness and injury, alleviation of suffering, comfort, and well-being."[10] An example of a nurse using the principle of justice in mental health care settings is ensuring that quality care is provided to all clients, even those who do not have the cognitive ability to communicate their needs.

Fidelity

Role fidelity is defined as being responsible for providing competent nursing care. An example of role fidelity in nursing is remaining up-to-date with evidence-based practice and implementing effective mental health interventions.

Veracity

Veracity means telling the truth. An example of veracity in health care is informed consent. Nurses ensure that clients have a good understanding of the benefits and risks of a prescribed procedure or psychotropic medication.

Role of Caring

Nurses use a client-centered, care-based, ethical approach to nursing care that focuses on the specific circumstances of each situation. This approach aligns with the foundational nursing concepts of holism and caring in a nurse-client relationship rooted in dignity, respect, kindness, and compassion.[11]

---

8 American Nurses Association. (2015). *Code of ethics for nurses with interpretive statements.* American Nurses Association. https://www.nursingworld.org/practice-policy/nursing-excellence/ethics/code-of-ethics-for-nurses/coe-view-only/

9 American Nurses Association. (2015). *Code of ethics for nurses with interpretive statements.* American Nurses Association. https://www.nursingworld.org/practice-policy/nursing-excellence/ethics/code-of-ethics-for-nurses/coe-view-only/

10 American Nurses Association. (2021). *Nursing: Scope and standards of practice* (4th ed.). American Nurses Association.

11 Legal Information Institute. (n.d.). *Welcome to LII.* Cornell Law School. https://www.law.cornell.edu

My Notes

5.3 STANDARDS OF CARE

Standards of care in nursing are guidelines that provide a foundation as to how a nurse should act and what they should and should not do in their professional capacity. These guidelines establish a baseline of quality patient care and provide an objective standard of accountability within the profession. Standards of care are enforced by courts of law and state Boards of Nursing, who evaluate a nurse's practice against these standards. If a nurse's actions (or lack of actions) do not meet the accepted standard of care, their conduct may be found to be negligent.[1]

Standards for nursing care are set by several organizations, including the American Nurses Association (ANA), states' Nurse Practice Acts, agency policies and procedures, federal regulators, and professional nursing organizations.

American Nursing Association's Scope and Standards of Practice

In the United States, the American Nurses Association (ANA) publishes two resources that set standards and guide professional nursing practice: *Code of Ethics for Nurses* and *Nursing: Scope and Standards of Practice.* The *Code of Ethics for Nurses* establishes an ethical framework for nursing practice across all roles, levels, and settings.[2] It is discussed in greater detail in the "Ethical Principles" section of this chapter. *Nursing: Scope and Standards of Practice* describes a professional nurse's scope of practice and defines the who, what, where, when, why, and how of nursing. It also sets 18 standards of professional practice that all registered nurses are expected to perform competently.[3]

The ANA's **Standards of Professional Nursing Practice** are "authoritative statements of the actions and behaviors that all registered nurses, regardless of role, population, specialty, and setting, are expected to perform competently."[4] These standards define a competent level of nursing practice based on the critical thinking model known as the nursing process and include the components of assessment, diagnosis, outcomes identification, planning, implementation, and evaluation.[5] Each of these standards is further discussed in the "Application of the Nursing Process in Mental Health Care" chapter of this book.

The ANA's **Standards of Professional Performance** are 12 additional standards that describe a nurse's professional behavior, including activities related to ethics, advocacy, respectful and equitable practice, communication, collaboration, leadership, education, scholarly inquiry, quality of practice, professional practice evaluation, resource stewardship, and environmental health. All registered nurses are expected to engage in these professional role activities based on their level of education, position, and role. Registered nurses are accountable for their professional behaviors to themselves, health care consumers, peers, and ultimately to society.[6] The Standards of Professional Performance are as follows[7]:

---

1 Law Office of Nicole Irmer. (2019). *Nursing standards of care issues.* https://www.californialicensingdefense.com/practice-areas/professionals/nursing-license/standards-of-care-issues/#:~:text=Standards%20of%20care%20in%20nursing,that%20all%20nurses%20must%20follow.

2 American Nurses Association. (2015). *Code of ethics for nurses with interpretive statements.* American Nurses Association. https://www.nursingworld.org/practice-policy/nursing-excellence/ethics/code-of-ethics-for-nurses/coe-view-only/

3 American Nurses Association. (2021). *Nursing: Scope and standards of practice* (4th ed.). American Nurses Association.

4 American Nurses Association. (2015). *Code of ethics for nurses with interpretive statements.* American Nurses Association. https://www.nursingworld.org/practice-policy/nursing-excellence/ethics/code-of-ethics-for-nurses/coe-view-only/

5 American Nurses Association. (2021). *Nursing: Scope and standards of practice* (4th ed.). American Nurses Association.

6 American Nurses Association. (2021). *Nursing: Scope and standards of practice* (4th ed.). American Nurses Association.

7 American Nurses Association. (2021). *Nursing: Scope and standards of practice* (4th ed.). American Nurses Association.

My Notes

- **Ethics.** The registered nurse integrates ethics in all aspects of practice.
- **Advocacy.** The registered nurse demonstrates advocacy in all roles and settings.
- **Respectful and Equitable Practice.** The registered nurse practices with cultural humility and inclusiveness.
- **Communication.** The registered nurse communicates effectively in all areas of professional practice.
- **Collaboration.** The registered nurse collaborates with the health care consumer and other key stakeholders.
- **Leadership.** The registered nurse leads within the profession and practice setting.
- **Education.** The registered nurse seeks knowledge and competence that reflects current nursing practice and promotes futuristic thinking.
- **Scholarly Inquiry.** The registered nurse integrates scholarship, evidence, and research findings into practice.
- **Quality of Practice.** The registered nurse contributes to quality nursing practice.
- **Professional Practice Evaluation.** The registered nurse evaluates one's own and others' nursing practice.
- **Resource Stewardship.** The registered nurse utilizes appropriate resources to plan, provide, and sustain evidence-based nursing services that are safe, effective, financially responsible, and judiciously used.
- **Environmental Health.** The registered nurse practices in a manner that advances environmental safety and health.

American Psychiatric Nurses Association Standards of Practice

In addition to the ANA Standards of Professional Nursing Practice, the American Psychiatric Nurses Association establishes standards of practice for psychiatric-mental health nurse specialists in *Psychiatric-Mental Health Nursing: Scope and Standards of Practice.*[8] These standards are built on the ANA's Standards of Professional Nursing Practice, with additional activities included under the *Intervention* standard of care. These interventions are further discussed in the "Application of the Nursing Process in Mental Health Care" chapter.

Read more about the American Psychiatric Nurses Association.

Nurse Practice Act

In addition to the professional standards of practice, nurses must legally follow regulations set by the Nurse Practice Act and enforced by the Board of Nursing in the state where they are employed. The Board of Nursing is the state-specific licensing and regulatory body that sets standards for safe nursing care and issues nursing licenses to qualified candidates, based on the Nurse Practice Act enacted by that state's legislature. The Nurse Practice Act establishes regulations for nursing practice within that state and defines the scope of nursing practice. If nurses

8 American Nurses Association, American Psychiatric Nurses Association, and International Society of Psychiatric-Mental Health Nurses. (2014). *Psychiatric-Mental Health Nursing: Scope and Standards of Practice* (2nd ed.). Nursebooks.org

My Notes

do not follow the standards and scope of practice set forth by the Nurse Practice Act, they can have their nursing license revoked by the Board of Nursing.

Nursing students are legally accountable for the quality of care they provide to patients just as nurses are accountable. Students are expected to recognize the limits of their knowledge and experience and appropriately alert individuals in authority regarding situations that are beyond their competency. A violation of the standards of practice constitutes unprofessional conduct and can result in the Board of Nursing denying a license to a nursing graduate.

Employer Policies, Procedures, and Protocols

In addition to following professional nursing standards and the state Nurse Practice Act, nurses and nursing students must also practice according to agency policies, procedures, and protocols. For example, each agency has specific policies regarding the use of restraints. If a nurse did not follow this policy and a patient was injured or died, the nurse could be held liable in a court of law.

Agencies also have their own sets of procedures and protocols. For example, each agency has specific procedural steps for performing nursing skills, such as inserting urinary catheters. Agencies also have protocols that are precisely written plans for a regimen of therapy. For example, agencies typically have a hypoglycemia protocol that nurses automatically implement when a patient's blood sugar falls below a specific number and includes actions such as providing orange juice and rechecking the blood sugar. These agency-specific policies, procedures, and protocols supersede the information taught in nursing school, and nurses and nursing students can be held legally liable if they don't follow them. Therefore, it is vital for nurses and nursing students to review and follow current agency-specific procedures, policies, and protocols when providing patient care.

Federal Regulations

In addition to professional standards, state Nurse Practice Acts, and employer policies, procedures, and protocols, nursing practice is also influenced by federal regulations enacted by government agencies such as The Joint Commission and the Centers for Medicare and Medicaid.

The Joint Commission (TJC) is a national organization that accredits and certifies over 20,000 health care organizations in the United States. The mission of The Joint Commission is to continuously improve health care by setting standards for providing safe, high-quality health care. The Centers for Medicare & Medicaid Services (CMS) enforces quality standards in health care organizations that receive Medicare and Medicaid funding. Nurses must follow standards set by these agencies and implemented by their employers. For example, the expectation that a nurse checks medication rights three times before administering medication to a patient is based on a federal regulation.

The Joint Commission

Centers for Medicare & Medicaid Services website

5.4 LAWS, TORTS, MALPRACTICE, AND DISCIPLINARY ACTIONS

My Notes

In addition to following standards of care, nurses must also follow related federal and state laws. **Criminal law** is a system of laws that punishes individuals who commit crimes. Crimes are classified as felonies, misdemeanors, and infractions. Conviction for a crime requires evidence to show the defendant is guilty beyond a shadow of doubt. This means the prosecution must convince a jury there is no reasonable explanation other than guilty that can come from the evidence presented at trial. See Figure 5.1[1] for an illustration of a criminal case being tried in front of a jury. **Civil law** focuses on the rights, responsibilities, and legal relationships between private citizens, and involves compensation to the injured party. A person bringing the lawsuit is called the **plaintiff**, and the parties named in the lawsuit are called **defendants**.[2]

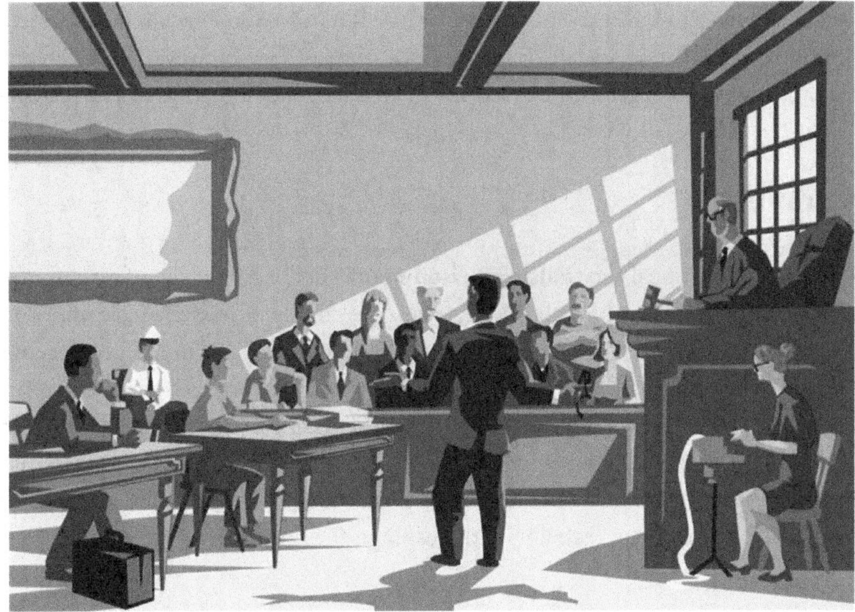

Figure 5.1 Criminal Trial by Jury

Civil law includes torts. A **tort** is an act of commission or omission that gives rise to injury or harm to another and amounts to a civil wrong for which courts impose liability. Tort law exists to compensate clients injured by negligent practice, provide corrective judgment, and deter negligence with consequences of action or inaction.[3]

Two categories of torts affecting nursing practice are intentional torts and unintentional torts. **Intentional torts** are wrongs that the defendant knew (or should have known) would be caused by their actions. Examples of intentional torts include assault, battery, false imprisonment, slander, libel, and breach of privacy or client confidentiality. **Unintentional torts** occur when the defendant's actions or inactions were unreasonably unsafe. Unintentional torts can result from acts of commission (i.e., doing something a reasonable nurse would not have

1 "Courtroom Trial with Judge, Jury - Vector Image" designed by WannaPik is licensed under CC0

2 Brous, E. (2019). The elements of a nursing malpractice case, part 1: Duty. *American Journal of Nursing, 119*(7), 64–67. https://doi.org/10.1097/01.NAJ.0000569476.17357.f5

3 Wis. JI—Civil 1005. (2016). https://wilawlibrary.gov/jury/civil/instruction.php?n=1005

My Notes

done) or omission (i.e., failing to do something a reasonable nurse would do). Examples of torts affecting nursing practice are discussed in further detail in the following subsections.[4]

Assault and Battery

Assault and battery are intentional torts. **Assault** is defined as intentionally putting another person in reasonable apprehension of an imminent harmful or offensive contact. **Battery** is defined as intentional causation of harmful or offensive contact with another person without that person's consent. Physical harm does not need to occur in order to be charged with assault or battery. Battery convictions are typically misdemeanors but can be felonies if serious bodily harm occurs.[5]

An example related to assault and battery in health care is the patient's right to refuse treatment. For example, a hospitalized patient can refuse to take prescribed medication. If a nurse forcibly administers medication without a patient's consent, it could be ruled assault or battery in a court of law. However, forcible administration of a medication based on a provider's order may be justified in an emergency situation to prevent imminent harm to oneself or others.[6]

False Imprisonment

False imprisonment is an intentional tort. **False imprisonment** is defined as an act of restraining another person and causing that person to be confined in a bounded area. An example of possible false imprisonment in health care is the use of restraints. See Figure 5.2[7] for an image of a simulated client in full physical medical restraints. Restraints can be physical, chemical, or verbal. Nurses must vigilantly follow agency policies related to the use of physical restraints and monitor clients who are restrained. Chemical restraints include administration of PRN medications such as benzodiazepines and require clear documentation supporting their use. Verbal threats to keep an individual in an inpatient environment can also qualify as false imprisonment and should be avoided. Additional information regarding the use of restraints is discussed in the "Patient Rights" section.

---

4 Brous, E. (2019). The elements of a nursing malpractice case, part 1: Duty. *American Journal of Nursing, 119*(7), 64–67. https://doi.org/10.1097/01.NAJ.0000569476.17357.f5

5 Brous, E. (2019). The elements of a nursing malpractice case, part 1: Duty. *American Journal of Nursing, 119*(7), 64–67. https://doi.org/10.1097/01.NAJ.0000569476.17357.f5

6 Fry, S. T. (1989). The role of caring in a theory of nursing ethics. *Hypatia, 4*(2), 87-103. https://doi.org/10.1111/j.1527-2001.1989.tb00575.x

7 "PinelRestaint.jpg" by James Heilman, MD is licensed under CC BY-SA 4.0

My Notes

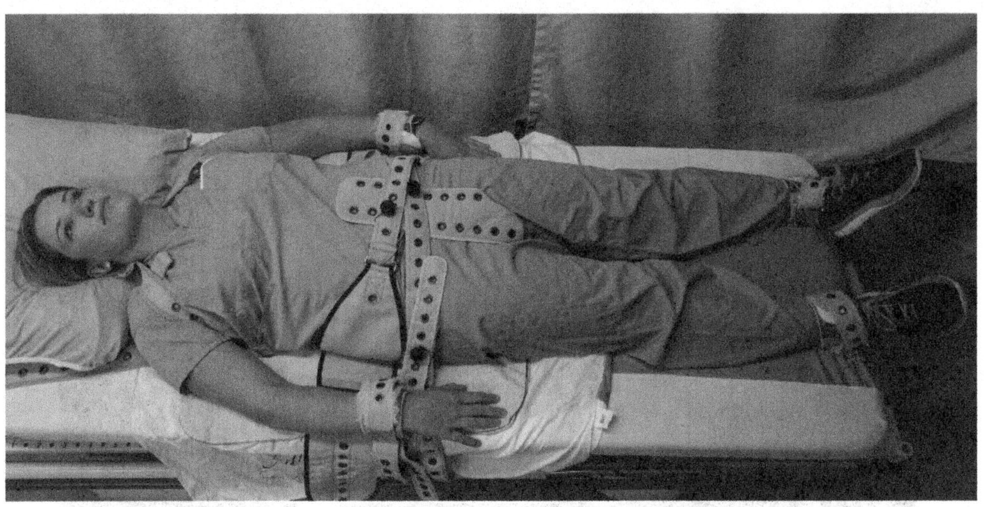

Figure 5.2 Full Physical Medical Restraints

Privacy and Confidentiality

Breaching privacy and confidentiality are intentional torts. **Confidentiality** is the right of an individual to have personal, identifiable medical information, referred to as protected health information, kept private. **Protected Health Information (PHI)** is defined as individually identifiable health information, including demographic data, that relates to the individual's past, present, or future physical or mental health or condition; the provision of health care to the individual; and the past, present, or future payment for the provision of health care to the individual.[8]

Confidentiality is a right protected by the **Health Insurance Portability and Accountability Act (HIPAA)**. HIPAA was enacted in 1996 and was prompted by the need to ensure privacy and protection of personal health records in an environment of electronic medical records and third-party insurance payers. There are two main sections of HIPAA law: the Privacy Rule and the Security Rule. The Privacy Rule addresses the use and disclosure of individuals' health information. The Security Rule sets national standards for protecting the confidentiality, integrity, and availability of electronically protected health information. HIPAA regulations extend beyond medical records and apply to client information shared with others. Therefore, all types of client information and data should be shared only with health care team members who are actively providing care to them. For example, when applying HIPAA to mental health inpatient settings, nurses may not answer in the affirmative if someone calls and asks if an individual has been admitted to the unit.[9] See Figure 5.3[10] for a depiction of confidentiality.

8 Wis. JI—Civil 1005. (2016). https://wilawlibrary.gov/jury/civil/instruction.php?n=1005

9 Wis. JI—Civil 1005. (2016). https://wilawlibrary.gov/jury/civil/instruction.php?n=1005

10 "Concept of Data Privacy And Policy Illustration" by Delesign Graphics at Iconscout is licensed under CC BY 4.0

My Notes

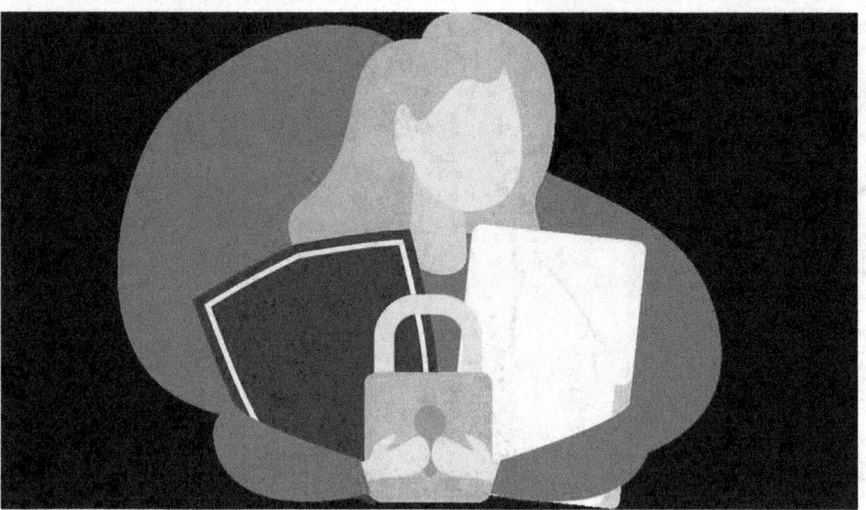

Figure 5.3 Confidentiality

There are specific circumstances in which HIPAA does not apply. For example, nurses have a duty to warn and protect, are mandated reporters of suspected abuse or neglect, and are required to share specific information reported by minors with authorities or their parents.

Duty to Warn and Protect

Most states have laws regarding the duty to protect third parties from potential life threats. Nurses and other mental health professionals have a duty to warn and protect third parties when they may be in danger from a patient. This duty falls outside of HIPAA regulations. This includes assessing and predicting the patient's threat of violence towards another person or groups of people and taking action to protect the identified victims.[11]

Mandatory Reporting of Suspected Abuse or Neglect

HIPAA does not apply to reporting the suspected neglect or abuse of children, adults at risk, or older adults. Many states require health professionals to report suspected neglect or abuse. State laws vary, but they generally include a definition of abuse, a list of people required to report abuse, and the government agency designated to receive and investigate the reports. Nurses and other health professionals are referred to as **mandated reporters** because they are required by state law to report suspected neglect or abuse of children, adults at risk, and the elderly. **Adults at risk** are adults who have a physical or mental condition that impairs their ability to care for their own needs.

For example, in Wisconsin, suspected neglect or abuse is reported to Child Protective Services (CPS), Adult Protective Services, or law enforcement. Nurses should be aware of the county or state agencies to whom they should report suspected abuse. See the following box for additional information.

---

11 Fry, S. T. (1989). The role of caring in a theory of nursing ethics. *Hypatia, 4*(2), 87-103. https://doi.org/10.1111/j.1527-2001.1989.tb00575.x

My Notes

Read additional information about signs of child and elder abuse in the "Trauma, Abuse, and Violence" chapter.

Read more about protective services in your state. For example, visit Wisconsin's Child Protective Services and Adult Protective Services.

Find resources in your area for reporting suspected child abuse at ChildHelp National Child Abuse Hotline or elder abuse at the National Adult Protective Services Association website.

Conditional Confidentiality for Minors

"Conditional confidentiality" applies to minors under the age of 18. State laws determine what information is considered confidential and what requires reporting to law enforcement or Child Protective Services, such as child abuse, gunshot or stabbing wounds, sexually transmitted infections, abortions, suicidal ideation, and homicidal ideation. Some state laws make it optional for clinicians to inform parents/guardians if their child is seeking services related to sexual health care, substance use, or mental health care. Nurses should be aware of the state laws affecting the confidentiality of child and adolescent care in the state in which they are practicing.[12]

View the Wisconsin Department of Health Services' Client Rights for Minors.

Slander and Libel

Slander and libel are intentional torts. **Defamation of character** occurs when an individual makes negative, malicious, and false remarks about another person to damage their reputation. Slander is spoken defamation and libel is written defamation. Nurses must take care in their oral communication and documentation to avoid defaming clients or coworkers.[13]

Fraud

Fraud is an intentional tort that occurs when an individual is deceived for personal gain. A nurse may be charged with fraud for documenting interventions not performed or for altering documentation to cover up an error. Fraud can result in civil and criminal charges, as well as suspension or revocation of a nurse's license.[14]

Negligence and Malpractice

Negligence and malpractice are unintentional torts. **Negligence** is the failure to exercise the ordinary care a reasonable person would use in similar circumstances. Wisconsin civil jury instruction states, "A person is not using ordinary care and is negligent, if the person, without intending to do harm, does something (or fails to do

---

12 Nurses Service Organization and CNA Financial. (2020, June). *Nurse professional liability exposure claim report* (4th ed.). https://www.nso.com/Learning/Artifacts/Claim-Reports/Minimizing-Risk-Achieving-Excellence

13 Wis. JI—Civil 1005. (2016). https://wilawlibrary.gov/jury/civil/instruction.php?n=1005

14 Wis. JI—Civil 1005. (2016). https://wilawlibrary.gov/jury/civil/instruction.php?n=1005

My Notes

something) that a reasonable person would recognize as creating an unreasonable risk of injury or damage to a person or property." **Malpractice** is a specific term used for negligence committed by a health professional with a license.

Elements of Malpractice

Clients bringing a malpractice lawsuit must be able to demonstrate to the court that their interests were harmed. Most malpractice lawsuits name physicians or hospitals as defendants, although nurses can be individually named. Employers can be held liable for the actions of their employees.

Malpractice lawsuits are concerned with the legal obligations nurses have to their patients to adhere to current standards of practice. These legal obligations are referred to as the duty of reasonable care. Nurses are required to adhere to standards of practice when providing care to patients they have been assigned. This includes following organizational policies and procedures, maintaining clinical competency, and confining their activities to the authorized scope of practice as defined by their state's Nurse Practice Act. Nurses also have a legal duty to be physically, mentally, and morally fit for practice. When nurses do not meet these professional obligations, they are said to have breached their duties to patients.[15]

All of the following elements must be established in a court of law to prove malpractice[16]:

- **Duty:** A nurse-client relationship exists.
- **Breach:** The standard of care was not met and harm was a foreseeable consequence of the action or inaction.
- **Cause:** Injury was caused by the nurse's breach.
- **Harm:** Injury resulted in damages.

Duty

In the work environment, a duty is created when the nurse accepts responsibility for a patient and establishes a nurse-patient relationship. This generally occurs during inpatient care upon acceptance of a handoff report from another nurse. Outside the work environment, a nurse-patient relationship is created when the nurse volunteers services. Mandatory reporting and duty to warn and protect are additional examples of a nurse's duty.[17]

Breach of Duty

The second element of malpractice is breach of duty. After a plaintiff has established the first element in a malpractice suit (i.e., the nurse owed a duty to the plaintiff), the plaintiff must demonstrate that the nurse breached that duty by failing to comply with the duty of reasonable care. To demonstrate that a nurse breached their duty to a patient, the plaintiff must prove the nurse deviated from acceptable standards of practice. The plaintiff must establish how a reasonably prudent nurse in the same or similar circumstances would act and then show how the defendant nurse departed from that standard of practice. The plaintiff must claim the nurse did something a reasonably prudent nurse would not have done (an act of commission) or failed to do something a reasonable nurse would have done (an act of omission).[18]

---

15 This work is a derivative of *StatPearls* by Teoli and Ghassemzadeh and is licensed under CC BY 4.0

16 This work is a derivative of *StatPearls* by Teoli and Ghassemzadeh and is licensed under CC BY 4.0

17 This work is a derivative of *StatPearls* by Teoli and Ghassemzadeh and is licensed under CC BY 4.0

18 This work is a derivative of *StatPearls* by Teoli and Ghassemzadeh and is licensed under CC BY 4.0

My Notes

Experts are needed during court hearings to explain things outside the knowledge of non-nurse jurors. In reaching their opinions, experts review many materials, including the state's Nurse Practice Act and organizational policies, to determine whether the nurse adhered to them. To qualify as a nurse expert, the person testifying must have relevant experience, education, skill, and knowledge. Medical malpractice trials take place primarily in state courts, so experts are deemed qualified based on state requirements.[19]

Cause

The third element of malpractice is cause. After the plaintiff has established that the nurse owed a duty to a patient and then breached that duty, they must then demonstrate that damages or harm were caused by that breach. Plaintiffs cannot prevail by only demonstrating the nurse departed from acceptable standards of practice, but also must prove that such departures were the cause of any injuries. Additionally, nurses are held accountable for foreseeability, meaning a nurse of ordinary skill, care, and diligence could anticipate the risk of harm of departing from standards of practice in similar circumstances.[20]

Plaintiffs must be able to link the defendant's acts or omissions to the harm for which they are seeking compensation. This requires expert testimony from a physician because it requires a medical diagnosis. Unlike criminal cases, where the standard of proof is "beyond reasonable doubt," the elements of a malpractice lawsuit must be proven by a "preponderance of evidence." Expert testimony is required to demonstrate "medical certainty" that the nurse's breach was the cause of an actual injury.[21]

Harm

The fourth element of malpractice is harm. In a civil lawsuit, after a plaintiff has established the nurse owed a duty to the patient, breached that duty, and injury was caused by the nurse's breach, they must prove the injury resulted in damages. They request compensation for what they have lost.[22]

There are several types of injuries for which patients or their representatives seek compensation. Injuries can be physical, emotional, financial, professional, marital, or any combination of these. Physical injuries include loss of function, disfigurement, physical or mental impairment, exacerbation of prior medical problems, the need for additional medical care, and death. Economic injuries can include lost wages, additional medical expenses, rehabilitation, durable medical expenses, the need for architectural changes to one's home, the loss of earning capacity, the need to hire people to perform tasks the plaintiff can no longer do, and the loss of financial support. Emotional injuries can include psychological damage, emotional distress, or other forms of mental suffering.[23]

Determining the specific amount a plaintiff needs can require expert witness testimony from a person known as a life care planner who is trained in analyzing and evaluating medical costs, as well as the subjective determination of a jury. Damages fall into several categories, including compensatory (economic) damages, noneconomic damages, and punitive damages.[24]

19 This work is a derivative of *StatPearls* by Teoli and Ghassemzadeh and is licensed under CC BY 4.0

20 This work is a derivative of *StatPearls* by Teoli and Ghassemzadeh and is licensed under CC BY 4.0

21 This work is a derivative of *StatPearls* by Teoli and Ghassemzadeh and is licensed under CC BY 4.0

22 This work is a derivative of *StatPearls* by Teoli and Ghassemzadeh and is licensed under CC BY 4.0

23 This work is a derivative of *StatPearls* by Teoli and Ghassemzadeh and is licensed under CC BY 4.0

24 This work is a derivative of *StatPearls* by Teoli and Ghassemzadeh and is licensed under CC BY 4.0

My Notes

Implications for Nurses

Nurses defending themselves against allegations of professional malpractice must demonstrate that their actions conformed with accepted standards of practice. They must convince a jury they acted as a reasonably prudent nurse would have in the same or similar circumstances. Nurses should follow these practices to avoid allegations of malpractice[25]:

- Practice according to current standards of practice.
- Adhere to organizational policies and procedures. The standard of practice is to adhere to agency policy. Failing to do so creates an assumption of departure from standards.
- Document in a manner that permits accurate reconstruction of patient assessments and the sequence of events, especially when notifying providers regarding clinical concerns.
- Maintain competence through continuing education, participation in professional conferences, membership in professional organizations, and subscriptions to professional journals.
- When using an interpreter, ensure that properly trained interpreters are used and document the name of the interpreter. The use of family, friends, or other untrained interpreters is unsafe practice and is not consistent with acceptable standards of practice.
- Maintain professional boundaries. Personal relationships with patients or their families can be red flags for juries and can be viewed as evidence of departure from professional standards.
- Engage the chain of command with patient concerns and pursuing concerns to resolution.

Read more about actual nursing malpractice cases in the "Frequent Allegations and SBON Investigations" section of the "Legal Implications" chapter in Open RN *Nursing Management and Professional Concepts.*

Disciplinary Action by the Board of Nursing

In addition to being held liable in a court of law, nurses can have their licenses suspended or revoked by the State Board of Nursing (SBON) for unsafe nursing practice. The SBON governs nursing practice according to that state's Nurse Practice Act to protect the public through licensure, education, legislation, and discipline. A nursing license is a contract between the state and the nurse in which the licensee agrees to provide nursing care according to that state's Nurse Practice Act. Deviation from the Nurse Practice Act is a breach of contract that can lead to limited or revoked licensure. Nurses must practice according to the Nurse Practice Act of the state in which they are providing client care.[26]

A nurse may be named in a board licensing complaint called an allegation. Allegations can be directly related to a nurse's clinical responsibilities, or they can be nonclinical (such as operating a vehicle under the influence of a substance, exhibiting unprofessional behavior, or committing billing fraud). A complaint can be filed against a nurse by anyone, such as a patient, a patient's family member, a colleague, or an employer. It can also be filed anonymously. After a complaint is filed, the SBON follows a disciplinary process that includes investigation,

---

25 This work is a derivative of *StatPearls* by Teoli and Ghassemzadeh and is licensed under CC BY 4.0

26 American Nurses Association. (2012). *Position statement: Reduction of patient restraint and seclusion in health care settings.* https://www.nursingworld.org/practice-policy/nursing-excellence/official-position-statements/id/reduction-of-patient-restraint-and-seclusion-in-health-care-settings/

My Notes

proceedings, board actions, and enforcement. The process can take months or years to resolve, and it can be costly to hire legal representation.[27]

Disciplinary actions by the SBON may include the following[28]:

- **Reprimand:** The licensee receives a public warning for a violation.
- **Limitation of License:** The licensee has conditions or requirements imposed upon their license, their scope of practice, or both.
- **Suspension:** The license is completely and absolutely withdrawn and withheld for a period of time, including all rights, privileges, and authority previously conferred by the credential.
- **Revocation:** The license is completely and absolutely terminated, as well as all rights, privileges, and authority previously conferred by the credential.
- **Administrative Warning:** A warning is issued if the violation is of a minor nature, or a first occurrence and the warning will adequately protect the public. The issuance of an administrative warning is public information but the reason for issuance is not.
- **Remedial Education Order:** A remedial education order is issued when there is reason to believe that the deficiency can be corrected with remedial education, while sufficiently protecting the public.

Find and review your state's Nurse Practice Act.

27 American Nurses Association. (2012). *Position statement: Reduction of patient restraint and seclusion in health care settings.* https://www.nursingworld.org/practice-policy/nursing-excellence/official-position-statements/id/reduction-of-patient-restraint-and-seclusion-in-health-care-settings/

28 American Nurses Association. (2012). *Position statement: Reduction of patient restraint and seclusion in health care settings.* https://www.nursingworld.org/practice-policy/nursing-excellence/official-position-statements/id/reduction-of-patient-restraint-and-seclusion-in-health-care-settings/

My Notes

5.5 PATIENT RIGHTS

When individuals with mental health disorders are admitted to a hospital, they may lose a number of abilities that we take for granted, such as the ability to come and go, schedule their time, and choose and control their activities of daily living. In many states, patients' rights associated with inpatient admission to a mental health unit are spelled out in state law. Patients must be specifically informed of their rights as described in the Patient Bill of Rights document.

Clients who are determined to be legally incompetent also lose the ability to manage their financial and legal affairs and make important decisions. The Patient Self-Determination Act was passed to protect patient rights.[1]

The Patient Self-Determination Act was passed in 1990 and is considered a landmark law for patient rights. This law requires hospitals, skilled nursing facilities, home health agencies, hospice programs, and health maintenance organizations to provide clear written information for patients concerning their legal rights to make health care decisions, including the right to accept or refuse treatment. It also requires agencies to ask patients about advanced directives and to document any wishes the patient has in regard to the care they do or do not want.[2] Interprofessional team members, including nurses, have an ethical duty to ensure that patients know and understand their health care-related rights.[3] See the following box for a list of patient rights included in this law. These rights are further discussed in the following subsections.

Patient Self-Determination Act[4]

1. The right to appropriate treatment and related services in a setting and under conditions that are the most supportive of a person's personal liberty and restrict such liberty only to the extent necessary consistent with the person's treatment needs, applicable requirements of law, and applicable judicial orders.
2. The right to an individualized, written treatment or service plan (developed promptly after admission), the right to treatment based on the plan, the right to periodic review and reassessment of treatment and related service needs, and the right to appropriate revision of the plan, including revisions necessary to provide a description of mental health services that may be needed after the person is discharged from the program or facility.
3. The right to ongoing participation, in a manner appropriate to the person's capabilities, in the planning of mental health services to be provided (including the right to participate in the development and periodic revision of the plan).
4. The right to be provided with a reasonable explanation, in terms and language appropriate to the person's mental and physical condition, the objectives of treatment, the nature and

1 Cady, R. F. (2010). A review of basic patient rights in psychiatric care. *JONA'S Healthcare Law, Ethics and Regulation, 12*(4), 117–127. https://doi.org/10.1097/NHL.0b013e3181f4d357

2 This work is a derivative of *Nursing Fundamentals* by Open RN and is licensed under CC BY 4.0

3 Middleman, A. B., & Olson, K. A. (2021, August 10). Confidentiality in adolescent health care. *UpToDate.* Retrieved February 22, 2022, from https://www.uptodate.com/

4 Cady, R. F. (2010). A review of basic patient rights in psychiatric care. *JONA'S Healthcare Law, Ethics and Regulation, 12*(4), 117–127. https://doi.org/10.1097/NHL.0b013e3181f4d357

My Notes

significance of possible adverse effects of recommended treatment, the reasons why the recommended treatment is considered appropriate, the reasons why access to certain visitors may not be appropriate, and any appropriate and available alternative treatments, services, and types of providers of mental health services.

5. The right not to receive a course of treatment in the absence of informed, voluntary, written consent to treatments except during an emergency situation or as permitted by law when the person is being treated as a result of a court order.
6. The right to not participate in experimentation in the absence of informed, voluntary, written consent.
7. The right to freedom from restraint or seclusion, other than as a course of treatment during an emergency situation with a written order by a mental health professional.
8. The right to a humane treatment environment that affords reasonable protection from harm and appropriate privacy with regard to personal needs.
9. The right to access, on request, one's mental health care records.
10. The right of a person admitted to residential or inpatient care to converse with others privately, to have convenient and reasonable access to the telephone and mail, and to see visitors during regularly scheduled hours.
11. The right to be informed promptly at the time of admission and in writing of these rights.
12. The right to assert grievances with respect to infringement of these rights.
13. The right to exercise these rights without reprisal.
14. The right of referral to other providers upon discharge.

Informed Consent

Informed consent is the fundamental right of an individual to accept or reject health care. Based on the Patient Self-Determination Act, clients have the right to give informed consent before receiving medical assessment or treatment (except in emergency situations when imminent harm may occur to themselves or others). Most states allow a client to sue for battery if consent is not obtained before medical treatment is given.[5] However, a client must be competent and have the legal capacity to give informed consent.

Competency is a legal term related to the degree of cognitive ability an individual has to make decisions or carry out specific acts. Individuals are considered competent until they have been declared incompetent in a formal legal proceeding. If found incompetent, the individual is appointed a legal guardian or representative who is responsible for providing or refusing consent (while considering the individual's wishes). Guardians are typically family

5 Cady, R. F. (2010). A review of basic patient rights in psychiatric care. *JONA'S Healthcare Law, Ethics and Regulation, 12*(4), 117–127. https://doi.org/10.1097/NHL.0b013e3181f4d357

My Notes

members such as spouses, adult children, or parents. If family members are unavailable or unwilling to serve in this role, the court may appoint a court-trained guardian.[6]

Capacity is a functional determination that an individual is or is not capable of making a medical decision within a given situation. It is outside the scope of practice for nurses to formally assess capacity, but nurses may initiate the evaluation of client capacity and contribute assessment information. Capacity may be a temporary or permanent state. The following box outlines situations where the nurse may question a client's decision-making capacity.[7,8]

Triggers for Questioning a Client's Decision-Making Capacity

- Unawareness of surroundings
- Absence of questions about the treatment being offered or provided
- New inability to perform activities of daily living
- Disruptive behavior or agitation
- Labile emotions
- Hallucinations
- Intoxication

When a client does not have the capacity to provide informed consent, health care providers must obtain substituted consent for treatments. Substituted consent is authorization that another person gives on behalf of the patient. For example, the activation of a client's health care power of attorney is an example of substituted consent. Substituted consent may also come from a court-appointed guardian or if state law permits, from next of kin.[9]

Read more about informed consent and capacity in the "Other Legal Issues" section of Open RN *Nursing Management and Professional Concepts.*

Protective Placement

Guardianships and protective orders are legal methods in states for appointing an alternative decision-maker and identifying required services for individuals who are legally incompetent. Legally incompetent individuals may have developmental disabilities, chronic and serious mental illness, severe substance use disorders, or other conditions that limit their decision-making ability. A court can issue orders for a person who has a guardian to be

6 Halter, M. (2022). *Varcarolis' foundations of psychiatric-mental health nursing* (9th ed.). Saunders.

7 Cady, R. F. (2010). A review of basic patient rights in psychiatric care. *JONA'S Healthcare Law, Ethics and Regulation, 12*(4), 117–127. https://doi.org/10.1097/NHL.0b013e3181f4d357

8 Halter, M. (2022). *Varcarolis' foundations of psychiatric-mental health nursing* (9th ed.). Saunders.

9 Cady, R. F. (2010). A review of basic patient rights in psychiatric care. *JONA'S Healthcare Law, Ethics and Regulation, 12*(4), 117–127. https://doi.org/10.1097/NHL.0b013e3181f4d357

My Notes

protectively placed. The legal standard basically states that without the protective placement, the individual is so incapable of providing for their own care and well-being that it creates a substantial risk of serious harm to themselves or others. Protective services may include case management, in-home care, nursing services, adult day care, or inpatient treatment. Protective placements must be the least restrictive setting necessary to meet the individual's needs and must be reviewed annually by the court.

Psychiatric Advance Directive

A **Psychiatric Advance Directive (PAD)** is a legal document that describes a person's preferences for future mental health treatment or names an individual to make treatment decisions for them if they are in a crisis and unable to make decisions. Many people with mental illness, their family members, and health professionals are not familiar with PADs.[10]

For states that do not have laws regarding PADs, an individual can still draft a PAD under the more general statutes connected to advance health care directives and living wills. However, a PAD is more beneficial because of the unique issues of mental health care and treatment, such as medication preferences and inpatient treatment considerations and the fact that a person with mental health disorders can experience recovery and wellness over time.[11]

Read more about Psychiatric Advance Directives on the National Alliance on Mental Illness website.

Restraints and Seclusion

Restraints are devices used in health care settings to prevent patients from causing harm to themselves or others when alternative interventions are not effective. A restraint is a device, method, or process that is used for the specific purpose of restricting a patient's freedom of movement without the permission of the person. Restraints include mechanical devices such as a tie wrist device, chemical restraints, or seclusion. The Joint Commission defines a chemical restraint as a drug used to manage a patient's behavior, restrict the patient's freedom of movement, or impair the patient's ability to appropriately interact with their surroundings that is not standard treatment or dosage for the patient's condition.[12] It is important to note that the definition states the medication "is not standard treatment or dosage for the patient's condition." For example, administering prescribed benzodiazepines as standard treatment to manage the symptoms of a diagnosed mental health disorder is not considered a chemical restraint, but administering benzodiazepines to limit a patient's movement is considered a chemical restraint.

Seclusion is defined as the confinement of a patient in a locked room or an area from which they cannot exit on their own. Seclusion should only be used for the management of violent or self-destructive behavior. Seclusion limits freedom of movement because, although the patient is not mechanically restrained, they cannot leave the area.[13,14]

---

10 The Joint Commission. https://www.jointcommission.org/

11 The Joint Commission. https://www.jointcommission.org/

12 The Joint Commission. https://www.jointcommission.org

13 Wood County, Wisconsin. (n.d.). *Guardianship and protective placements.* https://www.co.wood.wi.us/Departments/HumanServices/GuardianshipAndProtectivePlacement.aspx

14 Knox, D. K., & Holloman, G. H., Jr. (2012). Use and avoidance of seclusion and restraint: Consensus statement of the American Association for Emergency Psychiatry Project Beta Seclusion and Restraint Workgroup. *The Western Journal of Emergency Medicine 13*(1), 35-40. https://doi.org/10.5811/westjem.2011.9.6867

My Notes

Although restraints are used with the intention to keep a patient safe, they impact a patient's psychological safety and dignity and can cause additional safety issues and death. A restrained person has a natural tendency to struggle and try to remove the restraint and can fall or become fatally entangled in the restraint. Furthermore, immobility that results from the use of restraints can cause pressure injuries, contractures, and muscle loss. Restraints take a large emotional toll on the patient's self-esteem and may cause humiliation, fear, and anger.

Restraint Guidelines

The American Nurses Association (ANA) has established evidence-based guidelines that a restraint-free environment is the standard of care. The ANA encourages the participation of nurses to reduce patient restraints and seclusion in all health care settings. Restraining or secluding patients is viewed as contrary to the goals and ethical traditions of nursing because it violates the fundamental patient rights of autonomy and dignity. However, the ANA also recognizes there are times when there is no viable option other than restraints to keep a patient safe, such as during an acute psychotic episode when patient and staff safety are in jeopardy due to aggression or assault. The ANA also states that restraints may be justified in some patients with severe dementia or delirium when they are at risk for serious injuries such as a hip fracture due to falling.[15]

The ANA provides the following guidelines: "When restraint is necessary, documentation should be done by more than one witness. Once restrained, the patient should be treated with humane care that preserves human dignity. In those instances where restraint, seclusion, or therapeutic holding is determined to be clinically appropriate and adequately justified, registered nurses who possess the necessary knowledge and skills to effectively manage the situation must be actively involved in the assessment, implementation, and evaluation of the selected emergency measure, adhering to federal regulations and the standards of the The Joint Commission (2009) regarding appropriate use of restraints and seclusion." Nursing documentation typically includes information such as patient behavior necessitating the restraint, alternatives to restraints that were attempted, the type of restraint used, the time it was applied, the location of the restraint, and patient education regarding the restraint.[16]

Any health care facility that accepts Medicare and Medicaid reimbursement must follow federal guidelines for the use of behavioral restraints. These guidelines include the following[17]:

- When a restraint is the only viable option, it must be discontinued at the earliest possible time.
- Orders for the use of seclusion or restraint can never be written as a standing order or PRN (as needed).
- The treating physician must be consulted as soon as possible if the restraint or seclusion is not ordered by the patient's treating physician.
- A physician or licensed independent practitioner must see and evaluate the need for the restraint or seclusion within one hour after the initiation.
- After restraints have been applied, the nurse should follow agency policy for frequent monitoring and regularly changing the patient's position to prevent complications. Nurses must also ensure the patient's basic needs (e.g., hydration, nutrition, and toileting) are met. Range of motion

---

15 Moore, G. P., & Pfaff, J. A. (2022, January 12). Assessment and emergency management of the acutely agitated or violent adult. *UpToDate.* Retrieved February 23, 2022, from https://www.uptodate.com/

16 Moore, G. P., & Pfaff, J. A. (2022, January 12). Assessment and emergency management of the acutely agitated or violent adult. *UpToDate.* Retrieved February 23, 2022, from https://www.uptodate.com/

17 Moore, G. P., & Pfaff, J. A. (2022, January 12). Assessment and emergency management of the acutely agitated or violent adult. *UpToDate.* Retrieved February 23, 2022, from https://www.uptodate.com/

My Notes

exercises and circulatory checks are typically provided hourly. Some agencies require a 1:1 patient sitter or continuous monitoring when restraints are applied or seclusion is implemented.

- Each written order for a physical restraint or seclusion is limited to 4 hours for adults, 2 hours for children and adolescents ages 9 to 17, or 1 hour for patients under 9. The original order may only be renewed in accordance with these limits for up to a total of 24 hours. After the original order expires, a physician or licensed independent practitioner (if allowed under state law) must see and assess the patient before issuing a new order.

Review safe use of restraints and alternatives to restraints in the "Restraints" section of the "Safety" chapter in Open RN *Nursing Fundamentals.*

Admission for Care

When clients with mental health disorders are admitted for inpatient care, the type of admission dictates certain rights and aspects of their treatment plan. Admissions may be voluntary admissions, emergency admissions, or involuntary admissions.

Voluntary Admission

Individuals over age 16 who present to a psychiatric facility and request hospitalization are considered **voluntary admissions**. Clients admitted under voluntary admission have certain rights that differ from emergency and involuntary admissions. For example, they are considered competent with the capacity to make health care decisions (unless determined otherwise).

Therefore, they have the right to refuse treatment, including psychotropic medications, unless they become a danger to themselves or others.[18]

Clients with voluntary admission do not necessarily have an absolute right to discharge at any time but may be required to request discharge. This gives the health care team an opportunity to initiate a procedure to change the client's admission status to involuntary if needed and associated legal requirements are met.[19]

Emergency Admissions

Many states allow individuals to be admitted to psychiatric facilities under **emergency admission** status when they are deemed likely to harm themselves or others. State laws define the exact procedure for the initial evaluation, possible length of detainment, and treatment provided. All clients who are admitted as emergency admissions require diagnosis, evaluation, and emergency treatment according to state law. At the end of the admission period, the facility must either discharge the patient, change their status to voluntary admission, or initiate a civil court hearing to determine the need for continuing treatment on an involuntary basis.[20]

18 Cady, R. F. (2010). A review of basic patient rights in psychiatric care. *JONA'S Healthcare Law, Ethics and Regulation, 12*(4), 117–127. https://doi.org/10.1097/NHL.0b013e3181f4d357

19 Cady, R. F. (2010). A review of basic patient rights in psychiatric care. *JONA'S Healthcare Law, Ethics and Regulation, 12*(4), 117–127. https://doi.org/10.1097/NHL.0b013e3181f4d357

20 Cady, R. F. (2010). A review of basic patient rights in psychiatric care. *JONA'S Healthcare Law, Ethics and Regulation, 12*(4), 117–127. https://doi.org/10.1097/NHL.0b013e3181f4d357

My Notes

During an emergency admission, the client's right to come and go is restricted, but they have a right to consult with an attorney and prepare for a hearing. Clients may be forced to receive psychotropic medications if they continue to be a danger to themselves or others. However, invasive procedures like electroconvulsive therapy (ECT) are not permitted unless they are ordered by the court or consented to by the client or their legal guardian.[21]

Involuntary Admissions

There may be circumstances when a person becomes so mentally ill they are at risk of hurting themselves or others, and involuntary admission for care becomes necessary even though the individual does not desire care. An individual can have an **involuntary admission** to a psychiatric facility if they are diagnosed with a mental illness, pose a danger to themselves or others, are gravely disabled (e.g., unable to provide themselves basic necessities like food, clothing, and shelter), or are in need of treatment but their mental illness prevents voluntary help-seeking behaviors. The legal procedures are different in each state, but standards for involuntary admission are similar.[22,23]

Because involuntary commitment is a serious matter, there are strict legal protections established by the U.S. Supreme Court. The standard of proof of "mentally ill and dangerous to self or others" must be based on "clear and convincing evidence." Therefore, two physicians must certify the individual's mental health status. Additionally, the client has the right to legal counsel and can take the case to a judge who can order release. If not released, the client can be involuntarily committed to a state-specified number of days with interim court appearances. Most states permit a 72-hour admission followed by a formal hearing. If the client feels they are being held without just cause, they can file a writ of habeas corpus (i.e., a formal written order to free the person). The court makes a decision based on the "least restrictive alternative" doctrine, meaning the least drastic action is taken to achieve the purpose of care.[24,25] Review your state's laws regarding involuntary admissions.

> For example, Wisconsin state law, referred to as "Chapter 51," dictates the requirements for involuntary admissions and is further explained by NAMI Kenosha County.

Involuntary Admission of Minors

Special considerations apply to minors receiving psychiatric care. Many states grant minors aged 12-18 the right to provide consent for mental health treatment and to protest involuntary admission unless they are a risk to themselves or others. In many cases, a neutral mental health review officer is assigned to the case to ensure rights are upheld.[26] State laws are complex; therefore, nurses must be aware of legal protections of minors in the state in which they work.

---

21 Cady, R. F. (2010). A review of basic patient rights in psychiatric care. *JONA'S Healthcare Law, Ethics and Regulation, 12*(4), 117–127. https://doi.org/10.1097/NHL.0b013e3181f4d357

22 Cady, R. F. (2010). A review of basic patient rights in psychiatric care. *JONA'S Healthcare Law, Ethics and Regulation, 12*(4), 117–127. https://doi.org/10.1097/NHL.0b013e3181f4d357

23 Halter, M. (2022). *Varcarolis' foundations of psychiatric-mental health nursing* (9th ed.). Saunders.

24 Cady, R. F. (2010). A review of basic patient rights in psychiatric care. *JONA'S Healthcare Law, Ethics and Regulation, 12*(4), 117–127. https://doi.org/10.1097/NHL.0b013e3181f4d357

25 Halter, M. (2022). *Varcarolis' foundations of psychiatric-mental health nursing* (9th ed.). Saunders.

26 Cady, R. F. (2010). A review of basic patient rights in psychiatric care. *JONA'S Healthcare Law, Ethics and Regulation, 12*(4), 117–127. https://doi.org/10.1097/NHL.0b013e3181f4d357

My Notes

Read additional information about Clients' Rights for Minors in Wisconsin.

Criminal Cases and Pleas of Insanity

If a defendant pleads an insanity defense in a criminal case, they are involuntarily admitted to a mental health facility for an evaluation period determined by state law. During this time an interprofessional team of mental health professionals (including nurses) evaluates the individual's need for hospitalization and notifies the court of their treatment recommendations. This specialized mental health care is referred to as forensic psychiatry.[27]

Discharge

When clients with mental health disorders are hospitalized, their admission status may impact their rights related to discharge. There are four main types of discharge[28]:

- **Unconditional Discharge:** Unconditional discharge refers to unconditional termination of the legal patient and institution relationship. Discharge may be ordered by a psychiatrist, advanced practice provider, or the court.
- **Release Against Medical Advice (AMA):** Clients who were admitted voluntarily may elect to leave an institution against the advice of the health care provider.
- **Conditional Release:** Conditional release means the client is discharged from inpatient care but requires outpatient treatment for a specified period of time. If the client was involuntarily admitted, they can be readmitted based on the original commitment order if they don't participate in outpatient treatment.
- **Assisted Outpatient Treatment:** Assisted outpatient treatment means the conditional release is court-ordered. This treatment is tied to services and goods provided by social welfare agencies, such as disability benefits and housing.

Reporting Unsafe or Impaired Professionals

Patients have the right to humane treatment and reasonable protection from harm. For example, if a suicidal patient is admitted and left alone with the means of self-harm, the nurse has a duty to protect the patient and can be held liable for injuries or death that occurs.

Nurses also have a duty to protect patients from suspected negligence by a colleague. In many states, nurses have a legal duty to intervene and report risks of harm to patients. This may include reporting concerns to a supervisor, the institution, and/or the state Board of Nursing. For example, nurses must report suspected drug diversion by colleagues because it can impact safe and humane treatment of patients. Read more about drug diversion and substance use disorder in nursing in the "Substance Use Disorders" chapter.

View the NCSBN PDF pamphlet: A Nurse's Guide to Substance Use Disorder in Nursing.

---

27 Cady, R. F. (2010). A review of basic patient rights in psychiatric care. *JONA'S Healthcare Law, Ethics and Regulation, 12*(4), 117–127. https://doi.org/10.1097/NHL.0b013e3181f4d357

28 Halter, M. (2022). *Varcarolis' foundations of psychiatric-mental health nursing* (9th ed.). Saunders.

My Notes

5.6 LEARNING ACTIVITIES

Interactive Activities

An interactive H5P element has been excluded from this version of the text. You can view it online here: https://wtcs.pressbooks.pub/nursingmhcc/?p=944#h5p-29

An interactive H5P element has been excluded from this version of the text. You can view it online here: https://wtcs.pressbooks.pub/nursingmhcc/?p=944#h5p-30

An interactive H5P element has been excluded from this version of the text. You can view it online here: https://wtcs.pressbooks.pub/nursingmhcc/?p=944#h5p-31

V GLOSSARY

My Notes

Adults at risk: Adults who have a physical or mental condition that impairs their ability to care for their own needs and are at risk for neglect and/or abuse.

Assault: Intentionally putting another person in reasonable apprehension of an imminent harmful or offensive contact.

Autonomy: The capacity to determine one's own actions through independent choice, including demonstration of competence. The nurse's primary ethical obligation is client autonomy.

Battery: Intentional causation of harmful or offensive contact with another person without that person's consent.

Beneficence: Benefiting others by preventing harm, removing harmful conditions, or affirmatively acting to benefit another or others, often going beyond what is required by law.

Board of Nursing: The state-specific licensing and regulatory body that sets standards for safe nursing care and issues nursing licenses to qualified candidates based on the Nurse Practice Act enacted by that state's legislature.

Capacity: A functional determination that an individual is or is not capable of making a medical decision within a given situation.

Competency: A legal term related to the degree of cognitive ability an individual has to make decisions or carry out specific acts.

Confidentiality: The right of an individual to have personal, identifiable medical information kept private.

Civil law: The rights, responsibilities, and legal relationships between private citizens and involves compensation to the injured party.

Criminal law: A system of laws that punishes individuals who commit crimes.

Defamation of character: Actions when an individual makes negative, malicious, and false remarks about another person to damage their reputation.

Defendants: The parties named in the lawsuit.

Emergency admission: Individuals are admitted to psychiatric facilities under emergency admission status when they are deemed likely to harm themselves or others.

False imprisonment: An act of restraining another person and causing that person to be confined in a bounded area.

Fraud: An intentional tort that occurs when an individual is deceived for personal gain.

Health Insurance Portability and Accountability Act (HIPAA): Federal regulations to ensure the privacy and protection of personal records and information.

Informed consent: The fundamental right of an individual to receive information about the risks, benefits, and alternatives in order to make a health care decision.

Intentional tort: A wrong that the defendant knew (or should have known) would be caused by their actions.

Involuntary admission: Circumstances when a person becomes so mentally ill they are at risk of hurting themselves or others, and inpatient care becomes necessary even though the individual does not desire inpatient care.

Justice: A moral obligation to act on the basis of equality and equity and a standard linked to fairness for all in society.

Malpractice: A specific term used for negligence committed by a health professional with a license.

Mandated reporters: Nurses and other professionals required by state law to report suspected neglect and/or abuse of children, adults at risk, and the elderly.

Negligence: The failure to exercise the ordinary care a reasonable person would use in similar circumstances.

Nonmaleficence: The bioethical principle that specifies a duty to do no harm and balances avoidable harm with benefits of good achieved.

My Notes

Nurse Practice Act: Law enacted by that state's legislature that establishes regulations for nursing practice within that state and defines the scope of nursing practice.

Plaintiff: A person bringing a lawsuit.

Protected Health Information (PHI): Individually identifiable health information including demographic data that relates to the individual's past, present, or future physical or mental health or condition; the provision of health care to the individual; and the past, present, or future payment for the provision of health care to the individual.

Psychiatric Advance Directive (PAD): A legal document that describes a person's preferences for future mental health treatment or names an individual to make treatment decisions for them if they are in a crisis and unable to make decisions.

Restraints: Devices used in health care settings to prevent patients from causing harm to themselves or others when alternative interventions are not effective.

Role fidelity: Being responsible for providing competent nursing care.

Seclusion: The confinement of a patient in a locked room from which they cannot exit on their own. It is generally used as a method of discipline, convenience, or coercion.

Standards of Professional Nursing Practice: Authoritative statements from the American Nurses Association regarding the actions and behaviors that all registered nurses, regardless of role, population, specialty, and setting, are expected to perform competently.

Standards of Professional Performance: Twelve standards set by the American Nurses Association that describe a nurse's professional behavior, including activities related to ethics, advocacy, respectful and equitable practice, communication, collaboration, leadership, education, scholarly inquiry, quality of practice, professional practice evaluation, resource stewardship, and environmental health.

Tort: An act of commission or omission that gives rise to injury or harm to another and amounts to a civil wrong for which courts impose liability.

Unintentional tort: A wrong that occurs when the defendant's actions or inactions were unreasonably unsafe. Unintentional torts can result from acts of commission (i.e., doing something a reasonable nurse would not have done) or omission (i.e., failing to do something a reasonable nurse would do).

Veracity: Telling the truth.

Voluntary admission: An individual over age 16 who presents to a psychiatric facility and requests hospitalization. They are considered competent with the capacity to make health care decisions (unless determined otherwise).

Chapter 6

Psychotropic Medications

6.1 INTRODUCTION

My Notes

Learning Objectives

- Relate the anatomy and physiology of the central nervous system to mental health disorders and psychotropic medications
- Describe patient education for classes of psychotropic medications

Psychotropic medications are medications that affect the mind, emotions, and behavior. This chapter will review the anatomy and physiology of the central nervous system (CNS) as it relates to mental health disorders and medications and then discuss several classes of psychotropic medications.

Be aware that information about medications changes frequently, and it is vital for nurses to consult evidence-based resources for the latest drug information, warnings, and patient education guidelines when administering medications. Free reference information is provided by the National Library of Medicine (NLM) on the DailyMed and MedlinePlus websites. DailyMed is a database containing current information from the Food and Drug Administration on prescription and over-the-counter medications. It provides essential information to health professionals for the safe and effective use of medications, including indications, dosage and administration, contraindications, boxed warnings and precautions, adverse reactions, drug interactions, information about use in specific populations, and other important information for health care practitioners.[1] MedlinePlus is an online health information resource for clients and their loved ones with easy-to-understand medication information.[2]

Specific information can be found on the National Alliance on Mental Illness' Mental Health Medications web page.[3]

---

1 DailyMed. *About us*. https://dailymed.nlm.nih.gov/dailymed/about-dailymed.cfm

2 MedlinePlus. *About us*. https://medlineplus.gov/

3 National Alliance on Mental Illness. (n.d.). *Mental health medications*. https://nami.org/About-Mental-Illness/Treatments/Mental-Health-Medications

My Notes

6.2 REVIEW OF THE CENTRAL NERVOUS SYSTEM

To understand how psychotropic medications work, it is important to understand the anatomy and physiology of the central nervous system. The nervous system is divided into the central and peripheral nervous systems. The central nervous system (CNS) is the brain and spinal cord, and the peripheral nervous system includes everything else in the nervous system. See Figure 6.1[1] for an illustration of the central and peripheral nervous systems.

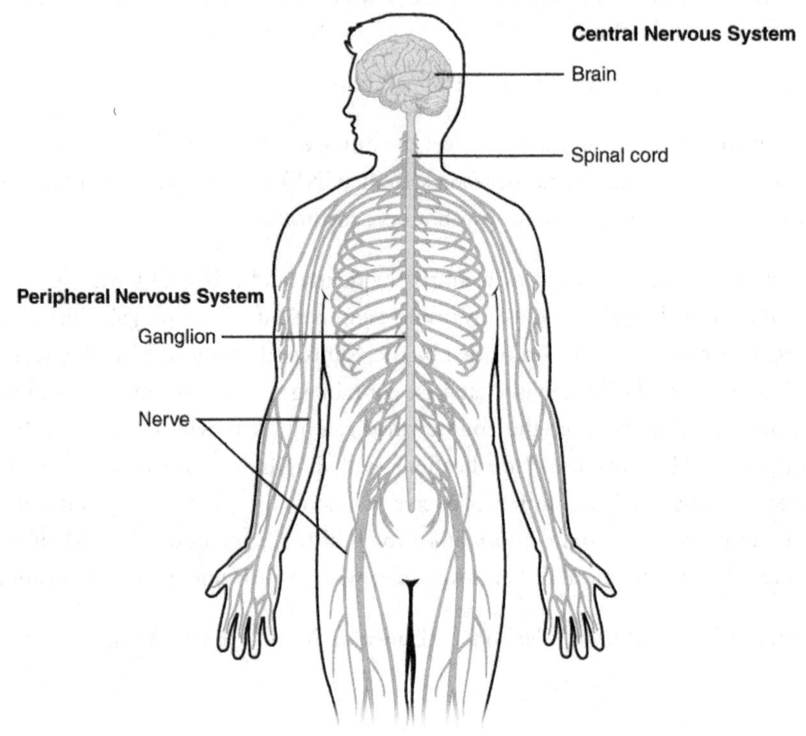

Figure 6.1 The Central and Peripheral Nervous Systems

The peripheral nervous system consists of sensory neurons and motor neurons. Sensory neurons sense the environment and conduct signals to the brain that become a person's conscious perception of that stimulus. This conscious perception may lead to a motor response that is conducted from the brain to the peripheral nervous system via motor neurons. Motor neurons are part of the somatic nervous system that stimulates voluntary movement of muscles and the autonomic nervous system that controls involuntary responses.

Sympathetic and Parasympathetic Nervous System

The autonomic nervous system is divided into the sympathetic nervous system (SNS) and the parasympathetic nervous system (PNS). Homeostatic mechanisms are regulated by the body through a balance of SNS and PNS stimulation. For example, stimulation of SNS receptors increases the heart rate, increases blood pressure via the constriction of blood vessels, and causes bronchodilation, whereas stimulation of the PNS slows the heart, lowers blood pressure due to vasodilation, and causes bronchoconstriction. Due to these effects, the SNS is associated

1 "1201 Overview of Nervous System.jpg" by OpenStax is licensed under CC BY 4.0. Access for free at https://openstax.org/books/anatomy-and-physiology/pages/12-1-basic-structure-and-function-of-the-nervous-system

My Notes

with the "fight-or-flight" response, and the PNS is often referred to as the "rest and digest" system. See Figure 6.2[2] to compare the effects of PNS and SNS stimulation on target organs.

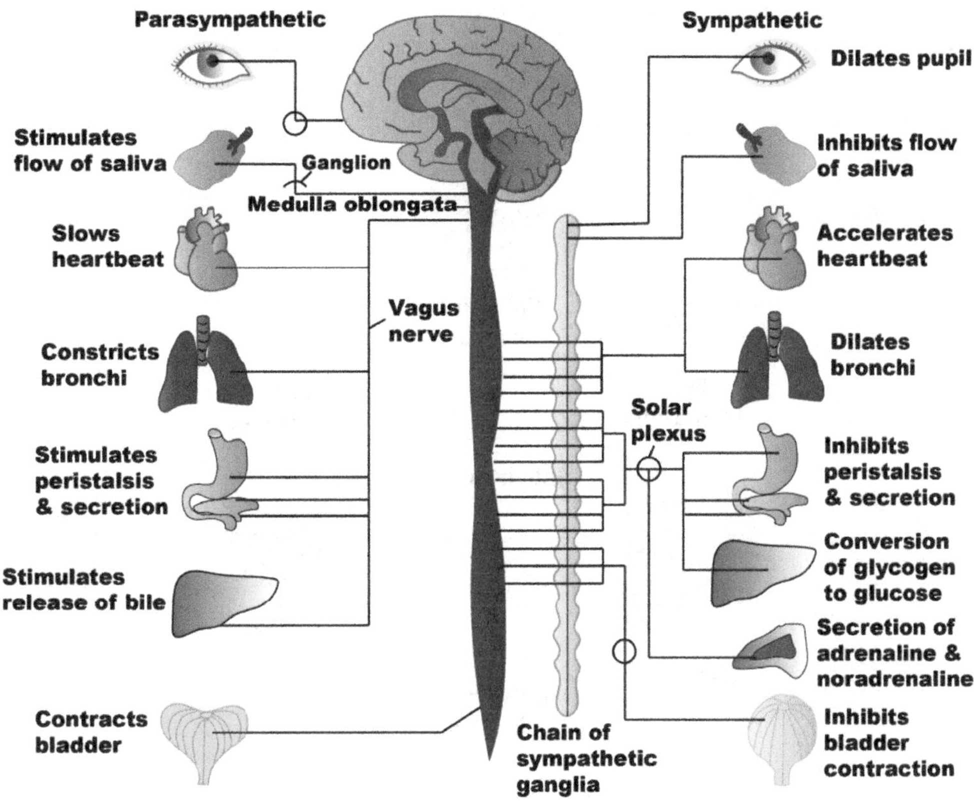

Figure 6.2 Effects of SNS and PNS Stimulation

SNS Receptors

SNS receptors include Alpha-1, Alpha-2, Beta-1, and Beta-2 receptors that are stimulated by epinephrine and norepinephrine. Medications that stimulate these receptors are referred to as **adrenergic agonists** because they mimic the effects of the body's natural SNS stimulation. For example, stimulants like methylphenidate are adrenergic agonists used to treat attention deficit hyperactivity disorder (ADHD). Conversely, **adrenergic antagonists** block SNS receptors. For example, propranolol is a Beta-2 antagonist used to treat the physical symptoms of severe anxiety (e.g., trembling, rapid heartbeat, and sweating).

PNS Receptors

PNS receptors include nicotinic and muscarinic receptors that are stimulated by acetylcholine (ACh). Drugs that stimulate nicotinic and muscarinic receptors are called **cholinergics**. For example, nicotine in tobacco products stimulates nicotinic receptors. Stimulation of muscarinic receptors primarily causes smooth muscle contraction. An example of a muscarinic agonist is bethanechol used to treat urinary retention by increasing the tone of the detrusor muscle to increase bladder emptying.[3] Drugs that block the effects of PNS receptors are called

2 "Updated SNS-PNS image.png" by Meredith Pomietlo for Open RN is licensed under CC BY 4.0

3 This work is a derivative of *StatPearls* by Padda and Derian and is licensed under CC BY 4.0

My Notes

anticholinergics. For example, benztropine is an anticholinergic used to treat muscle spasms associated with extrapyramidal symptoms from antipsychotic medications.[4] Many psychotropic medications cause anticholinergic adverse effects that can be especially hazardous for older adults. **SLUDGE** is a mnemonic for anticholinergic side effects: Salivation decreased, Lacrimation decreased, Urinary retention, Drowsiness/dizziness, GI upset, and Eyes (blurred vision/dry eyes). See Figure 6.3[5] for an illustration of the "SLUDGE" effects caused by anticholinergics.

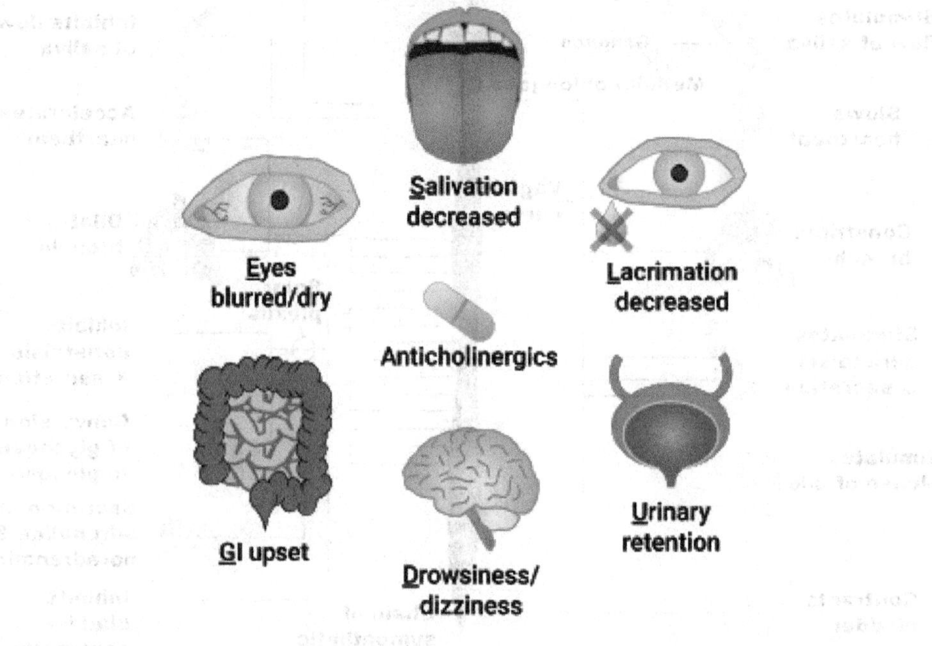

Figure 6.3 SLUDGE Effects of Anticholinergics

Opioid System

The opioid system in the brain controls pain, reward, and addictive behaviors. There are three types of **opioid receptors** called mu, delta, and kappa receptors. Opioid receptors are stimulated by endogenous peptides released by neurons (such as endorphins) and exogenous opiates. **Opiates** include powerful analgesics (such as morphine and oxycodone) prescribed to treat moderate to severe pain. Opiates also include illicit drugs (such as heroin). Chronic use of prescribed and illicit opiates can be highly addictive because of their actions on the reward system of the brain.[6] Read more about the addictive cycle in the "Substance Use Disorders" chapter.

---

4 This work is a derivative of *StatPearls* by Padda and Derian and is licensed under CC BY 4.0

5 "SLUDGE effects of Anticholinergics" by Dominic Slausen at Chippewa Valley Technical College is licensed under CC BY 4.0

6 This work is a derivative of *StatPearls* by Dhaliwal and Gupta and is licensed under CC BY 4.0

My Notes

Neurotransmitters

Neurotransmitters are chemical substances released at the end of a neuron by the arrival of an electrical impulse. They diffuse across the synapse and cause the transfer of the impulse to another nerve fiber, a muscle fiber, or other structure. Neurotransmitters interact with specific receptors like a key and a lock. See Figure 6.4[7] for an illustration of neuron communication with neurotransmitters and receptors.

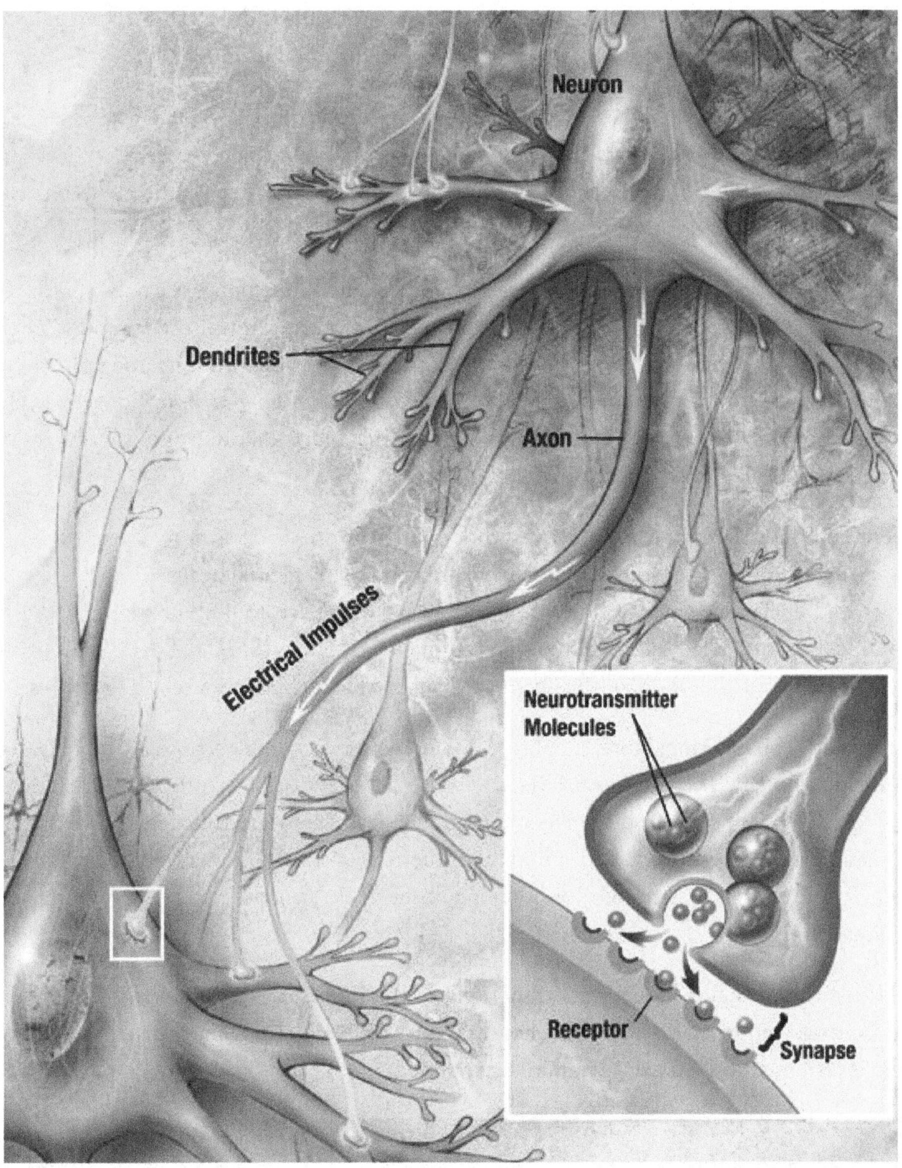

Figure 6.4 Neuron Communication With Neurotransmitters

7 "Chemical synapse schema cropped.jpg" by Looie496 is licensed under Public Domain. Access for free at https://med.libretexts.org/Bookshelves/Anatomy_and_Physiology/Book%3A_Anatomy_and_Physiology_(Boundless)/10%3A_Overview_of_the_Nervous_System/10.1%3A_Introduction_to_the_Nervous_System/10.1A%3A_Organization_of_the_Nervous_System

My Notes

There are several types of neurotransmitters associated with mental health disorders and psychoactive medications, including acetylcholine, glutamate, GABA, glycine, dopamine, serotonin, norepinephrine, and histamine[89]:

Acetylcholine: Acetylcholine stimulates nicotinic and muscarinic receptors in the parasympathetic nervous system. Other substances also bind to these receptors. For instance, nicotine (in tobacco products) binds to nicotinic receptors, and muscarine (products of specific mushrooms used as a hallucinogenic) binds to muscarinic receptors.

Glutamate: Glutamate is an excitatory neurotransmitter. Elevated levels of glutamate are associated with psychosis symptoms that can occur with schizophrenia, as well as with illicit drug use such as methamphetamines. Conversely, lamotrigine, a medication used to treat bipolar disorder, inhibits glutamate.

Gamma-Aminobutyric Acid and Glycine: Gamma-aminobutyric acid (GABA) and glycine are inhibitory neurotransmitters that act like brakes in a car by slowing down overexcited nerve cells. Low levels of GABA are associated with seizures, anxiety, mania, and impulse control. Pregabalin is an anticonvulsant that mimics the effects of GABA and is used to treat generalized anxiety disorder.

Dopamine: Dopamine plays an essential role in several brain functions, including learning, motor control, reward, emotion, and executive functions. It is associated with several mental health disorders and is targeted by many psychotropic medications. For example, bupropion is an antidepressant that inhibits dopamine reuptake, leading to increased dopamine levels in the synapse and relieving the symptoms of depression. Conversely, chlorpromazine blocks dopamine receptors and is used to treat psychosis, but this blockade can cause extrapyramidal side effects (involuntary and uncontrolled muscle movements).

Serotonin: Serotonin modulates multiple neuropsychological processes such as mood, sleep, libido, and temperature regulation. Abnormal levels of serotonin have been linked to many mental health disorders such as depression, bipolar disorder, and anxiety. Many psychotropic medications target serotonin. For example, fluoxetine belongs to a class of antidepressants called selective serotonin reuptake inhibitors (SSRIs). SSRIs prevent the reuptake of serotonin at the synapse, making more of the chemical available in the brain and relieving depression.

Norepinephrine and Epinephrine: Norepinephrine and epinephrine stimulate alpha- and beta-receptors in the sympathetic nervous system. Their release exerts effects on a variety of body processes, including stress, sleep, attention, and focus. Many psychotropic medications target these neurotransmitters. For example, venlafaxine belongs to a class of antidepressants called norepinephrine reuptake inhibitors (NRIs). NRIs are prescribed to treat depression by preventing the reuptake of norepinephrine at the synapse and boosting levels of norepinephrine in the brain.

Histamine: Histamine mediates homeostatic functions in the body, promotes wakefulness, modulates feeding behavior, and controls motivational behavior. For example, diphenhydramine, a histamine antagonist, causes drowsiness and is also used to treat extrapyramidal symptoms.

View a video that compares the effects of neurotransmitters: Receptor Debate.[10]

---

8 This work is a derivative of *Anatomy and Physiology* by OpenStax and is licensed under CC BY 4.0. Access for free at https://openstax.org/books/anatomy-and-physiology/pages/1-introduction

9 This work is a derivative of *StatPearls* by Sheffler, Reddy, and Pillarisetty and is licensed under CC BY 4.0

10 NEI Psychopharm. (2016, November 3). *Receptor debate* [Video]. YouTube. All rights reserved. https://youtu.be/GqX_J5h4aBw

6.3 ANTIDEPRESSANTS

My Notes

Antidepressants are commonly used to treat depression but are also used to treat other conditions, such as anxiety, chronic pain, and insomnia. According to a research review by the Agency for Healthcare Research and Quality, antidepressant medications work relatively equally as well to improve symptoms of depression and to keep depression symptoms from coming back.[1] For reasons not yet well understood, some people respond better to certain antidepressant medications than to others, so an individual may have to try different types of antidepressants before finding one that effectively treats their symptoms.[2] Additionally, it may take antidepressants two or more weeks to achieve peak effect.

There are several classes and types of antidepressants, including selective serotonin reuptake inhibitors (SSRIs), serotonin and norepinephrine reuptake inhibitors (SNRIs), norepinephrine and dopamine reuptake inhibitors (NDRIs), serotonin antagonist and reuptake inhibitors, tricyclic antidepressants (TCAs), and monoamine oxidase inhibitors (MAOIs). TCAs and MAOIs are often referred to as first-generation antidepressants because they were first marketed in the 1950s. They have many side effects and are not prescribed as frequently to treat depression as are SSRIs, SNRIs, and bupropion that have fewer side effects.

Selective Serotonin Reuptake Inhibitor (SSRI)

Selective serotonin reuptake inhibitors (SSRIs) prevent the uptake of serotonin at the synapse, causing the serotonin neurotransmitter to stay in the synapse longer and overall raise the level of serotonin in the brain. SSRIs are primarily used to treat depression but are also used to treat bipolar disorder, obsessive-compulsive disorder, bulimia, panic disorder, post-traumatic stress disorder, anxiety, premenstrual syndrome, and migraines. Examples of common SSRIs include fluoxetine, citalopram, sertraline, paroxetine, and escitalopram.[3]

Serotonin Norepinephrine Reuptake Inhibitor (SNRI)

Serotonin norepinephrine reuptake inhibitors (SNRIs) prevent the reuptake of serotonin and norepinephrine, with weak inhibition of dopamine reuptake. Examples of SNRIs are venlafaxine and duloxetine.[4]

Norepinephrine and Dopamine Reuptake Inhibitor (NDRI)

Bupropion is an example of a norepinephrine and dopamine reuptake inhibitor. It is used to treat depressive disorders, seasonal affective disorder, attention deficit disorder and to help people stop smoking.[5]

---

1 Volpi-Abadie, J., Kaye, A. M., & Kaye, A. D. (2013). Serotonin syndrome. *The Ochsner Journal, 13*(4), 533–540. https://dx.doi.org/10.1177%2F2045125311400779

2 National Institute of Mental Health. (2016, October). *Mental health medications.* U.S. Department of Health & Human Services.https://www.nimh.nih.gov/health/topics/mental-ealth-medications

3 National Institute of Mental Health. (2016, October). *Mental health medications.* U.S. Department of Health & Human Services. https://www.nimh.nih.gov/health/topics/mental-health-medications

4 National Institute of Mental Health. (2016, October). *Mental health medications.* U.S. Department of Health & Human Services. https://www.nimh.nih.gov/health/topics/mental-health-medications

5 MedlinePlus [Internet]. Bethesda (MD): National Library of Medicine (US); [updated 2022, Mar 16]. Bupropion; [reviewed 2018, Feb 15; cited 2022, Mar 25]. https://medlineplus.gov/druginfo/meds/a695033.html

My Notes

Serotonin Antagonist and Reuptake Inhibitor

Trazodone is an example of a serotonin antagonist and reuptake inhibitor. It is an antidepressant but most commonly prescribed off-label for anxiety or as a hypnotic. Trazodone reduces levels of the neurotransmitters associated with arousal effects, such as serotonin, noradrenaline, dopamine, acetylcholine, and histamine. Low-dose trazodone use exerts a sedative effect for sleep, so is typically administered in the evening.[6]

Tricyclic Antidepressants

Tricyclic antidepressants (TCAs) are older first-generation antidepressants that block the reuptake of serotonin and norepinephrine in the synapse, which leads to increased concentration of these neurotransmitters in the brain. They are now more commonly used to treat neuropathic pain and insomnia. An example of a TCA is amitriptyline.[7]

TCAs are often administered at bedtime due to sedating effects. Older adults are particularly sensitive to the anticholinergic side effects of tricyclic antidepressants (e.g., tachycardia, urinary retention, constipation, dry mouth, blurred vision, confusion, psychomotor slowing, sedation, and delirium).

Elderly clients should be started on low doses of amitriptyline and observed closely because they are at increased risk for falls. Blockage of adrenergic receptors can cause cardiac conduction disturbances and hypotension.[8]

Death may occur from overdosage with this class of drugs. Multiple drug ingestion (including alcohol) is common in deliberate tricyclic antidepressant overdose. If overdose occurs, call 911 in an outpatient setting or rapid response in an inpatient setting. Responders can consult with a Certified Poison Control Center (1-800-222-1222) or go to https://www.poisonhelp.org/help for the latest treatment recommendations.[9]

Monoamine Oxidase Inhibitor (MAOI)

Monoamine oxidase inhibitors (MAOIs) are an older first-generation antidepressant. MAOIs are contraindicated with all other classes of antidepressants. Monoamine oxidase is an enzyme that removes the neurotransmitters norepinephrine, serotonin, and dopamine from the brain. By inhibiting this enzyme, MAOIs cause the levels of these transmitters to increase. Tranylcypromine is an example of an MAOI.[10]

A significant disadvantage to MAOIs is their potential to cause a hypertensive crisis when taken with stimulant medications or foods or beverages containing tyramine. Examples of foods containing tyramine are aged cheese, cured or smoked meats, alcoholic beverages, and soy sauce. Older adults are at increased risk for postural hypotension and serious adverse effects.[11]

Read additional information about mechanism of action, potential adverse effects, and related patient education regarding antidepressants in the "Treatments for Depression" section of the "Depressive Disorders" chapter.

---

6 This work is a derivative of *StatPearls* by Shin and Saadabadi and is licensed under CC BY 4.0

7 This work is a derivative of *DailyMed* by U.S. National Library of Medicine and is available in the Public Domain

8 This work is a derivative of *DailyMed* by U.S. National Library of Medicine and is available in the Public Domain

9 This work is a derivative of *DailyMed* by U.S. National Library of Medicine and is available in the Public Domain

10 This work is a derivative of *DailyMed* by U.S. National Library of Medicine and is available in the Public Domain

11 This work is a derivative of *DailyMed* by U.S. National Library of Medicine and is available in the Public Domain

6.4 MOOD STABILIZERS

My Notes

Mood stabilizers are used primarily to treat bipolar disorder. They are also used to treat depression (usually in combination with an antidepressant), schizoaffective disorder, and disorders of impulse control. Lithium is an example of a mood stabilizer. Anticonvulsant medications are also used as mood stabilizers.[1] Antipsychotics, antianxiety, and antidepressants may also be used to treat bipolar disorders.

Lithium

Lithium reduces excitatory neurotransmission (dopamine and glutamate) and increases inhibitory neurotransmission (GABA). It also alters sodium transport in nerve and muscle cells and causes a shift in metabolism of catecholamines. When administered to a client experiencing a manic episode, lithium may reduce symptoms within 1 to 3 weeks. It also possesses unique antisuicidal properties that sets it apart from antidepressants. However, lithium toxicity can occur at doses close to therapeutic levels so lithium levels must be monitored regularly.[2,3]

Read additional information about mechanism of action and adverse effects of medications used to treat bipolar disorder in the "Treatments for Bipolar Disorder" in the "Bipolar Disorders" chapter.

1 National Institute of Mental Health. (2016, October). *Mental health medications.* U.S. Department of Health & Human Services. https://www.nimh.nih.gov/health/topics/mental-health-medications

2 This work is a derivative of *DailyMed* by U.S. National Library of Medicine and is available in the Public Domain

3 Malhi, G. S., Tanious, M., Das, P., Coulston, C. M., & Berk, M. (2013). Potential mechanisms of action of lithium in bipolar disorder. Current understanding. *CNS Drugs, 27*(2), 135–153. https://doi.org/10.1007/s40263-013-0039-0

My Notes

6.5 ANTIANXIETY MEDICATIONS

Antianxiety medications help reduce the symptoms of anxiety, panic attacks, or extreme fear and worry. The most common class of antianxiety medications is benzodiazepines. Benzodiazepines are used to treat generalized anxiety disorder, although SSRIs or other antidepressants are typically used to treat panic disorder or social phobia (i.e., social anxiety disorder). Beta-blockers and buspirone may also be prescribed for anxiety.[1]

Benzodiazepines

Benzodiazepines are used to treat anxiety and are also used for their sedation and anticonvulsant effects because they bind to GABA receptors and stimulate the effects of GABA (an inhibitory neurotransmitter). Benzodiazepines include clonazepam, alprazolam, and lorazepam. Benzodiazepines are a Schedule IV controlled substance because they have a potential for misuse and can cause dependence. Short-acting benzodiazepines (such as lorazepam) and beta-blockers are used to treat the short-term symptoms of anxiety. Lorazepam is available for oral, intramuscular, or intravenous routes of administration.[2]

Beta-Blockers

Beta-blockers (such as propranolol) block sympathetic nervous system stimulation of Beta-1 receptors. They may be prescribed to manage the physical symptoms of anxiety (such as trembling, rapid heartbeat, and sweating) for a short period of time or used "as needed" to reduce acute physical symptoms.[3]

Read additional information about medications used to treat anxiety in the "Treatments for Anxiety" section of the "Anxiety Disorders" chapter.

---

1 National Institute of Mental Health. (2016, October). *Mental health medications.* U.S. Department of Health & Human Services. https://www.nimh.nih.gov/health/topics/mental-health-medications

2 This work is a derivative of *DailyMed* by U.S. National Library of Medicine and is available in the Public Domain

3 National Institute of Mental Health. (2016, October). *Mental health medications.* U.S. Department of Health & Human Services. https://www.nimh.nih.gov/health/topics/mental-health-medications

6.6 ANTIPSYCHOTICS

My Notes

Antipsychotic medicines are primarily used to manage psychosis (i.e., a loss of contact with reality that may include delusions or hallucinations). Psychosis can be a symptom of a physical condition (such as a high fever, head injury, or substance intoxication) or a mental health disorder (such as schizophrenia, bipolar disorder, or severe depression). Antipsychotic medications may also be used in combination with other medications to treat the symptoms of other mental health conditions, including attention deficit hyperactivity disorder (ADHD), eating disorders, post-traumatic stress disorder (PTSD), obsessive-compulsive disorder (OCD), and generalized anxiety disorder.[1]

First-generation antipsychotics (also called typical antipsychotics) have several potential adverse effects, and medication is prescribed based on the client's ability to tolerate the adverse effects. Second-generation antipsychotics (also referred to as atypical antipsychotics) have fewer adverse effects and are generally better tolerated. Clients respond differently to antipsychotic medications, so it may take several trials of different medications to find the one that works best for their symptoms.[2]

First-Generation (Typical) Antipsychotics

Common first-generation antipsychotic medications (also called "typical" antipsychotics) include chlorpromazine, haloperidol, perphenazine, and fluphenazine.[3]

First-generation antipsychotics work by blocking dopamine receptors in certain areas of the CNS, such as the limbic system and the basal ganglia. These areas are associated with emotions, cognitive function, and motor function. As a result, blockage produces a tranquilizing effect in psychotic clients. However, several adverse effects are caused by this dopamine blockade, such as **extrapyramidal side effects** (e.g., involuntary or uncontrollable movements, tremors, and muscle contractions) and **tardive dyskinesia** (a syndrome of movement disorders that persists for at least one month and can last up to several years despite discontinuation of the medications).

Second-Generation (Atypical) Antipsychotics

Second-generation antipsychotics (also called atypical antipsychotics) work by blocking specific D2 dopamine receptors and serotonin receptors. Second-generation medications include risperidone, olanzapine, quetiapine, ziprasidone, aripiprazole, paliperidone, and lurasidone. Several atypical antipsychotics have a "broader spectrum" of action than the older medications and are used for treating bipolar depression or depression that has not responded to an antidepressant medication alone. They have a significantly decreased risk of extrapyramidal side effects but are associated with weight gain and the development of metabolic syndrome.[4] **Metabolic syndrome** increases the risk of heart disease, stroke, and type 2 diabetes. Clinical symptoms of metabolic syndrome include high blood glucose, symptoms of diabetes (i.e., increased thirst and urination, fatigue, and blurred vision), obesity with a large abdominal girth, hypertension, elevated triglyceride, and lower levels of HDL.

---

1 National Institute of Mental Health. (2016, October). *Mental health medications.* U.S. Department of Health & Human Services. https://www.nimh.nih.gov/health/topics/mental-health-medications#part_2362

2 National Institute of Mental Health. (2016, October). *Mental health medications.* U.S. Department of Health and Human Services. https://www.nimh.nih.gov/health/topics/mental-health-medications#part_2362

3 National Institute of Mental Health. (2016, October). *Mental health medications.* U.S. Department of Health and Human Services. https://www.nimh.nih.gov/health/topics/mental-health-medications#part_2362

4 This work is a derivative of *StatPearls* by Chokhawala and Stevens and is licensed under CC BY 4.0

My Notes

Clozapine

Clients with treatment-resistant schizophrenia may be prescribed clozapine, a specific atypical antipsychotic medication that binds to serotonin, as well as dopamine receptors. Clozapine also has strong anticholinergic, sedative, cardiac, and hypotensive properties and frequent drug-drug interactions.[5]

View a video explaining how clozapine binds to additional neuroreceptors compared to other antipsychotic medication: The pines, the dones, two pips, and a rip[6]

Read additional information about the mechanism of action, adverse side effects, and patient education regarding antipsychotic medications in the "Schizophrenia" section of the "Psychosis and Schizophrenia" chapter.

---

5 Jibson, M. D. (2021). Second-generation antipsychotic medications: Pharmacology, administration, and side effects. *UpToDate.* Retrieved January 14, 2022, from https://www.uptodate.com/

6 NEI Psychopharm. (2014, March 18). *The Pines, the Dones, Two Pips, and a Rip* [Video]. YouTube. All rights reserved. https://youtu.be/kuYGJOcloH8

6.7 STIMULANTS

My Notes

Stimulant medications are prescribed to treat children, adolescents, or adults diagnosed with attention deficit hyperactivity disorder (ADHD). Stimulants block the reuptake of norepinephrine and dopamine in the synapse and increase the overall level of these substances in the brain, but they have a paradoxical calming effect and improve the ability to focus and concentrate for individuals diagnosed with ADHD. Common stimulants used to treat ADHD include methylphenidate, amphetamine, dextroamphetamine, and lisdexamfetamine dimesylate. Stimulant medications are safe when prescribed with close supervision, but they are a Schedule II controlled substance because they have a high potential for misuse and dependence.

Read more information about medications used to treat attention deficit hyperactivity disorder (ADHD), adverse side effects, and patient education in the "Common Disorders and Disabilities in Children and Adolescents" section of the "Childhood and Adolescent Disorders" chapter.

My Notes

6.8 PSYCHOACTIVE SUBSTANCES AND MEDICATIONS TO TREAT SUBSTANCE USE AND WITHDRAWAL

Information about the effects of substances such alcohol, cannabis, and illicit drugs is discussed in the "Substances: Use, Intoxication, and Overdose" section of the "Substance Use Disorders" chapter.

Medications to treat alcohol use disorder and opioid disorder include buprenorphine-naloxone, methadone, naltrexone, acamprosate, and disulfiram. These medications are discussed in the "Treatment and Recovery Services" subsection of the "Substance Use Disorders" chapter.

Medications used to manage symptoms of substance withdrawal/detoxification include buprenorphine, methadone, and Alpha-2 adrenergic agonists (such as clonidine and lofexidine). Read more about these medications in the "Withdrawal Management/Detoxification" section of the "Substance Use Disorders" chapter.

My Notes

6.9 LEARNING ACTIVITIES

Interactive Activities

An interactive H5P element has been excluded from this version of the text. You can view it online here: https://wtcs.pressbooks.pub/nursingmhcc/?p=996#h5p-32

An interactive H5P element has been excluded from this version of the text. You can view it online here: https://wtcs.pressbooks.pub/nursingmhcc/?p=996#h5p-33

An interactive H5P element has been excluded from this version of the text. You can view it online here: https://wtcs.pressbooks.pub/nursingmhcc/?p=996#h5p-34

My Notes

VI GLOSSARY

Acetylcholine: A neurotransmitter that stimulates nicotinic and muscarinic receptors in the parasympathetic nervous system.

Adrenergic agonists: Substances that stimulate SNS receptors and cause effects similar to epinephrine and norepinephrine.

Adrenergic antagonists: Substances that block SNS receptors.

Agranulocytosis: Extremely low white blood cell count and an adverse effect of clozapine and antipsychotic medication.

Anticholinergics: Substances that block the effects of PNS receptors.

Black Box Warning: A significant warning from the Food and Drug Administration (FDA) that alerts the public and health care providers to serious side effects, such as injury or death.

Catecholamines: Substances that include epinephrine, norepinephrine, and dopamine and are responsible for the body's "fight-or-flight" response.

Central nervous system (CNS): The brain and spinal cord.

Cholinergics: Substances that stimulate nicotinic and muscarinic receptors and cause effects similar to acetylcholine (ACh).

Controlled substance: Drugs regulated by federal law that can cause dependence and abuse.

Dopamine: A neurotransmitter that plays an essential role in several brain functions, including learning, motor control, reward, emotion, and executive functions.

Extrapyramidal side effects: Involuntary or uncontrollable movements, tremors, and muscle contractions that can occur with antipsychotic medications.

Gamma-aminobutyric acid and Glycine: Inhibitory neurotransmitters that act like brakes in a car by slowing down overexcited nerve cells. Low levels of GABA are associated with seizures, anxiety, mania, and impulse control.

Pregabalin is an anticonvulsant that mimics the effects of GABA and is used to treat generalized anxiety disorder.

Glutamate: An excitatory neurotransmitter. Elevated levels of glutamate are associated with psychosis that can occur with schizophrenia, as well as with illicit drug use such as methamphetamines. Conversely, lamotrigine, a medication used to treat bipolar disorder, inhibits glutamate.

Histamine: A substance that mediates homeostatic functions in the body, promotes wakefulness, modulates feeding behavior, and controls motivational behavior. For example, diphenhydramine, a histamine antagonist, causes drowsiness.

Hypertensive crisis: A condition that can be caused by MAOIs with severe hypertension (blood pressure greater than 180/120 mm Hg) and evidence of organ dysfunction. Symptoms may include occipital headache (which may radiate frontally), palpitations, neck stiffness or soreness, nausea or vomiting, sweating, dilated pupils, photophobia, shortness of breath, or confusion.

Lithium toxicity: Lithium has a narrow therapeutic range of 0.8 to 1.2 mEq/L. Levels above this range cause lithium toxicity. Signs of early lithium toxicity include diarrhea, vomiting, drowsiness, muscular weakness, and lack of coordination. At higher levels, giddiness, ataxia, blurred vision, tinnitus, and a large output of dilute urine may occur.

Neuroleptic malignant syndrome (NMS): A rare but fatal adverse effect that can occur at any time during treatment with antipsychotics. It typically develops over a period of days to weeks and resolves in approximately nine days with treatment. Signs include increased temperature, severe muscular rigidity, confusion, agitation, hyperreflexia, elevation in white blood cell count, elevated creatinine phosphokinase, elevated liver enzymes, myoglobinuria, and acute renal failure.

Neurotransmitters: Chemical substances released at the end of a neuron by the arrival of an electrical impulse. They diffuse across the synapse and cause the transfer of the impulse to another nerve fiber, a muscle fiber, or other structure. Neurotransmitters interact with specific receptors like a key and a lock.

Norepinephrine and Epinephrine: Substances that stimulate alpha- and beta-receptors in the sympathetic nervous system.

Opiates: Powerful analgesics prescribed to treat moderate to severe pain (such as morphine and oxycodone). Opiates also include illicit drugs (such as heroin).

Opioid receptors: Mu, delta, and kappa receptors that are stimulated by endogenous peptides released by neurons (such as endorphins) and exogenous opiates.

Opioid system: A system in the brain that controls pain and reward and addictive behaviors.

Parasympathetic Nervous System (PNS) receptors: Nicotinic and muscarinic receptors that are stimulated by acetylcholine (ACh).

Serotonin: A neurotransmitter that modulates multiple neuropsychological processes such as mood, sleep, libido, and temperature regulation. Abnormal levels of serotonin have been linked to many mental health disorders such as depression, bipolar disorder, and anxiety. Many psychotropic medications target serotonin.

Serotonin syndrome: A syndrome caused by the combination of multiple medications that affect serotonin. It typically develops within 24 hours from the combination of medication and can range from mild to a life-threatening syndrome. Signs of serotonin syndrome include mental status changes (e.g., agitation, hallucinations, coma), autonomic instability (e.g., tachycardia, labile blood pressure, hyperthermia), incoordination, or gastrointestinal symptoms (e.g., nausea, vomiting, diarrhea). Serotonin syndrome, in its most severe form, can resemble neuroleptic malignant syndrome (NMS).

SLUDGE: A mnemonic for anticholinergic side effects: Salivation decreased, Lacrimation decreased, Urinary retention, Drowsiness/dizziness, GI upset, Eyes (blurred vision/dry eyes).

Sympathetic Nervous System (SNS) receptors: Alpha-1, Alpha-2, Beta-1, and Beta-2 receptors that are stimulated by epinephrine and norepinephrine.

Tardive dyskinesia: A syndrome of movement disorders associated with antipsychotic medications that persists for at least one month and can last up to several years despite discontinuation of the medications.

Chapter 7

Depressive Disorders

7.1 INTRODUCTION

My Notes

Learning Objectives

- Apply the nursing process to clients with depressive disorders
- Describe nursing assessments related to depressive disorders
- Identify common nursing problems/diagnoses related to depressive disorders
- Establish a safe environment
- Apply evidence-based practice when planning and implementing nursing care
- Describe common treatments for depressive disorders
- Identify appropriate referrals to community resources
- Evaluate the effectiveness of interventions
- Provide patient education to clients and their family members

Depression is a common illness affecting an estimated 8% of adults in the United States annually.[1] Approximately 280 million people in the world have depression.[2] This chapter will discuss causes and types of depression, treatments for depression, and steps for applying the nursing process when caring for clients with depressive disorders.

1 National Alliance on Mental Illness. (2017, August). *Depression*. https://nami.org/About-Mental-Illness/Mental-Health-Conditions/Depression

2 *Depression* by the World Health Organization is licensed under CC BY-NC-SA 3.0

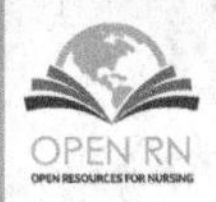

My Notes

7.2 CAUSES OF DEPRESSION

There are several possible causes of depression, including faulty mood regulation by the brain, genetic vulnerability, stressful life events, medications, and medical problems. Based on current research, it is believed that several of these forces interact to bring on depression.[1]

The Brain

Certain areas of the brain help regulate mood, including the hippocampus, amygdala, and hypothalamus. See Figure 7.1[2] for an image of these areas of the brain. Researchers believe that nerve cell connections, nerve cell growth, the functioning of nerve circuits, and levels of specific brain chemicals (called neurotransmitters) have a major impact on depression.[3]

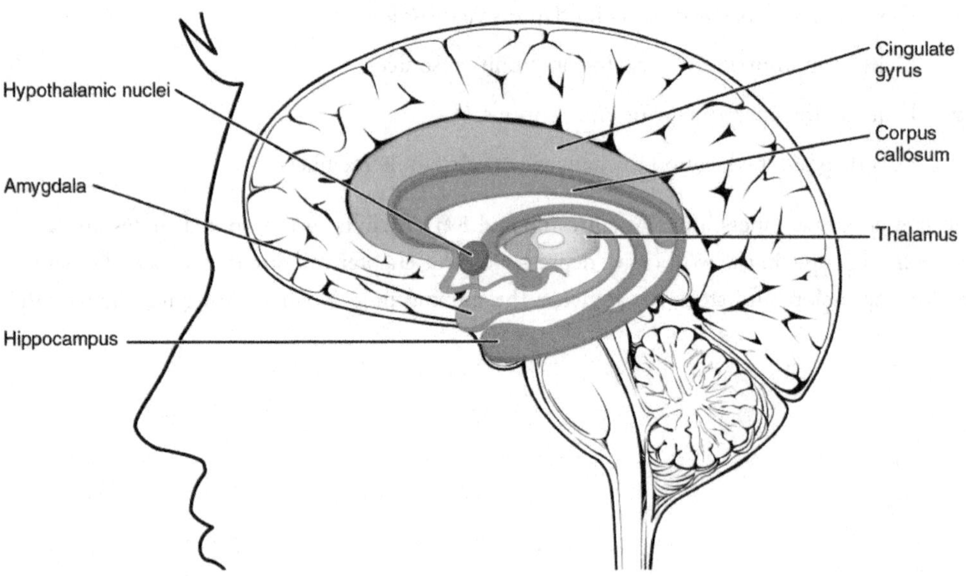

Figure 7.1 Areas of the Brain Regulating Mood

The hippocampus is part of the limbic system in the brain that has a central role in processing long-term memory and recollection. For example, this part of the brain registers fear when you are confronted by a frightening situation, like an aggressive dog, and the memory of such an experience may make you wary of dogs you come across later in life. The hippocampus is smaller in some depressed people, and research suggests that ongoing exposure to the stress hormone impairs the growth of nerve cells in this part of the brain.[4]

---

1 Harvard Health Publishing. (2019, June 24). *What causes depression?* Harvard Medical School. https://www.health.harvard.edu/mind-and-mood/what-causes-depression

2 "1511_The_Limbic_Lobe.jpg" by OpenStax College is licensed under CC BY 3.0. Access for free at http://cnx.org/content/col11496/1.6/

3 Harvard Health Publishing. (2019, June 24). *What causes depression?* Harvard Medical School. https://www.health.harvard.edu/mind-and-mood/what-causes-depression

4 Harvard Health Publishing. (2019, June 24). *What causes depression?* Harvard Medical School. https://www.health.harvard.edu/mind-and-mood/what-causes-depression

My Notes

The amygdala is also part of the limbic system and is a group of structures deep in the brain that are associated with emotions such as anger, pleasure, sorrow, fear, and sexual arousal. The amygdala is activated when a person experiences or recalls emotionally charged memories, such as a frightening situation, and sends signals to the hypothalamus to stimulate the sympathetic fight-or-flight response. Activity in the amygdala is higher when a person is sad or clinically depressed. This increased activity continues even after recovery from depression.[5]

The hypothalamus is involved in the stress response. The stress response starts with a signal from the hypothalamus. The hypothalamus, pituitary gland, and adrenal glands form the hypothalamic-pituitary-adrenal (HPA) axis, which governs a multitude of hormonal activities in the body and also plays a role in depression. When a physical or emotional threat looms, the hypothalamus secretes corticotropin-releasing hormone (CRH) that rouses the body. CRH follows a pathway to the pituitary gland, where it stimulates the secretion of adrenocorticotropic hormone (ACTH) into the bloodstream. When ACTH reaches the adrenal glands, it prompts the release of cortisol. The boost in cortisol readies the body to fight or flee by causing the heart to beat faster, the blood pressure to rise, and the respiratory rate to increase. CRH also affects the cerebral cortex, part of the amygdala, and the brain stem. It is thought to play a major role in coordinating one's thoughts and behaviors, emotional reactions, and involuntary responses. Working along a variety of neural pathways, it influences the concentration of neurotransmitters throughout the brain. Disturbances in hormonal systems affect neurotransmitters and vice versa.[6]

Neurotransmitters

There are many types of neurotransmitters that play a role in depression[7]:

- **Acetylcholine** enhances memory and is involved in learning and recall.[8]
- **Serotonin** helps regulate sleep, appetite, and mood and inhibits pain. Research supports the idea that some depressed people have reduced serotonin transmission. Low levels of a serotonin by-product have been linked to a higher risk for suicide.[9]
- **Norepinephrine** constricts blood vessels, raising blood pressure. It may trigger anxiety and be involved in some types of depression. It also seems to help determine motivation and reward.[10]
- **Dopamine** is essential to movement. It also influences motivation and plays a role in how a person perceives reality. Problems in dopamine transmission have been associated with psychosis, a

5 Harvard Health Publishing. (2019, June 24). *What causes depression?* Harvard Medical School. https://www.health.harvard.edu/mind-and-mood/what-causes-depression

6 Harvard Health Publishing. (2019, June 24). *What causes depression?* Harvard Medical School. https://www.health.harvard.edu/mind-and-mood/what-causes-depression

7 Harvard Health Publishing. (2019, June 24). *What causes depression?* Harvard Medical School. https://www.health.harvard.edu/mind-and-mood/what-causes-depression

8 Harvard Health Publishing. (2019, June 24). *What causes depression?* Harvard Medical School. https://www.health.harvard.edu/mind-and-mood/what-causes-depression

9 Harvard Health Publishing. (2019, June 24). *What causes depression?* Harvard Medical School. https://www.health.harvard.edu/mind-and-mood/what-causes-depression

10 Harvard Health Publishing. (2019, June 24). *What causes depression?* Harvard Medical School. https://www.health.harvard.edu/mind-and-mood/what-causes-depression

My Notes

severe form of distorted thinking characterized by hallucinations or delusions. It's also involved in the brain's reward system, so it is thought to play a role in substance abuse.[11]

- **Glutamate** is a small molecule believed to act as an excitatory neurotransmitter and to play a role in bipolar disorder and schizophrenia. Animal research suggests that lithium stabilizes glutamate reuptake and smooths out the highs of mania and the lows of depression in the long-term.[12]
- **Gamma-aminobutyric acid (GABA)** is an amino acid that researchers believe acts as an inhibitory neurotransmitter. It is thought to help subdue anxiety.[13]

See Figure 7.2[14] for an illustration of neurotransmitter communication between neurons at the synapse. Antidepressants immediately boost the concentration of chemical messengers in the brain (neurotransmitters), but people typically don't begin to feel better for several weeks or longer. Experts have long wondered why people don't improve as soon as the level of neurotransmitters increases. New theories explain that antidepressants spur the growth and enhanced branching of nerve cells in the hippocampus (a process called neurogenesis), and mood improves over several weeks as nerves grow and form new connections.[15]

11 Harvard Health Publishing. (2019, June 24). *What causes depression?* Harvard Medical School. https://www.health.harvard.edu/mind-and-mood/what-causes-depression

12 Harvard Health Publishing. (2019, June 24). *What causes depression?* Harvard Medical School. https://www.health.harvard.edu/mind-and-mood/what-causes-depression

13 Harvard Health Publishing. (2019, June 24). *What causes depression?* Harvard Medical School. https://www.health.harvard.edu/mind-and-mood/what-causes-depression

14 "1225_Chemical_Synapse.jpg" by Young, KA., Wise, JA., DeSaix, P., Kruse, DH., Poe, B., Johnson, E., Johnson, JE., Korol, O., Betts, JG., & Womble, M. is licensed under CC BY 4.0

15 Harvard Health Publishing. (2019, June 24). *What causes depression?* Harvard Medical School. https://www.health.harvard.edu/mind-and-mood/what-causes-depression

My Notes

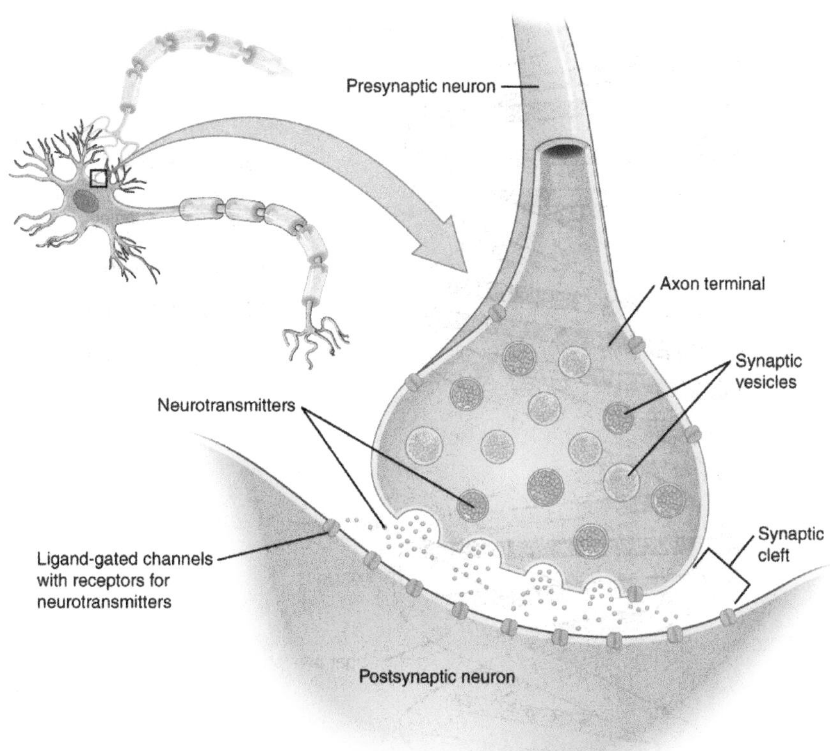

Figure 7.2 Neurotransmitters at the Synapse Level

Genes

Every part of our body, including our brain, is controlled by our genes. Humans have almost 22,000 genes in their DNA within 46 chromosomes inside the nucleus of each cell. The sequence of nitrogen-containing bases within a strand of DNA forms the genes that act as a molecular code instructing cells in the assembly of amino acids into proteins. See Figure 7.3[16] for an image of sequences of bases within a DNA strand that forms genes. Genes make proteins that are involved in biological processes. Throughout life, different genes turn on and off and make the right proteins at the right time. However, genes can alter biology in a way that results in a person's mood becoming unstable. In a person who is genetically vulnerable to depression, any stress (such as a missed deadline at work or a medical illness) can then push this system off balance.[17]

16 "229_Nucleotides-01.jpg" by OpenStax College is licensed under CC BY 3.0. Access for free at http://cnx.org/content/col11496/1.6/

17 Harvard Health Publishing. (2019, June 24). *What causes depression?* Harvard Medical School. https://www.health.harvard.edu/mind-and-mood/what-causes-depression

My Notes

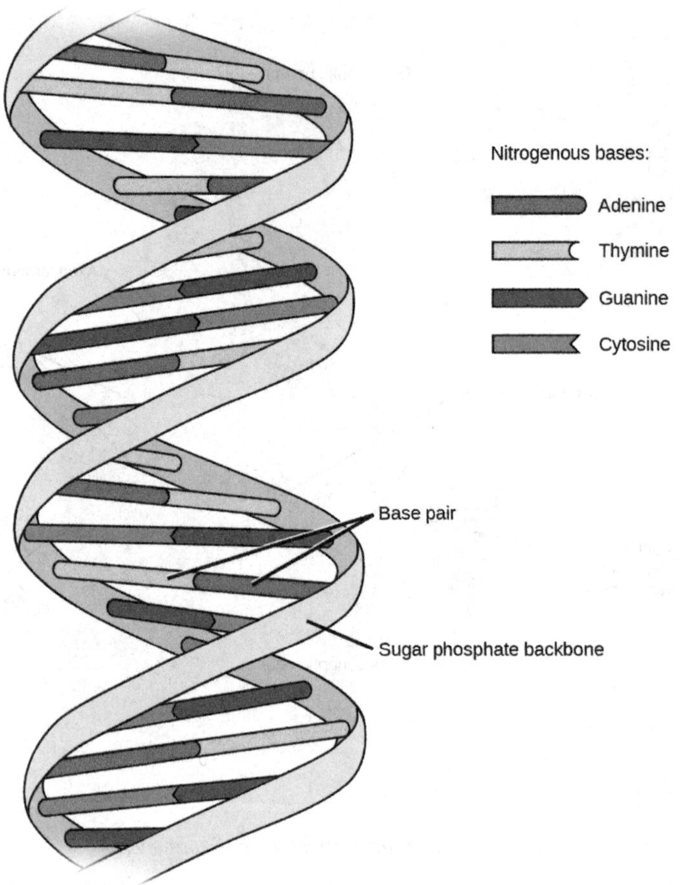

Figure 7.3 Sequence of Bases Within DNA That Form Genes

It is well-known that depressive and bipolar disorders run in families. Mood is affected by dozens of genes, and as our genes differ, so does depression. As researchers pinpoint specific genes involved in mood disorders and better understand their functions, it is hoped that treatment for depressive disorders can become more individualized and more successful as patients receive targeted medication for their specific type of depression.[18]

Genetics provides one perspective on how resilient an individual is in the face of difficult life events. Temperament is determined by a person's genetic inheritance and the experiences they have had in life. For example, one person may have the temperament of an introvert and tend to withdraw from social situations, whereas another person may have the temperament of an extrovert who seeks out social situations and feels energized by them. Cognitive psychologists believe that one's view of the world and assumptions about how the world works influence how a person feels. Individuals develop their assumptions about life early and automatically fall back on them when loss, disappointment, or rejection occurs. For example, a person who was continually criticized as a child may have the genetic inheritance and temperament where they become so self-critical they can't bear the slightest criticism from

---

18 Harvard Health Publishing. (2019, June 24). *What causes depression?* Harvard Medical School. https://www.health.harvard.edu/mind-and-mood/what-causes-depression

My Notes

others, which can slow or block their career progress and make intimate relationships more difficult. Therapy and medications can shift thoughts and attitudes that have developed over time.[19]

Stressful Life Events

At some point, nearly everyone encounters stressful life events such as the death of a loved one, the loss of a job, the diagnosis of a severe illness, or the end of a significant relationship. Many individuals have also experienced traumatic childhood experiences that continue to affect their coping and functioning into adulthood. It is estimated that 61% of adults have experienced early adverse childhood experiences (ACEs) such as abuse, neglect, or growing up in a household with violence, mental illness, substance use, incarceration, or divorce. See Figure 7.4[20] for an illustration of adverse childhood experiences. Toxic stress from ACEs can change brain development and affect how the body responds to stress. ACEs are linked to chronic health problems, mental illness, and substance misuse in adulthood.[21]

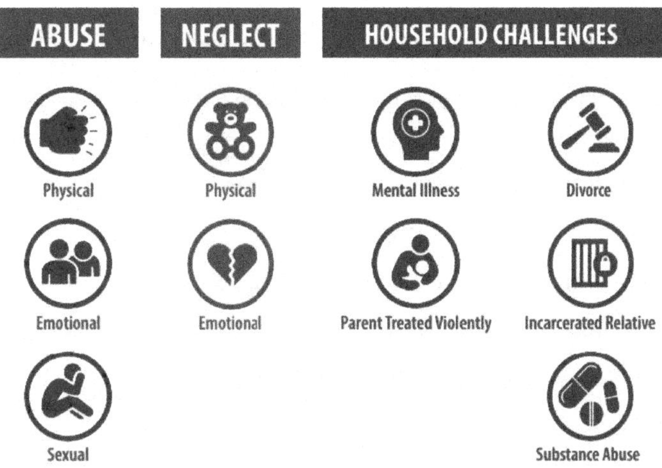

Figure 7.4 Adverse Childhood Experiences (ACEs)

Stress triggers a chain of chemical reactions and responses in the body. If the stress is short-lived, the body usually returns to normal. But when stress is chronic or the system gets stuck in overdrive, changes in the body and brain can be long-lasting. Every real or perceived threat to one's body triggers a cascade of stress hormones that produces physiological changes called the stress response. Normally, a feedback loop allows the body to turn off "fight-or-flight" defenses when the threat passes. In some cases, though, the floodgates never close properly, and cortisol levels rise too often or simply stay high. These elevated cortisol levels can contribute to problems such

19 Harvard Health Publishing. (2019, June 24). *What causes depression?* Harvard Medical School. https://www.health.harvard.edu/mind-and-mood/what-causes-depression

20 "ACEs.png" by unknown author for Centers for Disease Control and Prevention is licensed in the Public Domain. Access for free at https://www.cdc.gov/injury/pdfs/priority/ACEs-Strategic-Plan_Final_508.pdf

21 Centers for Disease Control and Prevention. (2021, April 2). *Adverse childhood experiences (ACEs)*. https://www.cdc.gov/violenceprevention/aces/index.html

My Notes

as high blood pressure, immune suppression, asthma, and depression. Studies have also shown that people who have depressive disorders typically have increased levels of CRH. Antidepressants and electroconvulsive therapy are both known to reduce these high CRH levels. As CRH levels return to normal, depressive symptoms recede. Research also suggests that trauma during childhood can negatively affect the functioning of CRH and the HPA axis throughout life.[22]

Read the Adverse Childhood Experiences Prevention Strategy PDF.

Medical Problems

Certain medical problems are linked to up to 10% to 15% of all depressions. For example, hypothyroidism, a condition where the body produces too little thyroid hormone, often leads to exhaustion and depression, whereas hyperthyroidism (excess thyroid hormone) can trigger manic symptoms. Heart disease has also been linked to depression, with up to half of heart attack survivors reporting feeling blue and many having significant depression. Another example of depression linked to a medical condition is postpartum depression that occurs after pregnancy.[23]

The following medical conditions have also been associated with depression and other mood disorders[24]:

- Degenerative neurological conditions, such as multiple sclerosis, Parkinson's disease, Alzheimer's disease, and Huntington's disease
- Cerebrovascular accidents (i.e., strokes)
- Some nutritional deficiencies, such as a lack of vitamin B12
- Endocrine disorders with the parathyroid or adrenal glands
- Immune system diseases, such as lupus
- Some viruses, such as mononucleosis, hepatitis, and HIV
- Cancer
- Erectile dysfunction in men

When considering the connection between health problems and depression, an important question to address is which came first, the medical condition or the mood changes. Stress of having certain illnesses can trigger depression, whereas in other cases, depression precedes the medical illness and may even contribute to it. If depression is caused by an underlying medical problem, the mood changes should disappear after the medical condition is treated. For example, after hypothyroidism is treated, lethargy and depression often lift. In many cases, however,

---

22 Harvard Health Publishing. (2019, June 24). *What causes depression?* Harvard Medical School. https://www.health.harvard.edu/mind-and-mood/what-causes-depression

23 Harvard Health Publishing. (2019, June 24). *What causes depression?* Harvard Medical School. https://www.health.harvard.edu/mind-and-mood/what-causes-depression

24 Harvard Health Publishing. (2019, June 24). *What causes depression?* Harvard Medical School. https://www.health.harvard.edu/mind-and-mood/what-causes-depression

My Notes

the depression is an independent problem, which means that in order to be successful, treatment must address depression directly.[25]

Symptoms of depression can be a side effect of certain drugs, such as steroids or some types of blood pressure medication. A health care provider can help sort out whether a new medication, a change in dosage, or interactions with other drugs or substances might be affecting an individual's mood.[26]

25 Harvard Health Publishing. (2019, June 24). *What causes depression?* Harvard Medical School. https://www.health.harvard.edu/mind-and-mood/what-causes-depression

26 Harvard Health Publishing. (2019, June 24). *What causes depression?* Harvard Medical School. https://www.health.harvard.edu/mind-and-mood/what-causes-depression

My Notes

7.3 TYPES OF DEPRESSION

Depression is different from the usual mood fluctuations and short-lived emotional responses to everyday life stressors. When it is recurrent with moderate or severe intensity, depression can become a serious health condition that causes the affected person to suffer greatly and function poorly at work and school and can affect relationships with family and friends. At its worst, depression can lead to suicide. Over 700,000 people die every year due to suicide. Barriers to effective care for depression include a lack of resources, lack of trained health care providers, and social stigma associated with mental health disorders.[1] See Figure 7.5[2] for an artistic depiction of an individual experiencing depression.

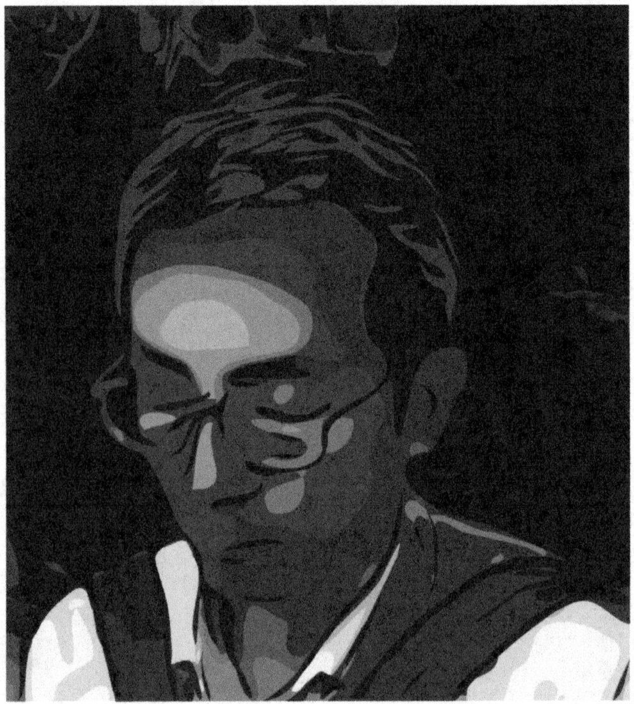

Figure 7.5 Depression

During a **depressive episode**, the person experiences a depressed mood (feeling sad, irritable, empty) or a loss of pleasure or interest in activities (anhedonia) for most of the day, nearly every day, for at least two weeks. Several other symptoms may also be present, which may include poor concentration, feelings of excessive guilt or low self-worth, hopelessness about the future, thoughts about dying or suicide, disrupted sleep, changes in appetite or weight, and feeling especially tired or low in energy. In some cultural contexts, some people may express their mood changes more readily in the form of bodily symptoms (such as pain, fatigue, or weakness) that are not due to another medical condition. During a depressive episode, the person experiences significant difficulty and/or impairment in important areas of personal, family, social, educational, and work functioning.[3]

---

1 World Health Organization. (2021, September 13). *Depression.* https://www.who.int/news-room/fact-sheets/detail/depression

2 "320531.png" by j4p4n at openclipart.org is licensed in the Public Domain.

3 World Health Organization. (2021, September 13). *Depression.* https://www.who.int/news-room/fact-sheets/detail/depression

My Notes

A depressive episode is categorized by a provider as mild, moderate, or severe depending on the number and severity of symptoms, as well as the impact on the individual's functioning.[4] Mild severity indicates the symptoms to make the diagnosis are present but result in minor impairment in social or occupational functioning. Moderate severity indicates symptoms and impairment are between mild and severe. Severe indicates the intensity is seriously distressing, unmanageable, and markedly interferes with social and occupational functioning. Read the full list of criteria for Major Depressive Disorder from the *DSM-5* in the following box.

DSM-5 Criteria for Major Depressive Disorder[5]

1. Five or more of the following symptoms have been present during the same two-week period and represent a change from previous functioning; at least one of the symptoms is either (1) depressed mood or (2) loss of interest or pleasure.

    - Depressed mood most of the day, nearly every day, as indicated by either subjective report (e.g., feels sad, empty, hopeless) or observation made by others (e.g., appears tearful). (Note: In children and adolescents, can be irritable mood.)
    - Markedly diminished interest or pleasure in all, or almost all, activities most of the day, nearly every day.
    - Significant weight loss when not dieting or weight gain (i.e., a change of more than 5% of body weight in a month) or decrease or increase in appetite nearly every day. (Note: In children, consider failure to make expected weight gain.)
    - Insomnia or hypersomnia nearly every day.
    - Psychomotor agitation or retardation nearly every day (observable by others, not merely subjective feelings of restlessness or being slowed down).
    - Fatigue or loss of energy nearly every day.
    - Feelings of worthlessness or excessive or inappropriate guilt (which may be delusional) nearly every day (not merely self-reproach or guilt about being sick).
    - Diminished ability to think or concentrate, or indecisiveness, nearly every day (either by subjective account or as observed by others).
    - Recurrent thoughts of death (not just fear of dying), recurrent suicidal ideation without a specific plan, or a suicide attempt or a specific plan for committing suicide.

2. The symptoms cause clinically significant distress or impairment in social, occupational, or other important areas of functioning.

---

4 World Health Organization. (2021, September 13). *Depression.* https://www.who.int/news-room/fact-sheets/detail/depression

5 Schreiber, J., & Culpepper, L. (2021). Suicidal ideation and behavior in adults. *UpToDate.* Retrieved November 16, 2021, from https://www.uptodate.com/

My Notes

3. The episode is not attributable to the physiological effects of a substance or another medical condition.

Types of Depression

According to the *DSM-5*, the types of depressive disorders include the following[6]:

- **Major Depressive Disorder:** Five or more symptoms are present during the same two-week period and represent a change from previous functioning and at least one of the symptoms is depressed mood or loss of interest or pleasure. Read the symptoms of depression in the previous box.
  - Specifiers may be attached to the diagnosis such as:
    - With anxious distress (tense and/or restless)
    - With mixed features (manic symptoms)
    - With psychotic features (delusions and/or hallucinations)
    - With peripartum onset (includes perinatal and postpartum depression)
    - With a seasonal pattern (includes seasonal affective disorder)
- **Persistent Depressive Disorder (Dysthymia):** Depressed mood for most of the day for at least two years.
- **Premenstrual Dysphoric Disorder:** In the majority of menstrual cycles, at least five symptoms are present in the week before the onset of menses, start to improve after the onset of menses, and become minimal or absent in the week postmenses.
- **Substance/Medication-Induced Depressive Disorder:** A persistent disturbance in mood that develops during or soon after substance intoxication or during withdrawal from a substance.
- **Depressive Disorder Due to Another Medical Condition:** A persistent period of depressed mood that is the direct consequence of another medical condition.

Seasonal Affective Disorder

Seasonal affective disorder (SAD) is a type of major depressive disorder that affects about 5% of adults in the United States. People with SAD experience mood changes and symptoms similar to depression. The symptoms usually occur during the fall and winter months when there is less sunlight and usually improve with the arrival

6 American Psychiatric Association. (2013). *Desk reference to the diagnostic criteria from DSM-5.*

My Notes

of spring. SAD is more than just "winter blues." The symptoms can be distressing and overwhelming and can interfere with daily functioning.[7]

SAD has been linked to a biochemical imbalance in the brain prompted by shorter daylight hours and less sunlight in winter. As seasons change, people experience a shift in their biological internal clock or circadian rhythm that can cause them to be out of step with their daily schedule. SAD is more common in people living far from the equator where there are fewer daylight hours in the winter.[8]

SAD can be effectively treated with light therapy, antidepressant medications, cognitive behavioral therapy, or some combination of these. While symptoms will generally improve on their own with the change of season, symptoms can improve more quickly with treatment. **Light therapy** involves sitting in front of a light therapy box that emits a very bright light (and filters out harmful ultraviolet [UV] rays). It usually requires 20 minutes or more per day, typically first thing in the morning during the winter months. Most people see some improvements from light therapy within one or two weeks of beginning treatment. For some people, increased exposure to natural sunlight can help improve symptoms of SAD by spending time outside or arranging their home or office space to increase exposure to windows during daylight hours. General wellness activities such as performing regular exercise, eating healthfully, getting enough sleep, and staying active and connected (such as volunteering, participating in group activities, and getting together with friends and family) can also help.[9]

Peripartum Depression

Pregnancy and the period after delivery can be a vulnerable time for women. Mothers can experience significant biological, emotional, financial, and social changes during this time. Up to 70 percent of new mothers experience the "baby blues," a short-term condition that does not interfere with their daily activities and does not require medical attention. Symptoms include crying for no reason, irritability, restlessness, and anxiety. These symptoms generally last up to two weeks and resolve on their own.[10]

However, as many as 3 to 6% of women experience a type of major depressive disorder during pregnancy (called **perinatal depression**) or after delivery (called postpartum depression).[11] See Figure 7.6[12] for an illustration of perinatal depression from the National Institutes of Health.

Postpartum depression includes feelings of extreme sadness, anxiety, and exhaustion that may make it difficult for these new mothers to complete daily care activities for themselves and/or for their babies. Untreated peripartum depression is not only a problem for the mother's health and quality of life but can also affect the well-being of the baby. Postpartum depression can cause bonding issues with the baby and also contribute to sleeping and feeding

---

7 American Psychiatric Association. (2020). *Seasonal affective disorder (SAD)*. https://www.psychiatry.org/patients-families/depression/seasonal-affective-disorder

8 American Psychiatric Association. (2020). *Seasonal affective disorder (SAD)*. https://www.psychiatry.org/patients-families/depression/seasonal-affective-disorder

9 American Psychiatric Association. (2020). *Seasonal affective disorder (SAD)*. https://www.psychiatry.org/patients-families/depression/seasonal-affective-disorder

10 American Psychiatric Association. (2020). *What is peripartum depression (formerly postpartum)?* https://www.psychiatry.org/patients-families/postpartum-depression/what-is-postpartum-depression

11 American Psychiatric Association. (2013). *Desk reference to the diagnostic criteria from DSM-5*.

12 This image is a derivative of "20-mh-8116-perinataldepression.pdf" by National Institute of Mental Health and is licensed in the Public Domain. Access for free at https://www.nimh.nih.gov/health/publications/perinatal-depression.

My Notes

problems for the baby. In the long-term, children of mothers with peripartum depression are at greater risk for cognitive, emotional, developmental and verbal deficits, and impaired social skills.[13]

Severe postpartum depression can lead to postpartum psychosis, a medical emergency. Women who have **postpartum psychosis** may have delusions (thoughts or beliefs that are not true), hallucinations (seeing, hearing, or smelling things that are not there), mania (a high, elated mood that often seems out of touch with reality), paranoia, and confusion. Women who have postpartum psychosis are at risk for harming themselves or their child and should receive help as soon as possible by calling 911 or taking the mother to the nearest emergency room.

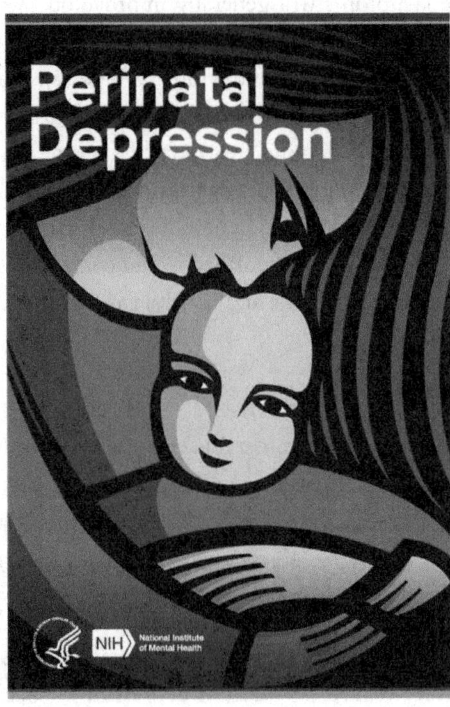

Figure 7.6 Perinatal Depression

Read more information about perinatal depression on the National Institute of Mental Health's Perinatal Depression web page.

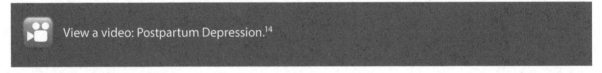

Mixed Features

Depressive episodes can also be classified as "mixed," meaning they alternate with periods of manic symptoms such as euphoria, irritability, increased activity, increased talkativeness, racing thoughts, increased self-esteem,

13 American Psychiatric Association. (2020, October). *What is peripartum depression (formerly postpartum)?* https://www.psychiatry.org/patients-families/postpartum-depression/what-is-postpartum-depression

14 National Institute of Mental Health. (2016, April 19). *Postpartum depression* [Video]. YouTube. All rights reserved. https://youtu.be/zbUl2hZNlKY

My Notes

decreased need for sleep, distractibility, and impulsive reckless behavior.[15] Characteristics and treatment of bipolar disorder are further discussed in the "Bipolar Disorders" chapter. See Figure 7.7[16] for a comparison of the features of different types of mood disorders.

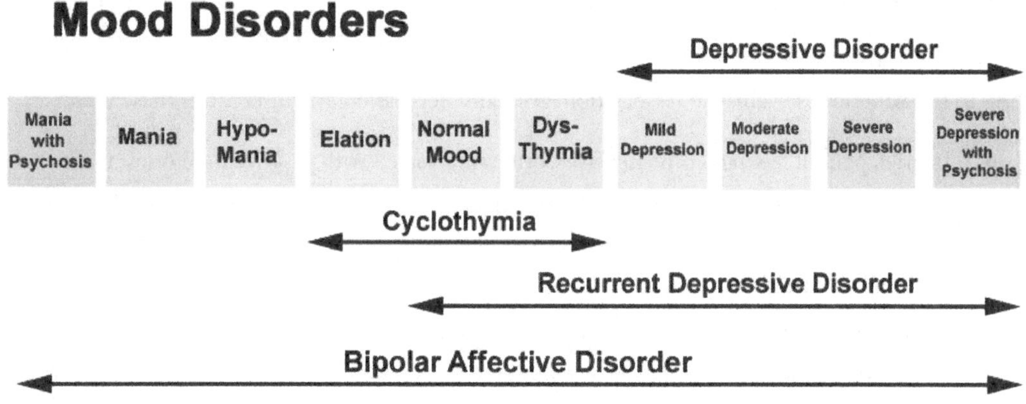

Figure 7.7 Mood Disorders. Used under Fair Use.

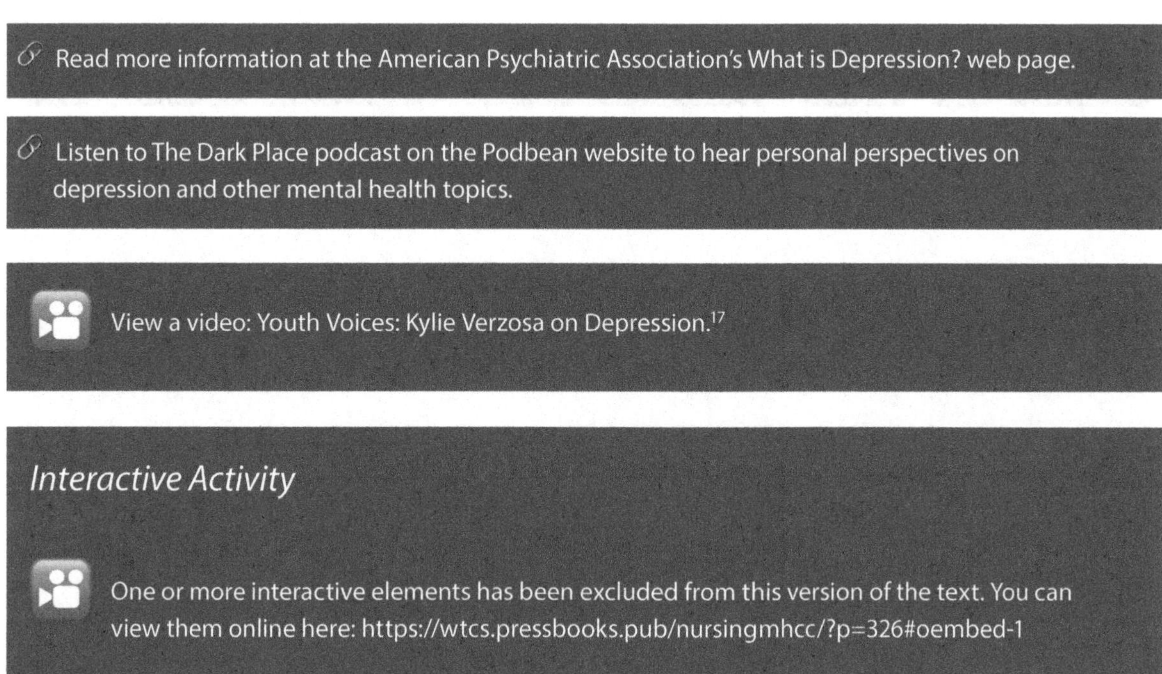

Read more information at the American Psychiatric Association's What is Depression? web page.

Listen to The Dark Place podcast on the Podbean website to hear personal perspectives on depression and other mental health topics.

View a video: Youth Voices: Kylie Verzosa on Depression.[17]

Interactive Activity

One or more interactive elements has been excluded from this version of the text. You can view them online here: https://wtcs.pressbooks.pub/nursingmhcc/?p=326#oembed-1

---

15 World Health Organization. (2021, September 13). *Depression.* https://www.who.int/news-room/fact-sheets/detail/depression

16 "mood-disorders.jpg" by Dr. Vipul Rastogi, MBBS; DCP (Ireland); MRCPsych (UK) Speciality Registrar, Hampshire Partnership Trust, UK for www.clinicaljunior.com. Image used under Fair Use. Access for free at http://www.clinicaljunior.com/psychmoodvipul.html

17 World Health Organization (WHO). (2018, September 19). *Youth voices: Kylie Verzosa on depression* [Video]. YouTube. Licensed in the Public Domain. https://youtu.be/tRc4XZXYTgY

My Notes

Depression Associated With Grief

People have difficulty coping with the death or loss of a loved one, job, or relationship. It is normal for feelings of sadness or grief to develop in response to such situations, but being sad is not the same as having depression. The grieving process is natural and unique to each individual and shares some of the same features of depression. Both grief and depression can involve intense sadness and withdrawal from usual activities with increased risk for suicide.

According to the American Psychiatric Association, grief and depression are different in these ways[18]:

- In grief, painful feelings come in waves, often intermixed with positive memories of the deceased. In major depression, mood and/or interest (pleasure) are decreased for most of two weeks.
- In grief, self-esteem is usually maintained. In major depression, feelings of worthlessness and self-loathing are common.
- In grief, thoughts of death may surface when thinking of or fantasizing about "joining" the deceased loved one. In major depression, thoughts are focused on ending one's life due to feeling worthless or undeserving of living or being unable to cope with the pain of depression.

Grief and depression can coexist. When grief and depression occur together, the grief is more severe and lasts longer than grief without depression. Nurses must be able to distinguish between symptoms of grief and depression and assist people in getting the help, support, or treatment they need.[19]

Read more information about grief in the "Grief and Loss" chapter in Open RN *Nursing Fundamentals*.

---

18 American Psychiatric Association. (2020). *What is depression?* https://www.psychiatry.org/patients-families/depression/what-is-depression

19 American Psychiatric Association. (2020). *What is depression?* https://www.psychiatry.org/patients-families/depression/what-is-depression

7.4 TREATMENTS FOR DEPRESSION

My Notes

Depression is one of the most treatable mental disorders. Between 80% and 90% percent of people with depression eventually respond well to treatment. Almost all patients gain some relief from their symptoms with effective treatment. Before a diagnosis is made or treatment planned, a mental health care provider should conduct a thorough diagnostic evaluation, including an interview, mental status examination, psychosocial assessment, and a physical examination performed by a primary care provider. In some cases, a blood test might be done to make sure the depression is not due to a medical condition like a thyroid problem or a vitamin deficiency. The evaluation also explores medical and family histories, cultural beliefs, and environmental factors as part of the psychosocial assessment with the goal of arriving at a diagnosis and planning a course of action. Treatments for depression include medications, psychotherapy, electroconvulsive therapy, transcranial magnetic stimulation, and encouraging self-care and effective coping strategies. Nurses should keep patient-centered care and client preferences in mind when implementing a client's treatment plan. For example, the client should be educated about the possible adverse effects associated with antidepressant medication, and their ability to pay for and obtain transportation to treatments like psychotherapy should be considered.[1]

Antidepressant Medications

Brain chemistry may contribute to an individual's depression and may factor into their treatment. Read more about the causes of depression in the "Causes of Depression" section of this chapter. For this reason, providers may prescribe antidepressants to help modify an individual's brain chemistry.

Antidepressants are used to regulate and increase neurotransmitters in the brain to improve mood. There are several classes of antidepressants with different mechanisms of action and potential adverse side effects. Classes of antidepressants, their mechanism of action, and common side effects are outlined in Table 7.4.[2] Common side effects are listed in this table by frequency of their occurrence. Some medications can cause QTc prolongation, which refers to delayed cardiac electrical conduction that can lead to dysrhythmias. Tricyclic antidepressants (TCAs) and monoamine oxidase inhibitors (MAOIs) often cause anticholingeric side effects (e.g., tachycardia, urinary retention, constipation, dry mouth, blurred vision, confusion, psychomotor slowing, sedation, and delirium). A specific medication class is typically initiated by the provider based on the individual's symptoms, potential side effects, cost, and family history of success with certain medications.

Review neurotransmitter actions and related central nervous system physiology in the "Psychotropics Medications" chapter.

---

1 American Psychiatric Association. (2020). *What is depression?* https://www.psychiatry.org/patients-families/depression/what-is-depression

2 Side effects of antidepressant medication. *UpToDate*. Retrieved July 14, 2022, from https://www.uptodate.com/

My Notes

Table 7.4 Antidepressants		
Medication Class	**Mechanism of Action**	**Common Side Effects** **(*Indicates medical emergency)**
Serotonin-Norepinephrine Reuptake Inhibitors (SNRIs) Common examples: Venlafaxine Duloxetine	Block the uptake of both serotonin and norepinephrine from the cell synapse. Similar to SSRIs but with two neurotransmitters.	■ Gastrointestinal upset ■ Sexual dysfunction ■ Drowsiness ■ Insomnia ■ Agitation ■ Weight gain
Selective Serotonin Reuptake Inhibitors (SSRIs) Common examples: Fluoxetine Sertraline Citalopram	Impact the receptors of the cell synapse to inhibit or prevent the uptake of serotonin, making the neurotransmitter serotonin stay in the synapse longer.	■ Sexual dysfunction ■ Gastrointestinal upset ■ QTc prolongation ■ Weight gain ■ Insomnia ■ Agitation ■ Drowsiness ■ Dizziness ■ Headache ■ Dry mouth ■ Constipation ■ Tremor ■ *Serotonin syndrome
Tricyclic Antidepressants (TCAs) Common examples: Amitriptyline Nortriptyline	Block the presynaptic receptor for norepinephrine and partially serotonin. This makes the neurotransmitter norepinephrine level increase in the synapse.	■ Anticholinergic side effects ■ Orthostatic hypotension ■ Drowsiness ■ QTc prolongation ■ Insomnia ■ Agitation ■ Weight gain ■ Sexual dysfunction

My Notes

Medication Class	Mechanism of Action	Common Side Effects (*Indicates medical emergency)
Monoamine Oxidase Inhibitors (MAOIs) Common examples: Phenelzine Tranylcypromine	Block the enzyme that breaks down monoamine, which causes an increase in the level of neurotransmitters serotonin and norepinephrine.	■ Sexual dysfunction ■ Orthostatic hypotension ■ Insomnia ■ Agitation ■ Anticholinergic side effects ■ Drowsiness ■ Gastrointestinal upset ■ Weight gain ■ *Hypertensive crisis
Norepinephrine and Dopamine Reuptake Inhibitor (NDRI) Bupropion	Blocks the uptake of both norepinephrine and dopamine from the cell synapse.	■ Tachycardia ■ Diaphoresis ■ Weight loss ■ Gastrointestinal upset ■ Agitation ■ Dizziness ■ Headache ■ Insomnia ■ Tremor ■ Blurred vision

Antidepressants may produce some improvement within the first week or two, but full benefits may not be seen for two to three months. If a patient feels little or no improvement after several weeks, the mental health care provider can alter the dose of the medication, add another medication, or substitute another antidepressant. In a similar manner, if a client develops ongoing bothersome side effects, the provider can switch them to a different medication. Nurses should encourage clients to contact their mental health care prescriber if a medication is not working within the expected time frame or if they are experiencing ongoing bothersome side effects. It is typically recommended that clients continue to take medication(s) for six or more months after the symptoms have improved. Long-term maintenance therapy may be suggested to decrease the risk of future episodes for people at high risk for recurrence.[3]

Black Box Warning

A **Black Box Warning** is a significant warning from the Food and Drug Administration (FDA) that alerts the public and health care providers to serious side effects, such as injury or death. Black Box Warnings are in place for all classes of antidepressants used with children, adolescents, and young adults due to a higher risk of suicide.

3 American Psychiatric Association. (2020). *What is depression?* https://www.psychiatry.org/patients-families/depression/what-is-depression

My Notes

All clients receiving antidepressants should be monitored for signs of worsening depression or changing behavior, especially when the medication is started or dosages changed.

Adverse/Side Effects

Nurses must monitor clients receiving antidepressants for side effects and report concerns to the prescribing provider. Clients should be instructed to immediately call their provider if they have any of the following symptoms, especially if they are new or worsening[4]:

- Thoughts about suicide or dying
- Attempts to commit suicide
- Worsening depression
- Anxiety
- Agitation or restlessness
- Panic attacks
- Trouble sleeping (insomnia)
- Irritability
- Aggression, anger, or violence
- Dangerous impulses
- Increased activity and talking (i.e., signs of mania)
- Other unusual changes in behavior or mood

Serotonin Syndrome

High doses of antidepressants or a combination of medications that affect serotonin, such as antidepressants or triptans (used to treat migraine headaches) can cause a medical emergency called serotonin syndrome. The presentation of **serotonin syndrome** is extremely variable, ranging from mild symptoms to a life-threatening syndrome. It typically develops within 24 hours from the increased dosage or combination of medications and can be fatal.

Symptoms of serotonin syndrome can be classified into three categories[5,6,7]:

- Mental status changes: Agitation, restlessness, or delirium
- Autonomic hyperactivity: Tachycardia, hypertension, hyperthermia, diaphoresis, shivering, vomiting, or diarrhea

---

4 National Institute of Mental Health. (2016, October). *Mental health medications.* U.S. Department of Health & Human Services. https://www.nimh.nih.gov/health/topics/mental-health-medications

5 A.D.A.M. Medical Encyclopedia [Internet]. Atlanta (GA): A.D.A.M., Inc.; c1997-2021. *Serotonin syndrome.* [updated 2021, November 30]. https://medlineplus.gov/ency/article/007272.htm

6 Boyer, E. W. (2021). Serotonin syndrome (serotonin toxicity). *UpToDate.* Retrieved on December 27, 2021, from https://www.uptodate.com/

7 Tanen, D. (2021, February). *Serotonin syndrome.* Merck Manual Professional Version. https://www.merckmanuals.com/professional/injuries-poisoning/heat-illness/serotonin-syndrome

- Neuromuscular hyperactivity: Tremor, muscle hypertonia or rigidity, myoclonus, hyperreflexia, or clonus (including rapid, horizontal eye movements)

A mnemonic commonly used to remember the symptoms of serotonin syndrome is **SHIVERS**:

- **S:** Shivering: A neuromuscular symptom similar to tremors specific to serotonin syndrome
- **H:** Hyperreflexia (and myoclonus): Hyperactive reflexes most prominent in the lower extremities
- **I:** Increased Temperature
- **V:** Vital Sign Abnormalities: Tachycardia, tachypnea, and labile blood pressure
- **E:** Encephalopathy: Mental status changes such as agitation, delirium, and confusion
- **R:** Restlessness
- **S:** Sweating

People may get slowly worse and can become severely ill if not quickly treated. Untreated serotonin syndrome can be deadly. With treatment, symptoms usually go away within 24 hours, but permanent kidney damage may result even with treatment. Uncontrolled muscle spasms can cause severe muscle breakdown called rhabdomyolysis. Myoglobin is released into the blood with muscle breakdown and clogs renal filtrations, which can cause severe kidney damage if serotonin syndrome isn't recognized promptly and treated.

Treatment of serotonin syndrome may include the following[8,9]:

- Stopping all serotonergic medications.
- Providing supportive care to normalize vital signs such as IV fluids, cooling measures, and medications to control heart rate and blood pressure.
- Sedating with benzodiazepines, such as diazepam or lorazepam, to decrease agitation, seizure-like movements, and muscle stiffness.
- If symptoms persist, administering cyproheptadine to block serotonin production.

Serotonin syndrome, in its most severe form, can resemble neuroleptic malignant syndrome (NMS) caused by antipsychotic medications. However, NMS develops over a period of days to weeks.

Hypertensive Crisis

Hypertensive crisis can occur when clients taking monoamine oxidase inhibitors (MAOIs) also take medications containing pseudoephedrine or eat foods containing tyramine (aged foods; fermented foods; cured meats; alcoholic beverages such as beer or red wine; or overripe fruits such as raisins, prunes, or bananas). MAOIs inhibit the breakdown of tyramine, causing elevated tyramine levels in the body that can lead to hypertensive crisis. **Hypertensive crisis** is a medical emergency defined as severe hypertension (blood pressure over 180/120 mm Hg) with acute end-organ damage such as stroke, myocardial infarction, or acute kidney damage. Symptoms may include a severe headache accompanied with confusion and blurred vision. Tachycardia or bradycardia may be present and associated with constricting chest pain. Other symptoms include neck stiffness or soreness, nausea or

---

8 Boyer, E. W. (2021). Serotonin syndrome (serotonin toxicity). *UpToDate.* Retrieved on December 27, 2021, from https://www.uptodate.com/

9 Tanen, D. (2021, February). *Serotonin syndrome.* Merck Manual Professional Version. https://www.merckmanuals.com/professional/injuries-poisoning/heat-illness/serotonin-syndrome

My Notes

vomiting, sweating, dilated pupils, photophobia, shortness of breath, severe anxiety, and unresponsiveness. Seizures may occur, as well as intracranial bleeding in association with the increased blood pressure. Hypertensive crisis is treated in the intensive care unit with intravenous medications that safely and quickly lower the blood pressure.[10,11]

Patient Education Regarding Antidepressants

Clients should be instructed it may take 4 to 6 weeks for antidepressants to achieve their full effectiveness. They should not suddenly stop taking antidepressants or they may experience withdrawal symptoms. When it is time to stop the medication, the provider will slowly and safely decrease the dose. If clients stop taking the medication before the provider advises, the depression may return. They may not feel better with the first antidepressant they try, and they may need to try several different classes of medications to find one that works best for them.

Psychotherapy

Psychotherapy may be used alone for treatment of mild depression or in combination with antidepressant medications for moderate to severe depression. Psychotherapy may involve only the individual, but it can include others such as family members or couples therapy to help address issues within these close relationships. Depending on the severity of the depression, significant improvement can be made in 10 to 15 sessions. **Group therapy** brings people with similar disorders together in a supportive environment to learn how others cope in similar situations.[12]

Cognitive Behavioral Therapy

Cognitive behavioral therapy (CBT) is a form of psychotherapy that is effective for a range of problems, including depression, anxiety disorders, alcohol and drug use problems, marital conflict, eating disorders, and severe mental illness. CBT helps a person to recognize distorted/negative thinking with the goal of changing thoughts and behaviors to respond to changes in a more positive manner.[13] Numerous research studies suggest that CBT leads to significant improvement in functioning and quality of life. Studies show that CBT has been demonstrated to be as effective as, or more effective than, other forms of psychological therapy or psychiatric medications.[14]

CBT is based on these core principles[15]:

- Psychological problems are based, in part, on faulty or unhelpful ways of thinking.

---

10 This work is a derivative of *DailyMed* by U.S. National Library of Medicine and is available in the Public Domain

11 Sheps, S. G. (2021, February 16). *Hypertensive crisis: What are the symptoms?* Mayo Clinic. https://www.mayoclinic.org/diseases-conditions/high-blood-pressure/expert-answers/hypertensive-crisis/faq-20058491#:~:text=A%20hypertensive%20crisis%20is%20a,higher%20%E2%80%94%20can%20damage%20blood%20vessels

12 American Psychiatric Association. (2020). *What is depression?* https://www.psychiatry.org/patients-families/depression/what-is-depression

13 American Psychiatric Association. (2020). *What is depression?* https://www.psychiatry.org/patients-families/depression/what-is-depression

14 Clinical Practice Guideline for the Treatment of Posttraumatic Stress Disorder. (2017, July). *What is cognitive behavioral treatment?* American Psychological Association. https://www.apa.org/ptsd-guideline/patients-and-families/cognitive-behavioral

15 Clinical Practice Guideline for the Treatment of Posttraumatic Stress Disorder. (2017, July). *What is cognitive behavioral treatment?* American Psychological Association. https://www.apa.org/ptsd-guideline/patients-and-families/cognitive-behavioral

My Notes

- Psychological problems are based, in part, on learned patterns of unhelpful behavior.
- People suffering from psychological problems can learn better ways of coping with them, thereby relieving their symptoms and increasing quality of life.

CBT treatment involves efforts to change thinking patterns. These strategies might include the following[16]:

- Learning to recognize one's distortions in thinking that are creating problems, and then reevaluating them in light of reality.
- Gaining a better understanding of the behavior and motivation of others.
- Using problem-solving skills to cope with difficult situations.
- Learning to develop a greater sense of confidence in one's own abilities.

CBT treatment also usually involves efforts to change behavioral patterns. These strategies might include facing one's fears instead of avoiding them, using role-playing to prepare for potentially problematic interactions with others, and learning to calm one's mind and relax one's body.[17]

CBT aims to help clients develop skills to manage their feelings in healthy ways. Through in-session exercises and "homework" between sessions, clients develop coping skills, whereby they learn ways to change their own thinking and behavior, ultimately changing how they feel. CBT therapists focus on current situations, thought patterns, and behaviors rather than past events. A certain amount of information about one's history is needed, but the focus is primarily on developing more effective ways of coping with life moving forward.[18]

Dialectic Behavior Therapy

Dialectical behavior therapy (DBT) is a type of cognitive behavioral therapy that provides clients with new skills to manage painful emotions and decrease conflict in relationships. It has been used successfully to treat people experiencing depression, bulimia, binge-eating, bipolar disorder, post-traumatic stress disorder, borderline personality disorder, and substance abuse. DBT focuses on providing therapeutic skills in four key areas[19]:

- Mindfulness focuses on improving an individual's ability to accept and be present in the current moment.
- Distress tolerance is geared toward increasing a person's tolerance of negative emotion, rather than trying to escape from it.
- Emotion regulation strategies are used to manage and change intense emotions that are causing problems in a person's life.

---

16 Clinical Practice Guideline for the Treatment of Posttraumatic Stress Disorder. (2017, July). *What is cognitive behavioral treatment?* American Psychological Association. https://www.apa.org/ptsd-guideline/patients-and-families/cognitive-behavioral

17 Clinical Practice Guideline for the Treatment of Posttraumatic Stress Disorder. (2017, July). *What is cognitive behavioral treatment?* American Psychological Association. https://www.apa.org/ptsd-guideline/patients-and-families/cognitive-behavioral

18 Clinical Practice Guideline for the Treatment of Posttraumatic Stress Disorder. (2017, July). *What is cognitive behavioral treatment?* American Psychological Association. https://www.apa.org/ptsd-guideline/patients-and-families/cognitive-behavioral

19 Psychology Today. (n.d.). *Dialectical behavior therapy.* https://www.psychologytoday.com/us/therapy-types/dialectical-behavior-therapy

My Notes

- Interpersonal effectiveness techniques allow a person to communicate with others in a way that is assertive, maintains self-respect, and strengthens relationships.

Electroconvulsive Therapy

Electroconvulsive therapy (ECT) is a medical treatment reserved for patients with severe major depression who have not responded to medications, psychotherapy, or other treatments. It involves a brief electrical stimulation of the brain while the patient is under anesthesia. A client typically receives ECT two to three times a week for a total of 6 to 12 treatments. It is usually managed by a team of trained medical professionals, including a psychiatrist, an anesthesiologist, and a nurse.[20] See Figure 7.8[21] for an image showing ECT electrode placement.

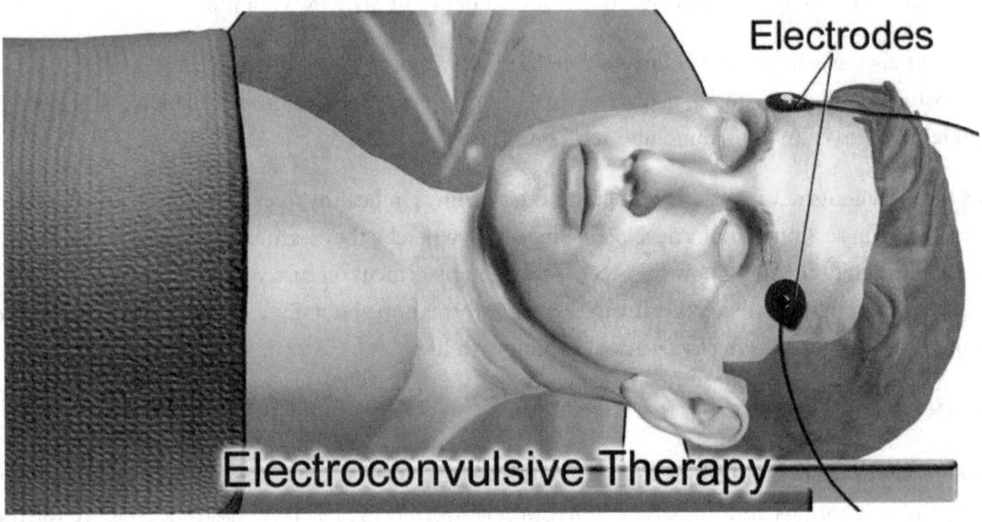

Figure 7.8 Electroconvulsive Therapy

Nursing considerations regarding ECT include the following:

- Pre-procedure education
- Securement of informed consent
- Pre-procedure preparation
- Screening tools used pre- and post-ECT to evaluate side effects, including memory loss
- Medication administration
- Post-ECT care, such as monitoring vital signs and for changes in airway, breathing, and circulation, and implementing fall risk precautions post-anesthesia

---

20 American Psychiatric Association. (2020). *What is depression?* https://www.psychiatry.org/patients-families/depression/what-is-depression

21 "Electroconvulsive_Therapy.png" by BruceBlaus is licensed under CC BY-SA 4.0

My Notes

A client must provide written informed consent before ECT is administered. In situations where a client is too ill to make decisions for themselves, the consent process is governed by state law (for example, a court-appointed guardian).[22]

Clients and their families should discuss all options for treatment with the psychiatrist before making a specific treatment decision. They should be provided with sufficient information to fully understand the procedure and the potential benefits, risks, and side effects of each treatment option before providing written consent.[23]

General anesthesia is provided during ECT, so presurgical preparation is provided with typical dietary restrictions before the procedure. Typically, this means no food or water after midnight and only a sip of water with morning medications. An intravenous line is inserted, and electrode pads are placed on the head.

A client typically receives ECT two or three times a week for a total of 6 to 12 treatments, depending on the severity of symptoms and the response to treatment. At the time of each treatment, a patient is given general anesthesia and a muscle relaxant, and electrodes are attached to the scalp at precise locations. The patient's brain is stimulated with a brief controlled series of electrical pulses. This causes a seizure within the brain that lasts for approximately one minute. The patient is asleep for the procedure and awakens after 5-10 minutes, much as from minor surgery.[24]

ECT treatment has been associated with some risks such as short-term memory loss and difficulty learning. Some people have trouble remembering events that occurred in the weeks before the treatment or earlier. In most cases, memory problems improve within a couple of months. Some patients may experience longer-lasting problems, including permanent gaps in memory.[25]

Transcranial Magnetic Stimulation

Transcranial Magnetic Stimulation (TMS) is a noninvasive procedure that uses magnetic fields to stimulate nerve cells in the brain to improve symptoms of depression. TMS is typically used when other depression treatments haven't been effective. It uses a magnet to activate the brain. Unlike electroconvulsive therapy (ECT), in which electrical stimulation is more generalized, TMS can be targeted to a specific site in the brain. A typical TMS session lasts 30 to 60 minutes and does not require anesthesia. During the procedure, an electromagnetic coil is held against the forehead near an area of the brain that is thought to be involved in mood regulation. Short electromagnetic pulses are administered through the coil. The magnetic pulses easily pass through the skull and cause small electrical currents that stimulate nerve cells in the targeted brain region. The magnetic field is about the same strength as that of a magnetic resonance imaging (MRI) scan. The person generally feels a slight knocking or tapping on the head as the pulses are administered. The muscles of the scalp, jaw, or face may contract or tingle during the procedure, and mild headaches or brief light-headedness may result after the procedure. It is also

---

22 American Psychiatric Association. (2019). *What is electroconvulsive therapy (ECT)?* https://www.psychiatry.org/patients-families/ect

23 American Psychiatric Association. (2019). *What is electroconvulsive therapy (ECT)?* https://www.psychiatry.org/patients-families/ect

24 American Psychiatric Association. (2019). *What is electroconvulsive therapy (ECT)?* https://www.psychiatry.org/patients-families/ect

25 American Psychiatric Association. (2019). *What is electroconvulsive therapy (ECT)?* https://www.psychiatry.org/patients-families/ect

My Notes

possible that the procedure could cause a seizure, although this adverse effect is uncommon. Because the treatment is relatively new, long-term side effects are unknown.[26]

Self-Care and Coping Strategies

Nurses can teach clients many coping strategies to reduce symptoms of depression. For example, regular exercise helps create positive feelings and improves mood. Getting enough quality sleep on a regular basis, eating a healthy diet, and avoiding alcohol (a depressant) can also reduce symptoms of depression.[27] Read more about coping strategies in the "Stress, Coping, and Crisis Intervention" chapter.

26 National Institute of Mental Health. (2016, June). *Brain stimulation therapies*. U.S. Department of Health and Human Services. https://www.nimh.nih.gov/health/topics/brain-stimulation-therapies/brain-stimulation-therapies

27 American Psychiatric Association. (2020). *What is depression?* https://www.psychiatry.org/patients-families/depression/what-is-depression

7.5 APPLYING THE NURSING PROCESS TO DEPRESSIVE DISORDERS

My Notes

Assessment

Assessing a client with a depressive disorder focuses on both verbal and nonverbal assessments. As the registered nurse conducts follow-up assessments, findings are compared to baseline admission assessments.

The role of the nurse in caring for clients with depression is related to primary nursing care, as well as collaboration with interprofessional team members. As a team member, the nurse may collaborate with psychiatrists, psychologists, licensed social workers, and other health care providers. The scope and practice of each team member is clearly defined within their professional licensure.

Psychiatric Interview

The registered nurse uses specific questions during the client's admission process based on agency policy. It is also important to consider the impact of culture on a client's perception of their illness. See suggested "Cultural Formulation Interview Questions" in the "Application of the Nursing Process in Mental Health Care" chapter.

Mental Status Examination

See Table 7.5a for common findings when assessing a client with a depressive disorder. (See expected findings for these components of a mental status examination in the "Assessment" section in Chapter 4.) Critical findings that require immediate notification of the provider are bolded with an asterisk.

My Notes

Table 7.5a Common Findings During Mental Status Examinations for Clients With Depressive Disorders

Mental Status Examination Component	Common Findings in Depressive Disorders (*Indicates immediately notify provider)
Level of Consciousness and Orientation	■ Disoriented/confused. The client may be very self-focused and may appear disoriented when others initiate conversation or talk about current events because they are unaware of what is occurring around them due to their depression.
Appearance and General Behavior	■ Disheveled. The client's hair may not be combed, and they may be unwashed with poor dental care. They may be wearing dirty clothing with food stains and have body odor with little or no attention to self-care. ■ Sleep disturbances. The client may exhibit too much sleep (i.e., 14-18 hours daily) or have insomnia (i.e., less than 4 hours of sleep or in intervals of sleep). ■ Psychomotor retardation. The client may have a slow response with walking, talking, and reacting; may tend to stay put on the couch or in bed. ■ Vegetative signs. The client may exhibit weight loss, insomnia, constipation, and self-care deficits. ■ Avolition (reduced motivation or goal-directed behavior). For example, the client states, "I just don't want to shower today." ■ Anergia (low energy). For example, the client states, "I have no energy; I cannot get out of bed." ■ Social isolation. ■ Aggressiveness and agitation. ■ ***Verbal and nonverbal threats of harm**. ■ ***Self-harming behaviors** such as cutting, picking at skin, knocking head against the wall, tightening string or items on wrists, or stabbing self with anything fashioned into a weapon. ■ ***"Cheeking pills"** (i.e., holding pills in mouth and not swallowing them). Clients may save medications for use in a later suicide attempt.
Speech	■ May speak slowly in a monotone. ■ May exhibit **latency** (i.e., a delayed response to a question or comment). However, be aware of the client's baseline because this may be their normal if they have a history of traumatic brain injuries, dementia, or are English language learners.
Motor Activity	■ Psychomotor retardation. ■ Motor restlessness and anxiety. ■ Inactive or not initiating self-activity or care.

My Notes

Mental Status Examination Component	Common Findings in Depressive Disorders (*Indicates immediately notify provider)
Mood and Affect	■ Apathy (a lack of interest in events that one previously found enjoyable). For example, the client is no longer interested in participating in pleasurable activities. This may be verbalized or observed. ■ Anxious, irritable, angry, euphoric, tearful, or depressed. ■ Labile mood (rapid, exaggerated changes in mood). For example, a client is crying uncontrollably but when asked about the reason for crying, they state, "I don't know, I have no reason but can't stop crying." ■ Dysphoria (a state of unease or dissatisfaction). For example, the client states, "I don't like it here." ■ Sadness. ■ Crying episodes. ■ Flat or blunted affect. ■ Constricted/restricted affect. For example, a client usually laughs at jokes and giggles at funny comments but now does neither. ■ Incongruency (a lack of alignment between response and actions). For example, a client responds that they are fine, yet their body language is curled in a fetal position with no eye contact, and they are mumbling. ■ Mood is inappropriate for the current situation. ■ ***Hopelessness**. For example, a client may feel there is no longer any hope for them getting better or for life improving. ■ ***Worthlessness**. For example, a client may have feelings of guilt regarding themselves and their depression. They may feel like a burden to others and are unable to recognize their own value. ■ ***Helplessness**. For example, a client does not feel in control of life events. ***Note: Hopelessness, worthlessness, and helplessness are related to an increased risk of self-injury behavior and suicide and must be reported to provider. Do not leave clients alone if statements such as these are being made.**

My Notes

Mental Status Examination Component	Common Findings in Depressive Disorders (*Indicates immediately notify provider)
Thought and Perception	■ Poverty of content (responds without saying anything substantive or says much more than is necessary to convey a message). For example, if a client is asked, "How did you sleep last night?," the client answers with a long response about different brands of bedsheets without answering the question. ■ Decreased attention span. ■ Obsessions/preoccupations/ruminations. For example, a client may dwell on negative aspects of self-concept or faults and failures because they are unable to focus on anything else and thus repeat these thoughts often. ■ ***Suicidal ideation.** ■ ***Homicidal ideation.** ■ ***Violence ideation.** ***Note: Suicidal, homicidal, and violence ideations are characteristics of depression with recurring thoughts of death. These types of comments indicate increased risk for self-injury, suicide, or injury to others and must be reported to provider. Do not leave clients alone if statements such as these are being made.**
Attitude and Insight	■ Unaware of the current situation. ■ Unable to relate to current trends or settings. ■ Lack of perception. ■ Low awareness outside of self. ■ Irritability.
Cognitive Abilities and Level of Judgment	■ The inability to make decisions, think clearly, or solve problems is common in clients with depression.

Psychosocial Assessment

As previously discussed in the "Application of the Nursing Process in Mental Health Care" chapter, psychosocial assessment obtains additional subjective data that detects risks and identifies treatment opportunities and resources. Agencies have specific forms used for psychosocial assessment that typically consist of these components[1,2]:

- Cultural assessment
- Reason for seeking health care (i.e., "chief complaint")
- Thoughts of self-harm or suicide (both current and historical)
- Current and past medical history

---

1 Clinical Practice Guideline for the Treatment of Posttraumatic Stress Disorder. (2017, July). *What is cognitive behavioral treatment?* American Psychological Association. https://www.apa.org/ptsd-guideline/patients-and-families/cognitive-behavioral

2 Halter, M. (2022). *Varcarolis' foundations of psychiatric-mental health nursing* (9th ed.). Saunders.

My Notes

- Current medications
- History of previously diagnosed mental health disorders
- Previous hospitalizations
- Educational background
- Occupational background
- Family dynamics
- History of exposure to psychological trauma, violence, and domestic abuse
- Substance use (tobacco, alcohol, recreational drugs, misused prescription drugs)
- Family history of mental illness
- Coping mechanisms
- Functional ability/Activities of daily living
- Spiritual assessment

Screening Tools

Screening tools assess characteristics of specific mental health disorders. The screening tools listed below are examples of screenings, assessments, and question/answer prompts designed to address depressive disorders. These screening tools may be used on admission and at different times throughout the hospital or treatment stay. The findings may be used to compare and contrast client progress within the hospital stay, from a previous admission, or periodically on an outpatient basis. The registered nurse often conducts these tools as a collaborative member of the health care team.

Common Screening Tools for Depressive Disorders

Columbia-Suicide Severity Rating Scale (C-SSRS) PDF: A rating scale for suicidal ideation and behaviors that rates the degree of risk or intent of harm. It can be a self-assessment or administered by the health care professional.

Patient Health Questionnaire-9 (PHQ-9): A quick screening tool with nine criteria for assessing a client's risk of depression.

Beck Depression Inventory (BDI): A 21-item self-assessment questionnaire that determines the severity of depression from none to severe.

Hamilton Depression Scale (HDRS) PDF: A 17-item questionnaire used to rate the severity of one's depression.

Geriatric Depression Scale (GDS) PDF: A self-report of depressive symptoms for older adults; the new version is 15 questions.

My Notes

Edinburgh Postnatal Depression Scale (EPDS): A self-report of ten statements by mothers to screen for postpartum depression.

Laboratory Testing

For patients with depressive symptoms in the absence of general medical symptoms or findings on examination, the utility of screening laboratory tests has not been demonstrated. Commonly performed screening laboratory tests for new onset or severe depression include complete blood count, serum chemistry panels, urinalysis, thyroid stimulating hormone, rapid plasma reagin (RPR) for syphilis, human chorionic gonadotropin (HCG) for pregnancy, and toxicology screening for drugs of abuse.[3]

Routine laboratory monitoring is performed for some clients based on the medications they are taking, such as the following:

- Kidney Function (Creatinine, BUN)
  - May be impaired from medications the client is taking
- Liver Function (AST, ALT, Bilirubin)
  - May be impaired from antidepressants
- Therapeutic Medication Blood Levels
  - Some medications require that drug levels be monitored to assess for toxicity and therapeutic ranges

Read more about laboratory monitoring required for specific medications in the "Treatments for Depression" section of this chapter.

Life Span Considerations

Life span considerations influence how the client is assessed, as well as the selection of appropriate nursing interventions. Depressive disorders can be found across the life span from the very young to the very old. Read more about specific disorders in the "Childhood and Adolescence Disorders" chapter or the "Vulnerable Populations" chapter. It is important to individualize all interventions to the age and developmental level of the client. Review developmental stages in the "Application of the Nursing Process in Mental Health Care" chapter.

Depression Associated With Dementia

Individuals with dementia are susceptible to depression. **Dementia** refers to a group of symptoms that lead to a progressive, irreversible decline in mental function severe enough to disrupt daily life caused by a group of conditions, including Alzheimer's disease, vascular dementia, frontal-temporal dementia, and Lewy body disease. Alzheimer's disease is one of the most common forms of dementia. Alzheimer's disease causes impaired memory and the ability to learn, reason, make judgments, communicate, and carry out daily activities. An early symptom of Alzheimer's disease can be subtle memory loss and personality changes that differ from normal age-related memory problems. They seem to tire or become upset or anxious more easily. They do not cope well with change. For

---

3 Lyness, J. M. (2021). Unipolar depression in adults: Assessments and diagnosis. *UpToDate.* Retrieved on December 27, 2021, from https://www.uptodate.com/

My Notes

example, they can follow familiar routes, but traveling to a new place confuses them, and they can easily become lost. In the early stages of the illness, people with Alzheimer's disease are particularly susceptible to depression.[4]

While changes in the brain that cause dementia are permanent and worsen over time, thinking and memory problems can be aggravated by untreated depression.[5] Nurses should report new symptoms of depression in clients who have been diagnosed with dementia.

Read more about dementia at the Alzheimer's Association's web page.

Reflective Questions

1. How does the nurse differentiate between depression, delirium, dementia, and psychosis?
2. What are some common underlying medical conditions that could potentially mimic the symptoms of depression or mania in those who are elderly?
3. What other symptoms might a client who is a child/ adolescent display that would indicate the need to assess for disorders other than depression?

Cultural Considerations

Review cultural considerations of care in the "Application of the Nursing Process in Mental Health Care" chapter.

Reflective Questions

1. Reflect on how a client's cultural values, beliefs, or preferences impact presenting symptoms, the nursing care plan, or treatment modalities. Consider the following components:
   - Religious/Spiritual beliefs
   - Language/Communication
   - Nutritional preferences
   - Fasting
   - Potential drug-food interactions

4 American Psychiatric Association. (2019). *What is Alzheimer's disease?* https://www.psychiatry.org/patients-families/alzheimers/what-is-alzheimers-disease

5 Alzheimer's Association. (n.d.) *What is dementia?* https://www.alz.org/alzheimers-dementia/what-is-dementia

My Notes

- Rituals/Customs/Practices
- Gender dysphoria

Diagnoses

Mental health disorders are diagnosed by mental health providers using the *DSM-5*, similar to how medical conditions are diagnosed by trained medical professionals. Nurses create individualized nursing care plans based on the client's response to mental health disorders. See common nursing diagnoses related to mental health disorders in the "Diagnosis" section of the "Application of the Nursing Process in Mental Health Care" chapter.

Risk for suicide is always evaluated for clients with depressive disorders because suicidal ideation is a symptom of depression. Other common nursing diagnoses and sample expected outcomes for clients with depressive disorders are discussed in the following section in Table 7.5b.

Outcomes Identification

SMART outcomes are identified in relation to the established nursing diagnoses for each client. SMART is an acronym for Specific, Measurable, Attainable/Actionable, Relevant, and Timely.

Read more about outcome identification in the "Application of the Nursing Process in Mental Health Care" chapter.

Table 7.5b. Common Expected Outcomes for Nursing Diagnoses Related to Depressive Disorders[6]

Nursing Diagnosis[7,8]	Sample Expected Outcomes
Risk for Suicide	The client will communicate feelings and thoughts of suicide to the health care team, prior to acting on thoughts, during their inpatient stay. ***Note: Clients with depression are at higher risk of suicide when experiencing sudden euphoric recovery from major depression.**[9]
Ineffective Coping/Readiness for Enhanced Coping	The client will identify effective coping strategies within 24 hours of admission. The client will engage in preferred stress management techniques by Day 3 of admission.

---

6 Halter, M. (2022). *Varcarolis' foundations of psychiatric-mental health nursing* (9th ed.). Saunders.

7 Ackley, B., Ladwig, G., Makic, M. B., Martinez-Kratz, M., & Zanotti, M. (2020). *Nursing diagnosis handbook: An evidence-based guide to planning care* (12th ed.). Elsevier.

8 Herdman, T. H., & Kamitsuru, S. (Eds.). (2018). *Nursing diagnoses: Definitions and classification, 2018-2020.* Thieme Publishers New York.

9 Ackley, B., Ladwig, G., Makic, M. B., Martinez-Kratz, M., & Zanotti, M. (2020). *Nursing diagnosis handbook: An evidence-based guide to planning care* (12th ed.). Elsevier.

My Notes

Self-Neglect	The client will increase participation in baseline personal care each day during their stay.
Fatigue/Sleep Deprivation	The client will, within one week, report feeling rested upon awakening.
Imbalanced Nutrition: Less than Body Requirements	The client will eat 50% or more on their meal tray at each meal.
Constipation	The client will have a soft, formed stool at least every three days during their inpatient stay.
Social Isolation	The client will communicate with others during their inpatient stay by participating in daily group offerings within the milieu.
Chronic Low Self-Esteem	The client will verbalize at least three personal strengths within three days of admission.
Hopelessness	The client will describe plans for a positive future by discharge.
Spiritual Distress	The client will identify a meaning and purpose in life within two weeks.
Readiness for Enhanced Knowledge	The client will verbalize three common side effects of their medications by the end of the shift.

Planning Interventions

Interventions are planned based on the client's nursing diagnoses, expected outcomes, and current status. Clients with depressive disorders are monitored closely for risk of suicide, and interventions are planned according to their level of risk. See interventions for clients at risk of suicide in the "Application of the Nursing Process in Mental Health Care" chapter.

Implementation

As discussed earlier in this chapter, a combination of pharmacological treatments and psychotherapies is often an effective approach to treating depressive disorders. There are three phases in treatment and recovery from major depression[10]:

- The active phase (6 to 12 weeks) is directed at reduction of depressive symptoms and restoration of psychosocial and work function. Hospitalization may be required, and medication and other biological treatments may be initiated.
- The continuation phase (4 to 9 months) is directed at prevention of relapse through pharmacotherapy, education, and depression-specific psychotherapy. This phase focuses on maintaining the client as a functional and contributing member of the community after recovery from the acute phase.
- The maintenance phase (1 year or more) is directed at preventing future episodes of depression. Medication may be phased out or continued.

10 Halter, M. (2022). *Varcarolis' foundations of psychiatric-mental health nursing* (9th ed.). Saunders.

My Notes

Nurses target interventions based on the client's current phase of treatment and recovery.

Interventions can be categorized based on the American Psychiatric Nurses Association (APNA) standard for *Implementation* that includes the *Coordination of Care; Health Teaching and Health Promotion; Pharmacological, Biological, and Integrative Therapies; Milieu Therapy;* and *Therapeutic Relationship and Counseling*. Read more about these subcategories in the "Application of the Nursing Process in Mental Health Care" chapter. See examples of interventions for each of these categories for clients with depressive disorders in Table 7.5c.

Table 7.5c Examples of Nursing Interventions by APNA Subcategories

Subcategory of the APNA Standard of Implementation	**The nurse will . . .**	**Rationale**
Coordination of Care	Communicate client trends, such as risk for suicide or cheeking of medications, with interprofessional team members.	All team members providing care must be aware of the client's suicide risk to maintain a safe environment.
Health Teaching and Health Promotion	Promote health by teaching about adaptive coping strategies such as journaling and daily exercise.	Nurses encourage resilience with adaptive coping strategies.
Pharmacological, Biological, and Integrative Therapies	Deliver patient education about antidepressants and expected time frames for improvement. Open all medications in front of the client.	Client understanding of their medications and potential side effects can increase medication compliance. Opening all medications in front of the client may decrease paranoia.
Milieu Therapy	Perform and document intentional rounding every 15 to 60 minutes on varied schedule.	Visually rounding on every client in the milieu creates a strong safety plan for all clients and staff.
Therapeutic Relationship and Counseling	Provide 1:1 therapeutic communication to encourage the client to develop adaptive coping strategies, use stress management techniques, develop supportive relationships, and seek spiritual supports. See the "Communication Tips" subsection below.	Providing effective therapeutic techniques for clients with depression can promote hope and positive self-esteem.

Nursing interventions are also planned that target common physiological signs of depression and associated self-care deficits. See common interventions for these conditions in Table 7.5d.

My Notes

Table 7.5d Nursing Interventions Targeting Physiological Signs of Depression and Self-Care Deficit[11]	
Problem/Intervention	**Rationale**
Nutrition ■ **Offer small, high-calorie, and high-protein snacks and fluids frequently.** ■ **When possible, encourage family or friends to join the client during meals.** ■ **Encourage the client to participate in selecting food and drinks.** ■ **Refer the client to a dietician if necessary.** ■ **Weigh the client weekly and monitor trends.** ■ **Observe the client's eating patterns.**	Poor nutrition increases the risk for physical illness. Small, frequent snacks are more easily tolerated than large portions of food if the client has a loss of appetite. Fluids prevent dehydration and minimize constipation. Eating is a social event. Eating with loved ones reinforces the idea that someone cares about them and can serve as an incentive to eat. The client is more likely to eat foods they prefer. A dietician can help create an individualized diet plan. Monitoring the patient's status provides data for evaluating effectiveness.
Sleep ■ **Provide periods of rest after activities.** ■ **Encourage the client to get up and dress and stay out of bed during the day.** ■ **Encourage relaxation measures in the evening, such as a warm bath, warm milk, or soothing music.** ■ **Avoid caffeinated beverages.**	Disturbances in one's sleep cycle can intensify feelings of depression. Minimizing sleep during the day and establishing routines increase the likelihood of restful sleep at night. Relaxation techniques induce sleep. Decreasing caffeine intake increases the possibility of sleep.
Elimination (Constipation) ■ **Monitor frequency of bowel movements.** ■ **Encourage fluids and foods high in fiber.** ■ **Provide periods of exercise.** ■ **Evaluate the need for a bowel management program with stool softeners and laxatives.**	Many depressed patients are constipated, so frequency of bowel movements should be monitored. Fluids, fiber, and exercise stimulate peristalsis and soften stools. Bowel management programs may be needed to avoid constipation or fecal impaction.
Self-Care Deficits ■ **Encourage the use of a toothbrush, washcloth, soap, and makeup or shaving supplies.** ■ **When appropriate, give step-by-step reminders, such as "Wash the right side of your face and now your left."**	Being clean and well-groomed can improve self-esteem. Slowed thinking and difficulty concentrating make organizing simple tasks difficult.

11 Halter, M. (2022). *Varcarolis' foundations of psychiatric-mental health nursing* (9th ed.). Saunders.

My Notes

Communication Tips

Some clients with depression are so withdrawn they are unwilling or unable to speak. Sitting with them in silence may feel like a waste of time, but nurses should be aware that providing therapeutic presence can be meaningful in supporting the client with depression. Helpful communication techniques for severely withdrawn clients and their rationale are described in the following box.

Guidelines for Communication With Severely Withdrawn Individuals[12]

- Use simple, concrete words and allow the client time to respond.
    - **Rationale:** Slowed thinking and difficulty concentrating impair comprehension and require time to formulate a response.
- Listen for covert messages and ask about suicide plans.
    - **Rationale:** People often experience relief and decreased feelings of isolation when they share thoughts of suicide.
- Avoid platitudes such as "Everyone feels down once in a while."
    - **Rationale:** Platitudes minimize the individual's feelings and can increase feelings of guilt or worthlessness because they cannot "snap out of it."
- When a client is silent, use the technique of making observations, such as "There are new pictures on the wall," or "You are wearing new shoes."
    - **Rationale:** When an individual is not ready to talk, direct questions can raise their anxiety levels. Pointing out objects in the environment draws the person into reality.

There are several guidelines for counseling individuals with depression, helping them identify current coping skills, and exploring new adaptive coping strategies:

- Encourage stress management techniques such as exercise, good sleep, and healthy food choices.
- Promote the formation of supportive relationships such as peer support and support groups to reduce social isolation and enable the individual to work on personal goals and relationship needs.
- Provide information about spiritual support as the individual defines it, such as chaplain or pastoral visits or spending time in nature; many people find strength and comfort in spiritual and/or religious activities.
- Help the client reconstruct a healthier and more hopeful attitude about the future (without providing false reassurance).[13]

12 Halter, M. (2022). *Varcarolis' foundations of psychiatric-mental health nursing* (9th ed.). Saunders.

13 Halter, M. (2022). *Varcarolis' foundations of psychiatric-mental health nursing* (9th ed.). Saunders.

My Notes

Collaborative Mental Health Treatments

Nurses assist in implementing collaborative interventions based on the client's treatment plan. Review collaborative mental health treatments and common medications used to treat depression in the "Treatments for Depression" section of this chapter.

Patient Education Regarding Antidepressant Medications

Nurses educate clients about their medications, including the manner in which they work, common side effects, and issues to report to their provider. Clients taking antidepressants should also be educated regarding the following considerations[14]:

- When taking antidepressants, it is important to follow the instructions on how much to take. Some people start to feel better a few days after starting the medication, but it can take four to eight weeks to feel the most benefit. Antidepressants work well and are safe for most people, but it is still important to talk with your mental health care provider if you have side effects such as sexual dysfunction, weight gain, dizziness, nausea, palpitations, drowsiness, insomnia, or anxiety. Side effects may go away as your body adjusts to the medication, but in some cases, switching to a different medication may be required.
- Don't stop taking an antidepressant without first talking to your mental health care provider. Stopping your medicine suddenly can cause symptoms or worsen depression.
- Antidepressants cannot solve all of your problems. Antidepressants work best when combined with psychotherapy and healthy coping strategies. If you notice that your mood is getting worse or if you have thoughts about hurting yourself, it is important to call your provider right away.
- Some people who are depressed may think about hurting themselves or committing suicide (taking their own life). If you are having thoughts about committing suicide, please seek immediate help by calling your provider, 911, or 1-800-273-TALK to reach a 24-hour crisis center that provides free, confidential help to people in crisis.
- Some antidepressants may cause risks to the baby during pregnancy. Talk with your provider if you are pregnant or might be pregnant or if you are planning to become pregnant.
- For individuals who are very depressed or suicidal, it is important to provide close monitoring when the individual first starts taking an antidepressant medication. Often an individual may have increased energy to make a suicidal attempt when they first begin a medication, whereas previously they may have had suicidal thoughts but lacked the energy to make an attempt.

Supporting Family Members

It is important to support the family members and significant others who are living with an individual with a depressive disorder. Read tips on living with someone with depression in Figure 7.9.[15]

---

14 Centers for Disease Control and Prevention. (2021, February 15). *Mental health conditions: Depression and anxiety.* https://www.cdc.gov/tobacco/campaign/tips/diseases/depression-anxiety.html

15 "2_living_with_someone_with_depression.png" by unknown author for World Health Organization is in the Public Domain. Access for free at https://www.who.int/campaigns/world-mental-health-day/2021/campaign-materials

My Notes

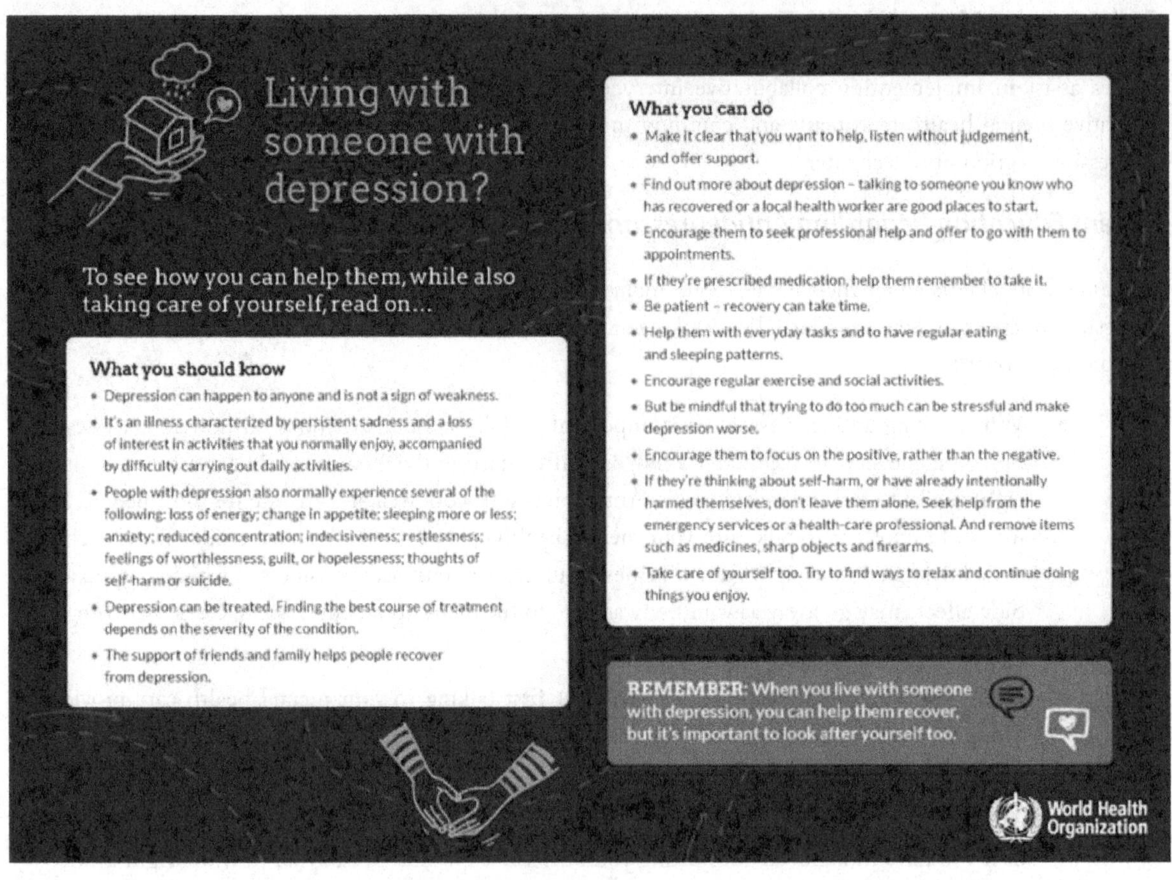

Figure 7.9 Supporting Family Members and Significant Others

Evaluation

Evaluation of the client's progress towards meeting expected outcomes occurs continuously throughout the treatment phase. Evaluation includes comparing results from screening tools, reviewing laboratory results, and monitoring the effectiveness of prescribed medications, treatments, and nursing interventions. Based on the evaluation findings, the nursing care plan may be modified, or new interventions or outcomes may be added.

My Notes

7.6 SPOTLIGHT APPLICATION

Patient Story: Postpartum Depression[1]

Maya is a healthy 32-year-old woman who has been married for over two years and is expecting her first child, a baby boy. She had a history of depression and generalized anxiety disorder.

She had been doing well with a combination of medication and cognitive behavioral therapy (CBT) for many years. Maya had decided in the months leading up to getting pregnant that she wanted to be off medication and worked with her psychiatrist to carefully accomplish this. She continued weekly therapy. She was mostly active, upbeat, and cheerful during her pregnancy. She gave birth to a healthy 7.3-pound baby boy. After the delivery, she started to feel sad, overwhelmed, and consistently tearful. She frequently felt irritable and on edge. This feeling persisted for the first ten weeks after the baby was born. She had limited support—her parents were divorced, and her mother was living in another state. Her in-laws were much older with numerous health complications and couldn't help regularly.

Maya and her husband went to see her psychiatrist. She was quite tearful and felt she was a "failure as a mom." Her baby cried incessantly, and she could barely get any sleep. Maya felt utterly incapable of soothing her baby and would get frustrated and tearful. She was so afraid of what she had learned about sudden infant death (SIDS) that she would barely allow herself to sleep. She felt that it was a constant race against the clock—with nursing, pumping, and changing. She was always cleaning bottles and diapers. She felt horrified with how she looked. She had expected to wear pre-pregnancy clothes immediately after childbirth. She hadn't had a meal in peace or gotten her hair or nails done and couldn't even think about having sex with her husband. He tried to be supportive, but also felt overwhelmed by it all. He felt she was inconsolable, and they both felt at a loss.

The psychiatrist talked about a variety of tools, including participating in cognitive behavioral therapy, incorporating 15-20 minutes of daily relaxation, practicing mindfulness skills, hiring help, getting her mom to stay with her for a few weeks, and seeking other support. Her husband understood the urgency of the situation and offered to take time off work and to do some of the overnight feedings. Maya decided to restart on her previous antidepressant and also joined a new moms' support group and continued CBT weekly therapy.

Over the next few months, she was exercising more and getting more sleep and support and had significant improvement in mood and energy. She received some sleep training tips from her pediatrician as well. Maya and her husband shared with her psychiatrist that they were feeling significantly better. They were excited to share that they found a series of self-help parenting books to be particularly helpful and had gotten some helpful tips from others in the moms' group.

"Wow, it really does take a village to raise a child, doesn't it?" Maya commented to her psychiatrist. They spoke about how in previous generations new couples could rely on extended family support and how that support often doesn't exist now. Also, inaccurate beliefs, such as babies are easy and infancy should be a happy time for parents, add to stress, conflict, and guilt. Being able to normalize the stress of adjusting to parenthood was extremely helpful for Maya and her husband.

---

1 American Psychiatric Association. (n.d.). *Patient story: Postpartum depression.* https://www.psychiatry.org/patients-families/postpartum-depression/patient-story

My Notes

Reflective Questions

1. What educational tips and strategies may have been of benefit to Maya as part of her prenatal care?
2. How have cultural and societal norms impacted families in relation to child rearing?
3. What support strategies and education might be offered to birth partners to help them anticipate challenges and recognize early signs of post-partum depression?

7.7 LEARNING ACTIVITIES

My Notes

Interactive Activities

An interactive H5P element has been excluded from this version of the text. You can view it online here: https://wtcs.pressbooks.pub/nursingmhcc/?p=313#h5p-17

An interactive H5P element has been excluded from this version of the text. You can view it online here: https://wtcs.pressbooks.pub/nursingmhcc/?p=313#h5p-18

An interactive H5P element has been excluded from this version of the text. You can view it online here: https://wtcs.pressbooks.pub/nursingmhcc/?p=313#h5p-19

My Notes

VII GLOSSARY

Cognitive behavioral therapy (CBT): A type of psychotherapy that helps a person recognize distorted/negative thinking with the goal of changing thought and behaviors to respond to changes in a more positive manner.[1]

Depressive episode: An episode where the person experiences a depressed mood (feeling sad, irritable, empty) or a loss of pleasure or interest in activities for most of the day, nearly every day, for at least two weeks. Several other symptoms are also present, which may include poor concentration, feelings of excessive guilt or low self-worth, hopelessness about the future, thoughts about dying or suicide, disrupted sleep, changes in appetite or weight, and feeling especially tired or low in energy.

Electroconvulsive therapy (ECT): A medical treatment reserved for patients with severe major depression who have not responded to medications, psychotherapy, or other treatments. It involves a brief electrical stimulation of the brain while the patient is under anesthesia.

Group therapy: A type of psychotherapy that brings people with similar disorders together in a supportive environment to learn how others cope in similar situations.[2]

Hypertensive crisis: An acute rise and significantly elevated blood pressure, typically over 180/120 mm Hg, that causes acute end-organ damage such as stroke, myocardial infarction, or acute kidney damage. It can be caused by MAOIs, a class of antidepressants.

Light therapy: Therapy for seasonal affective disorder (SAD) that involves sitting in front of a light therapy box that emits a very bright light. It usually requires 20 minutes or more per day, typically first thing in the morning during the winter months. Most people see some improvements from light therapy within one or two weeks of beginning treatment.

Perinatal depression: Depressive disorder that occurs during pregnancy.

Postpartum depression: Feelings of extreme sadness, anxiety, and exhaustion that may make it difficult for mothers of newborns to complete daily care activities for themselves and/or for their babies. Severe postpartum depression can lead to postpartum psychosis.

Postpartum psychosis: Severe postpartum depression can cause delusions (thoughts or beliefs that are not true), hallucinations (seeing, hearing, or smelling things that are not there), mania (a high, elated mood that often seems out of touch with reality), paranoia, and confusion. Women who have postpartum psychosis are at risk for harming themselves or their child and should receive help as soon as possible by calling 911 or taking the mother to the emergency room.

Seasonal affective disorder (SAD): A type of depression causing symptoms during the fall and winter months when there is less sunlight and usually improves with the arrival of spring. SAD is more than just "winter blues." The symptoms can be distressing and overwhelming and can interfere with daily functioning.[3]

---

1 American Psychiatric Association. (2020). *What is depression?* https://www.psychiatry.org/patients-families/depression/what-is-depression

2 American Psychiatric Association. (2020). *What is depression?* https://www.psychiatry.org/patients-families/depression/what-is-depression

3 American Psychiatric Association. (2020). *Seasonal affective disorder (SAD).* https://www.psychiatry.org/patients-families/depression/seasonal-affective-disorder

My Notes

Serotonin syndrome: A medical emergency that can occur in clients taking medications that affect serotonin levels.

Transcranial Magnetic Stimulation (TMS): A noninvasive procedure that uses magnetic fields to stimulate nerve cells in the brain to improve symptoms of depression when other depression treatments haven't been effective.

Chapter 8

Bipolar Disorders

8.1 INTRODUCTION

My Notes

Learning Objectives

- Apply the nursing process to clients with bipolar disorders
- Describe nursing assessments related to bipolar disorders
- Identify common nursing problems/diagnoses related to bipolar disorders
- Establish a safe environment
- Apply evidence-based practice when planning and implementing nursing care
- Describe common treatments for bipolar disorders
- Identify appropriate referrals to community resources
- Evaluate the effectiveness of interventions
- Provide patient education to clients and their family members

Bipolar disorder is a mental illness that causes dramatic shifts in a person's mood, energy, and ability to think clearly. Moods shift from abnormally elevated moods called manic episodes to abnormal low moods of depression. See Figure 8.1[1] for a depiction of the shifts in mood that occur with bipolar disorder. Severe bipolar episodes of mania can also include hallucinations or delusions, which can be confused with symptoms of schizophrenia.[2] This chapter will discuss the signs, symptoms, and treatments for bipolar disorder and explain how to apply the nursing process when caring for clients with bipolar disorder.

Figure 8.1 Bipolar Disorder

---

1 "P_culture.svg" by he:משתמש:נעמה מ is licensed under CC BY-SA 3.0

2 National Alliance on Mental Illness. (2017, August). *Bipolar disorder.* https://www.nami.org/About-Mental-Illness/Mental-Health-Conditions/Bipolar-Disorder

My Notes

8.2 BASIC CONCEPTS OF BIPOLAR DISORDERS

Manic Episodes

Bipolar disorders include shifts in mood from abnormal highs (called manic episodes) to abnormal lows (i.e., depressive episodes). A **manic episode** is a persistently elevated or irritable mood with abnormally increased energy lasting at least one week. The mood disturbance is severe and causes marked impairment in social or occupational function. Severe episodes often require hospitalization to prevent harm to self or others. As the manic episode intensifies, the individual may become psychotic with hallucinations, delusions, and disturbed thoughts. The episode is not caused by the physiological effects of a substance (such as drug abuse, prescribed medication, or other treatment) or by another medical condition.[1]

According to the *DSM-5*, three or more of the following symptoms are present during a manic episode[2]:

- Inflated self-esteem or grandiosity
- Decreased need for sleep (i.e., feels rested after only three hours of sleep)
- More talkative than usual or pressure to keep talking
- Flight of ideas or subjective experience that thoughts are racing
- Distractibility (i.e., attention is too easily drawn to unimportant or irrelevant stimuli)
- Increase in goal-directed activity (either socially, at work or school, or sexually) or psychomotor agitation
- Excessive involvement in activities that have a high potential for painful consequences (e.g., engaging in unrestrained buying sprees, sexual indiscretions, or foolish business investments)

People experiencing a manic episode may become physically exhausted. Depressive episodes associated with bipolar disorder can lead to suicide. The mortality ratio due to suicide for people with bipolar disorder is 20 times above the general population rate and exceeds rates for other mental health disorders.[3]

Hypomanic episodes have similar symptoms to a manic episode but are less severe and do not cause significant impairment in social or occupational functioning or require hospitalization.[4]

Bipolar Disorders

There are three major types of bipolar and related disorders called Bipolar I, Bipolar II, and Cyclothymia. See Figure 8.2[5] for an illustration comparing these three types of bipolar disorders.

---

1 American Psychiatric Association. (2013). *Desk reference to the diagnostic criteria from DSM-5.*

2 American Psychiatric Association. (2013). *Desk reference to the diagnostic criteria from DSM-5.*

3 Baldessarini, R.J., Vázquez, G.H. & Tondo, L. (2020, January 6). Bipolar depression: A major unsolved challenge. *International Journal of Bipolar Disorders 8*, (1). https://doi.org/10.1186/s40345-019-0160-1

4 American Psychiatric Association. (2013). *Desk reference to the diagnostic criteria from DSM-5.*

5 "Bipolar_mood_shifts.png" by Osmosis is licensed under CC BY-SA 4.0

My Notes

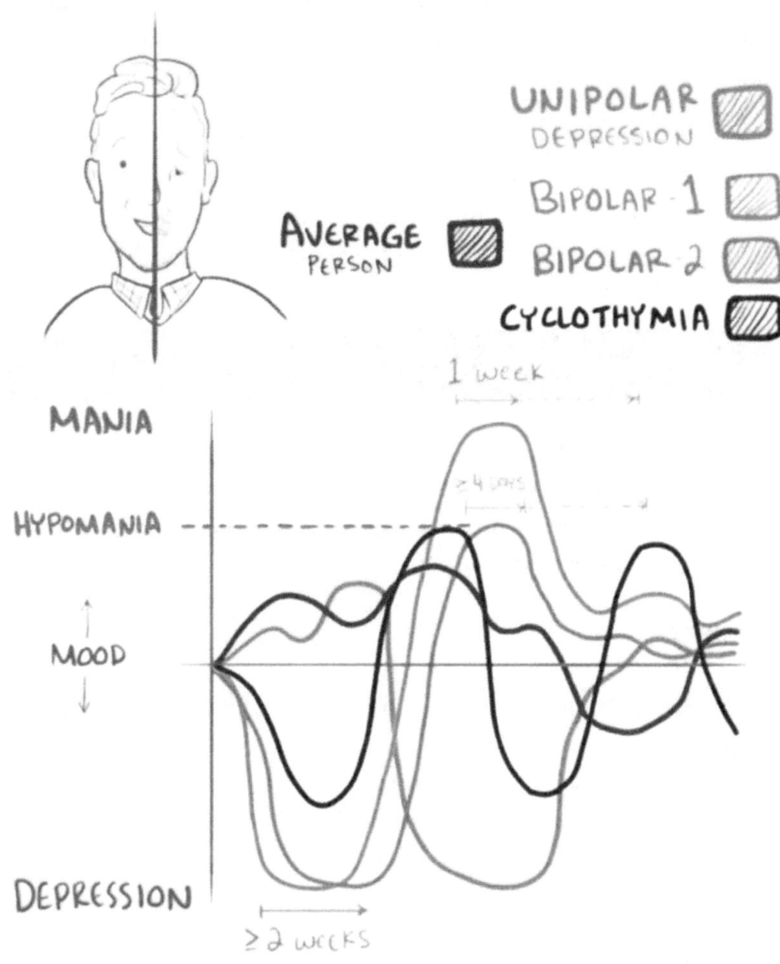

Figure 8.3 Bipolar Disorders

Bipolar I Disorder is the most severe bipolar disorder. Individuals with Bipolar 1 Disorder have had at least one manic episode and often experience additional hypomanic and depressive episodes. (Read about the symptoms of depressive episodes in the "Depressive Disorders" chapter of this book.) One manic episode in the course of an individual's life can change an individual's diagnosis from depression to bipolar disorder. Manic episodes last at least one week and present for most of the day, nearly every day. They can be so severe that the person requires hospitalization. Depressive episodes typically last at least two weeks. Episodes of depression with mixed features (having depressive symptoms and manic symptoms at the same time) are also possible.[6,7]

---

6 National Institute of Mental Health. (2020, January). *Bipolar disorder.* National Institutes of Health. https://www.nimh.nih.gov/health/topics/bipolar-disorder

7 American Psychiatric Association. (2013). *Desk reference to the diagnostic criteria from DSM-5.*

My Notes

Bipolar II Disorder is defined by a pattern of depressive episodes and hypomanic episodes, but individuals have never experienced a full-blown manic episode typical of Bipolar I Disorder. Individuals with Bipolar II Disorder often have higher productivity when they are hypomanic and may exhibit increased irritability.[8]

Cyclothymia is defined by periods of hypomanic symptoms and depressive symptoms lasting for at least two years (1 year in children and adolescents). However, the symptoms do not meet the diagnostic requirements for hypomanic episodes or depressive episodes.[9] Individuals with cyclothymia do not experience the same severity or impairment in functioning as seen in individuals with bipolar disorder. Individuals with cyclothymia are often able to maintain work, personal relationships, etc.

Read more on the National Institute of Mental Health's Bipolar Disorder web page.

Some people with Bipolar I or Bipolar II disorders experience rapid cycling with at least four mood episodes in a 12-month period. These mood episodes can be manic episodes, hypomanic episodes, or major depressive episodes. Cycling can also occur within a month or even a 24-hour period. **Rapid cycling** is associated with severe symptoms and poorer functioning and is more difficult to treat.[10]

Coexisting Disorders

It is common for people with bipolar disorder to also have an anxiety disorder or attention deficit hyperactivity disorder. Sometimes, a person with severe episodes of mania or depression may experience psychotic symptoms, such as hallucinations or delusions, resulting in an incorrect diagnosis of schizophrenia. People with bipolar disorder may misuse alcohol or drugs and engage in other high-risk behaviors in times of impaired judgment during manic episodes. In some cases, people with bipolar disorder also have an eating disorder, such as binge eating or bulimia.[11]

Causes of Bipolar Disorder

Researchers continue to study the possible causes of bipolar disorder. Similar to depressive disorders, most experts agree there is no single cause, and there are many factors that contribute to bipolar disorder. Research shows that people who have a parent or sibling with bipolar disorder have an increased chance of having the disorder. Some studies indicate that the brains of people with bipolar disorder may differ from the brains of people who do not have bipolar disorder. People with certain genes are more likely to develop bipolar disorder. Newer research indicates altered intracellular calcium signaling occurs in people with bipolar disorders, and anti-seizure medications can provide effective treatment.[12,13]

---

8 National Institute of Mental Health. (2020, January). *Bipolar disorder.* National Institutes of Health. https://www.nimh.nih.gov/health/topics/bipolar-disorder

9 National Institute of Mental Health. (2020, January). *Bipolar disorder.* National Institutes of Health. https://www.nimh.nih.gov/health/topics/bipolar-disorder

10 Halter, M. (2022). *Varcarolis' foundations of psychiatric-mental health nursing* (9th ed.). Saunders.

11 National Institute of Mental Health. (2020, January). *Bipolar disorder.* National Institutes of Health. https://www.nimh.nih.gov/health/topics/bipolar-disorder

12 National Institute of Mental Health. (2020, January). *Bipolar disorder.* National Institutes of Health. https://www.nimh.nih.gov/health/topics/bipolar-disorder

13 *The Emerging Neurobiology of Bipolar Disorder* by Harrison, Geddes, & Tunbridge is licensed under CC BY 4.0

My Notes

Stress is a common trigger for mania and depression in adults, and previous adverse childhood events (ACEs) are significantly associated with bipolar disorder.[14] For example, a person with an unstable, chaotic childhood may experience bipolar disorder later in adulthood that is triggered by extreme stress. Read more about ACEs in the the "Mental Health and Mental Illness" section in Chapter 1.

Physiological causes can also cause mania-like symptoms. For example, hyperthyroidism can cause difficulty sleeping, irritability, anxiety, and unintentional weight loss. Individuals can also experience substance-induced bipolar symptoms that develop during intoxication by a substance or withdrawal from a substance. For example, alcohol, sedatives, cocaine, methamphetamines, and phencyclidine (PCP) can cause bipolar-like symptoms.[15] For these reasons, on initial evaluation of a client experiencing a manic episode, screening is often typically performed for thyroid disorders and substance use.

---

14 Halter, M. (2022). *Varcarolis' foundations of psychiatric-mental health nursing* (9th ed.). Saunders.

15 American Psychiatric Association. (2013). *Desk reference to the diagnostic criteria from DSM-5*.

My Notes

8.3 TREATMENTS FOR BIPOLAR DISORDERS

Bipolar disorder is often a lifelong illness, and episodes of mania and depression typically recur. Between episodes, many people with bipolar disorder are free of mood disruption, but some people have lingering symptoms. Long-term, continuous treatment can help people manage symptoms and prevent relapse. An effective treatment plan for bipolar disorder typically includes a combination of medications and psychotherapy.[1]

Medications

Medications used to treat bipolar disorder include mood stabilizers, anti-seizure medications, and second-generation ("atypical") antipsychotics. Treatment plans may also include medications that target sleep disruption or anxiety. Antidepressant medication may be used to treat depressive episodes in bipolar disorder in combination with a mood stabilizer and/or antipsychotic to prevent precipitating a manic episode.[2] See Table 8.3 for a list of common medications used to treat bipolar disorders.[3] Review information about the associated neurotransmitters in the "Psychotropic Medications" chapter.

1 National Institute of Mental Health. (2020, January). *Bipolar disorder.* National Institutes of Health. https://www.nimh.nih.gov/health/topics/bipolar-disorder

2 National Institute of Mental Health. (2020, January). *Bipolar disorder.* National Institutes of Health. https://www.nimh.nih.gov/health/topics/bipolar-disorder

3 Post, R. M. (2022, May 17). Bipolar treatment in adults: Choosing maintenance treatment. *UpToDate.* Retrieved July 13, 2022, from https://www.uptodate.com/

My Notes

Table 8.3 Common Medications Used to Treat Bipolar Disorders		
Medication Class	**Nursing Considerations**	**Common Side Effects** **(*Indicates medical emergency)**
Mood Stabilizers	**Used to treat symptoms of mania and mood lability.**	
Lithium	Used as a first-line mood stabilizing agent to treat mania when symptoms are acute or as maintenance therapy Improved tolerance with food and better drug absorption Recommended water intake is 1.5 – 3 liters/day Given in divided doses if gastrointestinal distress occurs NSAIDs are not recommended because they increase lithium levels Therapeutic blood levels are required. Blood levels are drawn 10-12 hours after the last dose taken. The therapeutic lithium serum level is 0.6-1.2 mEq/L	Lithium blocks ADH, so monitor for symptoms of diabetes insipidus (i.e., excessive thirst and urination) Long-term use increases risk for hypothyroidism, hyperparathyroidism, and impaired kidney functioning ***Lithium toxicity** (notify the health care provider) Early signs (<1.5 mEq/L): nausea, vomiting, diarrhea, thirst, polyuria, slurred speech, muscle weakness, or fine tremors Moderate signs (1.6-1.9 mEq/L): coarse hand tremors, mental confusion, persistent GI complaints, muscle hyperirritability, EEG changes, or uncoordinated movements Severe signs (>2.0 mEq/L): ataxia, blurred vision, large output of dilute urine, severe hypotension, clonic movements, overt confusion, cardiac dysrhythmias, proteinuria, or death secondary to pulmonary complications ***Lithium levels > 2.5 mEq/L constitute a medical emergency, even if the client is asymptomatic.** Treatments for toxicity: ■ Notify the health care provider for any level of toxicity ■ Hold the lithium ■ Encourage fluids; IV fluids may be required ■ Gastric lavage ■ May require urea, mannitol, aminophylline, or dialysis to hasten the excretion of the drug in severe cases

My Notes

Medication Class	Nursing Considerations	Common Side Effects (*Indicates medical emergency)
Anti-seizure Medications	**Used to treat mania and other symptoms.**	
Valproic Acid (Depakote)	Used for rapid cycling in acute manic phase when not responding to other mood stabilizers Require periodic therapeutic serum valproic acid blood levels. Therapeutic range is 50-125 mcg/mL Require laboratory monitoring, including liver function tests, amylase, and lipase and platelet levels due to higher risk for blood dyscrasias and pancreatitis	■ Weight gain ■ Sedation ■ Nausea and/or vomiting ■ Hair loss ■ Tremors ■ Gastrointestinal discomfort ***Signs of toxicity** (notify the health care provider): ■ **Abdominal pain** ■ **Dark-colored urine** ■ **Jaundice**
Carbamazepine (Tegretol)	Used in combination with lithium and antipsychotic drugs for resistive symptoms Used when treatment resistant due to rapid cycling, paranoia, and extreme hyperactivity Requires routine laboratory monitoring, including white blood cells and liver function tests because it can cause bone marrow suppression and liver damage Therapeutic serum blood levels are 4-12 mcg/mL	■ Risk for hyponatremia ■ Fatigue ■ Blurred vision ■ Nausea ■ Ataxia Risk for toxicity if tegretol blood level is >20 mcg/mL. If suspect toxicity, hold the drug and notify the health care provider.
Lamotrigine (Lamictal)	Used with acute mania or as maintenance therapy Therapeutic serum blood level is 2.5 to 15 mcg/mL Improved tolerance in divided doses	■ Stevens-Johnson syndrome (A rare but potentially life-threatening reaction to medication that starts with flu-like symptoms, followed by a painful rash that spreads and blisters.)
Topiramate (Topamax) **Oxcarbazepine (Oxtellar)**	Used for treatment-resistant mania	Topiramate ■ Weight loss ■ Fatigue ■ Visual disturbances Oxcarbazepine ■ Hyponatremia

My Notes

Medication Class	Nursing Considerations	Common Side Effects (*Indicates medical emergency)
Antipsychotics Medications	**Used to treat symptoms of psychosis, agitation, insomnia, or anxiety.**	
Olanzapine (Zyprexa) **Risperidone (Risperdal)** **Quetiapine (Seroquel)** **Ziprasidone (Geodon)** **Aripiprazole (Abilify)** **Clozapine (Clozaril)**	Help stabilize mood and slow down hyperactive motor activity Several drugs come in oral, parental, liquid, oral disintegrating tablets, and long-acting injections	Review common adverse effects in the "Schizophrenia" section of the "Psychosis and Schizophrenia" chapter.
Antianxiety Medications	**Used to treat symptoms of anxiety and irritability.**	
Benzodiazepines **Lorazepam (Ativan)** **Alprazolam (Xanax)** **Other** **Gabapentin (Neurontin)** **Buspirone (Buspar)**	Help reduce the level of hyperactivity during an acute manic phase as a supplement with mood stabilizing drugs Avoid in patients with substance use disorders due to high risk of addiction	Review common adverse effects in the "Treatments for Anxiety" section of the "Anxiety Disorders" chapter.
Antidepressants Medications	**Used to treat symptoms of depressive episodes.**	
Medication Classes: **SSRIs** **SNRIs** **TCAs** **MAOIs**	Can precipitate a manic episode if not used in combination with a mood stabilizer and/or antipsychotic.	Review common adverse effects in the "Treatments for Depression" section of the "Depressive Disorders" chapter.

My Notes

Lithium

When administered to a client experiencing a manic episode, lithium may reduce symptoms within 1 to 3 weeks. It also possesses unique antisuicidal properties that sets it apart from antidepressants.[4,5]

Black Box Warning

A Black Box Warning for lithium states that lithium toxicity is closely related to serum lithium levels and can occur at doses close to therapeutic levels. Facilities for prompt and accurate serum lithium determinations should be available before initiating therapy.[6]

Adverse/Side Effects

Lithium must be closely monitored with routine blood work because it has a narrow therapeutic range of 0.8 to 1.2 mEq/L. Levels above this range cause **lithium toxicity**. Lithium levels > 2.5 mEq/L constitute a medical emergency, even if the client is asymptomatic. Signs of early lithium toxicity include diarrhea, vomiting, drowsiness, muscular weakness, and lack of coordination. At higher levels giddiness, ataxia, blurred vision, tinnitus, and a large output of dilute urine may be seen. Treatment of lithium toxicity includes withholding the lithium and pushing fluids; IV fluids may be required. In severe cases, gastric lavage, mannitol, urea, aminophylline, or dialysis may be used to hasten the excretion of the drug. Lithium is contraindicated in clients with renal or cardiovascular disease, severe dehydration or sodium depletion, and those receiving diuretics because these conditions increase the risk of lithium toxicity.[7,8]

Fine hand tremor, polyuria, and mild thirst may persist throughout treatment. Lithium can cause abnormal electrocardiographic (ECG) findings and risk of sudden death. Clients should be advised to seek immediate emergency assistance if they experience fainting, light-headedness, abnormal heartbeats, or shortness of breath.[9]

Renal function is adversely affected by lithium and requires routine laboratory testing including urinalysis, blood urea nitrogen, and creatinine. Thyroid and parathyroid functioning can also be adversely affected by lithium, requiring routine laboratory testing including thyroid function studies and calcium levels.[10]

Lithium can cause fetal harm in pregnant women. Safety has not been established for children under 12 and is not recommended.[11]

---

4 This work is a derivative of *DailyMed* by U.S. National Library of Medicine and is available in the Public Domain

5 Malhi, G. S., Tanious, M., Das, P., Coulston, C. M., & Berk, M. (2013). Potential mechanisms of action of lithium in bipolar disorder. Current understanding. *CNS Drugs, 27*(2), 135–153. https://doi.org/10.1007/s40263-013-0039-0

6 This work is a derivative of *DailyMed* by U.S. National Library of Medicine and is available in the Public Domain

7 This work is a derivative of *DailyMed* by U.S. National Library of Medicine and is available in the Public Domain

8 Janicak, P. G. (2022). Bipolar disorder in adults and lithium: Pharmacology, administration, and management of adverse effects. *UpToDate*. Retrieved July 14, 2022, from https://www.uptodate.com

9 This work is a derivative of *DailyMed* by U.S. National Library of Medicine and is available in the Public Domain

10 Janicak, P. G. (2022). Bipolar disorder in adults and lithium: Pharmacology, administration, and management of adverse effects. *UpToDate*. Retrieved July 14, 2022, from https://www.uptodate.com

11 This work is a derivative of *DailyMed* by U.S. National Library of Medicine and is available in the Public Domain

Patient Education for Lithium

Lithium must be taken as prescribed or serious side effects can occur. Blood tests to measure lithium levels will be ordered regularly by the provider. The provider should be immediately notified of symptoms of elevated levels of lithium, including diarrhea, vomiting, drowsiness, muscular weakness, lack of coordination, ringing in the ears (tinnitus), or large amounts of dilute urine. Driving or operating heavy machinery should be avoided when first starting lithium because it can impair mental alertness. Lithium should not be taken during pregnancy or while breastfeeding unless it is determined that the benefits to the mother outweigh the potential risks to the baby.

Psychotherapy

Psychotherapy is a term for a variety of treatment techniques that help an individual identify and change troubling emotions, thoughts, and behaviors. Treatment may include therapies such as cognitive-behavioral therapy (CBT), dialectical behavior therapy (DBT), and psychoeducation. Read more information about CBT and DBT in the "Treatments for Depression" section in the "Depressive Disorders" chapter.

Treatment may also include newer therapies designed specifically for the treatment of bipolar disorder, including **Interpersonal and Social Rhythm Therapy (IPSRT)** and **family-focused therapy**. IPSRT emphasizes the importance of establishing stable daily routines such as sleeping, waking up, working, and eating meals. Family-focused therapy focuses on psychoeducation, communication enhancement training, and problem-solving skills. It includes attention to family dynamics and relationships as contributing factors to the client's mood.

Electroconvulsive Therapy

Electroconvulsive therapy (ECT) is used to treat bipolar disorders. ECT is a brain stimulation procedure delivered under general anesthesia. It can be effective in treating severe depressive and manic episodes when medication and psychotherapy are not effective. ECT can also be effective when a rapid response is needed, as in the case of suicide risk or **catatonia** (a state of unresponsiveness). Read more about electroconvulsive therapy (ECT) in the "Depressive Disorders" chapter.

Self-Help and Coping

Regular aerobic exercise, such as jogging, brisk walking, swimming, or bicycling, helps with depression and anxiety, promotes better sleep, and is healthy for the heart and brain. There is also some evidence that anaerobic exercise such as weightlifting, yoga, and Pilates can be helpful.[12]

Even with proper treatment, mood changes can occur. Treatment is more effective when a patient and health care provider work together and talk openly about concerns and choices. Keeping a life chart that records daily mood symptoms, treatments, sleep patterns, and life events can help clients and health care providers track and treat bipolar disorder over time. Clients can easily share data collected via smartphone apps – including self-reports, self-ratings, and activity data – with their health care providers and therapists.[13]

---

12 National Institute of Mental Health. (2020, January). *Bipolar disorder.* National Institutes of Health. https://www.nimh.nih.gov/health/topics/bipolar-disorder

13 National Institute of Mental Health. (2020, January). *Bipolar disorder.* National Institutes of Health. https://www.nimh.nih.gov/health/topics/bipolar-disorder

My Notes

Take the American Psychiatric Association's free course: The Treatment of Bipolar Depression: From Pills to Words.

8.4 APPLYING THE NURSING PROCESS TO BIPOLAR DISORDERS

My Notes

Assessment

Assessment of a client with a mood disorder focuses on both verbal and nonverbal assessments. People with a bipolar disorder experience periods of unusually intense emotion, grandiose delusions, changes in sleep patterns and activity levels, and impulsive behaviors, often without recognizing potential harmful effects.[1] See Figure 8.3[2] for an artistic depiction of grandiose delusions when a cat looking in a mirror sees a lion.

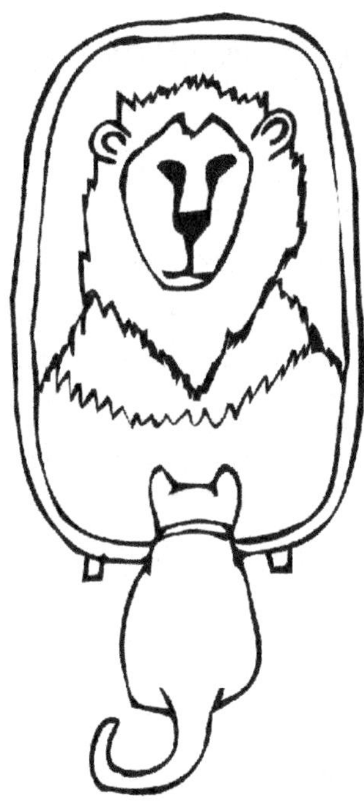

Figure 8.3 Grandiose Delusions

It is often helpful to interview family members or significant others of clients with mood disorders. Clients with mania, hypomania, or psychosis often have poor insight and may have difficulty providing an accurate history.[3]

Safety guidelines for assessing a client with a bipolar disorder include the following[4]:

- Assess if the client is a danger to self or others. The client may have suicidal or homicidal ideation. Poor impulse control may result in harm to self or others. Assess the need for protection from uninhibited behaviors. For example, external controls may be needed to protect the client from consequences such as bankruptcy.

---

1 National Institute of Mental Health. (2020, January). *Bipolar disorder.* National Institutes of Health. https://www.nimh.nih.gov/health/topics/bipolar-disorder

2 "Cat_and_lion_in_mirror_illustration.svg" by Arlo Barnes is licensed under CC BY 3.0

3 Suppes, T. (2021). Bipolar disorder in adults: Assessment and diagnosis. *UpToDate.* https://www.uptodate.com/contents/bipolar-disorder-in-adults-assessment-and-diagnosis?csi=6494a8a6-ebea-46a1-a6a3-aa9e1bafcb6d&source=contentShare

4 Halter, M. (2022). *Varcarolis' foundations of psychiatric-mental health nursing* (9th ed.). Saunders.

My Notes

- Assess physiological stability while obtaining vital signs and lab results including electrolytes. The client may not eat or sleep for days at a time with potential physiological consequences.

Mental Status Examination

Table 8.4a outlines typical assessment findings a nurse may observe in a client experiencing a manic episode. Typical findings relate to mood, behavior, thought processes, speech patterns, and cognitive function.

Table 8.4a Typical Mental Status Examination Findings for a Client Experiencing a Manic Episode[5,6,7]

Assessment	Typical Findings During a Manic Episode
Level of Consciousness and Orientation	May be disoriented/confused, but can be oriented to person, place, and time.
Mood and Affect	Exhibits an unstable, euphoric mood. Client may state they feel "up," "high," "jumpy," or "wired," but mood can quickly change to irritation and anger.[8]
Appearance and General Behavior	Typically exhibits a decreased need for sleep and a loss of appetite that may result in dehydration or poor nutritional status. May exhibit inappropriate dress or grooming or dress provocatively, sloppily, flamboyantly, or bizarrely. May change clothes frequently throughout the day. May use excessive makeup or demonstrate little attention to grooming. May demonstrate risky behaviors with poor impulse control and poor judgment, such as eating and drinking excessively, spending or giving away a lot of money, or having reckless sex.[9] Excessive spending can lead to financial hardship from credit card debt from buying items they don't need.
Speech	Typically talk very fast (e.g., pressured speech) about many different topics (hyperverbal).[10] May have difficulty in accurately communicating needs due to flight of ideas or slurred or garbled speech.
Motor Activity	Typically hyperactive with an inability to recognize need for rest or sleep.

---

5 National Institute of Mental Health. (2020, January). *Bipolar disorder.* National Institutes of Health. https://www.nimh.nih.gov/health/topics/bipolar-disorder

6 Halter, M. (2022). *Varcarolis' foundations of psychiatric-mental health nursing* (9th ed.). Saunders.

7 Suppes, T. (2021). Bipolar disorder in adults: Assessment and diagnosis. *UpToDate.* https://www.uptodate.com/contents/bipolar-disorder-in-adults-assessment-and-diagnosis?csi=6494a8a6-ebea-46a1-a6a3-aa9e1bafcb6d&source=contentShare

8 National Institute of Mental Health. (2020, January). *Bipolar disorder.* National Institutes of Health. https://www.nimh.nih.gov/health/topics/bipolar-disorder

9 National Institute of Mental Health. (2020, January). *Bipolar disorder.* National Institutes of Health. https://www.nimh.nih.gov/health/topics/bipolar-disorder

10 National Institute of Mental Health. (2020, January). *Bipolar disorder.* National Institutes of Health. https://www.nimh.nih.gov/health/topics/bipolar-disorder

My Notes

Assessment	Typical Findings During a Manic Episode
Thought and Perception	Client may state they feel as if their "thoughts are racing."[11] May feel as if they are unusually important, talented, or powerful.[12] May describe hallucinations, illusions, or paranoia. May exhibit flight of ideas, loose associations, and clang associations. (See definitions of terms in the "Application of the Nursing Process in Mental Health Care" chapter.) May exhibit suicidal, homicidal, or violence ideation.
Attitude and Insight	Typically exhibit limited insight with an inability to make sound decisions impacting their adherence to taking prescribed medications.
Cognitive Abilities	Typically exhibit decreased attention span, distraction, and impaired judgement.

Screening Tools

Many screening tools exist to assess mood disorders. Common examples include the following:

- Mood Disorder Questionnaire (MDQ) PDF: Thirteen questions with yes/no responses for assessing mania.
- Young Mania Rating Scale (YMRS) PDF: An 11-item assessment based on the client's subjective report of behaviors over the past 24 hours regarding manic symptoms. It is useful to evaluate baseline functioning and progress being made. There is also a parent version for assessing children and adolescents.
- Altman Self-Rating Mania Scale: A self-assessment questionnaire to evaluate the severity of mania or hypomania.

Laboratory Testing

Initial medical evaluation of clients with a possible or established diagnosis of bipolar disorder typically includes the following:

- Thyroid stimulating hormone
- Complete blood count
- Chemistry panel
- Urine toxicology to screen for substances of abuse

Thereafter, routine laboratory testing for clients with bipolar disorders can include these items:

- Therapeutic Medication Levels: Medication dosages may need adjustment based on blood levels to avoid toxicity and ensure they are in therapeutic range. Read more about therapeutic drug

---

11 National Institute of Mental Health. (2020, January). *Bipolar disorder.* National Institutes of Health. https://www.nimh.nih.gov/health/topics/bipolar-disorder

12 National Institute of Mental Health. (2020, January). *Bipolar disorder.* National Institutes of Health. https://www.nimh.nih.gov/health/topics/bipolar-disorder

My Notes

levels under the "Medications" subsection of the "Treatments for Bipolar Disorders" section of this chapter.

- Kidney or liver function tests, based on medications prescribed.
- Thyroid function studies and calcium levels.
- Nutrition or hydration status, such as serum sodium levels, hematocrit, albumin, and prealbumin levels, which can become impaired during manic episodes due to poor intake.

Reflective Questions

1. What are some common underlying medical conditions that could potentially mimic the symptoms of mania in older adults?
2. Why are some individuals with bipolar disorder misdiagnosed with schizophrenia?

Diagnoses

Mental health disorders are diagnosed by trained mental health professionals using the *Diagnostic and Statistical Manual of Mental Disorders (DSM-5).* Nurses create individualized nursing care plans using nursing diagnoses based on the client's response to their mental health disorders. Examples of common nursing diagnoses associated with bipolar disorders are listed in Table 8.4b.

Table 8.4b Common Nursing Diagnoses Related to Bipolar Disorder[13,14]

Nursing Diagnosis	Associated Behaviors and Characteristics
Safety: Risk for Injury Risk for Suicide Risk for Violence	Impulsive, risky behaviors with poor personal boundaries. Lack of insight into illness. May exhibit agitation, self-harm, or threatening behaviors.
Communication: Impaired Cognition Impaired Communication	Grandiose thinking with poor judgment, flight of ideas, or pressured speech with loose associations.
Self-Care Deficit: Bathing, Grooming, Hygiene, Dressing	Poor hygiene and distracted from tasks.
Impaired Nutrition	Unable to sit long enough to eat; poor appetite. May eat excessive amounts of food during hypomanic episodes.
Disturbed Sleep Patterns	Inability to rest or sleep without frequent awakenings; often hyperactive at night.
Fatigue r/t Psychological Demands	Hyperactive and restless.

13 Ackley, B., Ladwig, G., Makic, M. B., Martinez-Kratz, M., & Zanotti, M. (2020). *Nursing diagnosis handbook: An evidence-based guide to planning care* (12th ed.). Elsevier.

14 Halter, M. (2022). *Varcarolis' foundations of psychiatric-mental health nursing* (9th ed.). Saunders.

My Notes

Nursing Diagnosis	Associated Behaviors and Characteristics
Social Isolation r/t Ineffective Coping or Intrusive Behaviors	Feel different from others and preoccupied with own thoughts. Social behavior may be incongruent with norms. May demonstrate an excessive amount of verbal exchange or violation of personal boundaries. May engage in inappropriate sexual language or behavior.
Risk for Spiritual Distress	Demonstrate ineffective coping strategies, separation from support system, or hopelessness.

Outcomes Identification

Outcome criteria are based on the phase of bipolar illness the client is experiencing, either acute or maintenance phase.[15]

During an acute manic episode, the overall goals are symptom management, achieving remission of symptoms, preventing injury, and supporting physiological integrity. Examples of goals during the acute phase include the following[16]:

- Maintain stable cardiac status.
- Be well-hydrated.
- Get sufficient sleep and rest.
- Make no attempt at self-harm.
- Demonstrate thought control with the aid of staff and/or medication.
- Maintain tissue integrity.

The maintenance phase occurs after acute symptoms have been controlled and the goals become focused on preventing future exacerbations of manic episodes through education, support, and problem-solving skills. The following are examples of goals during the maintenance phase[17]:

- Identifying and avoiding triggers for developing acute mania
- Attending therapy sessions
- Developing new coping skills

SMART outcomes are Specific, Measurable, Attainable/Actionable, Relevant, and Timely. Read more about SMART outcomes in the "Application of the Nursing Process in Mental Health Care" chapter. The following are sample SMART outcomes for clients with bipolar disorders:

- The client will communicate feelings and thoughts of self-harm (self-injury) to the health care team, prior to acting on thoughts, during this shift.
- The client will eat breakfast within one hour of the arrival of the breakfast tray.

---

15 Halter, M. (2022). *Varcarolis' foundations of psychiatric-mental health nursing* (9th ed.). Saunders.

16 Halter, M. (2022). *Varcarolis' foundations of psychiatric-mental health nursing* (9th ed.). Saunders.

17 Halter, M. (2022). *Varcarolis' foundations of psychiatric-mental health nursing* (9th ed.). Saunders.

My Notes

- The client will attend one or more group meetings each day while in the outpatient setting.

Planning Interventions

When a client is hospitalized during an acute manic episode, planning focuses on stabilizing the client while maintaining safety. Nursing care focuses on managing medications, decreasing physical activity, increasing food and fluid intake, reinforcing a minimum of 4 to 6 hours of sleep per night, and ensuring self-care needs are met.[18]

During the maintenance phase, planning focuses on preventing relapse and limiting the severity and duration of future episodes. During this period, individuals with bipolar disorders often face multiple hardships resulting from their behaviors during previous acute manic episodes. Interpersonal, occupational, educational, and financial consequences may occur. Clients need support as they recover from acute illness and repair their lives.[19]

Individuals are often ambivalent about treatment, but bipolar disorders typically require medications to be taken over long periods of time or for a lifetime to prevent relapse. Self-medication through alcohol or other substances often complicates recovery and treatment. Nurses must establish a therapeutic nurse-client relationship to support continued treatment. Individuals are typically referred to community resources and outpatient mental health care settings. In addition to medication management, outpatient services provide structure and decrease social isolation.[20]

Implementation

Common nursing interventions for clients experiencing acute manic episodes are described in the following tables. Table 8.4c describes interventions according to categories in the APNA Standard of *Implementation*. (Read more about the APNA *Implementation* Standard in the "Application of the Nursing Process in Mental Health Care" chapter.) Table 8.4d describes nursing interventions to promote physiological integrity. See the "Treatments for Bipolar Disorders" section of this chapter for additional collaborative mental health interventions, including medications and psychotherapy.

18 Halter, M. (2022). *Varcarolis' foundations of psychiatric-mental health nursing* (9th ed.). Saunders.

19 Halter, M. (2022). *Varcarolis' foundations of psychiatric-mental health nursing* (9th ed.). Saunders.

20 Halter, M. (2022). *Varcarolis' foundations of psychiatric-mental health nursing* (9th ed.). Saunders.

My Notes

Table 8.4c Nursing Interventions for Mania Based on the Categories of the APNA Implementation Standard[21]		
Categories of Interventions Based on the APNA Standard ofImplementation	**What the nurse will do . . .**	**Rationale**
Coordination of Care	Plan for quality of life, independence, and optimal recovery. Refer to community resources and outpatient mental health care settings. Maintain safety by communicating safety precautions with interprofessional team members as needed to prevent self-harm, suicide, or homicide risks. Ensure consistency of behavioral expectations among all staff on the unit by including expectations in the nursing care plan.	The nurse coordinates care delivery during inpatient care and for after discharge. The client may exhibit high risk or impulsive behaviors that could pose a risk of harm to self/others. They may experience altered thought processes with poor insight and judgment. Consistent expectations help prevent manipulative behaviors and pushing of limits.
Health Teaching	Create, adapt, and deliver health teaching to clients, including self-care, self-awareness activities, and milieu group therapy topics. See "Patient Education" topics for bipolar disorder in the box following these tables.	Nurses encourage resilience by promoting adaptive coping strategies.
Pharmacological, Biological, and Integrative Therapies	Deliver patient education about mood stabilizers and other medications with expected time frames for improvement. Open all medications in front of the client. Observe for signs of medication toxicity, such as lithium.	The client's understanding of their medications and potential side effects can increase medication adherence. Opening all medications in front of the client may decrease paranoia. There is a small margin of safety between therapeutic and toxic doses of lithium.

21 Halter, M. (2022). *Varcarolis' foundations of psychiatric-mental health nursing* (9th ed.). Saunders.

My Notes

Categories of Interventions Based on the APNA Standard ofImplementation	What the nurse will do . . .	Rationale
Milieu Therapy	Manage the milieu by reducing environmental stimuli and excess noise. The client may require a private room. Provide structured 1:1 activities with the nurse or other staff. Avoid competitive activities or games. Encourage frequent rest periods and "down time." Promote physical exercise to redirect aggressive behavior. During acute mania, use prescribed medications, seclusion, or restraint to minimize physical harm. Store valuables in the hospital safe until safe judgment returns. Encourage participation in group therapy after acute manic episode has resolved addressing social skills, personal grooming, mindfulness, and stress management.	Reducing stimuli may prevent escalation of anxiety and agitation. Structured activities provide security and focus. However, avoid group and/or competitive activities because they may be too stimulating and can cause escalation of anxiety and agitation. Resting can prevent exhaustion that can result from constant physical activity. Physical exercise can decrease tension and provide focus. The nurse's priority is to protect the patient and others from harm. Storing valued items protects the patient from giving away money and possessions. Group therapy can encourage effective coping skills.
Therapeutic Relationship and Counseling	Use a firm and calm approach with short and concise statements. For example, "John, come with me. Eat this sandwich." Be consistent in approach and expectations. Identify expectations in simple, concrete terms with consequences. For example, "John, do not yell at or hit Peter. If you cannot control your behaviors, you will be escorted to the seclusion room to prevent harm to yourself and others." Listen to and act on legitimate complaints. Redirect energy into appropriate and constructive channels. Set limits with personal boundaries. See additional "Communication Tips" in the box below.	Structure and control can improve feelings of security for a client who is feeling out of control. Consistent limits and expectations minimize the potential for the client's manipulation of staff and provide feelings of security. Clear expectations help the patient experience outside controls and understand reasons for medication, seclusion, or restraints if they are not able to control their behaviors. Listening to legitimate complaints can reduce underlying feelings of helplessness and can minimize acting-out behaviors. Distraction is an effective tool with clients experiencing mania. Clients may be impulsive and hyperverbal and interrupt, blame, ridicule, or manipulate others.

My Notes

Table 8.4d Nursing Interventions to Promote Physiological Integrity[22]

Problem/ Intervention	Rationale
Nutrition ■ **Monitor intake, output, and vital signs.** ■ **Offer frequent, high-calorie, high-protein snacks, drinks, and finger foods.** ■ **Frequently remind the client to eat.** ■ **Monitor laboratory results.**	Ensure adequate intake and minimize development of dehydration. "Finger foods" allow for "eating on the run." The client experiencing mania is unaware of bodily needs and is easily distracted.
Sleep ■ **Encourage frequent rest periods during the day and adequate sleep during manic episodes.** ■ **Keep patient in areas of low stimulation to induce relaxation.** ■ **Before bedtime, provide warm baths, soothing music, and prescribed medication if needed.** ■ **Avoid caffeine.**	Lack of sleep can lead to exhaustion and increased mania. Relaxation techniques induce sleep. Encouraging bedtime routines and decreasing caffeine intake increases the possibility of sleep.[23]
Elimination (Constipation) ■ **Monitor frequency of bowel movements.** ■ **Encourage fluids and foods high in fiber.** ■ **Encourage the client to go to the bathroom.** ■ **Evaluate the need for a bowel management program with stool softeners and laxatives.**	Fluids and fiber stimulate peristalsis and soft stools. The client experiencing acute mania is easily distracted and not aware of bodily needs. Bowel management programs may be needed to avoid fecal impaction.
Self-Care Deficits ■ **Encourage the use of a toothbrush, washcloth, soap, and makeup or shaving supplies.** ■ **Encourage appropriate clothing choices.** ■ **Provide step-by-step reminders for hygiene and dress, such as "Wash the right side of your face and now your left."**	Distractibility and poor concentration are countered through simple, concrete instructions. The client is helped to maintain dignity and avoid potential for ridicule that can lower self-esteem.

22 Halter, M. (2022). *Varcarolis' foundations of psychiatric-mental health nursing* (9th ed.). Saunders.

23 Centers for Disease Control and Prevention. (2016, July 15). *Tips for a better sleep.* https://www.cdc.gov/sleep/about_sleep/ sleep_hygiene.html

My Notes

Effective Communication Tips for Clients With Bipolar Disorder

- Use a firm and matter-of-fact tone and calm approach (client needs structure).
- Use simple, concise, very short explanations (client has short attention span and difficulty focusing).
- Reinforce verbal limit setting on behaviors with personal boundaries (client is impulsive and distractible with limited insight and inappropriate behaviors towards others).
- Utilize therapeutic communication techniques, such as redirecting, active listening, distraction, clarification, or restating; avoid exploring because client's thought process is too expansive.
- Avoid the use of jargon, jingles, jokes, proverbs, or cliches (client is already overstimulated).
- Remain neutral with careful choice of words to avoid "power struggles." (A client experiencing a severe manic episode can be manipulative and lack personal boundaries.)
- If a client demonstrates agitation with escalation of manic behavior, review interventions described in the "Crisis and Crisis Intervention" section of the "Stress, Coping, and Crisis Intervention" chapter. Additional de-escalation techniques to maintain safety are described in the "Workplace Violence" section of the "Trauma, Abuse, and Violence" chapter.

Patient Education: Bipolar Disorder

Living with bipolar disorder can be challenging, but there are ways to control symptoms and enable oneself, a client, a friend, or a loved one to live a healthy life. The client may be resistant to teaching during the acute phase of a manic episode, so it is beneficial to wait until manic symptoms begin to resolve. Patient education regarding bipolar disorder includes the following guidelines[24]:

- Get treatment and stay committed to it. Recovery from a manic episode takes time and it's not easy, but treatment is the best way to start feeling better.
- Keep medical and therapy appointments and talk with the provider about treatment options.
- Take all medicines as directed.
- Maintain a structure for daily activities; keep a routine for eating, getting enough sleep, and exercising.
- Learn to recognize mood swings and warning signs for manic episodes such as decreased need for sleep.
- Ask for help when experiencing barriers or challenges for treatment. Social support helps coping.

---

24 National Institute of Mental Health. (2020, January). *Bipolar disorder.* National Institutes of Health. https://www.nimh.nih.gov/health/topics/bipolar-disorder

My Notes

- Be patient; improvement takes time.
- Avoid using alcohol and illicit drugs.
- Encourage participation in cognitive behavioral therapy (CBT) or dialectical behavioral therapy (DBT).
- Use stress management, relaxation techniques, and coping strategies to minimize anxiety.
- Participate in support groups such as those sponsored by the National Alliance on Mental Illness (NAMI) and the Depression and Bipolar Support Alliance (DBSA).

Implementing Seclusion or Restraints

Controlling escalating agitation during the acute phase of a manic episode may include immediate administration of a prescribed antipsychotic and benzodiazepine. A combination of haloperidol (Haldol) and lorazepam (Ativan) that can be injected for rapid onset of action is commonly used. The nurse must monitor for respiratory depression, hypotension, and oversedation after administering this type of medication.

De-escalation techniques should be attempted at early signs of escalating agitation to avoid the need for seclusion or restraints. However, if a client is escalating out of control to a point where they pose an immediate risk of injury to themselves or others, the use of a seclusion room or restraints may become necessary to maintain a safe environment. Most state laws prevent the use of unnecessary restraint or seclusion, so their use is associated with complex ethical, legal, and therapeutic issues.[25]

Agency policy must be closely followed when implementing seclusion or restraints. Documentation is required that indicates the need for seclusion and/or restraint[26]:

- There is a clear substantial risk of harm to self or others.
- The client is unable to control their actions.
- Other interventions have not been effective (e.g., reducing stimuli, providing distraction, setting limits, verbally de-escalating with therapeutic techniques, or offering PRN medications).

Each agency establishes a proper reporting procedure through the chain of command. For example, seclusion and restraint are only permitted with a written order from an authorized provider (e.g., physician, nurse practitioner, or physician assistant) and rewritten every 24 hours or more frequently according to hospital policy and state regulations. The order must include the type of restraint (e.g., physical or chemical) to be used. In an emergency, the charge nurse may place a client in seclusion or restraints and obtain a written order within a specified period of time (typically 15-30 minutes).[27]

25 Halter, M. (2022). *Varcarolis' foundations of psychiatric-mental health nursing* (9th ed.). Saunders.

26 Halter, M. (2022). *Varcarolis' foundations of psychiatric-mental health nursing* (9th ed.). Saunders.

27 Halter, M. (2022). *Varcarolis' foundations of psychiatric-mental health nursing* (9th ed.). Saunders.

My Notes

Established agency protocols specify associated nursing responsibilities to maintain client safety while in seclusion or restraints, such as the following[28]:

- 1:1 supervision or visual monitoring
- How often to offer the client food and fluids (e.g., every 30-60 minutes)
- How often the client can use the restroom (e.g., every 1-2 hours)
- How often to measure vital signs (e.g., every 1-2 hours)

Read more details about the legal implications of seclusion and restraints in the "Legal and Ethical Considerations in Mental Health Care" chapter.

Evaluation

Evaluation occurs continuously throughout the treatment of bipolar disorders. The registered nurse individualizes assessments based on the established goals and SMART outcomes for each client. The effectiveness of nursing and collaborative interventions is evaluated and revised as needed. Questions used to guide the evaluation process include the following:

- Is the client medically stable with nutritional intake, sleep patterns, labs, or activity levels?
- Is the client engaging in own self-care measures?
- Is the client safe with no self-harm behaviors, statements, gestures, or threats of harm towards others?
- Is the client engaging appropriately in unit-based activities and the therapeutic milieu?
- Is the client able to maintain appropriate personal boundaries with others?
- Is the client able to engage appropriately in verbal conversations and interactions with others?
- Is the client able to demonstrate insight into own illness?
- Is the client tolerating prescriptive medications at therapeutic serum levels and without key side effects?
- Is the client at or near baseline optimal functioning without manic symptoms?
- Is the client able to participate in their own plan of care including discharge planning?

---

28 Halter, M. (2022). *Varcarolis' foundations of psychiatric-mental health nursing* (9th ed.). Saunders.

My Notes

8.5 SPOTLIGHT APPLICATION

Sample Nursing Documentation

Here is a sample nursing narrative note for a client recently admitted who is currently experiencing an acute phase of a manic episode.

S: Patient reports feeling "very happy" with "high energy"' and "no need for sleep." She states, "I've got lots to accomplish today; now move out of my way."

O: Euphoric mood with full range affect. Denies suicidal or homicidal ideation. Is skipping in the hallways and singing loudly with rapid, pressured speech. Is easily distracted and unable to focus on the current conversation. Is intrusive with others with a poor sense of personal boundaries; she is giving away clothing items and going into other patients' rooms and taking their belongings. Dressing in multiple layers of clothes and unable to sit to eat or finish meals. She has experienced weight loss of four pounds in the past three days.

A: Acute mania nearing exhaustion with disruptive behaviors.

P: Reduce stimuli with calming milieu and redirect firmly to maintain appropriate personal boundaries with others. Encourage nutritional intake with hydration and finger foods, along with rest periods twice a day. Refrain from large group activities with short 1:1 time for unit programming needs.

My Notes

8.6 LEARNING ACTIVITIES

Interactive Activities

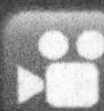

An interactive H5P element has been excluded from this version of the text. You can view it online here: https://wtcs.pressbooks.pub/nursingmhcc/?p=380#h5p-20

An interactive H5P element has been excluded from this version of the text. You can view it online here: https://wtcs.pressbooks.pub/nursingmhcc/?p=380#h5p-21

An interactive H5P element has been excluded from this version of the text. You can view it online here: https://wtcs.pressbooks.pub/nursingmhcc/?p=380#h5p-23

VIII GLOSSARY

My Notes

Bipolar I Disorder: The most severe bipolar disorder with at least one manic episode; most individuals experience additional hypomanic and depressive episodes.

Bipolar II Disorder: A pattern of depressive episodes and hypomanic episodes, but individuals have never experienced a full-blown manic episode typical of Bipolar I Disorder.

Catatonia: A state of unresponsiveness due to a person's mental state.

Cyclothymia: A disorder defined by periods of hypomanic symptoms and periods of depressive symptoms lasting for at least two years (1 year in children and adolescents). However, the symptoms do not meet the diagnostic requirements for hypomanic episodes or depressive episodes.[1]

Family-focused therapy: Psychotherapy that focuses on psychoeducation, communication enhancement training, and problem-solving skills. It includes attention to family dynamics and relationships as contributing factors to the client's mood.

Grandiose delusions: A symptom associated with bipolar disorders of feeling unusually important, talented, or powerful.

Hypomanic episode: Episodes similar to symptoms of a manic episode, but they are less severe and do not cause significant impairment in social or occupational functioning or require hospitalization.[2]

Interpersonal and social rhythm therapy (IPSRT): Psychotherapy that emphasizes the importance of establishing stable daily routines such as sleeping, waking up, working, and eating meals.

Manic episode: A persistently elevated or irritable mood with abnormally increased energy lasting at least one week. The mood disturbance is severe and causes marked impairment in social or occupational function. Severe episodes often require hospitalization to prevent harm to self or others.

Psychotherapy: A variety of treatment techniques that help an individual identify and change troubling emotions, thoughts, and behaviors.

Rapid cycling: At least four mood episodes associated with bipolar disorder occurring in a 12-month period.

1 National Institute of Mental Health. (2020, January). *Bipolar disorder.* National Institutes of Health. https://www.nimh.nih.gov/health/topics/bipolar-disorder

2 American Psychiatric Association. (2013). *Desk reference to the diagnostic criteria from DSM-5.*

Chapter 9

Anxiety Disorders

9.1 INTRODUCTION

My Notes

Learning Objectives

- Apply the nursing process to clients with anxiety disorders, obsessive-compulsive disorder, and post-traumatic stress disorder
- Describe nursing assessments related to anxiety disorders, obsessive-compulsive disorder, and post-traumatic stress disorder
- Identify common nursing problems/diagnoses related to anxiety disorders
- Establish a safe environment
- Apply evidence-based practice when planning and implementing nursing care
- Describe common treatments for anxiety disorders, obsessive-compulsive disorder, and post-traumatic stress disorder
- Identify appropriate referrals to community resources
- Evaluate the effectiveness of interventions
- Provide patient education to clients and their family members

Anxiety is a part of everyday life and can be experienced to varying degrees from helpful to harmful. Anxiety is a response to stress, whether the stressor is experienced as a positive or negative. Positive stressors might be cleaning the house before family and friends arrive for a holiday gathering or studying for an exam whereas negative stressors can be losing one's car keys or getting into a fight with a loved one. For example, mild anxiety can provide energy and concentration needed to complete important tasks or provide motivation to make healthy behavioral changes. However, excessive anxiety can cause distress and impair an individual's functioning in social, educational, occupational, or other areas of functioning.

This chapter will describe levels of anxiety and common anxiety disorders such as generalized anxiety disorder, panic disorder, and various phobias. It will also describe how anxiety is related to obsessive-compulsive disorder (OCD), post-traumatic stress disorder (PTSD), and some medical conditions. The nursing process will be applied to caring for individuals experiencing anxiety.

My Notes

9.2 BASIC CONCEPTS

Anxiety is a universal human experience that includes feelings of apprehension, uneasiness, uncertainty, or dread resulting from a real or perceived threat.[1] Fear is a reaction to a specific danger, whereas anxiety is a vague sense of dread to a specific or unknown danger. However, the body reacts physiologically with the stress response to both anxiety and fear.[2] See an artistic depiction of a person facing their feelings of anxiety from a perceived threat in Figure 9.1.[3] Review the stress response in the "Stress, Coping, and Crisis Intervention" chapter.

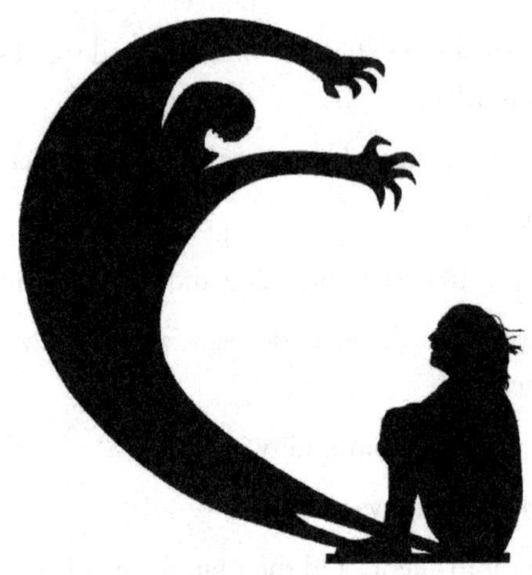

Figure 9.1 Anxiety

Levels of Anxiety

Hildegard Peplau, a psychiatric mental health nurse theorist, developed a model describing four levels of anxiety: mild, moderate, severe, and panic. Behaviors and characteristics can overlap across these levels, but it can be helpful to tailor interventions based on the level of anxiety the client is experiencing.[4]

Mild

Mild anxiety is part of everyday living and can help an individual use their senses to perceive reality in sharp focus. Symptoms of mild anxiety include restlessness, irritability, or mild tension-relieving behaviors such as finger tapping, fidgeting, or nail biting.[5]

Moderate Anxiety

As anxiety increases, the perceptual field narrows, and the ability of the individual to fully observe their surroundings is diminished/reduced. The person experiencing moderate anxiety may demonstrate selective inattention

1 Halter, M. (2022). *Varcarolis' foundations of psychiatric-mental health nursing* (9th ed.). Saunders.

2 Halter, M. (2022). *Varcarolis' foundations of psychiatric-mental health nursing* (9th ed.). Saunders.

3 "fear-g84d457182_1280" by mohamed_hassan on Pixabay.com is licensed under CC0

4 Halter, M. (2022). *Varcarolis' foundations of psychiatric-mental health nursing* (9th ed.). Saunders.

5 Halter, M. (2022). *Varcarolis' foundations of psychiatric-mental health nursing* (9th ed.). Saunders.

My Notes

where only certain things in the environment are seen or heard unless they are pointed out. The individual's ability to think clearly, learn, and problem solve is hampered, but can still take place. The physiological stress response kicks in with symptoms such as perspiration, elevated heart rate, and elevated respiratory rate. The individual may also experience headaches, gastric discomfort, urinary urgency, voice tremors, and shakiness; however, they may not be aware these symptoms are related to their level of stress and anxiety.[6]

Severe Anxiety

The perceptual field of a person experiencing severe anxiety is greatly reduced. They may either focus on one particular detail or on many scattered details. They often have difficulty noticing what is going on in their environment, even if it is pointed out; they may appear dazed or confused with automatic behavior. Learning, problem-solving, and critical thinking are not possible at this level. Symptoms of the stress response intensify and may include hyperventilation, a pounding heart, insomnia, and a sense of impending doom.[7] See Figure 9.2[8] for an artist's rendition of severe anxiety.

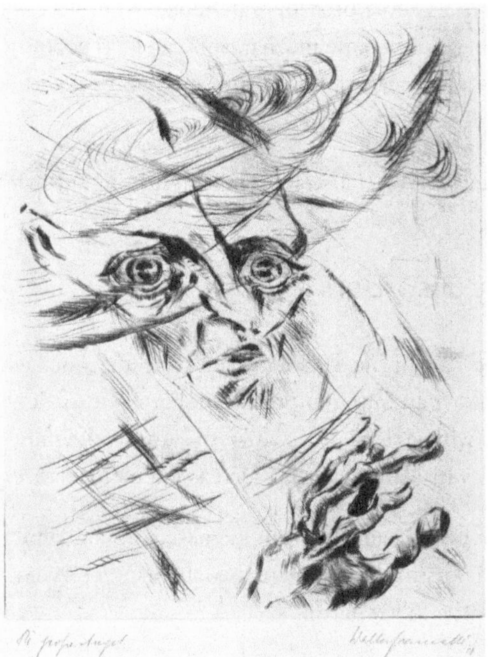

Figure 9.2 Severe Anxiety

Panic

Panic is the most extreme level of anxiety that results in significantly dysregulated behavior. The individual is unable to process information from the environment and may lose touch with reality. They may demonstrate

6 Halter, M. (2022). *Varcarolis' foundations of psychiatric-mental health nursing* (9th ed.). Saunders.

7 Halter, M. (2022). *Varcarolis' foundations of psychiatric-mental health nursing* (9th ed.). Saunders.

8 "Walter_Gramatté,_Die_Grosse_Angst_(The_Great_Anxiety),_1918,_NGA_71292.jpg" by Walter Gramatté is licensed in the Public Domain

My Notes

behavior such as pacing, running, shouting, screaming, or withdrawal, and hallucinations may occur. Acute panic can lead to exhaustion.[9]

Coping With Anxiety

Individuals may use several strategies to cope with anxiety. **Coping strategies** are an action, a series of actions, or a thought process used to address a stressful or unpleasant situation or modify one's reaction to such a situation. Coping strategies are classified as adaptive or maladaptive. Adaptive coping strategies include problem-focused coping and emotion-focused coping. Problem-focused coping typically focuses on seeking treatment such as counseling or cognitive behavioral therapy. Emotion-focused coping includes strategies such as engaging in mindfulness, meditation, or yoga; using humor and jokes; seeking spiritual or religious pursuits; engaging in physical activity or breathing exercises; and seeking social support. Maladaptive coping responses include responses such as avoidance of the stressful condition, withdrawal from a stressful environment, disengagement from stressful relationships, and misuse of alcohol or other substances.

Defense mechanisms are reaction patterns used by individuals to protect themselves from anxiety that arises from stress and conflict. Adaptive use of defense mechanisms can help people achieve their goals, but excessive or maladaptive use of defense mechanisms can be unhealthy.[10] Excessive use of defense mechanisms are associated with specific mental health disorders.

Read more about coping strategies and defense mechanisms in the "Stress, Coping, and Crisis Intervention" chapter.

Risk Factors for Anxiety Disorders

Occasional anxiety is an expected part of life. It is common to feel anxious when faced with a problem at work, before taking a test, or before making an important decision. However, anxiety disorders involve more than temporary worry or fear. For a person with an anxiety disorder, the anxiety does not go away and can worsen over time, and their symptoms can interfere with daily activities such as job performance, schoolwork, and relationships.[11]

Researchers have found that both genetic and environmental factors contribute to the risk of developing an anxiety disorder. Although the risk factors for each type of anxiety disorder can vary, some general risk factors for all types of anxiety disorders include the following[12]:

- Temperamental traits of shyness or behavioral inhibition in childhood
- Exposure to traumatic life or environmental events in early childhood or adulthood
- A history of anxiety or other mental health disorders in biological relatives

Review information about adverse childhood events in the "Mental Health and Mental Illness" section in Chapter 1.

---

9 Halter, M. (2022). *Varcarolis' foundations of psychiatric-mental health nursing* (9th ed.). Saunders.

10 Halter, M. (2022). *Varcarolis' foundations of psychiatric-mental health nursing* (9th ed.). Saunders.

11 Herdman, T. H., & Kamitsuru, S. (Eds.). (2018). *Nursing diagnoses: Definitions and classification, 2018-2020.* Thieme Publishers New York.

12 National Institute of Mental Health. (n.d.). *Any anxiety disorder.* U.S. Department of Health and Human Services. https://www.nimh.nih.gov/health/statistics/any-anxiety-disorder

Some medical conditions (such as thyroid problems, chronic obstructive pulmonary disease, and angina) or substances (such as caffeine, certain prescribed medications, or illicit drugs) can also cause symptoms of anxiety. When a client is initially evaluated for anxiety, a physical health examination is performed to rule out other potential causes of their anxiety symptoms.

My Notes

My Notes

9.3 ANXIETY - RELATED DISORDERS

Anxiety disorders are a common mental health problem. Research indicates 19% of adults and 31% of adolescents have an anxiety disorder in the United States.[1] The percentage of adults with an anxiety disorder associated with various levels of anxiety are estimated as mild (43%), moderate (33%), and severe (23%).[2]

There are several types of anxiety-related disorders, including generalized anxiety disorder, social anxiety disorder, panic disorder, phobia-related disorders, separation anxiety, and selective mutism.[3]

Generalized Anxiety Disorder

The *Diagnostic and Statistical Manual of Mental Disorders (DSM-5)* defines **generalized anxiety disorder (GAD)** as "excessive anxiety and worry, occurring on more days than not for at least six months, about a number of events or activities (such as work or school performance)." The individual finds it difficult to control the anxiety and worry, and it is associated with at least three of the following symptoms[4]:

- Restless or feeling keyed up or on edge
- Being easily fatigued
- Difficulty concentrating or going mentally blank
- Irritability
- Muscle tension
- Sleep disturbance (difficulty falling or staying asleep or restless, unsatisfying sleep)

The anxiety, worry, or physical symptoms cause clinically significant distress or impairment in social, occupational, or other areas of functioning and are not attributable to the physiological effects of a substance, medical condition, or other mental disorder.[5] See Figure 9.3[6] for an artist's depiction of feelings of anxiety.

---

1 National Institute of Mental Health. (n.d.). *Any anxiety disorder.* U.S. Department of Health and Human Services. https://www.nimh.nih.gov/health/statistics/any-anxiety-disorder

2 National Institute of Mental Health. (n.d.). *Any anxiety disorder.* U.S. Department of Health and Human Services. https://www.nimh.nih.gov/health/statistics/any-anxiety-disorder

3 National Institute of Mental Health. (n.d.). *Any anxiety disorder.* U.S. Department of Health and Human Services. https://www.nimh.nih.gov/health/statistics/any-anxiety-disorder

4 American Psychiatric Association. (2013). *Desk reference to the diagnostic criteria from DSM-5.*

5 American Psychiatric Association. (2013). *Desk reference to the diagnostic criteria from DSM-5.*

6 "Edvard_Munch_-_Anxiety_-_Google_Art_Project.jpg" by Edvard Munch is licensed in the Public Domain

My Notes

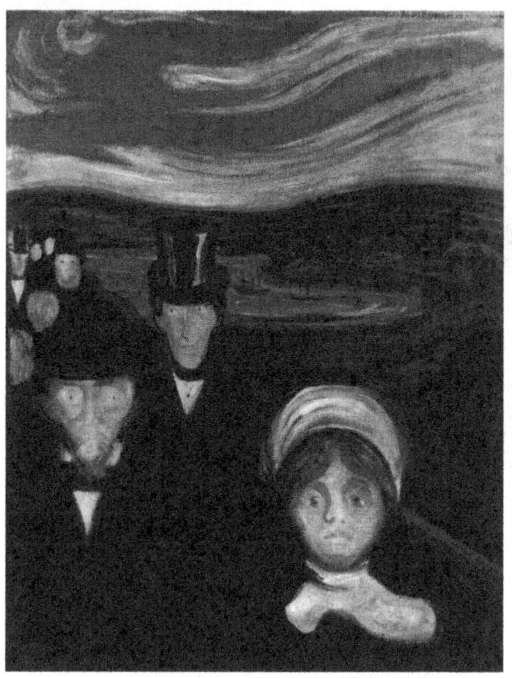

Figure 9.3 Anxiety

Social Anxiety Disorder

Social anxiety disorder was previously called social phobia. The *DSM-5* defines **social anxiety disorder** as marked fear or anxiety about one or more social situations in which the individual is exposed to possible scrutiny by others. Examples include social interactions (e.g., having a conversation, meeting unfamiliar people), being observed (e.g., eating or drinking), and performing in front of others (e.g., giving a speech). The individual fears they will act in a way or show anxiety symptoms that will be negatively evaluated by others, so social situations are avoided or endured with intense fear or anxiety. This fear, anxiety, or avoidance is persistent and typically lasts for six months or more and is not related to a substance, another mental health disorder, or medical condition. It results in clinically significant impairment in social, occupational, or other important areas of functioning. In children, the fear or anxiety may be expressed by crying, tantrums, freezing, clinging, shrinking, or failing to speak in social situations.[7]

Panic Disorder

People with panic disorder have recurrent unexpected panic attacks. **Panic attacks** are sudden periods of intense fear that come on quickly and reach their peak within minutes. Attacks can occur unexpectedly or can be brought on by a trigger, such as a feared object or situation. A panic attack can be caused solely by the fear of having a panic attack.[8] See Figure 9.4.[9]

---

7 American Psychiatric Association. (2013). *Desk reference to the diagnostic criteria from DSM-5.*

8 American Psychiatric Association. (2013). *Desk reference to the diagnostic criteria from DSM-5.*

9 "A_subjective_impression_of_a_panic_attack.png" by Yitzilitt is licensed under CC BY-SA 4.0

My Notes

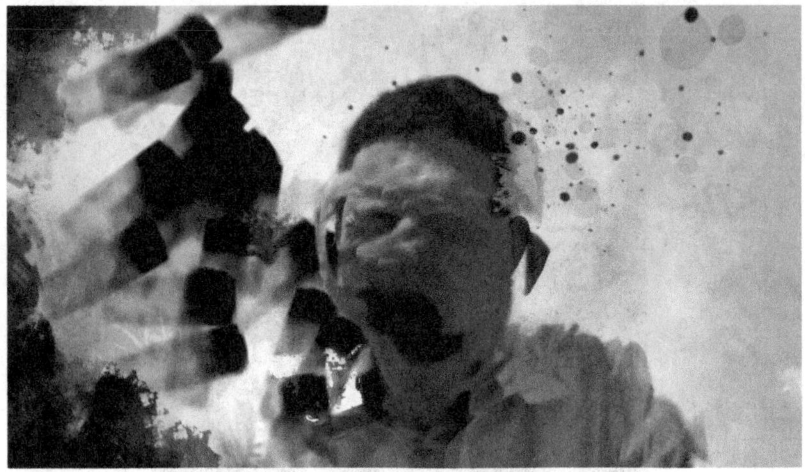

Figure 9.4 Panic Attack

The *DSM-5* defines a panic attack when four or more of the following symptoms occur[10]:

- Palpitations, a pounding heartbeat, or an accelerated heart rate
- Sweating
- Trembling or shaking
- Sensations of shortness of breath or smothering
- Feelings of choking
- Chest pain or discomfort
- Nausea or abdominal distress
- Feeling dizzy, unsteady, light-headed, or faint
- Chills or heat sensations
- Paresthesia (numbness or tingling sensations)
- Derealization (feelings of unreality) or depersonalization (being detached from oneself)
- Feelings of losing control or "going crazy"
- Fear of dying

A panic attack is not related to the physiological effects of a substance, medical condition, or another mental disorder. Culture-specific symptoms may also be seen, such as physical symptoms of anxiety of tinnitus, soreness, headache, and uncontrollable screaming or crying, but these should not be counted as one of the four symptoms.[11]

To be diagnosed as a panic disorder, at least one of the panic attacks has been followed by one month (or more) of one or both of the following characteristics[12]:

- Persistent concern or worry about additional panic attacks or their consequences

---

10 American Psychiatric Association. (2013). *Desk reference to the diagnostic criteria from DSM-5.*

11 American Psychiatric Association. (2013). *Desk reference to the diagnostic criteria from DSM-5.*

12 American Psychiatric Association. (2013). *Desk reference to the diagnostic criteria from DSM-5.*

- A significant maladaptive change in behavior related to the attacks (such as avoiding unfamiliar situations)

People with panic disorder often worry about when the next attack will happen and actively try to prevent future attacks by avoiding places, situations, or behaviors they associate with panic attacks. Worry about panic attacks and the effort spent trying to avoid attacks cause significant problems in various areas of the person's life, including the potential development of agoraphobia.[13] Read more about agoraphobia in the following "Phobia-Related Disorders" section.

Phobia-Related Disorders

A **phobia** is an intense fear or aversion to specific objects or situations (e.g., flying, heights, animals, receiving an injection, or seeing blood).[14] Although it can be realistic to feel anxious about certain objects or circumstances, the fear felt by people with phobias is out of proportion to the actual danger caused by the situation or object.[15] See Figure 9.5[16] for an illustration of a phobia called arachnophobia (fear of spiders).

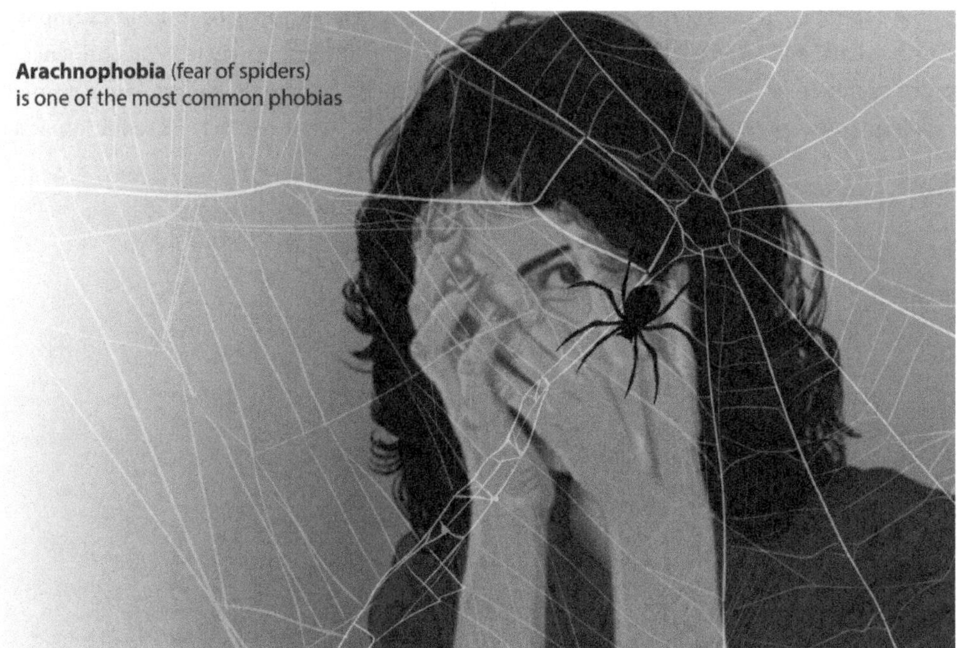

Figure 9.5 Arachnophobia

13 American Psychiatric Association. (2013). *Desk reference to the diagnostic criteria from DSM-5.*

14 American Psychiatric Association. (2013). *Desk reference to the diagnostic criteria from DSM-5.*

15 National Institute of Mental Health. (n.d.). *Any anxiety disorder.* U.S. Department of Health and Human Services. https://www.nimh.nih.gov/health/statistics/any-anxiety-disorder

16 "Depiction_of_a_person_living_with_a_phobia.png" by https://www.myupchar.com/en is licensed under CC BY-SA 4.0

My Notes

The phobic object almost always provokes immediate fear or anxiety and is actively avoided or endured with intense fear or anxiety. This fear, anxiety, or avoidance is persistent and typically lasts for six months or more.[17]

There are several types of phobias and phobia-related disorders. Three common phobias are social anxiety disorder, agoraphobia, and separation anxiety disorder.[18]

Agoraphobia

The *DSM-5* defines **agoraphobia** as intense fear of two or more of the following situations:

- Using public transportation
- Being in open spaces (e.g., parking lots, marketplaces, or bridges)
- Being in enclosed spaces (e.g., shops or theaters)
- Standing in line or being in a crowd
- Being outside of the home alone

People with agoraphobia often avoid these situations because they think it may be difficult or impossible to leave in the event they have a panic-like reaction or other embarrassing symptoms such as incontinence. In the most severe form of agoraphobia, the individual can become housebound. Agoraphobia can be diagnosed in an individual, in addition to the presence of a panic disorder.[19] See Figure 9.6[20] for an artistic rendition of agoraphobia.

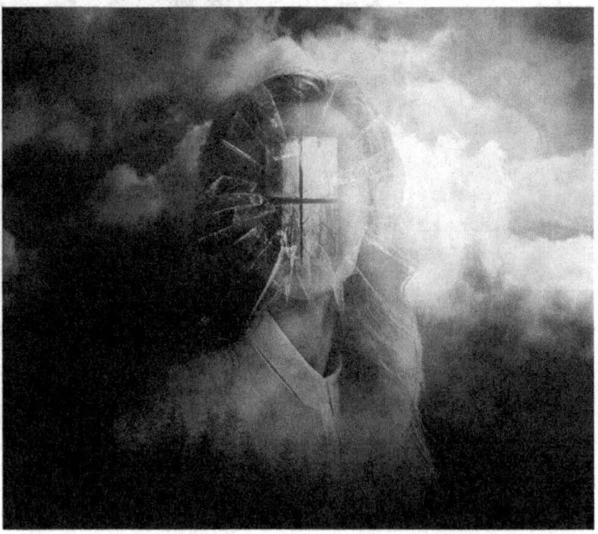

Figure 9.6 Agoraphobia

17 American Psychiatric Association. (2013). *Desk reference to the diagnostic criteria from DSM-5.*

18 National Institute of Mental Health. (n.d.). *Any anxiety disorder*. U.S. Department of Health and Human Services. https://www.nimh.nih.gov/health/statistics/any-anxiety-disorder

19 National Institute of Mental Health. (n.d.). *Any anxiety disorder.* U.S. Department of Health and Human Services. https://www.nimh.nih.gov/health/statistics/any-anxiety-disorder

20 “Agoraphobia” by Ali Emad is licensed under CC BY-NC-ND 4.0

My Notes

Separation Anxiety Disorder

Separation anxiety is often thought of as something that occurs in children, but adults can also be diagnosed with separation anxiety disorder. People who have **separation anxiety disorder** have fears about being separated from people to whom they are attached. They often worry that some sort of harm will happen to those to whom they are attached while they are separated. This fear leads them to avoid being separated from their attachment figures and to avoid being alone. People with separation anxiety may have nightmares about being separated from attachment figures or experience physical symptoms when separation occurs or is anticipated. The fear, anxiety, or avoidance is persistent, lasting at least four weeks in children and typically six months or more in adults, causing significant distress or impairment to social, occupational, or other important areas of functioning.[21,22]

Selective Mutism

Selective mutism is a rare disorder associated with anxiety. **Selective mutism** occurs when people fail to speak in specific social situations despite having normal language skills. Selective mutism usually occurs before the age of five and is often associated with extreme shyness and fear of social embarrassment. It can also be a symptom of post-traumatic stress syndrome. Individuals who are diagnosed with selective mutism are often also diagnosed with other anxiety disorders, and their symptoms are not related to a communication disorder, autism, schizophrenia, or other psychotic disorder.[23,24]

View a video: Mental Health Minute: Anxiety Disorders in Adults.[25]

---

21 American Psychiatric Association. (2013). *Desk reference to the diagnostic criteria from DSM-5.*

22 National Institute of Mental Health. (n.d.). *Any anxiety disorder.* U.S. Department of Health and Human Services. https://www.nimh.nih.gov/health/statistics/any-anxiety-disorder

23 American Psychiatric Association. (2013). *Desk reference to the diagnostic criteria from DSM-5.*

24 National Institute of Mental Health. (n.d.). *Any anxiety disorder.* U.S. Department of Health and Human Services. https://www.nimh.nih.gov/health/statistics/any-anxiety-disorder

25 National Institute of Mental Health (NIMH). (2021, December 20). *Mental health minute: Anxiety disorders in adults* [Video]. YouTube. All rights reserved. https://youtu.be/UjPRVKS4OBg

My Notes

9.4 TREATMENTS FOR ANXIETY

Anxiety disorders are generally treated with psychotherapy, medication, or a combination of both treatments.[1] Support groups, coping strategies, and psychoeducation can also help individuals manage their anxiety.

Psychotherapy

Psychotherapy or "talk therapy" can help people with anxiety disorders. To be effective, psychotherapy must be directed at the person's specific anxieties and tailored to their needs. Examples of psychotherapy include cognitive behavioral therapy (CBT) and dialectal behavior therapy (DBT). CBT teaches people different ways of thinking, behaving, and reacting to anxiety-producing situations and fearful objects. It can also help people learn and practice social skills, which is vital for treating social anxiety disorder. DBT assists individuals to develop distress tolerance skills and emotional regulation skills in managing their anxiety. CBT and DBT can be conducted individually or with a group of people who have similar difficulties.[2] Read more about CBT and DBT in the "Depressive Disorders" chapter.

Exposure therapy may be used alone or with CBT to treat social anxiety disorder. Exposure therapy focuses on confronting the fears underlying an anxiety disorder to help people engage in activities they have been avoiding. Exposure therapy can be used in combination with relaxation exercises and/or imagery.[3] A similar therapy that is particularly helpful with phobias is systematic desensitization. Systematic desensitization is a graduated exposure therapy conducted at a very slow pace used in combination with relaxation techniques and imagery.[4]

Medications

Medications do not cure anxiety disorders but are used to help relieve symptoms of anxiety, panic attacks, extreme fear, and worry. The most common classes of medications used to combat anxiety disorders are antianxiety drugs (such as benzodiazepines), antidepressants, and beta-blockers.

Review information regarding the effects of benzodiazepines and beta-blockers on neurotransmitters in the "Antianxiety Medications" section of the "Psychotropic Medications" chapter.[5]

Benzodiazepines

Benzodiazepines are prescribed for their immediate effect in relieving anxiety. For long-term use, benzodiazepines are considered a second-line treatment for anxiety (with antidepressants or buspirone considered first-line treatment), as well as an "as-needed" treatment for any distressing flare-ups of symptoms. However, people can build up

---

1 National Institute of Mental Health. (2018, July). *Anxiety disorders.* U.S. Department of Health and Human Services. https://www.nimh.nih.gov/health/topics/anxiety-disorders

2 National Institute of Mental Health. (2018, July). *Anxiety disorders.* U.S. Department of Health and Human Services. https://www.nimh.nih.gov/health/topics/anxiety-disorders

3 National Institute of Mental Health. (2018, July). *Anxiety disorders.* U.S. Department of Health and Human Services. https://www.nimh.nih.gov/health/topics/anxiety-disorders

4 Udayangani, S. (2021, November 24). *What is the difference between systematic desensitization and exposure therapy.* Difference Between. https://www.differencebetween.com/what-is-the-difference-between-systematic-desensitization-and-exposure-therapy/#Systematic%20Desensitization

5 National Institute of Mental Health. (2018, July). *Anxiety disorders.* U.S. Department of Health and Human Services. https://www.nimh.nih.gov/health/topics/anxiety-disorders

My Notes

a tolerance if taken over a long period of time, and they may need higher and higher doses to get the same effect. Benzodiazepines are a Schedule IV controlled substance because they have a potential for misuse and can cause dependence. To avoid these problems, benzodiazepines are typically prescribed for short periods of time, especially for people who have a history of substance use disorders. Short-acting benzodiazepines (such as lorazepam) and beta-blockers are used to treat the short-term symptoms of anxiety. Lorazepam is available for oral, intramuscular, or intravenous routes of administration.[6,7]

If people suddenly stop taking benzodiazepines after taking them for a long period of time, they may have withdrawal symptoms, or their anxiety may return. Withdrawal symptoms include sleep disturbances, irritability, increased tension and anxiety, hand tremors, sweating, difficulty concentrating, nausea and vomiting, weight loss, palpitations, headaches, muscular pain, and perceptual changes.[8] Therefore, benzodiazepines should be tapered off slowly.[9]

Black Box Warning

A Black Box Warning states that concurrent use of benzodiazepines and opioids may result in profound sedation, respiratory depression, coma, and death. The use of benzodiazepines exposes users to risks of misuse, substance use disorder, and addiction. Misuse of benzodiazepines commonly involves concomitant use of other medications, alcohol, and/or illicit substances, which is associated with an increased frequency of serious adverse outcomes. Additionally, the continued use of benzodiazepines may lead to clinically significant physical dependence. The risks of dependence and withdrawal increase with longer treatment duration and higher daily doses, and abrupt discontinuation or rapid dosage reduction may precipitate life-threatening withdrawal reactions. To reduce the risk of withdrawal reactions, a gradual taper should be used to stop or reduce the dosage.[10]

Adverse/Side Effects

Children and older adults are more susceptible to the sedative and respiratory depressive effects of lorazepam and may experience paradoxical reactions such as tremors, agitation, or visual hallucinations. Debilitated clients should be monitored frequently and have their dosage adjusted carefully according to their response; the initial dosage should not exceed 2 mg. Dosage for clients with severe hepatic insufficiency should be adjusted carefully according to client response. Benzodiazepines may cause fetal harm when administered to pregnant women.[11]

Overdosage

Overdosage of benzodiazepines is manifested by varying degrees of central nervous system depression, ranging from drowsiness to coma. If overdose occurs, call 911 or the rapid response team during inpatient care. Treatment of overdosage is mainly supportive until the drug is eliminated from the body. Vital signs and fluid balance should be carefully monitored in conjunction with close observation of the client. An adequate airway should be

---

6 National Institute of Mental Health. (2018, July). *Anxiety disorders.* U.S. Department of Health and Human Services. https://www.nimh.nih.gov/health/topics/anxiety-disorders

7 This work is a derivative of *DailyMed* by U.S. National Library of Medicine and is available in the Public Domain

8 Pétursson, H. (1994). The benzodiazepine withdrawal syndrome. *Addiction*, 89(11):1455-9. https://doi: 10.1111 /j.1360-0443.1994.tb03743.x

9 National Institute of Mental Health. (2018, July). *Anxiety disorders.* U.S. Department of Health and Human Services. https://www.nimh.nih.gov/health/topics/anxiety-disorders

10 This work is a derivative of *DailyMed* by U.S. National Library of Medicine and is available in the Public Domain

11 This work is a derivative of *DailyMed* by U.S. National Library of Medicine and is available in the Public Domain

My Notes

maintained; intubation and mechanical ventilation may be required. The benzodiazepine antagonist flumazenil may be used to manage benzodiazepine overdose. There is a risk of seizure in association with flumazenil treatment, particularly in chronic users of benzodiazepines.

Patient Education

Clients should be cautioned that driving a motor vehicle, operating machinery, or engaging in hazardous or other activities requiring attention and coordination should be delayed for 24 to 48 hours following administration of benzodiazepines or until the effects of the drug, such as drowsiness, have subsided. Alcoholic beverages should not be consumed for at least 24 to 48 hours after receiving lorazepam due to the additive effects on central nervous system depression. Hospitalized patients should be advised that benzodiazepines increase fall risk, and getting out of bed unassisted may result in falling and potential injury if undertaken within eight hours of taking lorazepam.

Antidepressants

Selective serotonin reuptake inhibitors (SSRIs) and serotonin-norepinephrine reuptake inhibitors (SNRIs) are commonly used as first-line treatments for anxiety. Less commonly used treatments for anxiety disorders are older classes of antidepressants, such as tricyclic antidepressants and monoamine oxidase inhibitors (MAOIs).[12] Read more about antidepressants in the "Depressive Disorders" chapter.

Buspirone

Buspirone is a non-benzodiazepine medication indicated for the treatment of chronic anxiety. It is included in the class of medications called anxiolytics, but it is not chemically related to benzodiazepines, barbiturates, or other sedatives. Buspirone should not be taken concurrently with a monoamine oxidase inhibitor (MAOI) due to the risk of fatal side effects. It can also cause serotonin syndrome if used in combination with MAOIs, SSRIs, or SNRIs.[13]

Buspirone increases serotonin and dopamine levels in the brain. In contrast to benzodiazepines, buspirone must be taken every day for a few weeks to reach its full effect; it is not useful on an "as-needed" basis. A common side effect of buspirone is dizziness.[14]

Beta-Blockers

Although beta-blockers are typically used to treat high blood pressure and other cardiac conditions, they can also be used to help relieve the physical symptoms of anxiety, such as rapid heartbeat, shaking, trembling, and flushing. These medications, when taken for a short period of time, can help people keep their physical symptoms under control. Beta-blockers can also be used "as needed" to reduce acute anxiety or as a preventive intervention for predictable forms of performance anxieties.[15] For example, some students who experience severe test anxiety that impairs their exam performance may take prescribed beta-blockers before their exams.

---

12 National Institute of Mental Health. (2018, July). *Anxiety disorders.* U.S. Department of Health and Human Services. https://www.nimh.nih.gov/health/topics/anxiety-disorders

13 This work is a derivative of *DailyMed* by U.S. National Library of Medicine in the Public Domain

14 This work is a derivative of *StatPearls* by Wilson and Tripp and is licensed under CC BY 4.0

15 National Institute of Mental Health. (2018, July). *Anxiety disorders.* U.S. Department of Health and Human Services. https://www.nimh.nih.gov/health/topics/anxiety-disorders

My Notes

Common side effects of beta-blockers are fatigue, hypotension, dizziness, weakness, and cold hands. Beta-blockers are typically avoided in clients with asthma or diabetes.[16]

Hydroxyzine

Hydroxyzine may be prescribed to alleviate anxiety for individuals for whom benzodiazepines are not appropriate. It causes sedation, so it must be used cautiously if used in combination with opioids or barbiturates.[17]

Support Groups

Support groups can be helpful for individuals experiencing anxiety disorders by sharing their problems and achievements with others experiencing similar symptoms. Talking with a trusted family member, friend, chaplain, or clergy member can also provide support.

Stress Management and Coping Strategies

Stress management techniques and coping strategies can help people with anxiety disorders calm themselves and enhance the effects of therapy. Research suggests that aerobic exercise can help some people manage their anxiety. Read more about stress management and coping strategies in the "Stress, Coping, and Crisis Intervention" chapter.

Psychoeducation

Clients should be educated about symptoms of their diagnosed anxiety disorder and techniques to manage it with psychotherapy and medications. For some individuals, even being aware that something is a symptom of anxiety, naming it, and connecting it to anxiety can help reduce the intensity of the anxiety. If antidepressants are prescribed, they can take several weeks to reach their optimal effectiveness, so it is important to teach clients to give the medication appropriate time before reaching a conclusion about its effectiveness. They should be advised to not stop taking them suddenly or without talking to their prescribing provider. Antidepressants should be tapered off slowly to safely decrease the dose because stopping them abruptly can cause withdrawal symptoms.

Certain substances such as caffeine, some over-the-counter cold medicines, illicit drugs, and herbal supplements may aggravate the symptoms of anxiety disorders or interact with prescribed medications. Clients should be advised to avoid these substances.

View a video: Mental Health Minute: Stress and Anxiety in Adolescents.[18]

16 National Institute of Mental Health. (2016, October). *Mental health medications.* U.S. Department of Health & Human Services. https://www.nimh.nih.gov/health/topics/mental-health-medications

17 This work is a derivative of *DailyMed* by U.S. National Library of Medicine and is available in the Public Domain

18 National Institute of Mental Health (NIMH). (2021, September 21). *Mental health minute: Stress and anxiety in adolescents* [Video]. YouTube. All rights reserved. https://youtu.be/wr4N-SdekqY

My Notes

9.5 OBSESSIVE-COMPULSIVE DISORDER

Obsessive-compulsive disorder (OCD) is a common chronic disorder in which a person has uncontrollable, reoccurring thoughts (obsessions) and/or behaviors (compulsions) they feel the urge to repeat over and over. These compulsions often temporarily relieve the stress/tension of the obsession.[1]

Historically, the relationship of OCD with anxiety disorders was strongly emphasized. The *Diagnostic and Statistical Manual of Mental Disorders, 5th edition (DSM-5)* classifies OCD under a separate group of disorders called "Obsessive-Compulsive and Related Disorders" due to the presence of obsessions and compulsions.[2] A systematic review found that lifetime psychiatric comorbidities were present in 69% of individuals with OCD, with anxiety disorders the most common comorbidity in children and depressive disorders being the most common comorbidity in adults.[3]

Signs and Symptoms

Symptoms of OCD can interfere with all aspects of life, such as work, school, and personal relationships. Symptoms may come and go, ease over time, or worsen.[4] See Figure 9.7[5] for an artist's depiction of obsessive thoughts related to OCD.

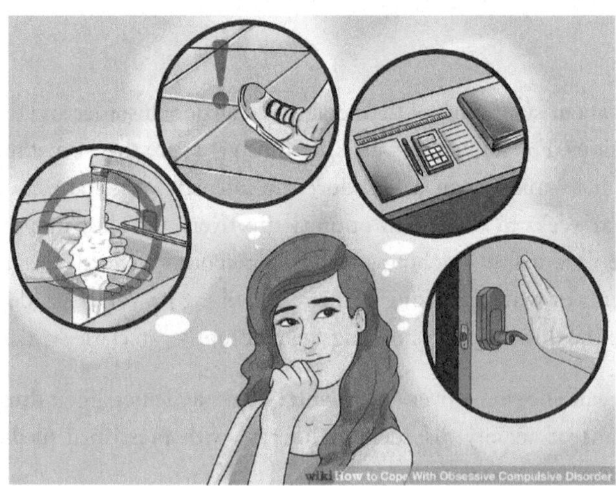

Figure 9.7 Obsessive Compulsive Disorder

---

1 National Institute of Mental Health. (2019, October). *Obsessive-compulsive disorder.* U.S. Department of Health and Human Services. https://www.nimh.nih.gov/health/topics/obsessive-compulsive-disorder-ocd

2 American Psychiatric Association. (2013). *Desk reference to the diagnostic criteria from DSM-5.*

3 Sharma, E., Sharma, L. P., Balachander, S., Lin, B., Manohar, H., Khanna, P., Lu, C., Garg, K., Thomas, T. L., Au, A. C. L., Selles, R. R., Højgaard, D. R. M. A., Skarphedinsson, G., & Stewart, S. E. (2021). Comorbidities in obsessive-compulsive disorder across the lifespan: A systematic review and meta-analysis. *Frontiers in Psychiatry, 12*:703701. https://doi.org/10.3389%2Ffpsyt.2021.703701

4 National Institute of Mental Health. (2019, October). *Obsessive-compulsive disorder.* U.S. Department of Health and Human Services. https://www.nimh.nih.gov/health/topics/obsessive-compulsive-disorder-ocd

5 "Cope-With-Obsessive-Compulsive-Disorder-Step-15.jpg" by unknown author at wikihow.com is licensed under CC BY-NC-SA 3.0

My Notes

Obsessions are repeated thoughts, urges, or mental images that cause anxiety. Common obsessions are as follows[6]:

- Fear of germs or contamination
- Unwanted forbidden or taboo thoughts involving sex, religion, or harm
- Aggressive thoughts towards self or others
- Having things symmetrical or in a perfect order

Compulsions are repetitive behaviors that a person with OCD feels the urge to do in response to an obsessive thought. Compulsions often match the obsession and include the following[7]:

- Excessive cleaning and/or handwashing
- Ordering and arranging things in a particular, precise way
- Repeatedly checking on things, such as repeatedly checking to see if the door is locked or that the oven is off
- Compulsive counting

Not all rituals or habits are compulsions; everyone double-checks things sometimes. For example, many people double-check that their doors are locked as they exit the vehicle. However, a person with OCD generally exhibits the following characteristics[8]:

- Spends at least one hour a day on these thoughts
- Can't control their thoughts or behaviors, even when those thoughts or behaviors are recognized as excessive
- Does not experience pleasure when performing the behaviors or rituals, but may feel relief from the anxiety the obsessive thoughts cause
- Experiences significant problems in their daily life due to these thoughts or behaviors

Sometimes compulsions are accompanied by a fear of potential consequences if they are not carried out. For this reason, an individual with OCD may become distressed if not able to complete a compulsive act.

Some individuals with OCD also have a tic disorder. Motor tics are sudden, brief, repetitive movements, such as eye blinking and other eye movements, facial grimacing, shoulder shrugging, and head or shoulder jerking. Vocal tics include repetitive throat-clearing, sniffing, or grunting sounds.[9]

People with OCD may try to cope by avoiding situations that trigger their obsessions or use alcohol or drugs to calm themselves. Although most adults with OCD have good insight and recognize what they are doing doesn't make sense, some may not realize that their behavior is out of the ordinary (i.e., they demonstrate "poor insight").

---

6 National Institute of Mental Health. (2019, October). *Obsessive-compulsive disorder.* U.S. Department of Health and Human Services. https://www.nimh.nih.gov/health/topics/obsessive-compulsive-disorder-ocd

7 National Institute of Mental Health. (2019, October). *Obsessive-compulsive disorder.* U.S. Department of Health and Human Services. https://www.nimh.nih.gov/health/topics/obsessive-compulsive-disorder-ocd

8 National Institute of Mental Health. (2019, October). *Obsessive-compulsive disorder.* U.S. Department of Health and Human Services. https://www.nimh.nih.gov/health/topics/obsessive-compulsive-disorder-ocd

9 National Institute of Mental Health. (2019, October). *Obsessive-compulsive disorder.* U.S. Department of Health and Human Services. https://www.nimh.nih.gov/health/topics/obsessive-compulsive-disorder-ocd

My Notes

Most children do not have good insight into their thoughts and behaviors, so parents or teachers typically recognize OCD symptoms in children.

Risk Factors

The causes of OCD are unknown, but risk factors include genetics, brain structure and functioning, and environmental factors such as adverse childhood events (ACEs).[10]

Genetics

Twin and family studies have shown that people with first-degree relatives (such as a parent, sibling, or child) who have OCD are at a higher risk for developing OCD. The risk is higher if the first-degree relative developed OCD as a child or teen.[11]

Brain Structure and Functioning

Imaging studies have shown differences in the frontal cortex and subcortical structures of the brain in patients with OCD, but the connection with symptoms is not clear. Research is still underway because understanding potential causes may help determine specific, personalized treatments to treat OCD.[12]

Environment

Research has found an association between childhood trauma, otherwise known as adverse childhood events (ACEs), and obsessive-compulsive symptoms. Some studies also found that children may develop OCD symptoms following a streptococcal infection, referred to as Pediatric Autoimmune Neuropsychiatric Disorders Associated with Streptococcal Infections (PANDAS). Children with PANDAS have a very sudden onset or worsening of their symptoms after a streptococcal infection, followed by a slow, gradual improvement.[13]

Review information about adverse childhood events (ACEs) in the "Mental Health and Mental Illness" section in Chapter 1.

Read more at the National Institute of Mental Health (NIMH) PANDAS – Questions and Answers web page.

Treatment

OCD is typically treated with medication, psychotherapy, or a combination of both. Although most patients with OCD improve with treatment, some patients continue to experience symptoms. Individuals with OCD may also have other mental health disorders, such as anxiety, depression, and body dysmorphic disorder (a disorder in

---

10 National Institute of Mental Health. (2019, October). *Obsessive-compulsive disorder.* U.S. Department of Health and Human Services. https://www.nimh.nih.gov/health/topics/obsessive-compulsive-disorder-ocd

11 National Institute of Mental Health. (2019, October). *Obsessive-compulsive disorder.* U.S. Department of Health and Human Services. https://www.nimh.nih.gov/health/topics/obsessive-compulsive-disorder-ocd

12 National Institute of Mental Health. (2019, October). *Obsessive-compulsive disorder.* U.S. Department of Health and Human Services. https://www.nimh.nih.gov/health/topics/obsessive-compulsive-disorder-ocd

13 National Institute of Mental Health. (2019, October). *Obsessive-compulsive disorder.* U.S. Department of Health and Human Services. https://www.nimh.nih.gov/health/topics/obsessive-compulsive-disorder-ocd

My Notes

which someone mistakenly believes that a part of their body is abnormal). It is important to consider these other comorbid disorders when planning interventions related to treatment.[14]

Medication

Selective serotonin reuptake inhibitors (SSRIs) are used to help reduce OCD symptoms. SSRIs often require higher daily doses in the treatment of OCD than of depression and may take 8 to 12 weeks to start working. If symptoms do not improve with SSRIs, research shows that some patients may respond well to an antipsychotic medication, especially if they also have a tic disorder.[15]

Read more about SSRIs in the "Depressive Disorders" chapter and antipsychotics in the "Psychosis and Schizophrenia" chapter.

Psychotherapy

Psychotherapy can be an effective treatment for adults and children with OCD. Research shows that certain types of psychotherapy, including cognitive behavior therapy (CBT) and other related therapies (such as habit reversal training), can be as effective as medication for many individuals. Research also shows that a type of CBT called **Exposure and Response Prevention (EX/RP)** is effective in reducing compulsive behaviors in clients with OCD. EX/RP includes spending time in the very situation that triggers compulsions (for example, touching dirty objects) but then being prevented from undertaking the usual resulting compulsion (handwashing). For many clients, EX/RP is an add-on treatment when SSRIs do not effectively treat OCD symptoms.[16]

Other Treatment Options

In 2018 the FDA approved transcranial magnetic stimulation as an adjunct in the treatment of OCD in adults. **Repetitive Transcranial Magnetic Stimulation (rTMS)** uses a magnet to activate the brain. Unlike electroconvulsive therapy (ECT), in which electrical stimulation is more generalized, rTMS can be targeted to a specific site in the brain. A typical rTMS session lasts 30 to 60 minutes and does not require anesthesia. During the procedure, an electromagnetic coil is held against the forehead near an area of the brain that is thought to be involved in mood regulation. Short electromagnetic pulses are administered through the coil. The magnetic pulses easily pass through the skull and cause small electrical currents that stimulate nerve cells in the targeted brain region. The magnetic field is about the same strength as that of a magnetic resonance imaging (MRI) scan. The person generally feels a slight knocking or tapping on the head as the pulses are administered. The muscles of the scalp, jaw, or face may contract or tingle during the procedure, and mild headaches or brief light-headedness may result after the procedure. It is also possible that the procedure could cause a seizure, although this adverse effect is uncommon. Because the treatment is relatively new, long-term side effects are unknown.[17]

---

14 National Institute of Mental Health. (2019, October). *Obsessive-compulsive disorder.* U.S. Department of Health and Human Services. https://www.nimh.nih.gov/health/topics/obsessive-compulsive-disorder-ocd

15 National Institute of Mental Health. (2019, October). *Obsessive-compulsive disorder.* U.S. Department of Health and Human Services. https://www.nimh.nih.gov/health/topics/obsessive-compulsive-disorder-ocd

16 National Institute of Mental Health. (2019, October). *Obsessive-compulsive disorder.* U.S. Department of Health and Human Services. https://www.nimh.nih.gov/health/topics/obsessive-compulsive-disorder-ocd

17 National Institute of Mental Health. (2016, June). *Brain stimulation therapies.* U.S. Department of Health and Human Services. https://www.nimh.nih.gov/health/topics/brain-stimulation-therapies/brain-stimulation-therapies

My Notes

Psychoeducation

In addition to teaching clients about the symptoms of OCD, prescribed medications, and other treatments, nurses should teach clients how to manage stress and anxiety associated with OCD:

- Create a consistent sleep schedule
- Make regular exercise a part of your routine
- Eat a healthy, balanced diet
- Seek support from trusted family and friends

9.6 POST-TRAUMATIC STRESS DISORDER

My Notes

Post-traumatic stress disorder (PTSD) is diagnosed in individuals who have been exposed to a traumatic event with chronic stress symptoms lasting more than one month that are so severe they interfere with relationships, school, or work. PTSD was formerly classified as an anxiety disorder but was placed in a new diagnostic category in the *DSM-5* called "Trauma and Stressor-Related Disorders."

Post-traumatic stress disorder has similar characteristics to severe anxiety and phobia-related disorders because of the physiological stress response that occurs. **Post-traumatic stress disorder (PTSD)** can develop in some people who have experienced a shocking, frightening, or dangerous event. It is natural to feel afraid during and after a traumatic situation, and the "fight-or-flight" stress response is a physiological reaction intended to protect a person from harm. Most people recover from the range of reactions that can occur after experiencing trauma. However, people who do not recover from these reactions and continue to experience problems are diagnosed with PTSD. People who have PTSD may feel stressed or frightened, even when they are not in danger.[1]

Symptoms

Symptoms of PTSD typically begin three months of the traumatic incident, but they may also begin years afterward. If symptoms occur within one month of the traumatic event, it is diagnosed as acute stress disorder. Symptoms must last more than a month and be severe enough to interfere with social or occupational functioning to be considered PTSD. The course of the illness varies; some people recover within six months, while others have symptoms that last much longer. In some people, the condition becomes chronic.[2,3]

To be diagnosed with PTSD, an adult must have the following types of symptoms for at least one month[4,5]:

- At least one "re-experiencing" symptom
- At least one "avoidance" symptom
- At least two "arousal and reactivity" symptoms
- At least two "cognition and mood" symptoms

Re-Experiencing Symptoms

Re-experiencing symptoms include the following[6]:

- Flashbacks—reliving the trauma over and over, including physical symptoms like a racing heart or sweating

---

1 National Institute of Mental Health. (2019, May). *Post-traumatic stress disorder.* U.S. Department of Health and Human Services. https://www.nimh.nih.gov/health/topics/post-traumatic-stress-disorder-ptsd

2 National Institute of Mental Health. (2019, May). *Post-traumatic stress disorder.* U.S. Department of Health and Human Services. https://www.nimh.nih.gov/health/topics/post-traumatic-stress-disorder-ptsd

3 American Psychiatric Association. (2013). *Desk reference to the diagnostic criteria from DSM-5.*

4 National Institute of Mental Health. (2019, May). *Post-traumatic stress disorder.* U.S. Department of Health and Human Services. https://www.nimh.nih.gov/health/topics/post-traumatic-stress-disorder-ptsd

5 American Psychiatric Association. (2013). *Desk reference to the diagnostic criteria from DSM-5.*

6 National Institute of Mental Health. (2019, May). *Post-traumatic stress disorder.* U.S. Department of Health and Human Services. https://www.nimh.nih.gov/health/topics/post-traumatic-stress-disorder-ptsd

My Notes

- Bad dreams
- Frightening thoughts

Re-experiencing symptoms can start from the person's own thoughts and feelings. Words, objects, or situations that are reminders of the event can also trigger re-experiencing symptoms. Re-experiencing symptoms may cause problems in a person's everyday routine and relationships.[7]

Avoidance Symptoms

Avoidance symptoms are as follows[8]:

- Staying away from places, events, or objects that are reminders of the traumatic experience
- Avoiding thoughts or feelings related to the traumatic event

These symptoms may cause a person to change their personal routine. For example, after a car accident, a person who usually drives may avoid driving or riding in a car.

Arousal and Reactivity Symptoms

Arousal and reactivity symptoms include the following[9]:

- Being easily startled
- Feeling tense or "on edge"
- Having difficulty sleeping
- Having angry outbursts

Arousal symptoms are usually constant instead of being triggered by things that remind one of the traumatic events. These symptoms can make the person feel stressed and angry and can make it hard to do daily tasks, such as sleeping, eating, or concentrating.[10]

Cognition and Mood Symptoms

Cognition and mood symptoms are as follows[11]:

- Trouble remembering key features of the traumatic event
- Negative thoughts about oneself or the world
- Distorted feelings like guilt or blame

---

7 National Institute of Mental Health. (2019, May). *Post-traumatic stress disorder.* U.S. Department of Health and Human Services. https://www.nimh.nih.gov/health/topics/post-traumatic-stress-disorder-ptsd

8 National Institute of Mental Health. (2019, May). *Post-traumatic stress disorder.* U.S. Department of Health and Human Services. https://www.nimh.nih.gov/health/topics/post-traumatic-stress-disorder-ptsd

9 National Institute of Mental Health. (2019, May). *Post-traumatic stress disorder.* U.S. Department of Health and Human Services. https://www.nimh.nih.gov/health/topics/post-traumatic-stress-disorder-ptsd

10 National Institute of Mental Health. (2019, May). *Post-traumatic stress disorder.* U.S. Department of Health and Human Services. https://www.nimh.nih.gov/health/topics/post-traumatic-stress-disorder-ptsd

11 National Institute of Mental Health. (2019, May). *Post-traumatic stress disorder.* U.S. Department of Health and Human Services. https://www.nimh.nih.gov/health/topics/post-traumatic-stress-disorder-ptsd

My Notes

- Loss of interest in enjoyable activities

Cognition and mood symptoms can begin or worsen after the traumatic event and make the person feel alienated or detached from friends or family members.[12]

It is natural to have some of these types of symptoms for a few weeks after a traumatic event. However, when the symptoms last more than a month, seriously affect a person's functioning, and are not related to substance use, medical illness, or anything except the event itself, they can be symptoms of PTSD. PTSD is also often accompanied by depression, substance abuse, or other anxiety disorders.[13]

Life Span Considerations

Children and teens can have extreme reactions to trauma, but they may exhibit different symptoms than adults. Symptoms of PTSD can be seen in young children (less than six years old) and may include the following:

- Bedwetting after having learned to use the toilet
- Forgetting how to talk or being unable to talk (i.e., selective mutism)
- Acting out the scary event during playtime
- Being unusually clingy with a parent or other adult

Older children and teens are more likely to show symptoms similar to those seen in adults. They may also develop disruptive, disrespectful, or destructive behaviors. Hypersexual behavior may occur if the trauma was related to a sexual assault. Older children and teens may also feel guilty for not preventing injury or death in certain traumatic situations and may have thoughts of revenge.[14]

Risk and Resilience Factors

Anyone can develop PTSD at any age, including war veterans; children who have experienced trauma; or adults who have experienced a physical or sexual assault, abuse, accident, disaster, being a refugee, or some other serious event. According to the National Center for PTSD, about 6 out of every 100 people will experience PTSD symptoms at some point in their lives. Women are more likely to develop PTSD than men, and genes may make some people more likely to develop PTSD than others.[15]

Not everyone with PTSD has directly experienced a dangerous event. Some people develop PTSD after a friend or family member experiences danger or harm. The sudden, unexpected death of a loved one can also lead to

---

12 National Institute of Mental Health. (2019, May). *Post-traumatic stress disorder.* U.S. Department of Health and Human Services. https://www.nimh.nih.gov/health/topics/post-traumatic-stress-disorder-ptsd

13 National Institute of Mental Health. (2019, May). *Post-traumatic stress disorder.* U.S. Department of Health and Human Services. https://www.nimh.nih.gov/health/topics/post-traumatic-stress-disorder-ptsd

14 National Institute of Mental Health. (2019, May). *Post-traumatic stress disorder.* U.S. Department of Health and Human Services. https://www.nimh.nih.gov/health/topics/post-traumatic-stress-disorder-ptsd

15 National Institute of Mental Health. (2019, May). *Post-traumatic stress disorder.* U.S. Department of Health and Human Services. https://www.nimh.nih.gov/health/topics/post-traumatic-stress-disorder-ptsd

My Notes

PTSD.[16] PTSD is triggered by events that are perceived to be life-threatening, and this can vary from individual to individual. It disrupts the general sense of safety that allows individuals to function in the world.

It is important to remember that not everyone who lives through a dangerous event develops PTSD. In fact, most people will not develop the disorder. Many factors play a part in whether a person will develop PTSD. Risk factors make a person more likely to develop PTSD, but other factors, called resilience factors, can help reduce the risk of developing the disorder or promote recovery from the disorder.[17]

These factors increase the risk for developing PTSD[18]:

- Living through dangerous events and traumas
- Being injured from a traumatic event
- Seeing another person hurt or seeing a dead body
- Experiencing childhood trauma or adverse childhood events (ACEs)
- Feeling horror, helplessness, or extreme fear
- Having little or no social support after the event
- Dealing with extra stress after the event, such as loss of a loved one, pain and injury, or loss of a job or home
- Having a history of mental illness or substance abuse

Review information about adverse childhood events (ACEs) in the "Mental Health and Mental Illness" section of Chapter 1.

Resilience factors that may promote recovery after trauma include the following[19]:

- Receiving support from other people, such as friends and family
- Finding a support group after a traumatic event
- Learning to feel good about one's own actions in the face of danger, recognizing that we controlled what we could in an uncontrollable situation
- Having a positive coping strategy or a way of getting through the bad event and learning from it
- Being able to act and respond effectively despite feeling fear

If a child or adolescent discloses traumatic events to caregivers, teachers, or other adults, it is important for them to feel their concerns are validated by the adult in order to develop resilience.

Researchers are studying the importance of risk and resilience factors, as well as the impact of genetics and neurobiology. With more research, it may be possible to someday predict who is likely to develop PTSD and how

---

16 National Institute of Mental Health. (2019, May). *Post-traumatic stress disorder.* U.S. Department of Health and Human Services. https://www.nimh.nih.gov/health/topics/post-traumatic-stress-disorder-ptsd

17 National Institute of Mental Health. (2019, May). *Post-traumatic stress disorder.* U.S. Department of Health and Human Services. https://www.nimh.nih.gov/health/topics/post-traumatic-stress-disorder-ptsd

18 National Institute of Mental Health. (2019, May). *Post-traumatic stress disorder.* U.S. Department of Health and Human Services. https://www.nimh.nih.gov/health/topics/post-traumatic-stress-disorder-ptsd

19 National Institute of Mental Health. (2019, May). *Post-traumatic stress disorder.* U.S. Department of Health and Human Services. https://www.nimh.nih.gov/health/topics/post-traumatic-stress-disorder-ptsd

My Notes

to prevent it from occurring.[20] See Figure 9.8[21] for an image of a veteran with PTSD using a service dog as an effective coping strategy.

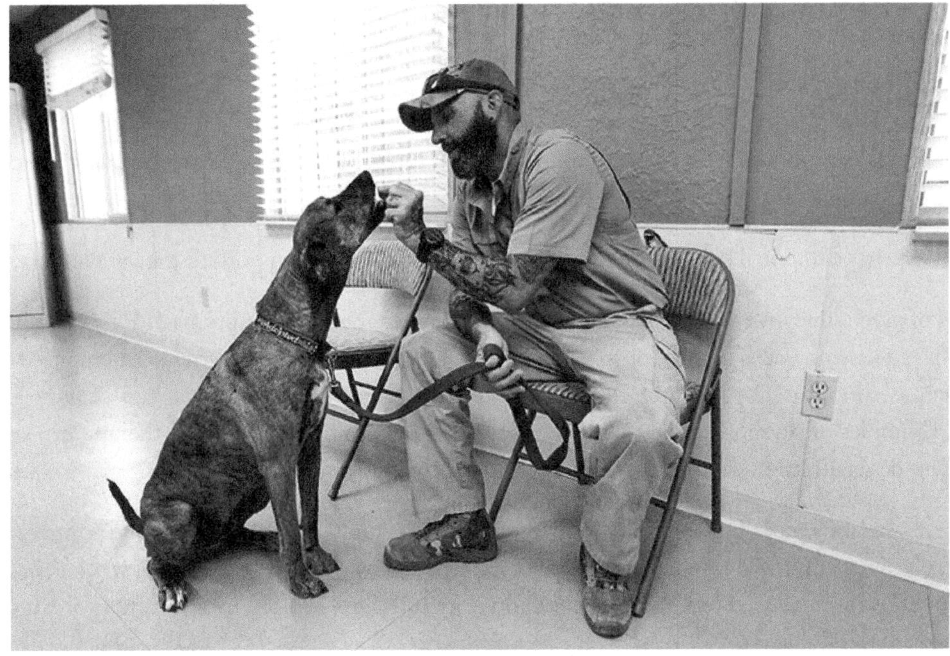

Figure 9.8 A Veteran With PTSD Using a Service Dog as a Coping Strategy

Treatments

For people with PTSD, treatments include medications, psychotherapy, or a combination of both. Everyone is different, and PTSD affects people differently, so a treatment that works for one person may not work for another. It is important for anyone with PTSD to be treated by a mental health provider who has experience treating PTSD.[22]

If someone with PTSD is also experiencing an ongoing trauma, such as an abusive relationship, both of the problems need to be addressed. Other ongoing problems can include panic disorder, depression, substance use disorder, and suicidal ideation.[23]

---

20 National Institute of Mental Health. (2019, May). *Post-traumatic stress disorder.* U.S. Department of Health and Human Services. https://www.nimh.nih.gov/health/topics/post-traumatic-stress-disorder-ptsd

21 "Local_veterans_group_gets_national_exposure_141127-F-ZZ999-001.jpg" by unknown author is licensed in the Public Domain

22 National Institute of Mental Health. (2019, May). *Post-traumatic stress disorder.* U.S. Department of Health and Human Services. https://www.nimh.nih.gov/health/topics/post-traumatic-stress-disorder-ptsd

23 National Institute of Mental Health. (2019, May). *Post-traumatic stress disorder.* U.S. Department of Health and Human Services. https://www.nimh.nih.gov/health/topics/post-traumatic-stress-disorder-ptsd

My Notes

Medications

Antidepressants can help control PTSD symptoms such as sadness, worry, anger, and feeling numb inside. For example, two FDA-approved medications for PTSD are sertraline and paroxetine. Other medications may be helpful for treating specific PTSD symptoms, such as sleep problems and nightmares.[24]

Psychotherapy

Psychotherapy can occur one-on-one or in a group setting. It typically lasts 6 to 12 weeks, but it can continue for as long as the individual finds it helpful.

Research shows that additional support from family and friends can be an important part of recovery.[25]

Many types of psychotherapy can help people with PTSD. Some target the symptoms of PTSD directly, whereas other therapies focus on social, family, or job-related problems. Effective psychotherapies emphasize key components such as education about symptoms, identification of triggers or symptoms, and skills to manage the symptoms. Examples of psychotherapies used to treat PTSD are cognitive behavioral therapy, exposure therapy, eye movement desensitization and reprocessing, and animal therapy programs.

Cognitive behavioral therapy (CBT) combined with exposure therapy helps people face and control their fear by gradually exposing them to the trauma they experienced in a safe way. It uses imagining, writing, or visiting the place where the event happened to help reduce the intensity of PTSD symptoms. Read more about CBT in the "Depressive Disorders" chapter.

Cognitive restructuring helps individuals create new thought patterns about the trauma. Sometimes events are remembered differently than how they truly happened, and individuals may experience feelings of guilt or shame in relation to the trauma, regardless of whether they played an active role or not. They may feel guilt or shame about something that is not their fault.Therapists can help individuals assess the trauma through a variety of lenses to process and continue the healing journey.

Eye movement desensitization and reprocessing (EMDR) is a psychotherapy treatment that was originally designed to alleviate the distress associated with traumatic memories. During EMDR therapy, the client attends to emotionally disturbing material in brief sequential doses while simultaneously focusing on an external stimulus. Therapist-directed lateral eye movements are the most commonly used external stimulus, but a variety of other stimuli such as hand-tapping and audio stimulation are also used. It is hypothesized that EMDR therapy facilitates the individual's access of their traumatic memory network so that new associations can be forged between the traumatic memory and more adaptive memories or information. These new associations are thought to result in elimination of emotional distress and development of cognitive insights.[26,27]

---

24 National Institute of Mental Health. (2019, May). *Post-traumatic stress disorder.* U.S. Department of Health and Human Services. https://www.nimh.nih.gov/health/topics/post-traumatic-stress-disorder-ptsd

25 National Institute of Mental Health. (2019, May). *Post-traumatic stress disorder.* U.S. Department of Health and Human Services. https://www.nimh.nih.gov/health/topics/post-traumatic-stress-disorder-ptsd

26 EDMR Institute. (n.d.) *What is EDMR?* https://www.emdr.com/what-is-emdr/

27 American Psychological Association. (2017, July 31). *Clinical practice guidelines for the treatment of post-traumatic stress disorder: Eye Movement Desensitization and Reprocessing (EMDR) Therapy.* https://www.apa.org/ptsd-guideline/treatments/eye-movement-reprocessing

My Notes

Animal assisted intervention (AAI), also referred to as animal therapy, is a commonly used complementary treatment for PTSD. It most often includes dogs or horses. A systematic review examined the outcomes in studies using AAI with trauma survivors. Although the reviewed studies were diverse and limited, all reported positive outcomes of AAI, such as reduced depression, PTSD symptoms, and anxiety.[28]

In 2017 a new therapy called methylenedioxymethamphetamine (MDMA) – assisted psychotherapy received Breakthrough Therapy Designation from the FDA for the treatment of PTSD. MDMA (also referred to by the illicit drug name Ecstasy) is administered under direct observation with psychotherapy in three monthly eight-hour sessions. Due to the limited number of sessions with direct observation, there is less chance of diversion, overdose, or withdrawal symptoms upon discontinuation.[29]

View a video: NIMH-Funded Researcher Dr. Barbara Rothbaum Discusses Post-Traumatic Stress Disorder.[30]

---

28 O'Haire, M., Guerin, N., & Kirkham, A. (2015). Animal-Assisted Intervention for trauma: A systematic literature review. *Frontiers in Psychology, 6*. https://doi.org/10.3389/fpsyg.2015.01121

29 Feduccia, A. A., Jerome, L., Yazar-Klosinski, B., Emerson, A., Mithoefer, M. C., & Doblin, R. (2019). Breakthrough for trauma treatment: Safety and efficacy of MDMA-assisted psychotherapy compared to paroxetine and sertraline. *Frontiers in Psychiatry, 10,* 650. https://doi.org/10.3389/fpsyt.2019.00650

30 National Institute of Mental Health (NIMH). (2021, June 21). *NIMH-funded researcher Dr. Barbara Rothbaum discusses post-traumatic stress disorder* [Video]. YouTube. All rights reserved. https://youtu.be/wIcWIbM4hLE

My Notes

9.7 APPLYING THE NURSING PROCESS TO ANXIETY DISORDERS

People with anxiety disorders rarely require hospitalization unless they are suicidal, although anxiety can occur with other mental disorders requiring hospitalization. As a nurse working with individuals with diagnosed anxiety disorders, be aware of your self-reaction. It is not uncommon to have feelings of frustration, especially if you feel as if the symptoms are a matter of choice or under the client's control. The client often acknowledges the fear is unrealistic or exaggerated but continues to engage in avoidant behavior. Recall that avoidant behavior is a symptom, and behavioral changes are accomplished slowly with treatment.[1]

It is also important to be aware that hospitalized patients may develop anxiety in association with other medical conditions (i.e., chronic obstructive pulmonary disease [COPD], angina, or hyperthyroidism) or medical procedures. Anxiety is a nursing diagnosis, as well as a potential mental health disorder. While implementing interventions that address medical conditions, often the nurse must also implement interventions that address associated anxiety.

Assessment

When assessing clients with anxiety, assess for the symptoms associated with the "fight or flight" stress response including the following[2]:

- Restlessness
- Altered concentration, attention, or memory
- Diminished ability to learn or problem solve
- Hypervigilance
- Fear
- Irritability or nervousness
- Hand tremors
- Increased perspiration
- Quivering voice
- Increased respiratory rate, heart rate, and blood pressure
- Palpitations
- Weakness
- Abdominal pain, nausea, or diarrhea
- Urinary urgency
- Altered sleep pattern

Determine the client's current level of anxiety (mild, moderate, severe, or panic) and assess for risk of suicide or self-harm. Perform a psychosocial assessment and focus on what factors could be contributing to the anxiety. For

1 Halter, M. (2022). *Varcarolis' foundations of psychiatric-mental health nursing* (9th ed.). Saunders.

2 Ackley, B., Ladwig, G., Makic, M. B., Martinez-Kratz, M., & Zanotti, M. (2020). *Nursing diagnosis handbook: An evidence-based guide to planning care* (12th ed.). Elsevier.

My Notes

example, the client may identify a problem such as a relationship issue, stressful job, or school challenges that could be addressed by counseling.[3]

Screening Tools

The Severity Measure for Generalized Anxiety Disorder in Adults is a common tool for measuring anxiety. High scores may indicate generalized anxiety disorder or panic disorder, although it can also be associated with major depressive disorder.

View the Severity Measure for Generalized Anxiety Disorder—Adult PDF screening tool.

Diagnostic and Lab Work

When assessing for anxiety disorders, the provider will typically order lab work to rule out common medical causes of anxiety, such as hyperthyroidism, hypoglycemia, hypercalcemia, hyperkalemia, hyponatremia, or hypoxia. Review and/or monitor the results of these tests as part of the nursing assessment.

Cultural Considerations

Cultural beliefs can affect an individual's expression of their feelings of anxiety. An example of a culture-mediated response related to anxiety and panic disorder is ataque de nervios (ADN) or "attack of the nerves" that may be exhibited in Hispanic populations. Symptoms of ADNs can vary widely but are typically described as an experience of distress characterized by a general sense of being out of control. The most common symptoms include uncontrollable shouting, attacks of crying, trembling, and heat in the chest rising into the head. Suicidal gestures, seizures, or fainting episodes may be observed. These symptoms are reported to typically occur following a distressing event such as an interpersonal conflict or the death of a loved one.[4]

Diagnoses

Anxiety is a NANDA-I nursing diagnosis and described as "vague, uneasy feeling of discomfort or dread accompanied by an autonomic response; a feeling of apprehension caused by anticipation of danger. It is an alerting sign that warns of impending danger and enables the individual to take measures to deal with the threat."[5] Read selected defining characteristics of anxiety in the preceding "Assessment" subsection or consult an evidence-based nursing care plan resource.

Outcomes Identification

The overall goal for anyone experiencing anxiety is to reduce the frequency and intensity of the anxiety symptoms. SMART outcomes are individualized to the client's diagnosed conditions, situational factors, and current status. Planning outcomes in small, attainable steps can help a client gain a sense of control over their anxiety.[6]

---

3 Halter, M. (2022). *Varcarolis' foundations of psychiatric-mental health nursing* (9th ed.). Saunders.

4 Keough, M. E., Timpano, K. R., & Schmidt, N. B. (2009). Ataques de nervios: Culturally bound and distinct from panic attacks? *Depression & Anxiety, 26*(1), 16-21. https://onlinelibrary.wiley.com/doi/10.1002/da.20498

5 Halter, M. (2022). *Varcarolis' foundations of psychiatric-mental health nursing* (9th ed.). Saunders.

6 Halter, M. (2022). *Varcarolis' foundations of psychiatric-mental health nursing* (9th ed.). Saunders.

My Notes

Examples of SMART outcomes include:

- The client's vital signs will return to baseline within one hour.
- The client will identify and verbalize symptoms of anxiety by the end of the shift.
- The client will verbalize three preferred stress management and coping strategies for controlling their anxiety by the end of Week 1.

Planning Interventions

The client should be encouraged to participate in planning outcomes and interventions tailored to their situation and needs. This will increase the likelihood that the interventions will be successful. Keep in mind that clients with severe anxiety or panic may not be able to participate in planning and rely on the nurse to take a directive role.[7]

Implementing Interventions

Safety

If a client is diagnosed with risk for suicide, interventions to maintain their safety receive priority. Review interventions for clients with a risk for suicide in the "Application of the Nursing Process in Mental Health Care" chapter.

If a client's anxiety continues to escalate and they become agitated, measures must be taken to keep them and others safe. The nurse may find that administering prescribed medications, initiating time in a quiet room, seclusion, or restraints is required. Review crisis intervention in the "Stress, Coping, and Crisis Intervention" chapter. Review information regarding the use of seclusion and restraints in the "Psychosis and Schizophrenia" chapter.

Mild to Moderate Anxiety

The nurse can reduce a client's anxiety level and prevent escalation by providing a calm presence in a quiet environment, acknowledging their feelings of distress, and actively listening. Using therapeutic techniques like open-ended questions, distraction, exploring, and seeking clarification can be used to relieve the client's feelings of tension and focus on previously successful coping strategies.[8] Review therapeutic communication techniques in the "Therapeutic Communication and the Nurse-Client Relationship" chapter.

It may be helpful to encourage the client to participate in physical activities that may provide relief from tension and increase endorphin levels. For example, the nurse can encourage the mildly anxious client to walk or play ping-pong.[9]

Severe Anxiety to Panic

A person experiencing severe anxiety to panic is often unable to solve problems or grasp what is going on in the environment. The nurse should also remain with a client experiencing acute, severe, or panic levels of anxiety.

---

7 Halter, M. (2022). *Varcarolis' foundations of psychiatric-mental health nursing* (9th ed.). Saunders.

8 Halter, M. (2022). *Varcarolis' foundations of psychiatric-mental health nursing* (9th ed.). Saunders.

9 Halter, M. (2022). *Varcarolis' foundations of psychiatric-mental health nursing* (9th ed.). Saunders.

My Notes

Therapeutic communication should focus on helping the client feel safe. Firm, short, simple statements using a slow, low-pitched voice are helpful.[10]

In addition to keeping the client and others safe, priority nursing interventions for a client experiencing severe anxiety focus on the client's physical needs, such as fluids to prevent dehydration, blankets for warmth, and rest to prevent exhaustion. If a person continues to constantly move or pace despite interventions, high-calorie finger foods may be offered to maintain their nutrition.[11] Read additional interventions related to crisis intervention in the "Stress, Coping, and Crisis Intervention" chapter.

Evaluation

Refer to the individualized SMART outcomes established for each client when evaluating the effectiveness of interventions in the care plan. In general, evaluation of outcomes with clients with anxiety disorders includes the following questions[12]:

- Is the client experiencing a reduced level of anxiety?
- Does the client recognize their symptoms are related to anxiety?
- Is the client successfully implementing adaptive coping strategies to manage their anxiety?
- Is the client adequately performing self-care activities (e.g., hygiene, eating, and elimination)?
- Is the client able to maintain satisfying interpersonal relationships?
- Is the client able to successfully function socially, occupationally, or in other important areas of functioning?

---

10 Halter, M. (2022). *Varcarolis' foundations of psychiatric-mental health nursing* (9th ed.). Saunders.

11 Halter, M. (2022). *Varcarolis' foundations of psychiatric-mental health nursing* (9th ed.). Saunders.

12 Halter, M. (2022). *Varcarolis' foundations of psychiatric-mental health nursing* (9th ed.). Saunders.

My Notes

9.8 SPOTLIGHT APPLICATION

Melissa is a 20-year-old nursing student who visits her primary care provider for a refill on her birth control pills. During the admission assessment, Melissa shares with the intake nurse that her "anxiety has gotten much worse" during nursing school. She states, "I always feel tired, but I can't sit down and relax. I feel like there is always more studying that I should be doing for my classes. Even though I'm tired at night, I don't sleep well and wake up frequently throughout the night. If I can't go back to sleep, I turn on my computer and study. I have also been getting headaches every day, and I think it is from being on the computer so much every day. My boyfriend keeps asking me why I am so crabby. Lately I have had a lot of test anxiety, and sometimes my mind goes blank during an exam even though I have memorized all of the material."

The primary care provider diagnoses Melissa with Generalized Anxiety Disorder and encourages her to attend a local support group with other people experiencing anxiety. A beta-blocker is prescribed on an "as needed" basis for before exams or other types of performance assessments, and a referral is made to a psychotherapist for cognitive behavioral therapy. The discharge nurse encourages Melissa to talk about her anxieties with a close personal friend or family member, as well as implement other stress management strategies like daily exercise, healthy food choices, and journaling. She encourages Melissa to decrease her screen time before bedtime and to avoid studying in bed.

Melissa returns to the clinic in one month for a follow-up appointment. She reports that the stress management techniques have helped her to sleep better and improve her concentration. She took a beta-blocker before a recent exam and reports it helped reduce her anxiety, and she did not experience her mind going blank. She plans on seeing a psychotherapist after the semester ends if she still needs assistance with managing her anxiety.

9.9 LEARNING ACTIVITIES

My Notes

Interactive Activities

An interactive H5P element has been excluded from this version of the text. You can view it online here: https://wtcs.pressbooks.pub/nursingmhcc/?p=492#h5p-24

An interactive H5P element has been excluded from this version of the text. You can view it online here: https://wtcs.pressbooks.pub/nursingmhcc/?p=492#h5p-25

An interactive H5P element has been excluded from this version of the text. You can view it online here: https://wtcs.pressbooks.pub/nursingmhcc/?p=492#h5p-27

My Notes

IX GLOSSARY

Agoraphobia: Intense fear of two or more of the following situations: using public transportation, being in open spaces (e.g., parking lots, marketplaces, or bridges), being in enclosed spaces (e.g., shops or theaters), standing in line or being in a crowd, or being outside of the home alone.

Anxiety: A universal human experience that includes feelings of apprehension, uneasiness, uncertainty, or dread resulting from a real or perceived threat.

Compulsions: Repetitive behaviors that a person with OCD feels the urge to do in response to an obsessive thought.

Coping strategies: An action, a series of actions, or a thought process used to address a stressful or unpleasant situation or modify one's reaction to such a situation.

Defense mechanisms: Reaction patterns used by individuals to protect themselves from anxiety that arises from stress and conflict.

Exposure and response prevention (EX/RP): A type of psychotherapy effective in reducing compulsive behaviors in clients with OCD. EX/RP includes spending time in the very situation that triggers compulsions (for example, touching dirty objects) but then being prevented from undertaking the usual resulting compulsion (handwashing).

Exposure therapy: A type of psychotherapy that focuses on confronting the fears underlying an anxiety disorder to help people engage in activities they have been avoiding.

Generalized anxiety disorder (GAD): Excessive anxiety and worry occurring for at least six months about a number of events or activities (such as work or school performance).

Obsessions: Repeated thoughts, urges, or mental images that cause anxiety.

Obsessive-compulsive disorder (OCD): A common chronic disorder in which a person has uncontrollable, reoccurring thoughts (obsessions) and/or behaviors (compulsions) they feel the urge to repeat over and over. Performing the compulsive behaviors often brings the person brief relief from the anxiety the obsessive thoughts cause them.

Panic: The most extreme level of anxiety that results in significantly dysregulated behavior. The individual is unable to process information from the environment and may lose touch with reality.

Panic attacks: Sudden periods of intense fear that come on quickly and reach their peak within minutes. Attacks can occur unexpectedly or can be brought on by a trigger, such as a feared object or situation.

Phobia: An intense fear or aversion to specific objects or situations (e.g., flying, heights, animals, receiving an injection, or seeing blood).

Post-traumatic stress disorder (PTSD): A disorder that develops in some people who have experienced a shocking, frightening, or dangerous event where they feel stressed or frightened even when they are not in danger.

Repetitive Transcranial Magnetic Stimulation (rTMS): Treatment that uses a magnet to activate specific sites in the brain.

Selective mutism: A condition when people fail to speak in specific social situations despite having normal language skills.

Separation anxiety disorder: A condition where an individual has a fear about being separated from people to whom they are attached.

Social anxiety disorder: Significant fear or anxiety about one or more social situations in which the individual is exposed to possible scrutiny by others.

Chapter 10

Personality Disorders

10.1 INTRODUCTION

My Notes

Learning Objectives

- Apply the nursing process to clients with personality disorders
- Describe nursing assessments related to personality disorders
- Identify common nursing problems/diagnoses related to personality disorders
- Establish a safe environment
- Apply evidence-based practice when planning and implementing nursing care
- Describe common treatments for personality disorders
- Identify appropriate referrals to community resources
- Evaluate the effectiveness of interventions
- Provide patient education to clients and their family members

Research studies have demonstrated that nine percent of Americans have a personality disorder. A large proportion of this population also has one or more other mental health disorders.[1] This chapter will describe the signs and symptoms of ten personality disorders and associated treatments. The nursing process will be applied to caring for a client with borderline personality disorder.

---

1 National Institute of Mental Health. (n.d.). *Personality disorders.* U.S. Department of Health and Human Services. https://www.nimh.nih.gov/health/statistics/personality-disorders

My Notes

10.2 BASIC CONCEPTS

A person's **personality** is a relatively stable pattern of thinking, feeling, and behaving that evolves over their lifetime. It is unique to each individual and influenced by their experiences, environment (surroundings and life situations), and inherited characteristics. **Personality traits** are characteristics, whether considered positive or negative, that make up one's personality. Healthy personality traits include characteristics such as the following:

- Demonstrating healthy personal boundaries
- Accepting responsibility for personal actions
- Communicating in a healthy and effective manner
- Obeying laws
- Showing mutual respect in relationships
- Being independent
- Displaying confidence
- Behaving in a non-impulsive manner

Review healthy personal boundaries in the "Foundational Mental Health Concepts" chapter. An individual's personality is considered unhealthy and classified as a disorder when it impacts their interpersonal relationships and results in impaired functioning in social, occupational, or other important areas of their life.[1]

The *Diagnostic and Statistical Manual of Mental Disorders (DSM-5)* defines a **personality disorder** as an enduring pattern of inner experience and behavior that deviates significantly from the expectations of one's culture. Its onset can be traced back to adolescence or early adulthood and is present in a variety of contexts. This abnormal pattern of behavior is manifested in two or more of the following areas[2]:

- Cognition (i.e., ways of perceiving and interpreting self, other people, and events)
- Affect (i.e., the range, intensity, lability, and appropriateness of emotional response)
- Interpersonal functioning
- Impulse control

There are ten different personality disorders that are categorized into three clusters (A, B, and C) in the *DSM-5.* Personality disorders within each cluster have similar patterns of behavior. The ten disorders include Cluster A (paranoid, schizoid, schizotypal), Cluster B (antisocial, narcissistic, borderline, histrionic), and Cluster C (dependent, avoidant, and obsessive-compulsive personality disorder).[3]

Based on several research studies, obsessive-compulsive personality disorder is the most common personality disorder in the United States, followed by narcissistic and borderline personality disorders. However, the most common personality disorder varies from country to country.[4]

---

1 American Psychiatric Association. (2013). *Desk reference to the diagnostic criteria from DSM-5.*

2 American Psychiatric Association. (2013). *Desk reference to the diagnostic criteria from DSM-5.*

3 American Psychiatric Association. (2013). *Desk reference to the diagnostic criteria from DSM-5.*

4 Sansone, R. A., & Sansone, L. A. (2011). Personality disorders: A nation-based perspective on prevalence. *Innovations in Clinical Neuroscience, 8*(4), 13-18. https://www.ncbi.nlm.nih.gov/pmc/articles/PMC3105841/

My Notes

Each personality disorder is further described in the following sections. As you read through each section, keep in mind that these disorders are more than just personality traits; they are diagnosed based on patterns of behaviors that significantly impair a person's functioning.

Cluster A Personality Disorders

Cluster A personality disorders include paranoid personality disorder, schizoid personality disorder, and schizotypal personality disorder. Cluster A is characterized as the odd, eccentric cluster. Individuals with these types of disorders often experience social awkwardness.

Paranoid Personality Disorder

The *DSM-5* defines **paranoid personality disorder** as a "pervasive distrust and suspiciousness of others such that their motives are interpreted as malevolent."[5] It is diagnosed in individuals with four or more of the following characteristics[6]:

- Suspects without evidence that others are exploiting, harming, or deceiving them
- Preoccupied with unjustified doubts about the loyalty or trustworthiness of friends or associates
- Reluctant to confide in others because of unwarranted fear that the information will be used maliciously against them
- Reads hidden meaning or threatening meanings into benign remarks or events
- Persistently bears grudges (i.e., is unforgiving of insults, injuries, or slights)
- Perceives attacks on their character or reputation that are not apparent to others and is quick to react angrily or to counterattack
- Has recurrent suspicions without justification regarding fidelity of spouse or sexual partner

See Figure 10.1[7] for a word cloud image representing paranoid personality disorder.

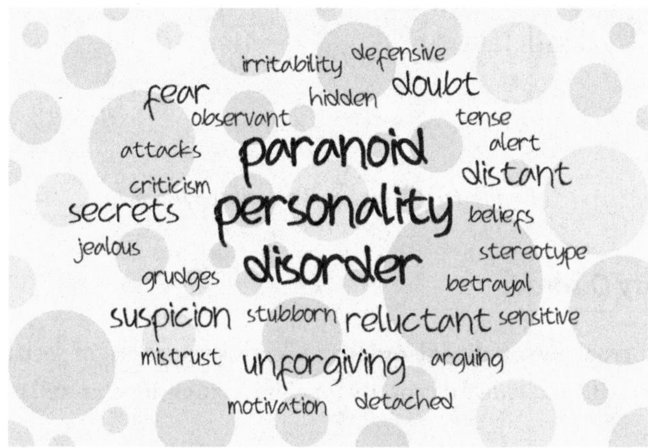

Figure 10.1 Paranoid Personality Disorder

5 American Psychiatric Association. (2013). *Desk reference to the diagnostic criteria from DSM-5.*

6 American Psychiatric Association. (2013). *Desk reference to the diagnostic criteria from DSM-5.*

7 "Word_Cloud_PPD.png" by MissLunaRose12 is licensed under CC BY-SA 4.0

My Notes

Schizoid Personality Disorder

The *DSM-5* defines **schizoid personality disorder** as a "pervasive pattern of detachment from social relationships and a restricted range of expression of emotions in interpersonal settings."[8] It is diagnosed in individuals with four or more of the following characteristics[9]:

- Neither desires nor enjoys close relationships including being part of a family
- Almost always chooses solitary activities
- Has little, if any, interest in having sexual experiences with another person
- Takes pleasure in few, if any, activities
- Lacks close friends other than first-degree relatives
- Appears indifferent to the praise or criticism of others
- Shows emotional coldness, detachment, or flat affect

See Figure 10.2[10] for a word cloud image representing schizoid personality disorder.

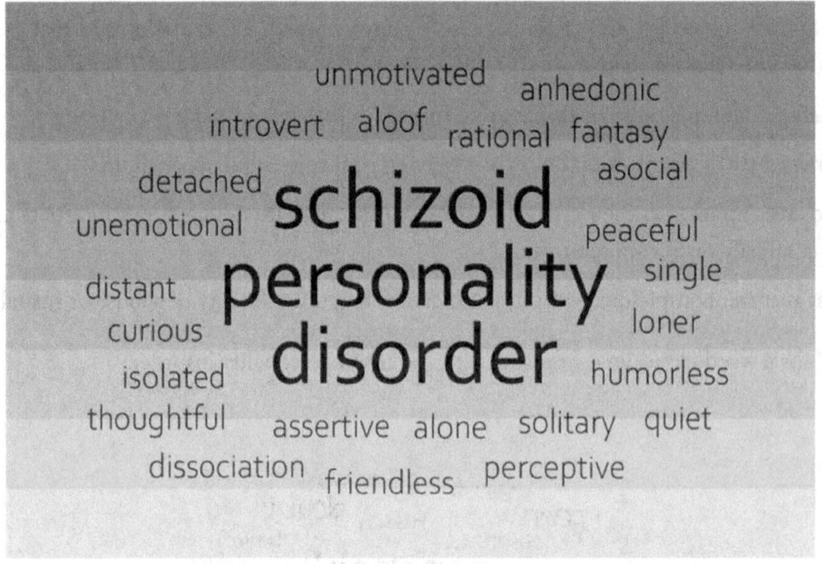

Figure 10.2 Schizoid Personality Disorder

Schizotypal Personality Disorder

The *DSM-5* defines **schizotypal personality disorder** as a "pervasive pattern of social and interpersonal deficits marked by acute discomfort with and reduced capacity for close relationships, as well as by cognitive or perceptual

8 American Psychiatric Association. (2013). *Desk reference to the diagnostic criteria from DSM-5.*

9 American Psychiatric Association. (2013). *Desk reference to the diagnostic criteria from DSM-5.*

10 "Word_Cloud_SzPD.png" by MissLunaRose12 is licensed under CC BY-SA 4.0

My Notes

distortions and eccentricities of behavior."[11] It is diagnosed in individuals with five or more of the following characteristics[12]:

- **Ideas of reference** (i.e., the false belief that coincidental events relate to oneself). For example, a person shopping in a store sees two strangers laughing and believes that they are laughing at them, when, in reality, the other two people do not even notice them.
- Odd beliefs or magical thinking that influence behavior and are inconsistent with cultural norms (**Magical thinking** refers to the idea that one can influence the outcome of specific events by doing something that has no bearing on the circumstances. For example, a person watching a baseball game exhibits magical thinking when believing that holding the remote control in a certain position caused their favorite player to hit a home run.)
- Unusual perceptual experiences including bodily illusions (A **body illusion** refers to a perception that one's body is significantly different from its actual configuration. For example, a person lying in bed feels as if they are levitating.)
- Odd thinking and speech
- Suspiciousness or paranoid ideation
- Inappropriate or constricted affect
- Behavior or appearance that is odd, eccentric, or peculiar
- Lack of close friends or confidants other than first-degree relatives
- Excessive social anxiety that does not diminish with familiarity and tends to be associated with paranoid fears rather than negative judgments about self

See Figure 10.3[13] for a word cloud image representing schizotypal personality disorder.

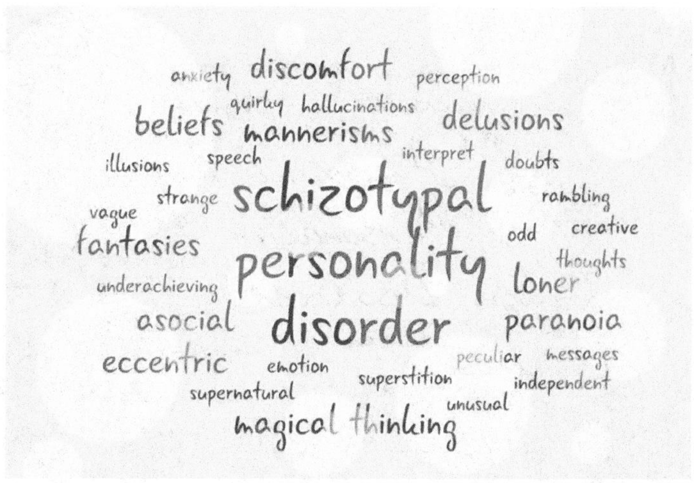

Figure 10.3 Schizotypal Personality Disorder

---

11 American Psychiatric Association. (2013). *Desk reference to the diagnostic criteria from DSM-5.*

12 American Psychiatric Association. (2013). *Desk reference to the diagnostic criteria from DSM-5.*

13 "Word_Cloud_SzPD.png" by MissLunaRose12 is licensed under CC BY-SA 4.0

My Notes

Cluster B Personality Disorders

Cluster B personality disorders include antisocial, borderline, histrionic, and narcissistic personality disorders. Cluster B personality disorders are characterized by dramatic, overly emotional, or unpredictable thinking or behavior.

Antisocial Personality Disorder

The *DSM-5* defines **antisocial personality disorder** as a "pervasive pattern of disregard for and violation of the rights of others since age 15."[14] It is diagnosed in individuals with three or more of the following characteristics[15]:

- Failure to conform to social norms with respect to lawful behaviors, as indicated by repeatedly performing acts that are grounds for arrest
- Deceitfulness, as indicated by repeated lying, use of aliases, or conning others for personal profit or pleasure
- Impulsivity or failure to plan ahead
- Irritability and aggressiveness, as indicated by repeated physical fights and assaults
- Reckless disregard for the safety of self or others
- Consistent irresponsibility, as indicated by repeated failure to sustain consistent work behavior or honor financial obligations
- Lack of remorse, as indicated by being indifferent to or rationalizing having hurt, mistreated, or stolen from another person

See Figure 10.4[16] for a word cloud image representing antisocial personality disorder.

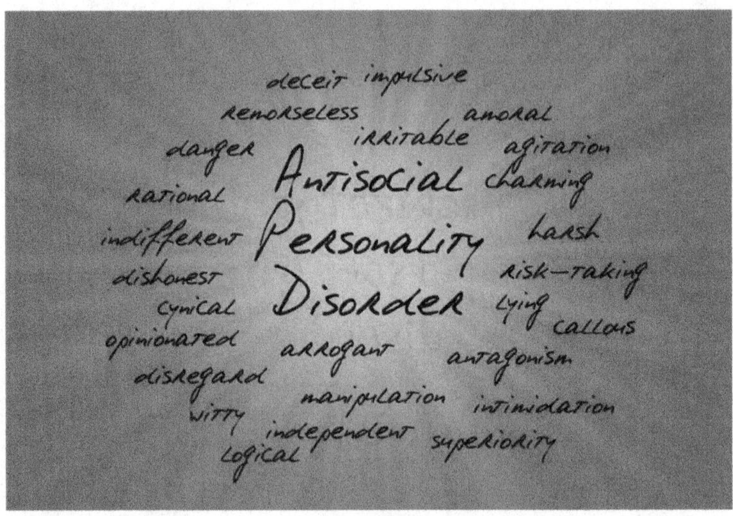

Figure 10.4 Antisocial Personality Disorder

---

14 American Psychiatric Association. (2013). *Desk reference to the diagnostic criteria from DSM-5.*

15 American Psychiatric Association. (2013). *Desk reference to the diagnostic criteria from DSM-5.*

16 "Word_Cloud_AsPD.png" by MissLunaRose12 is licensed under CC BY-SA 4.0

My Notes

Borderline Personality Disorder

The *DSM-5* defines **borderline personality disorder** as a "pervasive pattern of instability of personal relationships, self-image, and affect with significant impulsivity."[17] It is diagnosed in individuals with five or more of the following characteristics[18]:

- Frantic efforts to avoid real or imagined abandonment
- A pattern of unstable and intense personal relationships characterized by alternating between extremes of idealization and devaluation (referred to as **splitting**)
- Identity disturbance with significantly and persistently unstable self-image or sense of self
- Impulsivity in at least two areas that are potentially self-damaging (e.g., spending, sex, substance misuse, reckless driving, or binge eating)
- Recurrent suicidal behavior or self-mutilating behavior
- Unstable affect with significant mood reactivity (i.e., intense anxiety or irritability usually lasting only a few hours)
- Chronic feelings of emptiness
- Inappropriate, intense anger or difficulty controlling anger
- Transient, stress-related paranoid ideation or severe dissociative symptoms (**Dissociative symptoms** include the experience of detachment or feeling as if one is outside one's body. It is often associated with loss of memory of the experience. Dissociative disorders are associated with an individual's previous experience of trauma.)

See Figure 10.5[19] for a word cloud image representing borderline personality disorder.

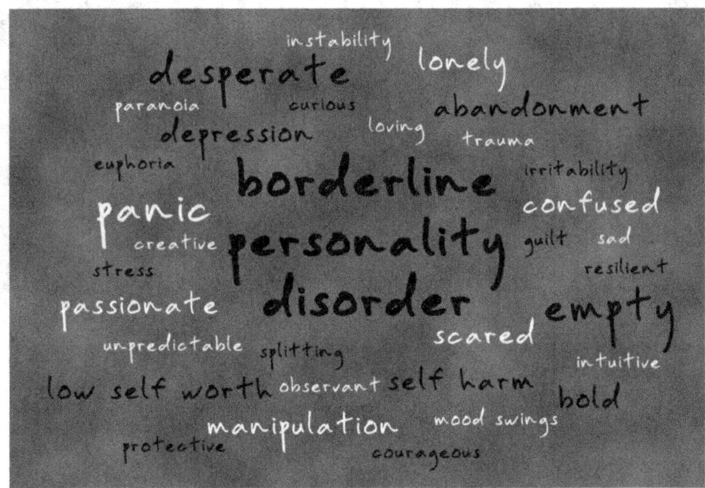

Figure 10.5 Borderline Personality Disorder

17 American Psychiatric Association. (2013). *Desk reference to the diagnostic criteria from DSM-5.*

18 American Psychiatric Association. (2013). *Desk reference to the diagnostic criteria from DSM-5.*

19 "Word_Cloud_BPD.png" by MissLunaRose12 is licensed under CC BY-SA 4.0

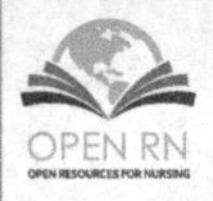

My Notes

Histrionic Personality Disorder

The *DSM-5* defines **histrionic personality disorder** as a "pervasive pattern of excessive emotionality and attention seeking."[20] It is diagnosed in individuals with five or more of the following characteristics[21]:

- Uncomfortable in situations in which they are not the center of attention
- Interaction with others is characterized by inappropriate sexually seductive or provocative behavior
- Rapidly shifting and shallow expression of emotion
- Consistently uses physical appearance to draw attention to oneself
- Excessively impressionistic speech that is lacking in detail
- Shows self-dramatization, theatricality, and exaggerated expression of emotion
- Suggestible (i.e., easily influenced by others)
- Considers relationships to be more intimate than they actually are

See Figure 10.6[22] for a word cloud image representing histrionic personality disorder.

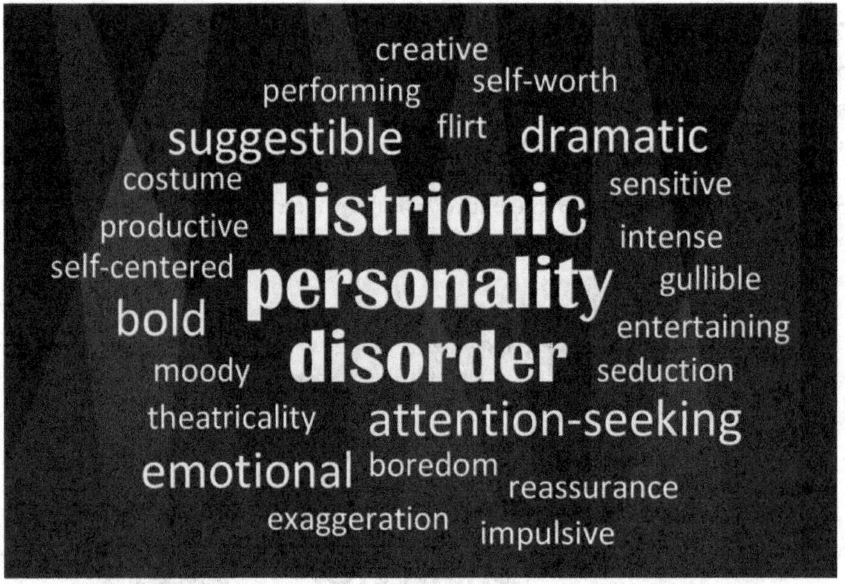

Figure 10.6 Histrionic Personality Disorder

20 American Psychiatric Association. (2013). *Desk reference to the diagnostic criteria from DSM-5.*

21 American Psychiatric Association. (2013). *Desk reference to the diagnostic criteria from DSM-5.*

22 "Word_Cloud_HPD.png" by MissLunaRose12 is licensed under CC BY-SA 4.0

My Notes

Narcissistic Personality Disorder

The *DSM-5* defines **narcissistic personality disorder** as a "pervasive pattern of grandiosity (in fantasy or behavior), need for attention, and lack of empathy."[23] It is diagnosed in individuals with five or more of the following characteristics[24]:

- Has a grandiose sense of self-importance (i.e., exaggerates achievements and talents)
- Is preoccupied with fantasies of unlimited success, power, brilliance, beauty, or ideal love
- Believes they are "special" and can only be understood by, or should only associate with, other "special" or high-status people (or institutions)
- Requires excessive admiration
- Has a sense of **entitlement** (i.e., unreasonable expectations of especially favorable treatment)
- Exploits others to achieve their own goals
- Lacks empathy and the ability to identify with the feelings and needs of others
- Is often envious of others or believes that others are envious of them
- Shows arrogant or haughty behaviors or attitudes

See Figure 10.7[25] for a word cloud image representing narcissistic personality disorder.

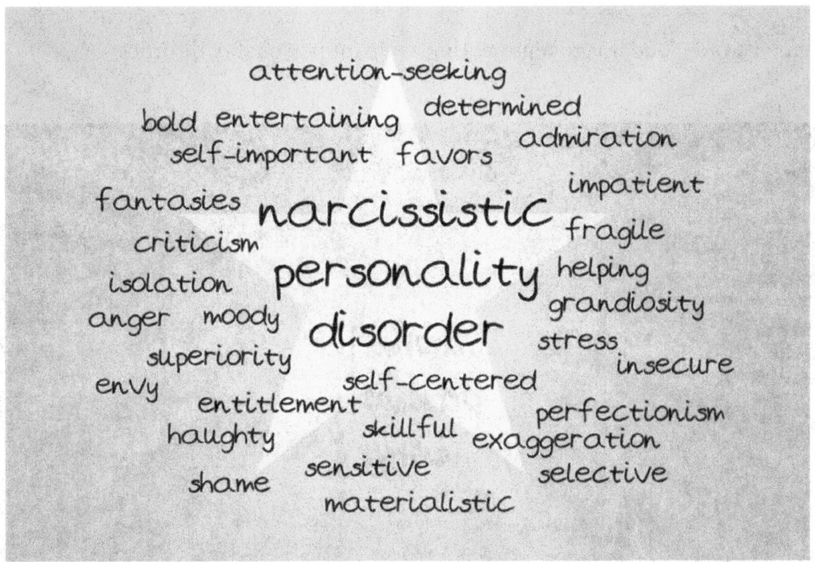

Figure 10.7 Narcissistic Personality Disorder

23 American Psychiatric Association. (2013). *Desk reference to the diagnostic criteria from DSM-5.*

24 American Psychiatric Association. (2013). *Desk reference to the diagnostic criteria from DSM-5.*

25 "Word_Cloud_NPD.png" by MissLunaRose12 is licensed under CC BY-SA 4.0

Cluster C Personality Disorders

Cluster C personality disorders include avoidant, dependent, and obsessive-compulsive personality disorders. Cluster C personality disorders are characterized by anxious, fearful thinking or behavior.

Avoidant Personality Disorder

The *DSM-5* defines **avoidant personality disorder** as a "pervasive pattern of social inhibition, feelings of inadequacy, and hypersensitivity to negative evaluation."[26] It is diagnosed in individuals with four or more of the following characteristics[27]:

- Avoids occupational activities that involve significant interpersonal contact because of fears or criticism, disapproval, or rejection
- Is unwilling to get involved with people unless certain of being liked
- Shows restraint within intimate relationships because of the fear of being shamed or ridiculed
- Is preoccupied with being criticized or rejected in social situations
- Is inhibited in new interpersonal situations because of feelings of inadequacy
- Views self as socially inept, personally unappealing, or inferior to others
- Is unusually reluctant to take personal risks or to engage in any new activities because they may prove embarrassing

See Figure 10.8[28] for a word cloud image representing avoidant personality disorders.

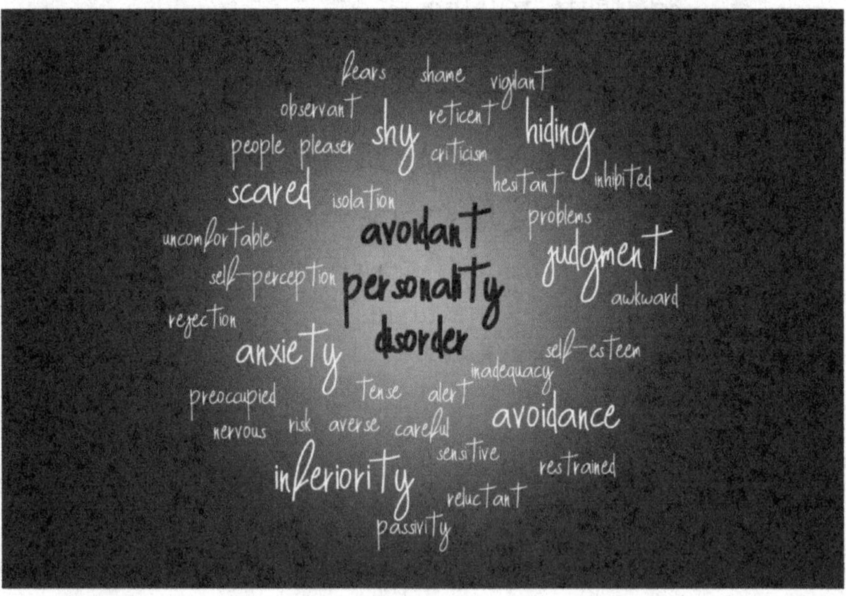

Figure 10.8 Avoidant Personality Disorder

---

26 American Psychiatric Association. (2013). *Desk reference to the diagnostic criteria from DSM-5.*

27 American Psychiatric Association. (2013). *Desk reference to the diagnostic criteria from DSM-5.*

28 "Word_Cloud_AvPD.png" by MissLunaRose12 is licensed under CC BY-SA 4.0

Dependent Personality Disorder

My Notes

The *DSM-5* defines **dependent personality disorder** as a "pervasive and excessive need to be taken care of that leads to submission and clinging behavior and fears of separation."[29] It is diagnosed by five or more of the following characteristics[30]:

- Has difficulty making everyday decisions without an excessive amount of advice and reassurance from others
- Needs others to assume responsibility for most major areas of their life
- Has difficulty expressing disagreement with others because of fear of loss or support or approval
- Has difficulty initiating projects or doing things on their own because of lack of self-confidence in judgment or abilities
- Goes to excessive lengths to obtain nurturance and support from others to the point of volunteering to do things that are unpleasant
- Feels uncomfortable or helpless when alone because of exaggerated fears of being unable to care for themselves
- Urgently seeks another relationship as a source of care and support when a close relationship ends
- Is unrealistically preoccupied with fears of being left to take care of themselves

See Figure 10.9[31] for a word cloud image representing dependent personality disorder.

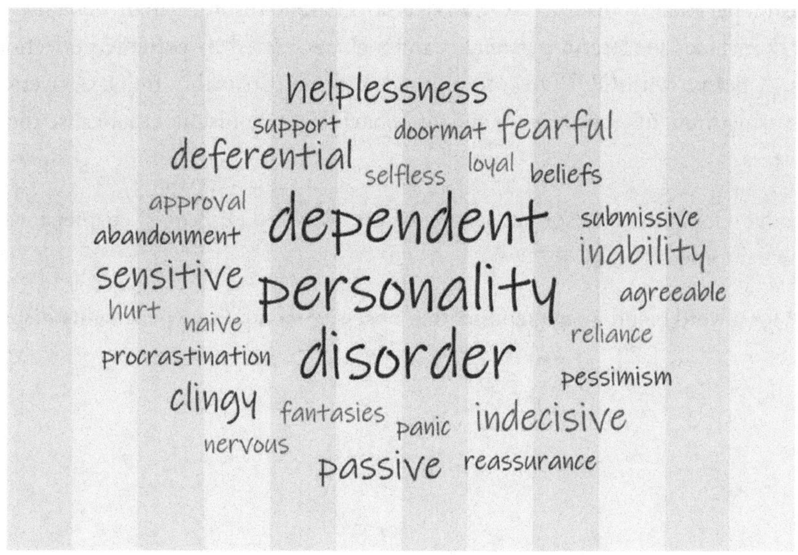

Figure 10.9 Dependent Personality Disorder

29 American Psychiatric Association. (2013). *Desk reference to the diagnostic criteria from DSM-5.*

30 American Psychiatric Association. (2013). *Desk reference to the diagnostic criteria from DSM-5.*

31 "Word_Cloud_DPD.png" by MissLunaRose12 is licensed under CC BY-SA 4.0

My Notes

Obsessive-Compulsive Personality Disorder

The *DSM-5* defines **obsessive-compulsive personality disorder** as a "pervasive pattern or preoccupation with orderliness, perfectionism, and mental and interpersonal control at the expense of flexibility, openness, and efficiency."[32] It is diagnosed in individuals with four or more of the following characteristics[33]:

- Is preoccupied with details, rules, lists, order, organization, or schedules to the extent that the major point of the activity is lost
- Shows perfectionism that interferes with task completion (i.e., is unable to complete a project because their overly strict standards are not met)
- Is excessively devoted to work and productivity to the exclusion of leisurely activities and friendships
- Is overconscientious, scrupulous, and inflexible about matters of morality, ethics, or values (not accounted for by cultural or religious identification)
- Is unable to discard worn-out or worthless objects even when they have no sentimental value
- Is reluctant to delegate tasks or work with others unless they submit to exactly their way of doing things
- Adopts a miserly spending style towards self and others; money is viewed as something to be hoarded for future catastrophes
- Shows rigidity and stubbornness

Obsessive-compulsive personality disorder (OCPD) is a different disorder than obsessive-compulsive disorder (OCD). OCPD includes long-term personality traits characterized by extreme perfectionism, rigidity, and adherence to rules. A person with OCPD is often proud of these personality traits. Conversely, OCD includes uncontrollable, recurring thoughts (obsessions) and/or behaviors (compulsions) that cause the individual significant emotional distress.

Review the "Obsessive-Compulsive Disorder" section of the "Anxiety Disorders" chapter for more details about obsessive-compulsive disorder.

See Figure 10.10[34] for a word cloud image representing obsessive-compulsive personality disorder.

---

32 American Psychiatric Association. (2013). *Desk reference to the diagnostic criteria from DSM-5.*

33 American Psychiatric Association. (2013). *Desk reference to the diagnostic criteria from DSM-5.*

34 "Word_Cloud_OCPD.png" by MissLunaRose12 is licensed under CC BY-SA 4.0

My Notes

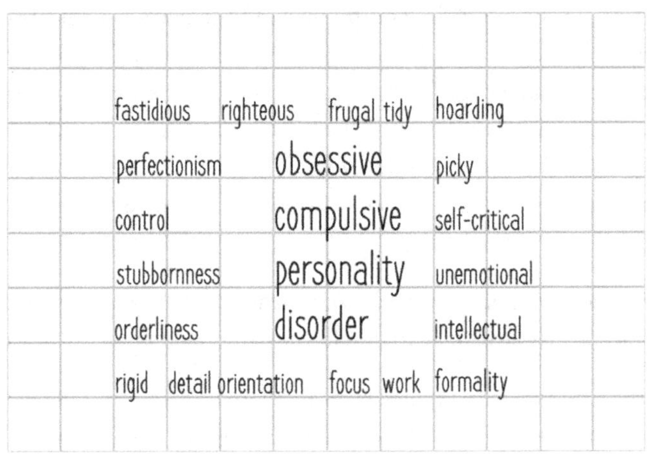

Figure 10.10 Obsessive-Compulsive Personality Disorder

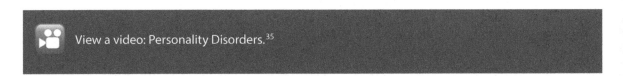

Reflective Question

1. When does one's personality become a disorder versus just personality traits?

Risk Factors for Personality Disorders

Research suggests that genetics, childhood trauma, peer influences, and other factors can contribute to the development of personality disorders.[36]

Genetics: Researchers have identified possible genetic factors behind personality disorders. One study identified a malfunctioning gene that may be a factor in obsessive-compulsive personality disorder. Research reveals the importance of gene-environment interactions in the development of antisocial behavior and psychopathic traits.[37,38]

35 khanacademymedicine. (2015, July 20). *Personality disorders | Behavior | MCAT | Khan Academy* [Video]. YouTube. https://youtu.be/-Xv593jgyJ4

36 American Psychological Association. (2010). *What causes personality disorders?* https://www.apa.org/topics/personality-disorders/causes

37 American Psychological Association. (2010). *What causes personality disorders?* https://www.apa.org/topics/personality-disorders/causes

38 Junewicz, A., & Billick, S.B. (2021). Preempting the development of antisocial behavior and psychopathic traits, *The Journal of American Academy of Psychiatry Law, 49*(1):66-76. https://doi: 10.29158/JAAPL.200060-20

My Notes

Childhood trauma: Research has linked childhood trauma and the development of personality disorders, especially if the individual's caregiver(s) do not validate the feelings associated with the trauma. People with borderline personality disorder, for example, had especially high rates of childhood sexual trauma.[39] In another study of 793 mothers and children, researchers asked mothers if they had screamed at their children, told them they didn't love them, or threatened to send them away. Children who had experienced such verbal abuse were three times as likely as other children to have borderline, narcissistic, obsessive-compulsive, or paranoid personality disorders in adulthood.[40]

Overactive or sensitive nervous system response: Overly sensitive children who have a high reactivity to light, noise, texture, and other stimuli are more likely to develop shy, timid, or anxious personalities.[41]

Certain positive factors can help prevent children from developing personality disorders. For example, a single strong relationship with a relative, teacher, or friend can offset negative influences. Strong resiliency factors contribute to health and development of a child.[42]

---

39 American Psychological Association. (2010). *What causes personality disorders?* https://www.apa.org/topics/personality-disorders/causes

40 American Psychological Association. (2010). *What causes personality disorders?* https://www.apa.org/topics/personality-disorders/causes

41 American Psychological Association. (2010). *What causes personality disorders?* https://www.apa.org/topics/personality-disorders/causes

42 American Psychological Association. (2010). *What causes personality disorders?* https://www.apa.org/topics/personality-disorders/causes

10.3 TREATMENT FOR PERSONALITY DISORDERS

My Notes

Clients with some types of personality disorders do not exhibity insight for their condition and are unlikely to seek treatment. They often go undiagnosed unless they seek treatment for another psychiatric or medical diagnosis. Some may also be forced to seek treatment at the influence of family members or as required by law if legal infractions have occurred. Personality disorders can be challenging for mental health professionals to treat. Individuals with personality disorders struggle to recognize that their difficulties in life are related to their personalities. They may truly believe their problems are a result of other people or outside factors. It is very common for clients with personality disorders to also have substance abuse, anxiety, depression, or eating disorders.[1]

Psychotherapy is the first line of treatment for personality disorders. Medications may also be prescribed to treat underlying co-occurring conditions such as anxiety or depression.

Psychotherapy

During psychotherapy, an individual can gain insight and knowledge about the personality disorder and what is contributing to their symptoms. They talk about their thoughts, feelings, and behaviors and ideally will develop an understanding of the impact of their thoughts and behaviors on themselves and others. They learn strategies for managing and coping with their symptoms. This treatment can help reduce problematic behaviors that impact an individual's relationships and functioning.[2]

Common types of psychotherapy used to treat personality disorders are as follows[3]:

- Cognitive behavior therapy
- Dialectical behavior therapy
- Interpersonal therapy
- Psychoanalytic/psychodynamic therapy
- Psychoeducation

Cognitive behavior therapy (CBT) teaches the client to become more aware of the way they think so they can ultimately change the way they behave.

Dialectical behavior therapy (DBT) is a type of cognitive behavioral therapy that was originally created for clients with borderline personality disorder to help them cope with stress, control emotions, and establish healthy relationships. It is considered the gold standard for treating borderline personality disorder and is also used for other types of disorders. The client learns how to be aware of how thoughts, feelings, behaviors link together. They learn how to use their senses to be aware of what is happening around them and how to use strategies (such as mindfulness, distress tolerance, interpersonal effectiveness, and emotion regulation) to react calmly in a crisis, avoid

1 Halter, M. (2022). *Varcarolis' foundations of psychiatric-mental health nursing* (9th ed.). Saunders.

2 American Psychiatric Association. (n.d.). *What are personality disorders?* https://www.psychiatry.org/patients-families/personality-disorders/what-are-personality-disorders

3 American Psychiatric Association. (n.d.). *What are personality disorders?* https://www.psychiatry.org/patients-families/personality-disorders/what-are-personality-disorders

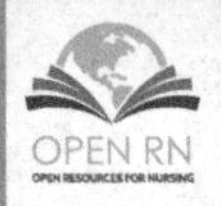

My Notes

negative impulsive behavior, and improve relationships.[4] See Figure 10.11[5] for an illustration of how thoughts, feelings and behaviors are linked together.

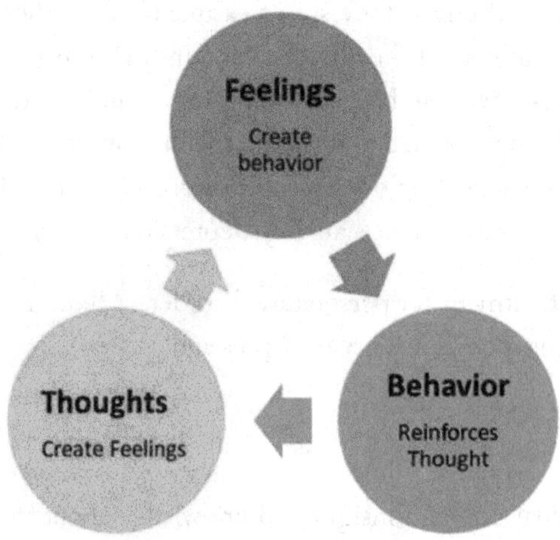

Figure 10.11 Dialectical Behavior Therapy

Interpersonal therapy focuses on developing healthy relationships with others. Negative aspects of relationships, such as social isolation and aggression, are identified, and strategies to improve relationships are discussed and planned.

Psychodynamic therapy promotes self-reflection and self-examination of problematic relationship patterns and unresolved conflicts. It can bring awareness of how one's past has an influence on one's present behavior.

Psychoeducation teaches the client about their medications, psychotherapies, and support groups available in the community. Wraparound services may be planned with an individualized plan of care that brings multiple services/supports together for the client.

Pharmacotherapy

There are no specific medications approved to treat personality disorders. However, clients who have severe symptoms may be prescribed medications as off-label use that are not necessarily approved by the U.S. Food and Drug administration (FDA) for personality disorders but are guided by expert opinion and experience. The decision to treat an individual with a personality disorder with medication should be made through shared decision-making with the client based on drug efficacy for their symptoms, potential adverse effects, and their degree of impairment.[6]

---

4 Schimelpfening, N. (2021, November 5). What is dialectical behavior therapy (DBT)? *Verywell Mind.* https://www.verywellmind.com/dialectical-behavior-therapy-1067402

5 "Dialectical Behavior Therapy by Kim Ernstmeyer.png" by Kim Ernstmeyer for Chippewa Valley Technical College is licensed under CC BY 4.0

6 Nelson, K. J. (2021). Pharmacotherapy for personality disorders. *UpToDate.* https://www.uptodate.com

My Notes

Symptom domains that cause impairment and distress across personality disorders and medications commonly used to treat them include the following[7]:

- Cognitive-perceptual symptoms (e.g., hallucinations and paranoid ideation): Treated with low-dose antipsychotics such as aripiprazole, risperidone, and quetiapine.
- Impulsive behaviors (e.g., self-injury, theft, interpersonal conflict): Treated with mood stabilizers (such as lithium and lamotrigine). Omega-3 is used as an adjunct to treat clients who demonstrate recurrent self-harm.
- Affective dysregulation (e.g., depressed mood, mood lability, anxiety, anger): Treated with low-dose antipsychotics and mood stabilizers.

Some guidelines apply to medications prescribed to clients with personality disorders for safety reasons. For example, medications that can be fatal in overdose should be avoided, as well as those that can induce physiological dependence and tolerance. Benzodiazepines can be especially toxic when combined with alcohol or opioids, and they can also cause behavioral disinhibition in patients with personality disorders.[8] Nurses should keep these safety guidelines in mind when teaching clients about their medications.

7 Nelson, K. J. (2021). Pharmacotherapy for personality disorders. *UpToDate.* https://www.uptodate.com

8 Nelson, K. J. (2021). Pharmacotherapy for personality disorders. *UpToDate.* https://www.uptodate.com

My Notes

10.4 APPLYING THE NURSING PROCESS TO PERSONALITY DISORDERS

This section will apply the nursing process to caring for a client diagnosed with borderline personality disorder who is hospitalized due to self-injurious behavior.

Assessment

Assessment includes interviewing the client, observing verbal and nonverbal behaviors, completing a mental status examination, and performing a psychosocial assessment. Review information about performing a mental status examination and psychosocial assessment in the "Application of the Nursing Process in Mental Health Care" chapter.

Assessment findings for clients hospitalized with borderline personality disorder may include the following[1]:

- Feelings of emptiness
- Self-mutilation and self-harm
- Suicidal behaviors, gestures, or threats
- Extreme mood shifts that occur in a matter of hours or days
- Impulsive behavior such as reckless driving, unsafe sex, substance use, gambling, overspending, or binge eating
- Intense feelings of abandonment
- A tendency towards anger, sarcasm, and bitterness
- Intense and unstable relationships

Review how to assess for suicide risk in the "Foundational Mental Health Concepts" chapter.

Diagnostic and Lab Work

There is no specific laboratory test that diagnoses personality disorders. Laboratory or diagnostic tests may be used to rule out other possible causes for the behaviors the client is exhibiting. For example, a thyroid stimulating hormone (TSH) test may be ordered because thyroid disorders can affect mood.

Diagnoses

Mental health disorders are diagnosed by mental health providers using the diagnostic criteria in the *DSM-5*. Personality disorder diagnoses are typically not made until late adolescence or over the age of 18 because it is important to determine if the symptoms are traits of a developmental stage or pervasive traits of a personality disorder in multiple contexts.

Nurses create individualized nursing care plans based on the client's response to their mental health disorder(s). Common nursing diagnoses related to the clusters of personality disorders include the following:

- **Cluster A:** Social Isolation, Disturbed Thought Process, Risk for Loneliness
- **Cluster B:** Risk for Suicide, Risk for Self-Directed Violence, Social Isolation, Chronic Low Self-Esteem, Ineffective Coping

---

1 Halter, M. (2022). *Varcarolis' foundations of psychiatric-mental health nursing* (9th ed.). Saunders.

My Notes

- **Cluster C:** Anxiety, Risk for Loneliness, Social Isolation

Common nursing diagnoses for clients diagnosed and hospitalized with borderline personality disorder are further described in Table 10.4.

Table 10.4 Common Nursing Diagnoses for Clients With Borderline Personality Disorder[2,3]

Nursing Diagnosis	Definition	Selected Defining Characteristics and/or Risk Factors
Risk for Suicide	Susceptible to self-inflicted, life-threatening injury.	■ Reports desire to die ■ Statements regarding killing self ■ Hopelessness ■ Social isolation
Risk for Self-Mutilation	Deliberate self-injurious behavior causing tissue damage with the intent of causing nonfatal injury to attain relief of tension.	■ Cuts or scratches on body ■ Ingestion or inhalation of harmful substances ■ Self-inflicted burns
Risk for Other-Directed Violence	Susceptible to behaviors in which an individual demonstrates they can be physically, emotionally, and/or sexually harmful to others.	■ History of childhood abuse ■ History of cruelty to animals ■ History of witnessing family violence ■ History of fire-setting
Ineffective Coping	A pattern of invalid appraisal of stressors, with cognitive and/or behavioral efforts, that fails to manage demands related to well-being.	■ Destructive behavior toward self or others ■ Ineffective coping strategies ■ Ineffective problem-solving skills
Defensive Coping	Repeated projection of falsely positive self-evaluation based on a self-protective pattern that defends against underlying perceived threats to positive self-regard.	■ Difficulty maintaining relationships ■ Hypersensitivity to criticism ■ Projection of blame ■ Projection of responsibility
Social Isolation	Aloneness experienced by the individual and perceived as imposed by others and as a negative or threatening state.	■ Hostility ■ Values incongruent with cultural norms ■ History of rejection

2 Halter, M. (2022). *Varcarolis' foundations of psychiatric-mental health nursing* (9th ed.). Saunders.

3 Ackley, B., Ladwig, G., Makic, M. B., Martinez-Kratz, M., & Zanotti, M. (2020). *Nursing diagnosis handbook: An evidence-based guide to planning care* (12th ed.). Elsevier.

My Notes

Nursing Diagnosis	Definition	Selected Defining Characteristics and/or Risk Factors
Ineffective Family Health Management r/t manipulative behavior	Aloneness experienced by the individual and perceived as imposed by others and as a negative or threatening state.	■ Impaired communication patterns ■ Disturbed thought processes ■ Delusional thinking
Risk for Spiritual Distress as manifested by poor relationships	A state of suffering related to the impaired ability to experience meaning in life through connections with self, others, the world, or a superior being.	■ Ineffective coping strategies ■ Perceived insufficient meaning in life ■ Hopelessness ■ Social alienation

Outcomes Identification

In the acute care setting, the focus for setting goals and outcomes is the reason for admission, which may include conditions such as suicidal ideation, self-injurious behavior, severe depression, or severe anxiety. Outcomes should address the acute nursing diagnoses with prioritization on safety. For example, if the client has a nursing diagnosis of *Risk for Self-Mutilation*, a SMART outcome could be, "The client will refrain from intentional self-inflicted injury during hospitalization." Read more information about setting SMART outcomes in the "Application of the Nursing Process in Mental Health Care" chapter.

Examples of other SMART outcomes for clients hospitalized with borderline personality disorder may include the following[4]:

- The client will remain safe and free of injury during their hospital stay.
- The client will seek help from staff when experiencing urges to self- mutilate during hospitalization.
- The client will identify three triggers to self-mutilation by the end of the shift.
- The client will describe two preferred healthy coping strategies by the end of the week.

Planning Interventions

Individuals diagnosed with borderline personality disorder may be suicidal, self-mutilating, impulsive, angry, manipulative, or aggressive. Nurses plan interventions according to the symptoms the client is currently exhibiting with the goal of keeping the client and others safe and free of injury. Review interventions for clients diagnosed with *Risk of Suicide* in the "Application of the Nursing Process in Mental Health Care" chapter.

Clear boundaries and limits should be set and consistently reinforced by the health care team. When behavioral problems emerge, the nurse should calmly review therapeutic goals, limits, and boundaries with the client.[5]

4 Ackley, B., Ladwig, G., Makic, M. B., Martinez-Kratz, M., & Zanotti, M. (2020). *Nursing diagnosis handbook: An evidence-based guide to planning care* (12th ed.). Elsevier.

5 Halter, M. (2022). *Varcarolis' foundations of psychiatric-mental health nursing* (9th ed.). Saunders.

Implementing Interventions

My Notes

Promoting Safety

When implementing planned interventions, the nurse must always consider safety. Develop a crisis/safety plan with the client that includes components such as these:

- Identifying thoughts or behaviors that increase the risk of harming self or others
- Identifying people, events, or situations that trigger those thoughts or behaviors
- Implementing coping strategies
- Reaching out to other coping resources

For example, if a client performs superficial self-injurious behavior, the nurse should act based on agency policy while remaining neutral and dressing the client's self-inflicted wounds in a matter-of-fact manner. The client may be asked to write down the sequence of events leading up to the injuries, as well as the consequences, before staff will discuss the event. This cognitive exercise encourages the client to think independently about their triggers and behaviors and facilitates discussion about alternative actions.[6]

Review information regarding developing a safety plan in the "Establishing Safety" section of the "Foundational Mental Health Concepts" chapter.

De-Escalating

The nurse should implement de-escalation strategies if the client exhibits early signs of increasing levels of anxiety or agitation. Strategies include the following:

- Speaking in a calm voice
- Avoiding overreacting
- Implementing active listening
- Expressing support and concern
- Avoiding continuous eye contact
- Asking how you can help
- Reducing stimuli
- Moving slowly
- Remaining patient and not rushing them
- Offering options instead of trying to take control
- Avoiding touching the client without permission
- Verbalizing actions before initiating them
- Providing space so the client doesn't feel trapped
- Avoiding arguing and judgmental comments

---

6 Halter, M. (2022). *Varcarolis' foundations of psychiatric-mental health nursing* (9th ed.). Saunders.

My Notes

- Setting limits early and enforcing them consistently across team members
- Addressing manipulative behaviors therapeutically

If the client continues to escalate, measures must be taken to keep the client and others safe. Review signs of crisis and crisis interventions in the "Stress, Coping, and Crisis Intervention" chapter. If interventions are not effective in de-escalating a client at risk to themselves or others, seclusion or restraints may be required. Review using seclusion and restraints in the "Psychosis and Schizophrenia" chapter.

Coping Strategies

Teaching self-care and coping strategies is helpful for people diagnosed with personality disorders and their loved ones.[7] Read about stress management and coping strategies in the "Stress, Coping, and Crisis Intervention" chapter.

For clients seeking immediate relief from intense symptoms such as panic or depersonalization, nurses can teach how to stimulate the parasympathetic nervous system. Stimulation of the vagal nerve can result in an immediate, direct relief of intense emotions. This can be accomplished by doing the following[8]:

- Applying ice or ice-cold water to the face.
- Performing paced-breathing techniques in which the exhalation phase is at least two to four counts longer than the inhalation phase. For example, advise the client to inhale while counting to four and then exhale while counting to eight.

Collaborative Interventions

Psychotherapy

First-line treatment for personality disorders is psychotherapy. Examples of psychotherapy used with clients with personality disorders are cognitive behavioral therapy, dialectical behavioral therapy, interpersonal therapy, mentalization-based therapy, psychodynamic psychotherapy, and psychoeducation. Read more about these treatments in the "Treatment for Personality Disorders" section of this chapter.

Pharmacotherapy

There are no specific medications approved to treat personality disorders. However, clients may be treated for symptoms associated with personality disorders that cause them significant impairment and distress. Read more information about common medications used to treat symptoms of personality disorders in the "Treatment for Personality Disorders" section of this chapter.

Evaluation

Refer to the SMART outcomes established for each individual client to evaluate the effectiveness of the planned interventions. Modification of the established nursing care plan may be required based on the effectiveness of the interventions.

---

7 American Psychiatric Association. (n.d.). *What are personality disorders?* https://www.psychiatry.org/patients-families/personality-disorders/what-are-personality-disorders

8 Nelson, K. J. (2021). Pharmacotherapy for personality disorders. *UpToDate.* https://www.uptodate.com

My Notes

10.5 SPOTLIGHT APPLICATION

Kay is a 27-year-old female who is admitted to the mental health unit for feelings of depression and suicidal ideations. She has a history of cutting her legs and arms since she was a teenager. She started psychiatric treatment at age 16 and has been admitted to the psychiatric hospital three times due to overdoses. She admits to a history of promiscuous behavior and occasional marijuana use. She is unmarried but reports having several relationships with male partners. However, she shares that the relationships "never worked out" because the partners didn't pay enough attention to her or text her as frequently as she expected, which made her angry. She describes feelings she experienced in relationships where one day she felt as if her partner was the "best thing ever," but the next day she "can't stand him." She admits to abusive behaviors toward her partners when she was angry, but states that afterwards she experiences anxiety fearing the loss of the relationship. She acknowledges having trouble getting along with others. She has very few close friends and refers to previous friends as "losers." She is unemployed with a history of several jobs from which she was terminated because of problems with anger control. There is evidence of scarring and recent cuts on bilateral lower arms. She related these injuries to self-cutting, which she reports "makes me feel better." She reports attending dialectical behavior therapy (DBT) in the past but hasn't attended therapy for over a year. She feels therapy helped her to learn how to feel more "in control of her extreme feelings."

Critical Thinking Questions

1. List the symptoms Kay is experiencing that supports the diagnosis of borderline personality disorder (BPD).
    - *Symptoms of BPD include anger, anxiety, impulsiveness, difficulty controlling emotions, self-injury, suicidal, intense/stormy relationships, and risky behaviors.*
2. Identify possible risk factors contributing to BPD.
    - *Possible risk factors include environmental factors that may contribute to BPD, including neglect, abuse, and genetics.*
3. Discuss two types of psychotherapy that may be prescribed for clients diagnosed with BPD.
    - *Cognitive behavioral therapy, dialectical behavioral therapy, interpersonal therapy, mentalization-based therapy, and psychodynamic therapy are types of psychotherapy that may be prescribed for clients.*
4. List at least three nursing interventions that should be included in this client's care plan.
    - *Explain policies, expectations, rules, and consequences upon admission.*
    - *Search the client's belongings and remove anything that could be used to inflict harm to self or others.*
    - *Implement suicide precautions based on a suicide risk screening tool.*
    - *Set and document clear boundaries and limits and share them with team members.*
    - *Encourage consistent implementation of limits by all team members; do not allow bargaining.*
    - *Call out manipulative behavior when it occurs.*
    - *If an episode of cutting occurs during hospitalization, remain neutral and dress the client's self-inflicted wounds in a matter-of-fact manner. Ask the client to write down the sequence of events leading up to the injuries before discussing the event. Encourage the client to think independently about her triggers and behaviors and facilitate discussion about alternative actions.*

My Notes

10.6 LEARNING ACTIVITIES

Learning Activities

(Answers to "Learning Activities" can be found in the "Answer Key" at the end of the book. Answers to the interactive activities are provided as immediate feedback.)

Please respond to the following questions.

1. Compare the difference between obsessive-compulsive personality disorder and the anxiety disorder of obsessive-compulsive disorder (OCD).
2. Name that personality disorder. Read each scenario and choose a personality disorder associated with the traits included in the scenario:
   a) Darla enters the breakroom at her job. She is dressed provocatively with excessive jewelry. She makes eye contact with everyone. She sits down and quickly interjects herself into the conversation. When one of her coworkers shares pictures of her new puppy, she pulls out her cell phone to show pictures of herself and tells the group how she had a romantic weekend with her handsome, rich boyfriend.
   b) Bob has been summoned to his supervisor's office. Despite his adequate job performance, he thinks to himself, "I knew it! She's out to get me and I am getting fired! She and others walk by my desk several times a day just to check up on me and see what I am doing. And that new employee has been trying to strike conversations with me, but I am not falling for that. I am sure he just wants something from me."
   c) Debbie is distraught after her boyfriend called her and told her their relationship was over. She began yelling on the phone, "I love you and can't live without you." The ex-boyfriend ends the phone call. Debbie begins calling him over and over; however, he doesn't answer the phone. She then leaves a message stating, "I hate you. I never want to see you again." Overcome with emotion, she begins to cut her wrist with a bobby pin.
   d) George is a loner and lives alone with his five cats. He has family members who live in the area, but he hasn't seen them in years, and that is okay with him. He has never been married or been in an intimate relationship. He does not have any close friends. He enjoys his job as a night security guard because there is little requirement for social interaction.
   e) Jordan is always trying to please others. She has trouble starting or completing projects because of a lack of self-confidence. She requires much reassurance and advice when making ordinary decisions. She allows her boyfriend to tell her what to wear, what kind of job to look for, and with whom to associate. She is afraid of him leaving her, so she is very careful not to get him mad at her.
   f) Roger has been arrested several times for domestic abuse and driving while intoxicated. He shows no remorse for any of his actions or the injuries he has caused others. He lies, breaks laws, and has no regard for the feelings of others. As a teenager, he was always in trouble and truant from school. He was incarcerated in the past but found it easy to manipulate the guards into breaking the rules for him.

My Notes

g) Deanna has very few friends. She is shy and avoids social interaction, even at work. She is worried that if she did get to know people better, she might say or do something embarrassing, and they might criticize or reject her. During her performance evaluation with her supervisor, she left the office crying because of minor constructive feedback she received. To prevent these painful experiences, she believes it is best to keep to herself.

h) Billy tells everyone how important he is to his company. He believes there is no way the company would be successful without him. During work meetings, he monopolizes the conversation and strives to be the center of attention. He often asks others, "Don't you think I did a great job with that?" Although he does not have any close relationships with coworkers, he does collaborate with a few of them because they are able to help him accomplish his goals.

i) Bobbi works as an administrative assistant. She is very organized and spends a lot of time making lists, scheduling, and reviewing details. Although she has several friends, she often passes on the opportunity to get together because she spends most of her time devoted to work. Sometimes, despite her efforts, she has difficulty finishing a project because she feels the need to check things "one more time."

j) Paul is loner and lacks close friends outside of his immediate family. Most view him as being very unusual, including his odd way of dressing. He wears ill-fitting and bizarre clothing combinations, such as winter boots with shorts. He is very superstitious and believes he is psychic. He believes prime numbers are unlucky and avoids objects (e.g., building floors and house numbers) that are prime numbers.

3. Check your medication knowledge. Select which medications are commonly used to treat severe symptoms of personality disorders.
   a) What medications are used to treat hallucinations and paranoia?
   b) What medications are used to treat depressed mood, mood lability, anger, and anxiety?
   c) What medications are used to treat self-injurious behavior?
4. Compare normal adolescent development with trait similarities of personality disorders.

Interactive Activities

An interactive H5P element has been excluded from this version of the text. You can view it online here: https://wtcs.pressbooks.pub/nursingmhcc/?p=413#h5p-35

An interactive H5P element has been excluded from this version of the text. You can view it online here: https://wtcs.pressbooks.pub/nursingmhcc/?p=413#h5p-36

An interactive H5P element has been excluded from this version of the text. You can view it online here: https://wtcs.pressbooks.pub/nursingmhcc/?p=413#h5p-37

My Notes

X GLOSSARY

Body illusion: A perception that one's own body is significantly different from its actual configuration. For example, a person lying in bed may feel as if they are levitating.

Dissociative symptoms: The experience of detachment or feeling as if one is outside one's body with loss of memory.

Entitlement: Unreasonable expectations of especially favorable treatment.

Ideas of reference: False beliefs that coincidental events relate to oneself. For example, a person shopping in a store sees two strangers laughing and believes they are laughing at them, when in reality the other two people do not even notice them.

Magical thinking: The idea that one can influence the outcome of specific events by doing something that has no bearing on the circumstances. For example, a person watching a baseball game exhibits magical thinking when believing that holding the remote control in a certain position caused their favorite player to hit a home run.

Personality: A relatively stable pattern of thinking, feeling, and behaving that evolves over a person's lifetime and is unique to each individual. It is influenced by one's experiences, environment (surroundings and life situations), and inherited characteristics.

Personality disorder: An enduring pattern of inner experience and behavior that deviates significantly from the expectations of one's culture. Its onset can be traced back to adolescence or early adulthood and is present in a variety of contexts. This pattern of behavior is manifested in two or more of the following areas: cognition/perceptions, affect, interpersonal functioning, and impulse control.

Personality traits: Characteristics, whether considered good or bad, that make up one's personality.

Splitting: A pattern of unstable and intense personal relationships characterized by alternating between extremes of idealization and devaluation.

Chapter 11

Psychosis and Schizophrenia

11.1 INTRODUCTION

My Notes

Learning Objectives

- Compare and contrast delirium and schizophrenia
- Apply the nursing process to clients with psychosis
- Describe nursing assessments related to psychosis, delirium, and schizophrenia
- Identify common nursing problems/diagnoses related to psychosis
- Establish a safe environment
- Apply evidence-based practice when planning and implementing nursing care
- Describe common treatments for psychosis and schizophrenia
- Identify appropriate referrals to community resources
- Evaluate the effectiveness of interventions
- Provide patient education to clients and their family members

Have you ever cared for a client who was confused, disoriented, had a change in mental status, or was experiencing delirium? These are considered "altered thought processes." There are several potential medical causes of altered thought processes referred to as delirium, such as a urinary tract infection in an elderly patient, hyperglycemia, or alcohol intoxication. There are also mental health disorders that can cause altered thought processes, such as schizophrenia. This chapter will discuss psychosis, delirium, and schizophrenia and explain how to care for clients experiencing hallucinations, delusions, and other symptoms of altered thought processes.

My Notes

11.2 PSYCHOSIS AND DELIRIUM

Psychosis

Approximately 3 percent of the people in the United States experience psychosis at some point in their lives. About 100,000 adolescents and young adults in the US experience their first episode of psychosis each year.[1]

The term **psychosis** describes conditions where there is a loss of contact with reality. When a person experiences psychosis, their thoughts and perceptions are disturbed, and the individual has difficulty understanding what is real and what is not real. Symptoms of psychosis include **delusions** and **hallucinations**, where the client is seeing, hearing, or experiencing other sensations and experiences that aren't real. See Figure 11.1.[2] for artwork titled *Hallucinations*. Other symptoms of psychosis include incoherent or nonsensical speech and behavior that is inappropriate for the situation. A person experiencing a psychotic episode may also experience depression, anxiety, sleep problems, social withdrawal, lack of motivation, and overall difficulty functioning. When someone experiences this condition, it is referred to as a psychotic episode.[3]

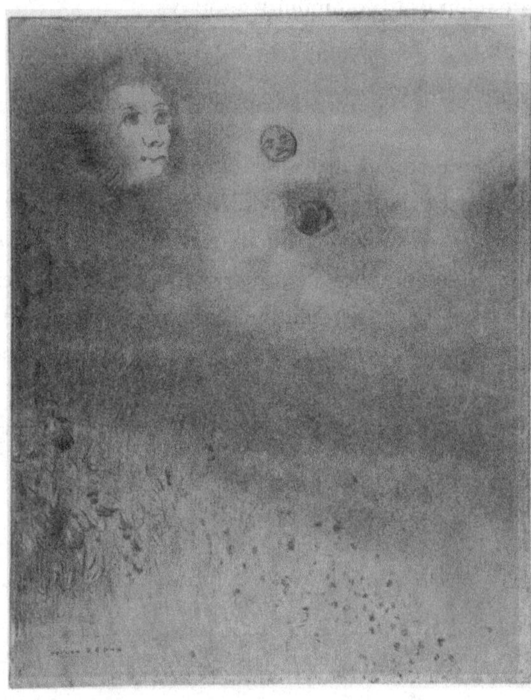

Figure 11.1 Hallucinations

Psychosis can be a symptom of various mental illnesses, such as schizophrenia, bipolar disorder, severe depression, or severe anxiety, but there are also other potential causes. Sleep deprivation, medical conditions such as

1 National Institute of Mental Health. (n.d.). *What is psychosis?* U.S. Department of Health and Human Services. https://www.nimh.nih.gov/health/topics/schizophrenia/raise/what-is-psychosis

2 "Hallucinations_MET_DP808068.jpg" by Odilon Redon is in the Public Domain

3 National Institute of Mental Health. (n.d.). *What is psychosis?* U.S. Department of Health and Human Services. https://www.nimh.nih.gov/health/topics/schizophrenia/raise/what-is-psychosis

hyperglycemia and hyperthyroidism, side effects of some prescription medications, and use of alcohol or other drugs can also cause psychotic symptoms.[4]

My Notes

Early Signs of Psychosis

Typically, a person will show changes in their behavior before psychosis develops. Behavioral warning signs for psychosis include the following[5]:

- Drop in grades or worsening job performance
- New trouble thinking clearly or concentrating
- Suspiciousness; paranoid ideas or uneasiness with others
- Withdrawing socially; spending a lot more time alone than usual
- Unusual, bizarre new ideas
- Strange feelings or having no feelings at all
- Decline in self-care or personal hygiene
- Difficulty telling reality from fantasy
- Confused speech or trouble communicating

Symptoms of a Psychotic Episode

See the following box for signs and symptoms of a psychotic episode according to the *Diagnostic and Statistical Manual of Mental Disorders (DSM–5)* by the American Psychiatric Association.

DSM-5 Symptoms of a Brief Psychotic Episode[6]

- Delusions
- Hallucinations
- Disorganized speech (e.g., frequent derailment or incoherence)
- Grossly disorganized or catatonic behavior (i.e., a pronounced increase or decrease in the rate and amount of movement; purposeless excessive movement)

A brief psychotic episode is defined by a psychotic event lasting at least one day but less than one month, with an eventual return to previous level of functioning. It does not include a culturally sanctioned response, such as a

4 National Institute of Mental Health. (n.d.). *What is psychosis?* U.S. Department of Health and Human Services. https://www.nimh.nih.gov/health/topics/schizophrenia/raise/what-is-psychosis

5 National Institute of Mental Health. (n.d.). *What is psychosis?* U.S. Department of Health and Human Services. https://www.nimh.nih.gov/health/topics/schizophrenia/raise/what-is-psychosis

6 American Psychiatric Association. (2013). *Desk reference to the diagnostic criteria from DSM-5.*

My Notes

person's response to the death of a loved one. The disturbance is not better explained by a major depressive disorder or bipolar disorder with psychotic features, another psychotic disorder, or the physiological effects of a substance or a medical condition. The mental health provider may specify if the symptoms are in response to significant stressors (i.e., significant events to anyone experiencing similar circumstances in the individual's culture) or as a peripartum onset (i.e., during pregnancy or within four weeks of delivery).[7]

Review information about delusions, hallucinations, and disorganized speech in the "Application of the Nursing Process in Mental Health Care" chapter.

Treatment of Psychosis

Treatment for psychosis is based on its cause. For example, if psychosis is caused by a medical condition, side effects of medication, or withdrawal from a substance, it will resolve as these conditions are treated. If psychosis is a symptom of mental illness, treatment typically includes a combination of antipsychotic medicines and psychological therapies. Read more about the treatment of psychosis associated with schizophrenia in the "Schizophrenia" section of this chapter.

Delirium

Psychosis caused by medical issues is often referred to as delirium. **Delirium** is a mental state in which the client becomes temporarily confused, disoriented, and not able to think or remember clearly. It usually starts suddenly and can indicate the onset of a life-threatening medical condition. Delirium resolves as the underlying condition is effectively treated. There are many common causes of delirium, including the following[8,9]:

- Dehydration and electrolyte imbalances
- Dementia
- Hospitalization, especially in intensive care
- Intoxication or withdrawal from alcohol or drugs
- Kidney or liver failure
- Medications, such as sedatives, opioids, anesthesia, antihistamines, anticholinergics, antidepressants, antipsychotics, or anticonvulsants
- Metabolic disorders, such as diabetic ketoacidosis (DKA)
- Serious infections, such as urinary tract infections, pneumonia, and influenza
- Severe pain
- Sleep deprivation

7 American Psychiatric Association. (2013). *Desk reference to the diagnostic criteria from DSM-5.*

8 MedlinePlus [Internet]. Bethesda (MD): National Library of Medicine (US); [updated 2021, Dec 2]. *Delirium*; [reviewed 2016, May 13; cited 2021, Dec 27]. https://medlineplus.gov/delirium.html

9 American Delirium Society. (n.d.). *About delirium.* https://americandeliriumsociety.org/

The symptoms of delirium usually start suddenly, over a few hours or a few days, and they often come and go. The most common symptoms are as follows[10]:

- Changes in alertness (usually more alert in the morning, less at night)
- Changing levels of consciousness
- Confusion
- Disorganized thinking or talking in a way that doesn't make sense
- Disrupted sleep patterns or sleepiness
- Emotional changes: anger, agitation, depression, irritability, or overexcitement
- Hallucinations and delusions
- Incontinence
- Memory problems, especially with short-term memory
- Trouble concentrating

The symptoms of delirium can often be managed with the following interventions[11]:

- Making sure the room is quiet and well-lit
- Having clocks and calendars within view
- Inviting family members to spend time in the room
- Ensuring hearing aids and glasses are worn
- Allowing for undisrupted sleep when possible
- Getting patients up and out of bed when possible
- Controlling pain with pain relievers (unless the pain medication is causing the psychosis)
- Administering prescribed medications to distressed clients at risk to themselves or to others to calm and settle them, such as haloperidol (However, administer medications with caution because oversedation can worsen delirium.)
- Avoiding the use of restraints

View the Confusion Assessment Method (CAM) PDF commonly used to detect delirium.

View a video: Managing Delirium Out of Hours.[12]

---

10 MedlinePlus [Internet]. Bethesda (MD): National Library of Medicine (US); [updated 2021, Dec 2]. *Delirium*; [reviewed 2016, May 13; cited 2021, Dec 27]. https://medlineplus.gov/delirium.html

11 MedlinePlus [Internet]. Bethesda (MD): National Library of Medicine (US); [updated 2021, Dec 2]. *Delirium*; [reviewed 2016, May 13; cited 2021, Dec 27]. https://medlineplus.gov/delirium.html

12 Association for Elderly Medicine Education. (2014, February 6). *Managing delirium out of hours* [Video]. YouTube. All rights reserved. https://youtu.be/1iKe-6lc5b0

My Notes

11.3 SCHIZOPHRENIA

There is a spectrum of psychotic disorders, and schizophrenia is one of the disorders on the spectrum. **Schizophrenia** is a serious mental illness that affects how a person thinks, feels, and behaves. It also affects the person's ability to recognize their symptoms as problematic, referred to as a "lack of insight." Continuous signs of the disturbance must be present for at least six months in order for schizophrenia to be diagnosed, and potential medical conditions that could be causing delirium must be ruled out.[1,2]

Schizophrenia is typically diagnosed in the late teen years to the early thirties and tends to emerge earlier in males than females. A diagnosis of schizophrenia often follows the first episode of psychosis when individuals first display symptoms of schizophrenia. Gradual changes in thinking, mood, and social functioning often begin before the first episode of psychosis, usually starting in mid-adolescence. (See "Early Signs of Psychosis" in the previous section.) Schizophrenia can occur in younger children, but it is rare for it to occur before late adolescence.[3]

Symptoms of Schizophrenia

Symptoms of schizophrenia are classified by three categories: positive, negative, and cognitive.[4]

- **Positive symptoms:** Positive symptoms include hallucinations, delusions, thought disorders, disorganized speech, and alterations in behaviors. Read more about delusions and hallucinations in the "Thoughts and Perceptions" subsection of the "Assessment" section of the "Application of the Nursing Process in Mental Health Care" chapter. The most common types of delusions experienced by individuals with schizophrenia are paranoia, persecutory, grandiose, or religious ideas. For example, an individual with persecutory delusions may feel the nursing staff is trying to poison them when they administer medications. People with psychotic symptoms lose a shared sense of reality and experience the world in a distorted way.[5]
- **Negative symptoms:** Negative symptoms refer to loss of motivation, disinterest or lack of enjoyment in daily activities, social withdrawal, difficulty showing emotions, and difficulty functioning normally. Individuals typically experience the following negative symptoms[6]:
  - Reduced motivation and difficulty planning, beginning, and sustaining activities (i.e., avolition)
  - Diminished feelings of pleasure in everyday life (i.e., anhedonia)
  - Flat affect (i.e., reduced expression of emotions via facial expression or voice tone)

---

1 National Institute of Mental Health. (2020, May). *Schizophrenia.* U.S. Department of Health and Human Services. https://www.nimh.nih.gov/health/topics/schizophrenia

2 American Psychiatric Association. (2013). *Desk reference to the diagnostic criteria from DSM-5.*

3 National Institute of Mental Health. (2020, May). *Schizophrenia.* U.S. Department of Health and Human Services. https://www.nimh.nih.gov/health/topics/schizophrenia

4 National Institute of Mental Health. (2020, May). *Schizophrenia.* U.S. Department of Health and Human Services. https://www.nimh.nih.gov/health/topics/schizophrenia

5 National Institute of Mental Health. (2020, May). *Schizophrenia.* U.S. Department of Health and Human Services. https://www.nimh.nih.gov/health/topics/schizophrenia

6 National Institute of Mental Health. (2020, May). *Schizophrenia.* U.S. Department of Health and Human Services. https://www.nimh.nih.gov/health/topics/schizophrenia

My Notes

- Reduced speaking

- **Cognitive symptoms:** Cognitive symptoms refer to problems in attention, concentration, and memory. For some individuals, the cognitive symptoms of schizophrenia are subtle, but for others, they are more prominent and interfere with activities like following conversations, learning new things, or remembering appointments. Individuals typically experience symptoms such as these[7]:
  - Difficulty processing information to make decisions
  - Problems using information immediately after learning it
  - Trouble focusing or paying attention

See the following box for signs and symptoms for the diagnosis of schizophrenia according to the *DSM-5*.

DSM-5: Symptoms of Schizophrenia[8]

Schizophrenia is diagnosed when two (or more) of the following characteristics are present for a significant portion of time during a one-month period (or less if successfully treated). At least one symptom is delusions, hallucinations, or disorganized speech:

- Delusions
- Hallucinations
- Disorganized speech (i.e., frequent derailment or incoherence)
- Grossly disorganized or catatonic behavior. (Catatonia is a state of unresponsiveness.)
- Negative symptoms (i.e., diminished emotional expression or avolition.) Avolition refers to reduced motivation or goal-directed behavior.

Additionally, for a significant portion of time, the client's level of functioning in one or more areas, such as work, interpersonal relations, or self-care, is significantly below their prior level of functioning. Continuous signs of schizophrenia persist for at least six months (or less if it is successfully treated). Depressive or bipolar disorders with psychotic features must have been previously ruled out, and the disturbance is not attributable to the physiological effects of a substance or other medical condition. The provider may specify if this is the first episode or multiple episodes and if it is an acute episode, in partial remission, or in full remission.[9]

7 National Institute of Mental Health. (2020, May). *Schizophrenia.* U.S. Department of Health and Human Services. https://www.nimh.nih.gov/health/topics/schizophrenia

8 American Psychiatric Association. (2013). *Desk reference to the diagnostic criteria from DSM-5.*

9 American Psychiatric Association. (2013). *Desk reference to the diagnostic criteria from DSM-5.*

My Notes

See Figure 11.2[10] for an artwork depiction of the thought disorders associated with schizophrenia.

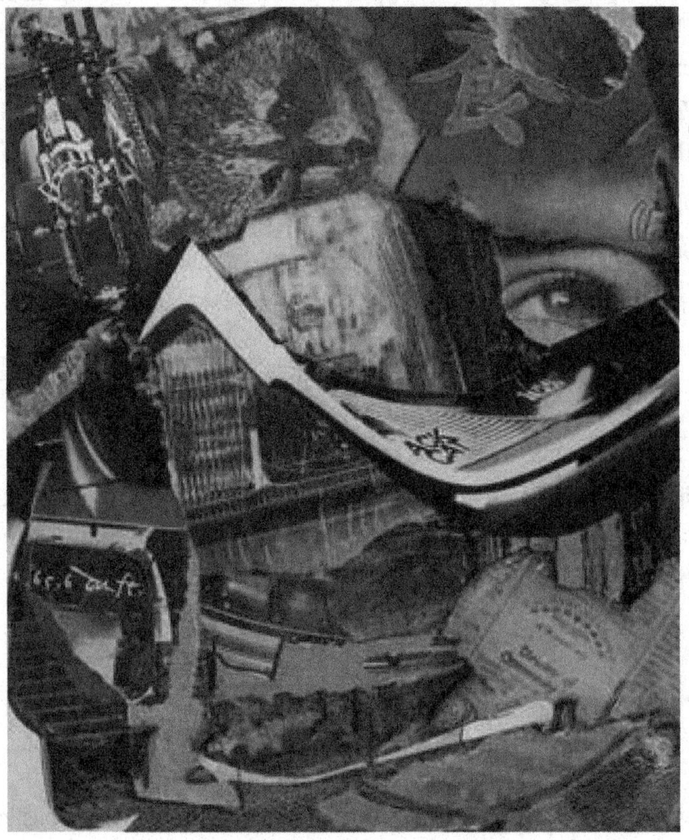

Figure 11.2 Schizophrenia

Risk Factors for Schizophrenia

It is believed that several factors contribute to the risk of developing schizophrenia, including genetics, environment, and brain structure and function.[11]

Genetics

Schizophrenia tends to run in families. Genetic studies strongly suggest that many different genes increase the risk of developing schizophrenia, but that no single gene causes the disorder by itself. It is not yet possible to use genetic information to predict who will develop schizophrenia.[12] A systematic review found that cannabis

10 "Schizophrenia.png" by William A. Ursprung is in the Public Domain

11 National Institute of Mental Health. (2020, May). *Schizophrenia.* U.S. Department of Health and Human Services. https://www.nimh.nih.gov/health/topics/schizophrenia

12 National Institute of Mental Health. (2020, May). *Schizophrenia.* U.S. Department of Health and Human Services. https://www.nimh.nih.gov/health/topics/schizophrenia

(marijuana) worsens symptoms of psychosis in genetically predisposed individuals and causes more relapses and hospitalizations.[13]

My Notes

Environment

Scientists think that interactions between genetic risk and aspects of an individual's environment play a role in the development of schizophrenia. Environmental factors that may be involved include adverse childhood experiences (ACE) or exposure to viruses or nutritional problems before birth.[14]

Brain Structure and Function

Scientists think that differences in brain structure, function, and interactions among neurotransmitters may contribute to the development of schizophrenia. For example, differences in the volumes of specific components of the brain, the manner in which regions of the brain are connected and work together, and neurotransmitters, such as dopamine, are found in people with schizophrenia. Differences in brain connections and brain circuits seen in people with schizophrenia may begin developing before birth. Changes to the brain that occur during puberty may trigger psychotic episodes in people who are already vulnerable due to genetics, environmental exposures, or the types of brain differences mentioned previously.[15]

View a video: What is Psychosis?[16]

Treatment

Early treatment of psychosis increases the chance of a successful remission.[17] Treatments focus on managing symptoms and solving problems related to day-to-day functioning and include antipsychotic medications, psychosocial treatments, family education and support, coordinated specialty care, and assertive community treatment.[18]

Antipsychotic Medications

Antipsychotic medications reduce the intensity and frequency of psychotic symptoms by inhibiting dopamine receptors. Certain symptoms of psychosis, such as feeling agitated and having hallucinations, resolve within days

13 Patel, S., Khan, M.S., & Hamid, P. (2020). The association between cannabis use and schizophrenia: Causative or curative? A systematic review, *Cureus, 12*(7), e9309. https://doi.org/10.7759/cureus.9309

14 National Institute of Mental Health. (2020, May). *Schizophrenia.* U.S. Department of Health and Human Services. https://www.nimh.nih.gov/health/topics/schizophrenia

15 National Institute of Mental Health. (2020, May). *Schizophrenia.* U.S. Department of Health and Human Services. https://www.nimh.nih.gov/health/topics/schizophrenia

16 Living Well with Schizophrenia. (2019, July 17). *What is psychosis?* [Video]. YouTube. All rights reserved. https://youtu.be/Pgsujx2UQl8

17 National Institute of Mental Health. (2020, May). *Schizophrenia.* U.S. Department of Health and Human Services. https://www.nimh.nih.gov/health/topics/schizophrenia

18 National Institute of Mental Health. (2020, May). *Schizophrenia.* U.S. Department of Health and Human Services. https://www.nimh.nih.gov/health/topics/schizophrenia

My Notes

of starting an antipsychotic medication. Symptoms like delusions usually resolve within a few weeks, but the full effects of the medication may not be seen for up to six weeks.[19]

Antipsychotic medicines are also used to treat other mental health disorders such as attention deficit hyperactivity disorder (ADHD), severe depression, eating disorders, post-traumatic stress disorder (PTSD), obsessive-compulsive disorder (OCD), and generalized anxiety disorder.[20]

First-generation antipsychotics (also called "typical antipsychotics") treat positive symptoms of schizophrenia and have several potential adverse effects due to their tight binding to dopamine receptors. Medication is prescribed based on the client's ability to tolerate the adverse effects. **Second-generation antipsychotics** (also referred to as "atypical antipsychotics") treat both positive and negative symptoms of schizophrenia. They have fewer adverse effects because they block selective dopamine D2 receptors, as well as serotonin, so they are generally better tolerated than first-generation antipsychotics. Clients respond differently to antipsychotic medications, so it may take several trials of different medications to find the one that works best for their symptoms.[21]

See Table 11.3 for a list of common antipsychotic medications. They are usually taken daily in pill or liquid form. Some antipsychotic medications can also be administered as injections twice a month, monthly, every three months, or every six months, which can be more convenient and improve medication adherence.

Review information on neuroreceptors affected by antipsychotic medications in the "Antipsychotics" section of the "Psychotropic Medications" chapter.

19 National Institute of Mental Health. (2016, October). *Mental health medications.* U.S. Department of Health and Human Services. https://www.nimh.nih.gov/health/topics/mental-health-medications#part_2362

20 National Institute of Mental Health. (2016, October). *Mental health medications.* U.S. Department of Health and Human Services. https://www.nimh.nih.gov/health/topics/mental-health-medications#part_2362

21 National Institute of Mental Health. (2016, October). *Mental health medications.* U.S. Department of Health and Human Services. https://www.nimh.nih.gov/health/topics/mental-health-medications#part_2362

My Notes

Table 11.3 Common Antipsychotic Medications[22,23,24]

Medication Class	Mechanism of Action	Adverse Effects
First-Generation (Typical) Examples: Chlorpromazine Haloperidol Perphenazine Fluphenazine	Postsynaptic blockade of dopamine receptors in the brain	■ Extrapyramidal side effects (EPS) ■ Tardive dyskinesia (TD) ■ Neuroleptic Malignant Syndrome (NMS)
Second-Generation (Atypical) Examples: Risperidone Olanzapine Quetiapine Ziprasidone Aripiprazole Paliperidone Lurasidone Clozapine	Postsynaptic blockade of dopamine receptors in the brain	■ Metabolic syndrome ■ Akathisia ■ Decreased risk for EPS, TD, and NMS

Clozapine

Patients with treatment-resistant schizophrenia may be prescribed clozapine, a specific type of atypical antipsychotic medication. However, people treated with clozapine must undergo routine blood testing to detect a potentially dangerous side effect called **agranulocytosis** (extremely low white blood cell count). Clozapine also has strong anticholinergic, sedative, cardiac, and hypotensive properties and frequent drug-drug interactions.[25]

Black Box Warning

A Black Box Warning states that elderly clients with dementia-related psychosis treated with antipsychotic drugs are at an increased risk of death.[26]

---

22 National Institute of Mental Health. (2016, October). *Mental health medications.* U.S. Department of Health and Human Services. https://www.nimh.nih.gov/health/topics/mental-health-medications#part_2362

23 This work is a derivative of *StatPearls* by Vasan and Padhy and is licensed under CC BY 4.0

24 Jibson, M. D. (2021). Second-generation antipsychotic medications: Pharmacology, administration, and side effects. *UpToDate.* Retrieved January 14, 2022, from www.uptodate.com

25 Jibson, M. D. (2021). Second-generation antipsychotic medications: Pharmacology, administration, and side effects. *UpToDate.* Retrieved January 14, 2022, from www.uptodate.com

26 This work is a derivative of *DailyMed* by U.S. National Library of Medicine and is available in the Public Domain

My Notes

Adverse Effects

Common side effects of both first- and second-generation antipsychotics include the following[27]:

- Anticholinergic symptoms: dry mouth, constipation, blurred vision, or urinary retention[28]
- Drowsiness
- Dizziness
- Restlessness
- Weight gain
- Nausea or vomiting
- Low blood pressure

First-generation antipsychotics, also known as neuroleptics or typical antipsychotics, have significant potential to cause extrapyramidal side effects and tardive dyskinesia due to their tight binding to dopamine receptors. The risk for developing these movement disorders is the primary difference between first-generation antipsychotics and second-generation antipsychotics (also known as atypical antipsychotics). In other respects, the two classes of medication have similar side effects and mechanisms of action.[29]

Extrapyramidal (EPS) side effects refer to **akathisia** (psychomotor restlessness), rigidity, **bradykinesia** (slowed movement), tremor, and **dystonia** (involuntary contractions of muscles of the extremities, face, neck, abdomen, pelvis, or larynx in either sustained or intermittent patterns that lead to abnormal movements or postures). See Figure 11.3[30] for an image of dystonia. Anticholinergic side effects (e.g., dry mouth, constipation, and urinary retention) are common, and histamine blockage causes sedation, with chlorpromazine being the most sedating.[31]

Acute dystonic reactions affecting the larynx can be a medical emergency requiring intubation and mechanical ventilation. EPS symptoms usually resolve dramatically within 10 to 30 minutes of administration of parenteral anticholinergics such as diphenhydramine and benztropine.[32]

Tardive dyskinesia (TD) is a syndrome of movement disorders that can occur in clients taking first-generation antipsychotics. Hallmark symptoms are smacking and puckering lips, eye blinking, grimacing, and twitching. TD persists for at least one month and can last up to several years despite discontinuation of the medications. Primary treatment of TD includes discontinuation of first-generation antipsychotics and may include the addition of another medication. Second-generation VMAT2 inhibitors such as deutetrabenazine and valbenazine are

---

27 National Institute of Mental Health. (2016, October). *Mental health medications.* U.S. Department of Health and Human Services. https://www.nimh.nih.gov/health/topics/mental-health-medications#part_2362

28 Jibson, M. D. (2021). Second-generation antipsychotic medications: Pharmacology, administration, and side effects. *UpToDate.* Retrieved January 14, 2022, from www.uptodate.com

29 Jibson, M. D. (2021). Second-generation antipsychotic medications: Pharmacology, administration, and side effects. *UpToDate.* Retrieved January 14, 2022, from www.uptodate.com

30 "Dystonia2010.JPG" by James Heilman, MD is licensed under CC BY-SA 3.0

31 This work is a derivative of *StatPearls* by Chokhawala and Stevens and is licensed under CC BY 4.0

32 This work is a derivative of *StatPearls* by Lewis and O'Day and is licensed under CC BY 4.0

considered first-line treatment for TD. Clonazepam and ginkgo biloba have also shown good effectiveness for improving symptoms of TD.[33,34]

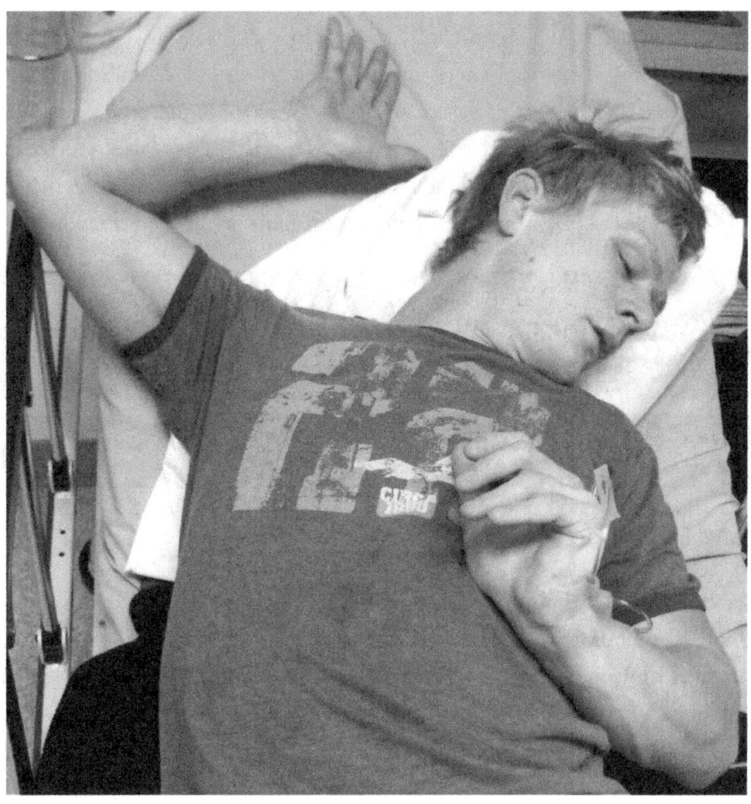

Figure 11.3 Dystonia

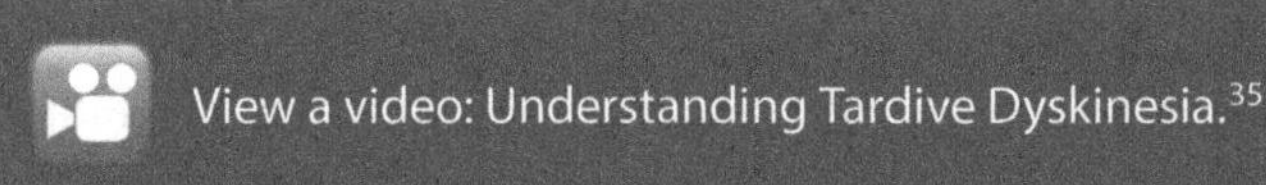

View a video: Understanding Tardive Dyskinesia.[35]

Neuroleptic malignant syndrome (NMS) is a rare but fatal adverse effect that can occur at any time during treatment with antipsychotics. It typically develops over a period of days to weeks and resolves in approximately nine days with treatment.[36] Signs include increased temperature, severe muscular rigidity, confusion, agitation, hyperreflexia, elevation in white blood cell count, elevated creatinine phosphokinase, elevated liver enzymes,

---

33 This work is a derivative of *StatPearls* by Vasan and Padhy and is licensed under CC BY 4.0

34 Pontone, G. (2020, January 3). Treating tardive dyskinesia: A clinical conundrum and new approaches. *Drug Induced Disorders: The Clinical Essentials.* Psychopharmacology Institute. https://psychopharmacologyinstitute.com/section/treating-tardive-dyskinesia-a-clinical-conundrum-and-new-approaches-2557-4810#:~:text=Clonazepam%20probably%20improves%20tardiv

35 Alliance for Patient Access. (2019, October 14). *Understanding tardive dyskinesia* [Video]. YouTube. All rights reserved. https://youtu.be/gBCiWt-4Cm4

36 Volpi-Abadie, J., Kaye, A. M., & Kaye, A. D. (2013). Serotonin syndrome. *The Ochsner Journal, 13*(4), 533–540. https://dx.doi.org/10.1177%2F2045125311400779

My Notes

myoglobinuria, and acute renal failure. The antipsychotic should be immediately discontinued when signs occur. Dantrolene is typically prescribed for treatment. Nursing interventions include adequate hydration, cooling, and close monitoring of vital signs and serum electrolytes.[37]

Second-generation antipsychotics have a significantly decreased risk of extrapyramidal side effects but are associated with weight gain and the development of metabolic syndrome.[38] **Metabolic syndrome** is a cluster of conditions that occur together, increasing the risk of heart disease, stroke, and type 2 diabetes. Symptoms include increased blood pressure; high blood sugar; excess body fat around the waist (also referred to as having an "apple waistline"); and abnormal cholesterol, triglyceride levels, and high-density lipoprotein (HDL) levels. Weight, glucose levels, and lipid levels should be monitored before treatment is initiated then annually.

 View a video: What Is Metabolic Syndrome?[39]

View this PDF: Adverse Effects of Antipsychotic Medications.

Patient Teaching and Education

Clients should be advised to contact their provider if involuntary or uncontrollable movements occur. They should be warned to not suddenly stop taking the medication because abrupt withdrawal can cause dizziness; nausea and vomiting; and uncontrolled movements of the mouth, tongue, or jaw. Clients should be warned to not consume alcohol or other CNS depressants because their ability to operate machinery or drive may be impaired.

Relapse

Some people may experience relapse, meaning their psychosis symptoms come back or get worse. Relapses typically occur when people stop taking their prescribed antipsychotic medication or when they take it sporadically. Some people stop taking prescribed medications because they feel better or they feel that they don't need it anymore, but medication should never be stopped suddenly. After talking with a prescriber, patients can gradually taper their medications in some situations. However, most people with schizophrenia must stay on an antipsychotic continuously for months or years for mental wellness.[40]

Psychosocial Treatments

Cognitive behavioral therapy, behavioral skills training, supported employment, and cognitive remediation interventions are types of psychosocial treatments that can help address the negative and cognitive symptoms of schizophrenia. A combination of these therapies and antipsychotic medication is a common treatment approach for schizophrenia. Psychosocial treatments can help improve an individual's coping skills with the everyday challenges of schizophrenia. Therapies can also help people pursue their life goals, such as attending school, working,

---

37 This work is a derivative of *StatPearls* by Chokhawala and Stevens and is licensed under CC BY 4.0

38 This work is a derivative of *StatPearls* by Chokhawala and Stevens and is licensed under CC BY 4.0

39 Health Link. (2019, December 31). *What is metabolic syndrome?* [Video]. YouTube. All rights reserved. https://youtu.be/fVMvY_Lsqzw

40 National Institute of Mental Health. (2016, October). *Mental health medications.* U.S. Department of Health and Human Services. https://www.nimh.nih.gov/health/topics/mental-health-medications#part_2362

My Notes

or forming relationships. Individuals who participate in regular psychosocial treatments are less likely to relapse or be hospitalized.[41]

Family Education and Support

Psychosis and schizophrenia can take a heavy toll on a client's family members, significant others, and friends. Educational programs offer instruction about schizophrenia symptoms, treatments, and strategies for assisting their loved one experiencing psychosis and schizophrenia. Increasing their understanding of psychotic symptoms, treatment options, and the course of recovery can lessen their distress, bolster their own coping strategies, and empower them to offer effective assistance to their loved one. Family-based services may be provided on an individual basis or through multi-family workshops and support groups.

For more information about family-based services in your area, visit the family education and support groups page on the National Alliance on Mental Illness website.[42]

Coordinated Specialty Care

Coordinated specialty care (CSC) is a general term used to describe recovery-oriented treatment programs for people with first-episode psychosis, an early stage of schizophrenia. A team of health professionals and specialists deliver CSC that includes psychotherapy, medication management, case management, employment and education support, and family education and support. The person with early psychosis and the team work together in a patient-centered and family-centered approach to make treatment decisions. Compared to typical care for early psychosis, CSC is more effective at reducing symptoms, improving quality of life, and increasing involvement in work or school.[43]

The goal is to link the individual with a CSC team as soon as possible after psychotic symptoms begin. There are many different programs that are considered CSC in the United States, including (but are not limited to) Comprehensive Community Support (CCS), Community Support Programs (CSP), NAVIGATE, Connection Program, OnTrackNY, Specialized Treatment Early in Psychosis (STEP) program, and Early Assessment and Support Alliance (EASA). Supported Employment/Education (SEE) is an important part of CSC that helps individuals return to work or school because it addresses the client's personal goals. A SEE specialist helps clients develop the skills they need to achieve school and work goals. In addition, the specialist can be a bridge between clients and educators or employers.[44]

Research from the RAISE project (Recovery After an Initial Schizophrenia Episode) has shown that treatments for psychosis work better when they are delivered closer to the time when psychotic symptoms first appear. The goal of the RAISE project is to help decrease the likelihood of future episodes of psychosis, reduce long-term disability, and help people to get their lives back on track so they can pursue their goals.[45]

---

41 National Institute of Mental Health. (2020, May). *Schizophrenia.* U.S. Department of Health and Human Services. https://www.nimh.nih.gov/health/topics/schizophrenia

42 National Institute of Mental Health. (2020, May). *Schizophrenia.* U.S. Department of Health and Human Services. https://www.nimh.nih.gov/health/topics/schizophrenia

43 National Institute of Mental Health. (2020, May). *Schizophrenia.* U.S. Department of Health and Human Services. https://www.nimh.nih.gov/health/topics/schizophrenia

44 National Institute of Mental Health. (n.d.). *What is psychosis?* U.S. Department of Health and Human Services. https://www.nimh.nih.gov/health/topics/schizophrenia/raise/what-is-psychosis

45 National Institute of Mental Health. (n.d.). *Raise researchers.* U.S. Department of Health and Human Services.

My Notes

Read more about the RAISE project at RAISE Questions and Answers web page.

With early diagnosis and appropriate treatment, it is possible to recover from psychosis. Many people who receive early treatment never have another psychotic episode. For other people, recovery means the ability to live a fulfilling and productive life, even if psychotic symptoms return at times. However, if untreated, psychotic symptoms can cause disruptions in school and work, strained family relations, and separation from friends. The longer the symptoms go untreated, the greater the risk for developing additional problems. These problems can include abusing substances, having legal trouble, or becoming homeless.[46]

Assertive Community Treatment

Assertive Community Treatment (ACT) is designed for individuals with schizophrenia who are at risk for repeated hospitalizations or homelessness. Research has demonstrated a prevalence of psychosis as high as 21% among homeless people living on the street.[47] See Figure 11.4[48] for an image of a homeless man. ACT is based on a multidisciplinary team approach, including a medication prescriber, a shared caseload among team members, direct service provision by team members, high frequency of patient contact, low patient to staff ratios, and outreach to patients in the community. ACT has been shown to reduce hospitalizations and homelessness among individuals with schizophrenia.[49]

---

46 National Institute of Mental Health. (n.d.). *What is psychosis?* U.S. Department of Health and Human Services. https://www.nimh.nih.gov/health/topics/schizophrenia/raise/what-is-psychosis

47 Ayano, G., Tesfaw, G., & Shumet, S. (2019). The prevalence of schizophrenia and other psychotic disorders among homeless people: A systematic review and meta-analysis. *BMC Psychiatry, 19*(370). https://doi.org/10.1186/s12888-019-2361-7

48 "HomelessParis_7032101.jpg" by Eric Pouhier is licensed under CC BY-SA 2.5

49 National Institute of Mental Health. (2020, May). *Schizophrenia.* U.S. Department of Health and Human Services. https://www.nimh.nih.gov/health/topics/schizophrenia

My Notes

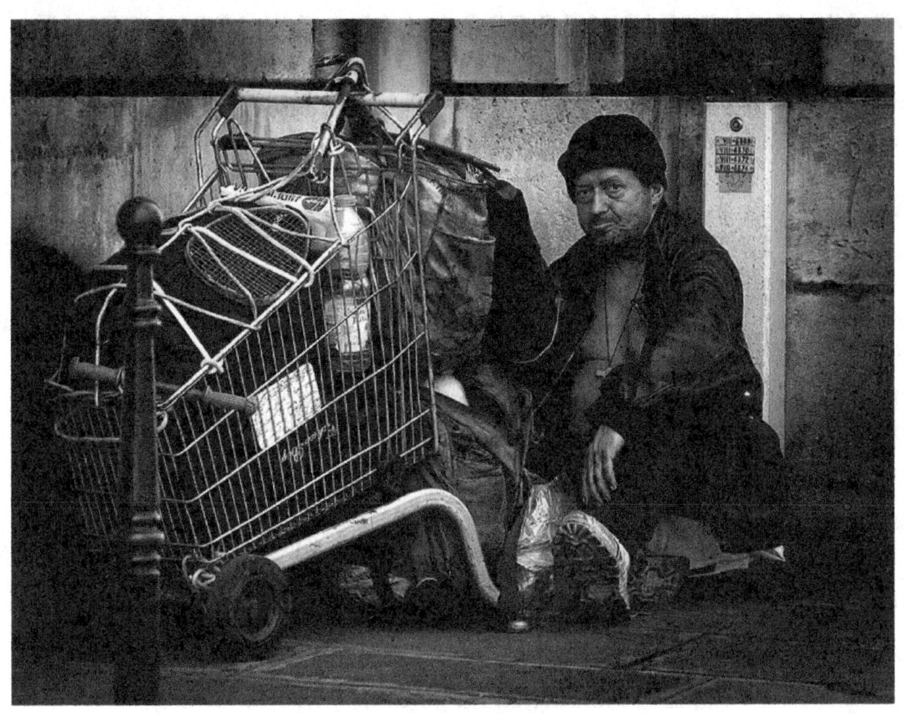

Figure 11.4 Homelessness

Read more information about ACT programs on the Substance Abuse and Mental Health Services Administration (SAMHSA) website.

My Notes

11.4 APPLYING THE NURSING PROCESS TO SCHIZOPHRENIA

Now that we have discussed the symptoms and treatments for psychosis and schizophrenia, we will explain how to apply the nursing process to a client experiencing an acute psychotic episode related to schizophrenia.

Assessment

Assessment includes interviewing the client, observing verbal and nonverbal behaviors, and completing a mental status examination and a psychosocial assessment. Common findings during a mental status examination for a client with schizophrenia experiencing an acute psychotic episode are described in Table 11.4a. Review information about performing a mental status examination and psychosocial assessment in the "Application of the Nursing Process in Mental Health Care" chapter. It is also important to assess for suicide risk for clients with psychosis. Review how to assess for suicide risk in the "Foundational Mental Health Concepts" chapter.

Table 11.4a Common Findings During a Mental Status Examination for Individual With Schizophrenia Experiencing an Acute-Psychotic Episode[1]

Assessment	Common Findings During Psychotic Episodes (*Indicates immediately the notify health care provider)
Level of Consciousness and Orientation	■ Unable to provide name, location, or day ■ Clouded consciousness
Appearance and General Behavior	■ Unkempt or poor hygiene ■ Not dressed appropriately for the weather and/or situation ■ Does not socialize with others ■ May demonstrate threatening behavior ■ Shows negativism (a tendency to resist or oppose requests of others) ■ Has impaired impulse control (which can increase the risk of assault) ■ Exhibits **boundary impairment**, an impaired ability to sense where one's influence ends and another person's begins (e.g., the person might walk up to a table and drink out of someone else's glass)
Speech	■ Does not respond to verbal questions ■ Does not appropriately follow instructions (based on development level) ■ Exhibits **alogia** (reduction or poverty in speech), rapid or pressured speech, or halting speech

1 Halter, M. (2022). *Varcarolis' foundations of psychiatric-mental health nursing* (9th ed.). Saunders.

My Notes

Assessment	Common Findings During Psychotic Episodes (*Indicates immediately the notify health care provider)
Motor Activity	■ **Catatonia** (a pronounced increase or decrease in the rate and amount of movement, where excessive movement is purposeless) ■ Motor retardation (a pronounced slowness of movement) ■ Motor agitation (running or pacing rapidly in response to internal or external stimuli) ■ **Echopraxia** (mimicking movements of another person)
Affect and Mood	■ Flat, blunted, constricted, or labile affect ■ Inappropriate or incongruent with the situation ■ **Anhedonia** (reduced ability to experience pleasure) ■ **Avolition** (reduced motivation or goal-directed behavior) ■ **Asociality** (decreased desire for social interaction) ■ **Apathy** (decreased interest in activities that would otherwise be interesting)
Thought and Perception	■ Hallucinations (false sensory perceptions not associated with real external stimuli that can include any of the five senses such as visual, auditory, tactile, gustatory, or olfactory) ■ Delusions (a fixed, false belief not held by cultural peers and persisting in the face of objective contradictory evidence) ■ **Illusions** (misperceptions of real stimuli) ■ Disorganized or bizarre thoughts ■ Flight of ideas ■ **Loose associations** (jumping from one idea to an unrelated idea in the same sentence) ■ **Clang associations** ■ **Echolalia** (pathological repetition of another person's words) ■ **Magical thinking** (falsely believing that reality can be changed simply by one's thoughts) ■ **Paranoia** (an irrational fear ranging from being suspicious to thinking someone is trying to kill you) ■ ***Suicidal or homicidal ideation that can result from command hallucinations or defensive actions in response to paranoia**
Attitude and Insight	■ **Anosognosia** (the inability to recognize that one is ill)
Cognitive Abilities	■ Concrete thinking (impaired ability to think abstractly) ■ Short-term memory impairment ■ Impaired information processing ■ Impaired reasoning

My Notes

Assessment	Common Findings During Psychotic Episodes (*Indicates immediately the notify health care provider)
Examiner's Reaction to Client	■ Frustration ■ Anxiousness ■ Countertransference

When assessing hallucinations, do not imply the perceptions are real. For example, a nurse should ask the client, "What do you hear?" not "What are the voices saying?" It is important to assess for command hallucinations, such as, "Are you hearing a voice that is telling you to do something," followed by, "Do you believe what you hear is real?" If the answer is "Yes," the client is at increased risk for acting on the command. Assess when the hallucinations began, their content, and the manner in which the client experiences them (i.e., Are they supportive or distressing? In the background or intrusive?). Ask what makes them worse or better, how the client responds, and what they do to cope with the hallucinations.[2]

When assessing delusions, determine if the client is capable of reality testing (i.e., questioning their thoughts and determining what is real). Ask the client if they believe there is any danger related to the delusion.[3]

Assess the client's ability to perform activities of daily living. Are they getting adequate food, fluid, sleep, and rest? Are they completing daily hygiene tasks and dressing safely for weather conditions? Are they able to control their impulses and make safe decisions?[4]

Determine if the client is taking their medications as prescribed, their effectiveness, and if they are experiencing side effects. Are there any barriers to medications or other treatment, such as cost, stigma, or mistrust of health care providers?[5]

Nurses also assess for adverse effects of medications, such as involuntary movements associated with the use of antipsychotic medications (e.g., extrapyramidal side effects or tardive dyskinesia). Clients are routinely assessed for these adverse effects using scales like the Abnormal Involuntary Movement Scale.

View a video: Mental Health AIMS Assessment.[6]

When possible, assess family members and significant others' knowledge of the client's illness and their response. Are they overprotective, frustrated, or anxious? Are they familiar with family support groups, respite, and other community resources?[7]

2 Halter, M. (2022). *Varcarolis' foundations of psychiatric-mental health nursing* (9th ed.). Saunders.

3 Halter, M. (2022). *Varcarolis' foundations of psychiatric-mental health nursing* (9th ed.). Saunders.

4 Halter, M. (2022). *Varcarolis' foundations of psychiatric-mental health nursing* (9th ed.). Saunders.

5 Halter, M. (2022). *Varcarolis' foundations of psychiatric-mental health nursing* (9th ed.). Saunders.

6 Banks, D. (2021, February 22). *Mental health AIMS assessment* [Video]. YouTube. All rights reserved. https://youtu.be/XuulM7G6T7A

7 Halter, M. (2022). *Varcarolis' foundations of psychiatric-mental health nursing* (9th ed.). Saunders.

My Notes

Diagnostic and Lab Work

Ensure the client has had a medical workup for other potential causes of psychosis. For example, dehydration, infection, electrolyte imbalances, abnormal blood glucose level, substance use, or withdrawal from substances can cause psychosis. Concurrent medical disorders are common and should be treated in addition to treating schizophrenia.

If the client is currently taking psychotropic medications, therapeutic drug levels of some types of medications are required. As always, review current information from a medication reference before administering medications.

Diagnoses

Mental health disorders like schizophrenia are diagnosed by mental health providers using the *DSM-5*. Nurses create individualized nursing care plans based on the client's responses to their mental health disorders. See Table 11.4b for a list of common nursing diagnoses and human responses related to schizophrenia.

Table 11.4b Common Nursing Diagnoses Related to Schizophrenia[8,9]

Nursing Diagnosis	Definition	Selected Defining Characteristics
Risk for Suicide	Susceptible to self-inflicted, life-threatening injury.	■ Reports desire to die ■ Threats of killing self ■ Hopelessness ■ Social isolation
Ineffective Coping	A pattern of invalid appraisal of stressors, with cognitive and/or behavioral efforts, that fails to manage demands related to well-being.	■ Alteration in concentration ■ Alteration in sleep pattern ■ Inability to meet basic needs ■ Ineffective coping strategies ■ Insufficient goal-directed behavior ■ Risk-taking behavior
Self-Neglect	A constellation of culturally framed behaviors involving one or more self-care activities in which there is a failure to maintain a socially accepted standard of health and well-being.	■ Insufficient personal hygiene ■ Insufficient environmental hygiene ■ Nonadherence to health activity
Impaired Communication	Decreased, delayed, or absent ability to receive, process, transmit, and/or use a system of symbols.	■ Inappropriate verbalizations ■ Difficulty comprehending communication ■ Difficulty expressing thoughts verbally

8 Halter, M. (2022). *Varcarolis' foundations of psychiatric-mental health nursing* (9th ed.). Saunders.

9 Ackley, B., Ladwig, G., Makic, M. B., Martinez-Kratz, M., & Zanotti, M. (2020). *Nursing diagnosis handbook: An evidence-based guide to planning care* (12th ed.). Elsevier.

My Notes

Nursing Diagnosis	Definition	Selected Defining Characteristics
Imbalanced Nutrition: Less than Body Requirements	Intake of nutrients insufficient to meet metabolic needs.	■ Food intake less than recommended daily allowance ■ Insufficient interest in food ■ Body weight 20% or more below ideal weight range ■ Read more in the "Nutrition" chapter in Open RN *Nursing Fundamentals*
Sleep Deprivation	Prolonged periods of time without sustained natural, periodic suspension of relative consciousness that provides rest.	■ Anxiety ■ Agitation ■ Transient paranoia ■ Intrusive thoughts ■ Read more in the "Sleep and Rest" chapter of Open RN *Nursing Fundamentals*
Social Isolation	Aloneness experienced by the individual and perceived as imposed by others and as a negative or threatening state.	■ Impaired communication patterns ■ Disturbed thought processes ■ Delusional thinking
Hopelessness	Subjective state in which an individual sees limited or no alternatives or personal choices available and is unable to mobilize energy on own behalf.	■ Long-term stress from mental illness
Spiritual Distress	A state of suffering related to the impaired ability to experience meaning in life through connections with self, others, the world, or a superior being.	■ Ineffective coping strategies ■ Perceived insufficient meaning in life ■ Hopelessness ■ Social alienation
Readiness for Enhanced Hope	A pattern of expectations and desires for mobilizing energy on one's own behalf, which can be strengthened.	■ Expresses desire to enhance connectedness with others ■ Expresses desires to enhance sense of meaning in life

Outcomes Identification

Outcomes should be consistent with the recovery model and emphasize hope, resilience, living a full and productive life, and recovery from illness. Expected outcomes are identified based on the client's current phase of their illness: acute, stabilization, or maintenance[10]:

10 Halter, M. (2022). *Varcarolis' foundations of psychiatric-mental health nursing* (9th ed.). Saunders.

My Notes

Acute: The overall goal in the acute phase of schizophrenia is patient safety and stabilization. An example of an expected outcome is, "The client will consistently be able to label their hallucinations as 'not real' and a symptom of their illness by discharge."[11]

Stabilization: Goals during the stabilization phase focus on understanding the illness and the prescribed treatment plan, as well as controlling and/or coping with symptoms using an optimal medication and psychosocial treatment regimen. Outcomes typically target negative and cognitive symptoms of schizophrenia during this phase because these symptoms respond less well to initial medication treatment than do positive symptoms.[12] An example of an expected outcome during the stabilization phase is, "The client will establish two goal-directed activities by the end of the shift."

Maintenance: Goals during the maintenance phase focus on maintaining and increasing symptom control and optimal functioning. Factors include treatment adherence, increasing independence, and a satisfactory quality of life.[13] An example of an expected outcome during the maintenance phase is, "The client will identify advantages for taking medications by the end of Week 2."

Planning Interventions

Hospitalization is indicated during the acute phase of schizophrenia if the client is considered a danger to self (e.g., refuses to eat or is too disorganized to function in the community) or to others (e.g., is behaving in a threatening manner to others).[14]

During the stabilization and maintenance phases, planning focuses on education, support, and skills training for the client and family. It also addresses how and where these needs can be met within the community. As explained previously in this chapter, relapse prevention efforts are vital. Each relapse can increase residual dysfunction and deterioration and can contribute to despair, hopelessness, and suicide risk. Additionally, recognizing early signs of relapse (e.g., reduced sleep, social withdrawal, and worsening concentration) and implementing intensive treatment are needed to minimize the disruption of the client's life.[15]

Implementation

During the acute phase of schizophrenia, hospitalization provides safety, structure, and support. As discussed earlier, anosognosia may impair the client's ability to recognize their mental illness. In this case, court-ordered hospitalization may be required.[16] Read more about court-ordered hospitalization in the "Legal and Ethical Considerations in Mental Health Care" chapter. Nursing interventions focus on providing safety, promoting hygiene and nutrition, improving socialization, encouraging hope and self-esteem, preventing falls, using specific therapeutic techniques, addressing physiological needs, and implementing collaborative interventions.

---

11 Halter, M. (2022). *Varcarolis' foundations of psychiatric-mental health nursing* (9th ed.). Saunders.

12 Halter, M. (2022). *Varcarolis' foundations of psychiatric-mental health nursing* (9th ed.). Saunders.

13 Halter, M. (2022). *Varcarolis' foundations of psychiatric-mental health nursing* (9th ed.). Saunders.

14 Halter, M. (2022). *Varcarolis' foundations of psychiatric-mental health nursing* (9th ed.). Saunders.

15 Halter, M. (2022). *Varcarolis' foundations of psychiatric-mental health nursing* (9th ed.). Saunders.

16 Halter, M. (2022). *Varcarolis' foundations of psychiatric-mental health nursing* (9th ed.). Saunders.

My Notes

Provide Safety

Clients with command hallucinations require close monitoring for suicide, homicide, and other violence risk. Implement interventions to reduce risk of suicide as described in the "Application of the Nursing Process in Mental Health Care" chapter.

Interpersonal conflict, paranoia, delusions, impaired judgment, limited impulse control, fear, and disagreement with unit rules increase the risk for aggressive behavior.[17] Nursing interventions addressing increased risk for violence to self and others are described in the following box. Read more about recognizing signs of crisis and crisis interventions in the "Stress, Coping, and Crisis Intervention" chapter.

Nursing Interventions Addressing Risk for Violence[18]

- Assess for suicide risk and increase supervision when risk is present. Make rounds at unpredictable intervals and adjust frequency based on risk. Read more about assessing suicide risk in the "Foundational Mental Health Concepts" chapter and interventions for risk of suicide in the "Application of the Nursing Process in Mental Health Care" chapter.
- Assess for paranoid thoughts, command hallucinations, impaired impulse control, interpersonal conflict, increasing tension and desperation, and other factors that increase the risk of violence.
- Establish trust and rapport. Engage regularly with the client. Promote communication in a safe manner regarding their concerns that contribute to risk of violence. Engender goodwill and a strong nurse-client relationship.
- Take actions to ensure the client feels safe and secure.
- Teach coping skills to reduce stressors.
- Provide constructive diversion and outlets for physical energy.
- Ensure clients are taking their medications as prescribed. Consider requesting long-acting injectable medications as indicated.
- If the client targets specific peers or staff, relocate individuals as needed.
- Search client belongings thoroughly on admission and repeat the search whenever circumstances suggest the client may have made or acquired a weapon.
- Use seclusion or restraints when other alternatives have not been successful in keeping the client or others safe.

17 Halter, M. (2022). *Varcarolis' foundations of psychiatric-mental health nursing* (9th ed.). Saunders.

18 Halter, M. (2022). *Varcarolis' foundations of psychiatric-mental health nursing* (9th ed.). Saunders.

My Notes

Promote Hygiene and Nutrition

Promote hygiene in clients experiencing psychosis by concisely and explicitly stating expected hygiene tasks. Break tasks into smaller, more manageable tasks and assist when needed. Use visual cues to prompt hygiene tasks, such as putting clean clothes on the bed or clean towels and a toothbrush in the bathroom. Share potential benefits of improved hygiene such as improved socialization with others. Reinforce progress in performing hygiene with verbal praise or concrete rewards like additional privileges on the unit.[19]

Clients who are experiencing catatonia require assistance with nutrition, as well as other activities of daily living.

Improve Socialization

Regularly engage with the client. Initially interact briefly about low-anxiety topics like the weather and gradually increase the duration and frequency of interactions as they become more comfortable. Encourage clients to participate in unit activities without pressure, such as "We would like to see you at the morning meeting." Reinforce the client's control in their choices, such as, "If you become uncomfortable in the group, you can leave and try again on another day." Provide positive reinforcement for attempts at socialization, such as, "It was nice to see you in the morning meeting today."[20]

Encourage Hope and Self-Esteem

Convey unconditional acceptance, empathy, and support. For example, say, "Sometimes it can feel very discouraging when experiencing a mental health disorder. I am wondering how you are feeling?" If the client cannot identify their feelings, suggest words that may apply, such as, "Sometimes it is hard to say what you are feeling. Do you feel sad, frustrated, or anxious?" Validate the client's feelings and assure them they are not alone. Help the client identify their positive traits or previous accomplishments. Suggest coping strategies such as journaling and attending a support group. Teach stress management techniques and coping strategies as outlined in the "Stress, Coping, and Crisis Intervention" chapter.

Prevent Falls

Fall risk may be increased due to orthostatic hypotension, impaired balance, bradykinesia, or other movement disorders. Assess the client's gait and for orthostatic hypotension. Teach the client to slowly change position from lying to sitting to standing and encourage the use of handrails or seeking assistance when feeling unsteady. Implement additional fall precautions as needed according to agency policy.

Read more information about fall precautions in the "Safety" chapter of Open RN *Nursing Fundamentals*.

Use Therapeutic Techniques for Delusions and Hallucinations

Recall that clients with schizophrenia may have memory and attention impairments. Repetition with visual and verbal reminders is helpful to promote task completion. Additionally, short but frequent interactions may be less stimulating to the client and better tolerated.[21] Additional techniques for helping clients who are experiencing delusions and hallucinations are described below.

---

19 Halter, M. (2022). *Varcarolis' foundations of psychiatric-mental health nursing* (9th ed.). Saunders.

20 Halter, M. (2022). *Varcarolis' foundations of psychiatric-mental health nursing* (9th ed.). Saunders.

21 Halter, M. (2022). *Varcarolis' foundations of psychiatric-mental health nursing* (9th ed.). Saunders.

My Notes

Helping Clients Who Are Experiencing Delusions

Delusions feel very real to the client and can be frightening. Nurses should acknowledge and accept the client's experience and feelings resulting from the delusion while conveying empathy. They can provide reassurance regarding their intentions to help the client feel safer.

Avoid questioning the delusion. Until the client's ability to test reality improves, trying to prove the delusion is incorrect can intensify it and cause the client to view the staff as people who cannot be trusted. Instead, focus on the fear and what would help the client feel safer. For example, if a client states, "The doctor is here. He wants to kill me," the nurse could respond, "Yes, the doctor is here and wants to see you. They talk with all of the patients about their treatment. Would you feel more comfortable if I stayed with you during your meeting with the doctor?" Focusing of events in the present keeps the client focused on reality and helps them distinguish what is real.[22]

If a client is exhibiting paranoia and is highly suspicious, it is helpful to maintain consistent staff assignments. Staff should avoid laughing, whispering, or talking quietly where the client can see these actions but cannot hear what is being said. Staff should ask permission before touching the client, such as before taking their blood pressure.

Read additional strategies for working with clients with delusions from the British Columbia Schizophrenia Society: Steps for Working With Delusions.

Helping Clients Who Are Experiencing Hallucinations

Hallucinations feel very real to the person experiencing them and can be distracting during their interactions with others. Hallucinations can be supportive or terrifying, faint or loud, or episodic or constant. For example, listen to simulations of auditory hallucinations in the following box. The nurse should focus on understanding the client's experiences and responses and convey empathy. Command hallucinations, suicidal ideation, or homicidal ideation requires safety measures as previously discussed in the "Provide Safety" subsection.

Simulations of Auditory Hallucinations

British Columbia Schizophrenia Society created music tracks simulating what auditory hallucinations can feel like to clients. Similar to auditory hallucinations experienced by people living with schizophrenia, when people listen to these songs, they hear voices that can be frightening. Listen to these simulations on YouTube with discretion because some people can find them disturbing:

Track 05: Mark Pelli – Everything (Songs of schizophrenia mix)[23]

Track 06: Cassandra Vasik – Sadly mistaken (Songs of schizophrenia mix)[24]

When working with a client who has a history of hallucinations, watch for hallucination indicators, such as eyes tracking an unheard speaker, muttering or talking to oneself, appearing distracted,

22 Halter, M. (2022). *Varcarolis' foundations of psychiatric-mental health nursing* (9th ed.). Saunders.

23 BC Schizophrenia. (2019, May 6). *Track 05: Mark Pelli - Everything (Songs of schizophrenia mix)* [Video]. YouTube. All rights reserved. https://youtu.be/pN-f6AEDNxY

24 BC Schizophrenia. (2019, May 6). *Track 06: Cassandra Vasik - Sadly mistaken (Songs of schizophrenia mix)* [Video]. YouTube. All rights reserved. https://youtu.be/HCewO3BL1qA

My Notes

suddenly stopping a conversation as if interrupted, or intently watching a vacant area of the room. Ask about the content of the hallucinations and if they are experiencing command hallucinations. Assess how the client is reacting to the hallucinations, especially if they are exhibiting anxiety, fear, or distress.[25]

Avoid referring to the hallucinations as if they were real to promote reality testing. For example, do not ask, "What are the voices saying to you," but instead ask, "You look as though you are hearing something. What do you hear?" Do not try to convince the client the hallucinations are not real, but instead offer your perception and convey empathy. For example, "I don't hear angry voices that you hear, but that must be very frightening for you." Address any underlying emotion, need, or theme indicated by the hallucination.[26]

Focus on reality-based activities in the "here and now," such as a conversation or simple project. Promote and guide reality testing. For example, guide the client to look around the room and see if others are frightened; if they are not, encourage them to consider what they are experiencing are hallucinations. Teach the client to compare their perceptions to trusted others.[27]

See the information in the following box for teaching clients how to manage their hallucinations.

Patient Education: Teaching Clients How to Manage Hallucinations[28]

- Manage stress and stimulation.
  - Avoid overly loud or stressful places or activities.
  - Avoid negative or overly critical people and seek out supportive people.
  - Use assertive communication skills so you can tell others "No" if they pressure or upset you.
  - When stressed, focus on your breathing and slow it down. Inhale slowly through your nose as you count from one to four, hold your breath, and then exhale slowly through your mouth.
  - Refer to other stress management and coping strategies in the "Stress, Coping, and Crisis Intervention" chapter.
- Use other sounds to compete with the hallucinations, such as talking with other people, listening to music or TV, reading aloud, singing, whistling, or humming.
- Determine what is real and unreal by looking at others. Do they seem to be hearing or seeing

25 Halter, M. (2022). *Varcarolis' foundations of psychiatric-mental health nursing* (9th ed.). Saunders.

26 Halter, M. (2022). *Varcarolis' foundations of psychiatric-mental health nursing* (9th ed.). Saunders.

27 Halter, M. (2022). *Varcarolis' foundations of psychiatric-mental health nursing* (9th ed.). Saunders.

28 Halter, M. (2022). *Varcarolis' foundations of psychiatric-mental health nursing* (9th ed.). Saunders.

My Notes

what you are? Ask trusted others if they are experiencing the same things you are. If the answers to these questions are "No," then although it feels real, it is not likely real and can be ignored.

- Engage in activities that can take your mind off the hallucinations, such as walking, taking a relaxing bath or shower, or going to a place you find enjoyable where others are present, such as a coffee shop, mall, or library.
- Talk out loud (or silently to yourself if others are nearby) and tell the voices or thoughts to go away. Tell yourself the voices or thoughts are a symptom and not real. Tell yourself that no matter what you hear, you are safe and can ignore what you hear.
- Seek contact with others. Visit a trusted friend or family member. Call a help line or go to a drop-in center. Visit a public place where you feel comfortable.
- Develop a plan with your provider for how to cope with hallucinations. Additional medications may be prescribed to use as needed.

Address Physiological Needs

The client may also be experiencing physiological problems related to nutritional status, sleep, and elimination due to their symptoms of psychosis. Review nursing interventions to address these physiological needs in the "Bipolar Disorders" chapter.

Implement Collaborative Interventions

See the "Treatment" subsection of this chapter for medications and therapies prescribed for clients with psychosis. Nurses often assist in implementing these collaborative interventions.

Categorizing Nursing Interventions According to the APNA Standard of Implementation

Interventions for clients experiencing psychosis previously discussed in this chapter can also be categorized by the standard of *Implementation* by the American Psychiatric Nursing Association (APNA). Read more about this standard in the "Application of the Nursing Process in Mental Health Care" chapter. See Table 11.4c for categorization of nursing interventions by this standard.

My Notes

Table 11.4c Nursing Interventions Based on the Categories of the APNA Implementation Standard[29]

Categories of Interventions Based on the APNA Standard of Implementation	What the nurse will do..	Rationale
Coordination of Care	Maintain safety by implementing safety precautions as needed to prevent self-harm, suicide, or homicide risks. Ensure consistency of behavioral expectations among all staff on the unit by including expectations in the nursing care plan. Plan for quality of life, independence, and optimal recovery by referring to local resources and support groups in the community on discharge.	The client may exhibit high risk for impulsive behaviors that could pose a risk of harm to self/others. They may experience altered thought processes with poor insight and judgment. Consistent expectations provide a feeling of structure and safety. The nurse coordinates care delivery during inpatient care, as well as for after discharge.
Health Teaching	Create, adapt, and deliver health teaching to clients, including stress management, coping strategies, and management of delusions and hallucinations. Deliver patient education about antipsychotics and expected time frames for improvement. Open all medications in front of the client. Observe for and promptly report symptoms of potential adverse effects of first-generation antipsychotics such as tardive dyskinesia (TD) and extrapyramidal side effects (EPS).	Nurses encourage resilience by promoting adaptive coping strategies. The client's understanding of their medications and potential side effects can increase medication compliance. Opening all medications in front of the client may decrease paranoia. Clients experiencing TD or new EPS symptoms should discontinue first-generation antipsychotics and start second-generation antipsychotics per provider order. Medications to treat symptoms may be required.

29 American Psychiatric Association. (2013). *Desk reference to the diagnostic criteria from DSM-5.*

My Notes

Categories of Interventions Based on the APNA Standard of Implementation	What the nurse will do..	Rationale
Milieu Therapy	Manage the milieu by reducing environmental stimuli and excess noise. The client may require a private room. Promote physical exercise to redirect aggressive behavior. During acute psychosis with agitation, use prescribed medications, seclusion, or restraint to minimize physical harm. Encourage participation in group therapy addressing social skills, personal grooming, mindfulness, and stress management. Avoid competitive activities or games if the client is agitated.	Reducing stimuli may prevent escalation of anxiety and agitation. Physical exercise can decrease tension and provide focus. The nurse's priority is to protect the patient and others from harm. Group therapy can encourage effective coping skills and socialization. Structured activities provide security and focus. However, avoid competitive activities because they may be too stimulating and can cause escalation of anxiety and agitation.
Therapeutic Relationship and Counseling	Use a firm and calm approach with short and concise statements. For example, "John, come with me. Eat this sandwich." Identify expectations in simple, concrete terms with consequences. For example, "John, do not yell at or hit Peter. If you cannot control yourself, the seclusion room will help you feel less out of control and prevent harm to yourself and others." Acknowledge feelings associated with delusions and hallucinations and convey empathy. Encourage and guide reality testing based on client status. Redirect excessive energy into appropriate and constructive channels. Set limits with personal boundaries.	Structure and control improve feelings of security for a client who is feeling out of control. Clear expectations help the patient experience outside controls and understand reasons for medication, seclusion, or restraints if they are not able to control their behaviors. Acknowledging emotion and conveying empathy build trust and a strong nurse-client relationship. Reality testing helps clients manage their delusions and hallucinations. Distraction and activity can be used to manage excessive movement. Clients may be impulsive and hyperverbal and interrupt, blame, ridicule, or manipulate others.

Evaluation

A client's progress is continually assessed using their individualized SMART outcomes and current status. Full recovery can take months. By setting small goals, it is easier to identify and recognize progress that may occur in small increments.[30]

---

30 Halter, M. (2022). *Varcarolis' foundations of psychiatric-mental health nursing* (9th ed.). Saunders.

11.5 SPOTLIGHT APPLICATION

My Notes

View a video: "Elyn Saks: A Tale of Mental Illness– From the Inside" [1]

Reflective Questions:

1. What strikes you most about Dr. Sak's journey with schizophrenia?
2. What are three takeaways points from Dr. Sak's presentation?

View a video: "What Living Well With Schizophrenia Means to Me"[2]

Reflective Questions:

1. How is X's journey with schizophrenia different from Dr. Sak's?
2. What are three things you learned from X's description of her journey with schizophrenia?

---

1 TEDGlobal. (2012). *A tale of mental illness -- From the inside* [Video]. TED. All rights reserved. https://www.ted.com/talks/elyn_saks_seeing_mental_illness

2 Living Well with Schizophrenia. (2020, March 7). *What living well with schizophrenia means to me* [Video]. YouTube. All rights reserved. https://youtu.be/VUhw64iEIQw

My Notes

11.6 LEARNING ACTIVITIES

Interactive Activities

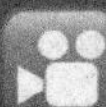

An interactive H5P element has been excluded from this version of the text. You can view it online here: https://wtcs.pressbooks.pub/nursingmhcc/?p=536#h5p-38

An interactive H5P element has been excluded from this version of the text. You can view it online here: https://wtcs.pressbooks.pub/nursingmhcc/?p=536#h5p-39

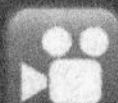

An interactive H5P element has been excluded from this version of the text. You can view it online here: https://wtcs.pressbooks.pub/nursingmhcc/?p=536#h5p-40

XI GLOSSARY

My Notes

Agranulocytosis: Extremely low white blood cell count.

Akathisia: Psychomotor restlessness (a feeling of being unable to sit still).

Alogia: Reduction or poverty in speech.

Anhedonia: The reduced ability to experience pleasure in daily activities.

Anosognosia: The inability to recognize that one is ill.

Apathy: A decreased interest in activities that would otherwise be interesting.

Asociality: A decreased desire for social interaction.

Avolition: Reduced motivation or goal-directed behavior.

Boundary impairment: An impaired ability to sense where one's influence ends and another person's begins. For example, the person might walk up to a table and drink out of someone else's glass.

Bradykinesia: Slowed movement.

Catatonia: A pronounced increase or decrease in the rate and amount of movement; excessive movement is purposeless.

Clang associations: Stringing words together that rhyme without logical association and do not convey rational meaning. For example, a client exhibiting clang associations may state, "Here she comes with a cat catch a rat match."

Cognitive symptoms: A category of symptoms of schizophrenia that refer to problems in attention, concentration, and memory, such as difficulty processing information to make decisions; problems using information immediately after learning it; and trouble focusing or paying attention.

Command hallucinations: Auditory hallucinations that command the individual to do something.

Coordinated specialty care (CSC): A general term used to describe recovery-oriented treatment programs for people with first-episode psychosis, an early stage of schizophrenia.

Delusion: A fixed, false belief not held by cultural peers and persisting in the face of objective contradictory evidence. For example, a client may have the delusion that the CIA is listening to their conversations via satellites.

Dystonia: Involuntary contractions of muscles of the extremities, face, neck, abdomen, pelvis, or larynx in either sustained or intermittent patterns that lead to abnormal movements or postures.

Echolalia: Pathological repetition of another person's words.

Echopraxia: Mimicking the movements of another person.

Extrapyramidal side effects (EPS): Adverse effects, such as akathisia, rigidity, bradykinesia, tremor, and acute-dystonic reactions, that can occur from first-generation antipsychotics.

First-generation antipsychotics: Also referred to as "typical antipsychotics"; this class of medications has several potential adverse effects due to the blockage of dopamine receptors. Medication is prescribed based on the client's ability to tolerate the adverse effects.

Flat affect: A reduced expression of emotions via facial expression or voice tone.

Hallucinations: False sensory perceptions not associated with real external stimuli that can include any of the five senses (auditory, visual, gustatory, olfactory and tactile). For example, a client may see spiders climbing on the wall or hear voices telling them to do things. These are referred to as "visual hallucinations" or "auditory hallucinations."

Illusions: Misperceptions of real stimuli. For example, a client may misperceive tree branches blowing in the wind at night to be the arms of monsters trying to grab them.

My Notes

Loose associations: Jumping from one idea to an unrelated idea in the same sentence. For example, the client might state, "I like to dance; my feet are wet."

Magical thinking: Falsely believing that reality can be changed simply by one's thoughts.

Metabolic syndrome: A cluster of conditions that occur together, increasing the risk of heart disease, stroke, and type 2 diabetes. Symptoms include increased blood pressure, high blood sugar, excess body fat around the waist, and abnormal cholesterol or triglyceride levels. Weight, glucose levels, and lipid levels should be monitored regularly.

Negative symptoms: A category of symptoms of schizophrenia that includes loss of motivation, diminished feelings of pleasure in everyday life, flat affect, and reduced speaking.

Neuroleptic malignant syndrome: A rare but fatal adverse effect that can occur at any time during treatment with antipsychotics. Signs include increased temperature, severe muscular rigidity, confusion, agitation, hyperreflexia, elevation in white blood cell count, elevated creatinine phosphokinase, elevated liver enzymes, myoglobinuria, and acute renal failure. The antipsychotic should be immediately discontinued if these signs occur.

Paranoia: An irrational fear that can range from being suspicious to thinking someone is trying to kill you.

Positive symptoms: A category of symptoms of schizophrenia that include hallucinations, delusions, thought disorders, disorganized speech, and alterations in behaviors.

Psychosis: Conditions where there is loss of contact with reality. Psychosis may be a symptom of a mental illness or other medical conditions. When a person experiences psychosis, their thoughts and perceptions are disturbed, and the individual has difficulty understanding what is real and what is not real. Symptoms of psychosis include delusions and hallucinations. Other symptoms include incoherent or nonsensical speech and behavior that is inappropriate for the situation.

Psychotic episode: An episode of psychosis that can include delusions, hallucinations, disorganized speech, and grossly disorganized or catatonic behavior.[1]

Schizophrenia: A severe mental illness characterized by periods of psychosis for at least six months.

Second-generation antipsychotics: Also referred to as "atypical antipsychotics"; this class of medication has fewer adverse effects because they block selective dopamine D2 receptors as well as serotonin. For this reason, they are generally better tolerated than first-generation antipsychotics.

Tardive dyskinesia (TD): A syndrome of movement disorders that can occur in clients taking first-generation antipsychotics, persisting for at least one month and up to several years despite discontinuation of the medications. The movement disorders include akathisia, dystonia, tics, and other abnormal involuntary movements.

1 American Psychiatric Association. (2013). *Desk reference to the diagnostic criteria from DSM-5.*

Chapter 12

Childhood and Adolescence Disorders

12.1 INTRODUCTION

My Notes

- Assess children or adolescents with mental health disorders, developmental disabilities, or disruptive behaviors
- Assess family dynamics and include family members in planning nursing care for children and adolescents
- Describe psychotherapy, behavioral therapy, and medical treatments for children or adolescents with mental health disorders, developmental disabilities, or disruptive behaviors
- Discuss conditional confidentiality and mandatory reporting related to caring for children and adolescents
- Apply the nursing process to children or adolescents with mental health disorders, developmental disabilities, or disruptive behaviors
- Identify community resources for children and adolescents with mental health disorders that enhance individual and family functioning
- Evaluate the effectiveness of interventions

Mental health disorders among children are described as "serious changes in the way children typically learn, behave, or handle their emotions, causing distress and problems getting through the day."[1] One in six children in the United States aged 2 to 8 years (17.4%) has a diagnosed mental, behavioral, or developmental disorder. Behavior problems are more common among children aged 6 to 11 years.[2]

This chapter will discuss common mental health disorders and disabilities in children and adolescents, as well as interprofessional treatments and related nursing plans of care.

---

1 Centers for Disease Control and Prevention. (2022, February 24). *Data and statistics on children's mental health.* https://www.cdc.gov/childrensmentalhealth/data.html

2 Centers for Disease Control and Prevention. (2022, February 24). *Data and statistics on children's mental health.* https://www.cdc.gov/childrensmentalhealth/data.html

My Notes

12.2 COMMON DISORDERS AND DISABILITIES IN CHILDREN AND ADOLESCENTS

The most commonly diagnosed mental health disorders in children aged 13-17 years are attention deficit hyperactivity disorder (ADHD), anxiety problems, behavioral problems, and depression[1]:

- ADHD: 9.8% (approximately 6.0 million)
- Anxiety: 9.4% (approximately 5.8 million)
- Behavioral problems: 8.9% (approximately 5.5 million)
- Depression: 4.4% (approximately 2.7 million)

For adolescents, depression, substance use, and suicide are important concerns. The following statistics demonstrate these concerns in adolescents aged 12-17 years in 2018-2019, prior to the COVID-19 pandemic[2]:

- 36.7% had persistent feelings of sadness or hopelessness.
- 18.8% seriously considered attempting suicide; 8.9% attempted suicide.
- 15.1% had a major depressive episode.
- 4.1% had a substance use disorder.
- 1.6% had an alcohol use disorder.

After the COVID-19 pandemic, the Centers for Disease Control and Prevention (CDC) found an 8% increase in persistent feelings of sadness in youth.[3]

These common disorders, as well as developmental disabilities, tics and Tourette syndrome, substance misuse, and gender dysphoria will be discussed in this section. Autism, another type of neurodevelopment disorder, is discussed in the "Autism Spectrum Disorder" section.

Attention Deficit Hyperactivity Disorder

Attention deficit hyperactivity disorder (ADHD) is one of the most common neurodevelopmental disorders of childhood. It is usually first diagnosed in childhood and often lasts into adulthood. Children with ADHD may have trouble paying attention, controlling impulsive behaviors, or are overly active.[4] See Figure 12.1[5] for an image depicting a child struggling with symptoms of ADHD in school.

---

1 Centers for Disease Control and Prevention. (2022, February 24). *Data and statistics on children's mental health.* https://www.cdc.gov/childrensmentalhealth/data.html

2 Centers for Disease Control and Prevention. (2022, February 24). *Data and statistics on children's mental health.* https://www.cdc.gov/childrensmentalhealth/data.html

3 Centers for Disease Control and Prevention. (2022, February 24). *Data and statistics on children's mental health.* https://www.cdc.gov/childrensmentalhealth/data.html

4 Centers for Disease Control and Prevention. (2022, February 24). *Data and statistics on children's mental health.* https://www.cdc.gov/childrensmentalhealth/data.html

5 Centers for Disease Control and Prevention. (2021, September 23). *What is ADHD?* https://www.cdc.gov/ncbddd/adhd/facts.html

My Notes

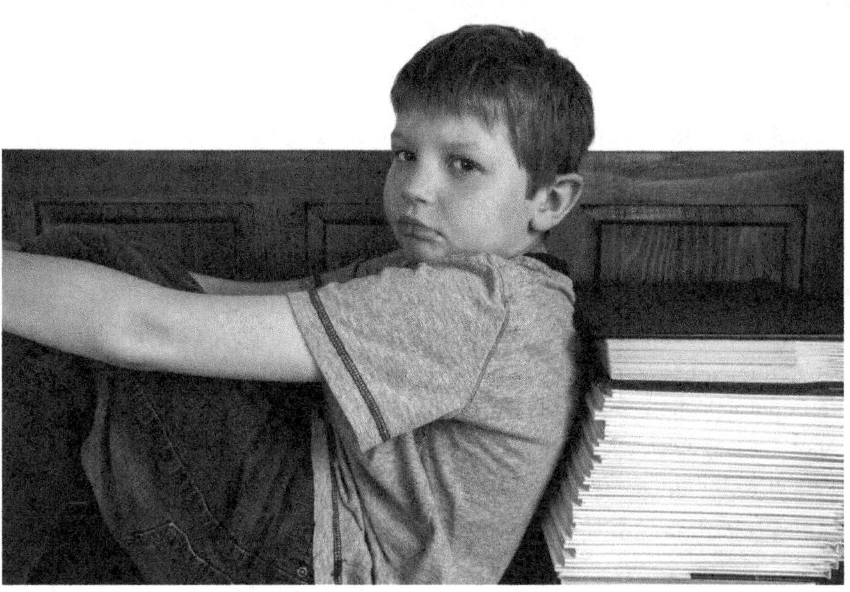

Figure 12.1 Child Struggling With Symptoms of ADHD in School

Signs and Symptoms

It is normal for children to exhibit challenging behaviors and have trouble focusing at certain times. However, children with ADHD often have more severe symptoms that cause difficulties at school, at home, or with friends[6]:

- Daydreaming
- Forgetting or losing things
- Squirming or fidgeting
- Talking too much
- Making careless mistakes or taking unnecessary risks
- Difficulty resisting temptation
- Difficulty getting along with others

Diagnosing a child with ADHD is a process requiring several steps by a mental health professional. There is no single test to diagnose ADHD, and many other problems such as anxiety, depression, sleep problems, and learning disorders can have similar symptoms as ADHD. The diagnostic process includes a medical exam; hearing and vision tests; and a checklist rating ADHD symptoms completed by parents, teachers, and the child.[7]

---

6 Centers for Disease Control and Prevention. (2021, September 23). *What is ADHD?* https://www.cdc.gov/ncbddd/adhd/facts.html

7 Centers for Disease Control and Prevention. (2021, September 23). *What is ADHD?* https://www.cdc.gov/ncbddd/adhd/facts.html

My Notes

Types of ADHD

There are three types of ADHD, depending on which types of symptoms are strongest in the individual[8]:

- **Predominantly Inattentive Presentation:** It is difficult for the individual to organize or finish a task, to pay attention to details, or to follow instructions or conversations. The person is easily distracted or forgets details of daily routines. The presentation of these symptoms can be missed or misinterpreted by others as "laziness" or "not paying attention."
- **Predominantly Hyperactive-Impulsive Presentation:** The person fidgets and talks a lot. It is hard for them to sit still for a length of time (such as during a meal or while doing homework). Young children may run, jump, or climb constantly. The individual feels restless and has trouble with impulsivity. Someone who is impulsive may interrupt others, grab things from other people, or speak at inappropriate times. It is hard for the person to wait their turn or listen to directions. A person with impulsiveness may also have more accidents and injuries than others.
- **Combined Presentation:** Symptoms of the above two types are equally present in the person.

A person's symptoms of ADHD can change over time, and their predominant presentation may change over time as well.

Causes of ADHD

The cause(s) and risk factors for ADHD are unknown, but current research shows that genetics plays an important role. In addition to genetics, other possible risk factors include the following[9]:

- Brain injury
- Exposure to environmental risks (e.g., lead) during pregnancy or at a young age
- Alcohol and tobacco use during pregnancy
- Premature delivery
- Low birth weight

Research does not support popularly held views that ADHD is caused by eating too much sugar, watching too much television, or ineffective parenting. Many of these factors may worsen symptoms, especially in genetically predisposed people, but the evidence is not strong enough to conclude that they are the main causes of ADHD.[10]

Treatments for ADHD

Behavioral Therapy and Psychotherapy

In most cases, ADHD is best treated with a combination of behavior therapy and medication. For preschool-aged children (4-5 years old) with ADHD, parent training with behavioral management is recommended as the first

---

8 Centers for Disease Control and Prevention. (2021, September 23). *What is ADHD?* https://www.cdc.gov/ncbddd/adhd/facts.html

9 Centers for Disease Control and Prevention. (2021, September 23). *What is ADHD?* https://www.cdc.gov/ncbddd/adhd/facts.html

10 Centers for Disease Control and Prevention. (2021, September 23). *What is ADHD?* https://www.cdc.gov/ncbddd/adhd/facts.html

line of treatment before medication is prescribed. ADHD affects a child's ability to pay attention and sit still at school, as well as relationships with family and other children due to disruptive behaviors. Psychotherapy can improve a child's behavior, self-control, and self-esteem.[11] Read more in the "Psychological Therapies and Behavioral Interventions" section of this chapter.

Parent Education About Behavioral Management

Nurses can teach parents strategies for improving the behavior of their child or adolescent with ADHD[12]:

- **Create a routine.** Try to follow the same schedule every day, from wake-up time to bedtime.
- **Get organized.** Encourage your child to put school bags, clothing, and toys in the same place every day so that they will be less likely to lose them.
- **Manage distractions.** Turn off the TV, limit noise, and provide a clean workspace when your child is doing homework. Some children with ADHD learn better if they are moving or listening to background music.
- **Limit choices.** To help your child not feel overwhelmed or overstimulated, offer choices with only a few options. For example, have them choose between this outfit or that one, this meal or that one, or this toy or that one.
- **Be clear and specific when you talk with your child.** Let your child know you are listening by describing what you heard them say. Use clear, brief directions when they need to do something.
- **Help your child plan.** Break down complicated tasks into simpler, shorter steps. For long tasks, starting early and taking breaks may help limit stress.
- **Use goals and praise or other rewards.** Use a chart to list goals and track positive behaviors, and then let your child know they have done well by telling them or by rewarding their efforts in other ways. Be sure the goals are realistic because progress towards small steps is important to maintain a child's self-esteem.
- **Discipline effectively.** Instead of scolding, yelling, or spanking, use effective directions, time-outs, or removal of privileges as consequences for inappropriate behavior.
- **Create positive opportunities.** Children with ADHD may find certain situations stressful. Finding out and encouraging what your child does well, whether it's school, sports, art, music, or play, can help create positive experiences.
- **Provide a healthy lifestyle.** Nutritious food, lots of physical activity, and sufficient sleep are important for preventing ADHD symptoms from getting worse.
- **Communicate regularly with teachers.** Clear, regular communication between teachers and parents helps reinforce behavior management strategies at school and at home.

Parents can also be referred to ADHD support groups in the following box.

---

11 Centers for Disease Control and Prevention. (2021, September 23). *What is ADHD?* https://www.cdc.gov/ncbddd/adhd/facts.html

12 Centers for Disease Control and Prevention. (2021, September 23). *What is ADHD?* https://www.cdc.gov/ncbddd/adhd/facts.html

My Notes

Support Groups for ADHD

- CHADD: Information and resources on ADHD, including treatment options, local support groups for clients and parents, and online support communities
- Attention Deficit Disorder Association (ADDA): Information and resources on ADD for adults living with the disorder, including support groups and workshops
- Psychology Today Support Groups: Support groups near you for ADHD and other conditions

Medications

Medication may be prescribed to help children aged six and older manage their ADHD symptoms and help them control behaviors that cause difficulties with family, friends, and at school.[13]

Before medications are initiated, a comprehensive medical exam including height, weight, blood pressure, heart rate, and cardiovascular history should be performed. A pretreatment baseline should be established for common side effects such as appetite, sleep, headaches, and abdominal pain.

Adolescent clients should also be assessed for substance use.[14]

The choice of medication by the prescriber depends on many factors, such as the following[15]:

- Duration of coverage (e.g., desired coverage for school day plus completion of homework)
- The desire to avoid medication administration at school
- The ability of the child to swallow pills or capsules
- Coexisting emotional or behavioral conditions
- History of substance abuse in the client or a household member (i.e., stimulants with less abuse potential are prescribed)
- Expense
- Preferences of the child and their caregivers

Stimulants

Stimulants such as methylphenidate (Ritalin), dextroamphetamine (Dexedrine), and dextroamphetamine-amphetamine (Adderall) are considered first-line treatment because of rapid onset of action and a long record of safety and efficacy. Stimulants are available in short-, intermediate-, and long-acting formulations. The exact

---

13 Centers for Disease Control and Prevention. (2021, September 23). *What is ADHD?* https://www.cdc.gov/ncbddd/adhd/facts.html

14 Krull, K. R. (2022, January 29). Attention deficit hyperactivity disorder in children and adolescents: Treatment with medications. *UpToDate.* Retrieved February 19, 2022, from www.uptodate.com

15 Krull, K. R. (2022, January 29). Attention deficit hyperactivity disorder in children and adolescents: Treatment with medications. *UpToDate.* Retrieved February 19, 2022, from www.uptodate.com

mechanism of action of stimulants in ADHD is unknown, but they are known to affect the dopaminergic and noradrenergic systems, causing a release of catecholamines. Stimulants have been found to improve caregiver-child interactions, aggressive behavior, and academic productivity.[16]

Stimulants are controlled substances and require a Schedule II prescription.

Black Box Warning

CNS stimulants, including methylphenidate and amphetamine-like substances, have a high potential for abuse and dependence. The risk of abuse by the client or their family members should be assessed prior to prescribing stimulants, and signs of abuse and dependence should be evaluated while the client is receiving therapy.[17]

Side Effects

Stimulants may cause minor side effects that resolve when dosage levels are lowered or a different stimulant is prescribed. The most common side effects include the following[18,19]:

- Difficulty falling asleep or staying asleep
- Loss of appetite and weight loss
- Stomach pain
- Headache

Less common side effects include motor or verbal tics (sudden, repetitive movements or sounds) or personality changes (such as appearing "flat" or without emotion).[20] Sudden death, stroke, and myocardial infarction have been reported in adults with CNS-stimulant treatment at recommended doses. Sudden death has been reported in pediatric clients with structural cardiac abnormalities and other serious heart problems taking CNS stimulants at recommended doses. If paradoxical worsening of symptoms or other adverse reactions occur, the provider should be contacted, and the dosage reduced or discontinued. Stimulants are contraindicated in clients using a monoamine oxidase inhibitor (MAOI) or using an MAOI within the preceding 14 days.[21]

Nurses should be aware there is a possibility of diversion or misuse of stimulants by adolescents or their caregivers. Up to 29 percent of school- and college-aged students with stimulant prescriptions have been asked to give, sell, or trade their medication.[22]

---

16 Krull, K. R. (2022, January 29). Attention deficit hyperactivity disorder in children and adolescents: Treatment with medications. *UpToDate.* Retrieved February 19, 2022, from www.uptodate.com

17 This work is a derivative of *DailyMed* by U.S. National Library of Medicine and is available in the Public Domain

18 National Institute of Mental Health. (2016, October). *Mental health medications.* U.S. Department of Health & Human Services. https://www.nimh.nih.gov/health/topics/mental-health-medications

19 This work is a derivative of *DailyMed* by U.S. National Library of Medicine and is available in the Public Domain

20 National Institute of Mental Health. (2016, October). *Mental health medications.* U.S. Department of Health & Human Services. https://www.nimh.nih.gov/health/topics/mental-health-medications

21 This work is a derivative of *DailyMed* by U.S. National Library of Medicine and is available in the Public Domain

22 Krull, K. R. (2022, January 29). Attention deficit hyperactivity disorder in children and adolescents: Treatment with medications. *UpToDate.* Retrieved February 19, 2022, from www.uptodate.com

My Notes

Selective Norepinephrine Reuptake Inhibitors

Selective norepinephrine reuptake inhibitors (SNRIs) such as atomoxetine (Strattera) are an alternative to stimulants for clients who experience side effects with stimulants. They may also be helpful in treating concurrent depressive or anxiety disorders. SNRIs are not controlled substances, so they may be prescribed for adolescents (or their family members) with substance use disorders. The dosage depends on the child's weight, and the duration of action is 10 to 12 hours. Atomoxetine has a Black Box Warning about increased risk of suicidal thinking in children and adolescents.[23]

Alpha-2 Adrenergic Agonists

Alpha-2 adrenergic agonists such as clonidine are typically used when children respond poorly to stimulants or SNRIs, have unacceptable side effects, or have significant coexisting conditions.

Patient and Parent Education

There are several important patient education topics to provide to clients and/or the parents of minor children[24]:

- **Controlled Substance Status/High Potential for Abuse and Dependence:** Stimulants are a controlled substance by the FDA and can be abused and lead to dependence. Stimulants should be stored in a safe (preferably locked) place to prevent misuse and should not be shared with anyone. Unused or expired stimulants should be disposed of based on state law and regulations or returned to a medicine take-back program if it is available in the community.
- **Cardiovascular Risks:** Stimulants can increase one's blood pressure and pulse rate. There is a potential serious cardiovascular risk, including sudden death, cardiomyopathy, myocardial infarction, stroke, and hypertension. Instruct clients to contact a health care provider immediately if they develop symptoms, such as exertional chest pain, dizziness, or passing out.
- **Suppression of Growth:** Stimulants may cause slowing of growth in children and weight loss.
- **Psychiatric Risks:** Stimulants can cause psychosis or manic symptoms, even in clients who have no prior history of these symptoms.
- **Priapism:** Painful or prolonged penile erections can occur; seek immediate medical attention.
- **Alcohol:** Alcohol should be avoided when taking extended-release capsules.

Nurses should reinforce with the client and their family members that the reason for the prescribed medication is to help with self-control and the ability to focus. Possible side effects should be reviewed, and clients and their family members should be reminded it may take one to three months to determine the best pharmacological treatment, dose, and frequency of medication administration. During this time, the child's symptoms and adverse effects will be monitored weekly and the medication dose adjusted accordingly.[25]

---

23 Krull, K. R. (2022, January 29). Attention deficit hyperactivity disorder in children and adolescents: Treatment with medications. *UpToDate.* Retrieved February 19, 2022, from www.uptodate.com

24 This work is a derivative of *DailyMed* by U.S. National Library of Medicine and is available in the Public Domain

25 Krull, K. R. (2022, January 29). Attention deficit hyperactivity disorder in children and adolescents: Treatment with medications. *UpToDate.* Retrieved February 19, 2022, from www.uptodate.com

My Notes

ADHD Into Adulthood

ADHD lasts into adulthood for at least one third of children with ADHD. Treatments for adults can include medication, psychotherapy, or a combination of treatments.[26]

Anxiety

All children experience some anxiety, and anxiety is expected at specific times of a child's development. For example, from approximately age 8 months through the preschool years, healthy youngsters may show anxiety when separated from their parents or caregivers. Young children also commonly have fears, such as fear of the dark, storms, animals, or strangers.[27] Anxiety is functional and normal when situational. Consider the fear of dangerous situations such as approaching a rattlesnake or standing on a steep cliff; at crucial times anxiety is important because it provides safety. Anxiety is also motivational as it drives adolescents to accomplish goals such as passing a test by working hard and studying.

When a child is overly worried or anxious, a nurse's initial assessment should determine if conditions in the child's environment are causing this feeling. For example, is the anxiety resulting from being bullied or from adverse childhood experiences (ACEs)? If so, protective interventions should be put into place. If no realistic threat exists and the anxiety causes significant life dysfunction, then the child should be referred to a mental health provider to determine if an anxiety disorder exists.[28]

Read more about "Adverse Childhood Experiences" in the "Trauma, Abuse, and Violence" chapter.

Symptoms of Anxiety Disorder in Children and Adolescents

Children with anxiety disorders are overly tense or fearful; some may seek lots of reassurance; and their worries may interfere with daily activities. Because anxious children may also be quiet, compliant, and eager to please, their feelings of anxiety can be easily missed. When a child does not outgrow the typical fears and anxieties in childhood or when there are so many fears and worries they interfere with school, home, or play activities, the child may be diagnosed with an anxiety disorder. Examples of symptoms related to different types of anxiety disorders in children and adolescents include the following[29]:

- Being very afraid when away from parents or caregivers (i.e., **separation anxiety**)
- Having extreme fear about a specific thing or situation, such as dogs, insects, or going to the doctor (i.e., phobias)
- Being very afraid of school and other places where there are people (i.e., social anxiety)

---

26 Centers for Disease Control and Prevention. (2021, September 23). *What is ADHD?* https://www.cdc.gov/ncbddd/adhd/facts.html

27 American Academy of Child & Adolescent Psychiatry. (2017, October). *Anxiety and children.* https://www.aacap.org/AACAP/Families_and_Youth/Facts_for_Families/FFF-Guide/The-Anxious-Child-047.aspx

28 Hilt, R. J., & Nussbaum, A. M. (Eds.). (2016). *DSM-5 pocket guide for child and adolescent mental health.* https://doi.org/10.1176/appi.books.9781615370511

29 Centers for Disease Control and Prevention. (2021, March 22). *Children's mental disorders.* https://www.cdc.gov/childrensmentalhealth/symptoms.html

My Notes

- Being very worried about the future and about bad things happening (i.e., general anxiety)
- Having repeated episodes of sudden, unexpected, intense fear associated with symptoms like fast heart rate, trouble breathing, dizziness, or shakiness (i.e., panic disorder)

Anxiety can also make children irritable and angry and can include physical symptoms like fatigue, headaches, stomachaches, or trouble sleeping.[30]

Treatment of Anxiety Disorders in Children and Adolescents

Early treatment of anxiety disorders in children can enhance friendships, social and academic potential, and self-esteem. Interprofessional treatments often include a combination of individual psychotherapy and behavioral therapy, family therapy, medications, and consultations with the child's school.[31] Read more about psychological and behavioral treatments for children and adolescents in the "Psychological Therapies and Behavioral Interventions" section.

Read additional information about anxiety disorders and associated treatments in the "Anxiety Disorders" chapter. Post-traumatic stress disorder (PTSD) can develop in children or adolescents who have experienced a shocking, frightening, or dangerous event. It has similar symptoms to severe anxiety. Read more in the "Post-Traumatic Stress Disorder" section of the "Anxiety Disorders" chapter. There is also an association between obsessive-compulsive disorder (OCD) and children who have been exposed to trauma. Read more in the "Obsessive-Compulsive Disorder" section of the "Anxiety Disorders" chapter.

Depression

Every child, adolescent, and adult feels sad occasionally. However, some children feel sad, hopeless, or uninterested in things they previously enjoyed. When a child appears withdrawn or sad for two or more weeks, they may be diagnosed with a depressive disorder.[32]

Symptoms of Depressive Disorders in Children and Adolescents

Examples of behaviors observed in children and adolescents with a depressive disorder are as follows[33]:

- Feeling sad, hopeless, or irritable most of the time
- Not wanting to do or enjoy fun things
- Showing changes in eating patterns (e.g., eating a lot more or a lot less than usual)
- Showing changes in sleep patterns (e.g., sleeping a lot more or a lot less than normal)
- Showing changes in energy (e.g., being tired and sluggish or tense and restless most of the time)
- Difficulty paying attention

30 Centers for Disease Control and Prevention. (2021, March 22). *Children's mental disorders.* https://www.cdc.gov/childrensmentalhealth/symptoms.html

31 Centers for Disease Control and Prevention. (2021, March 22). *Children's mental disorders.* https://www.cdc.gov/childrensmentalhealth/symptoms.html

32 Centers for Disease Control and Prevention. (2021, March 22). *Children's mental disorders.* https://www.cdc.gov/childrensmentalhealth/symptoms.html

33 American Academy of Child & Adolescent Psychiatry. (2017, October). *Anxiety and children.* https://www.aacap.org/AACAP/Families_and_Youth/Facts_for_Families/FFF-Guide/The-Anxious-Child-047.aspx

My Notes

- Feeling worthless, useless, or guilty
- Engaging in self-injury or self-destructive behavior
- Having suicidal thoughts or making a plan for suicide
- Exhibiting physical complaints, such as frequent headaches or stomachaches
- Using alcohol or drugs as a way of trying to feel better

Depression might also cause a child to appear unmotivated or act out, causing others to incorrectly label the child as "lazy" or a "trouble-maker."[34]

It is important to ask children and adolescents who are withdrawn or sad about self-harm risks. Adolescents may perceive a single disappointment (such as a relationship break-up) as so catastrophic they feel suicidal or begin to hurt themselves.[35]

The cause of depression is not always known. Depression can be hereditary but can also be situational or environmental. Some causes of depression are increased stress, death of a family member or close friend, social media, and bullying. Having other conditions such as attention problems, learning disorders, anxiety, or conduct disorders creates a higher risk for depression.[36]

Treatment of Depressive Disorders in Children and Adolescents

If a child or adolescent is suspected to have depression, a nurse or school counselor can refer them to a mental health professional to conduct a comprehensive assessment and plan effective treatments. Treatment may include psychotherapy, behavioral therapy with the child and their family members, and collaboration with the child's school. Cognitive behavioral therapy (CBT), interpersonal psychotherapy (IPT), and antidepressant medications are effective in treating depression in children. Read more about behavioral treatments in the "Psychological Therapies and Behavioral Interventions" section.

Read more about depression in the "Depressive Disorders" chapter.

Behavior Disorders

Children sometimes argue or act angry or defiant around adults. However, a behavior disorder is diagnosed when disruptive behaviors are uncommon for the child's age, persist over time, or are severe. Two types of behavior disorders are oppositional conduct disorder and conduct disorder.[37]

---

34 Centers for Disease Control and Prevention. (2021, March 22). *Children's mental disorders.* https://www.cdc.gov/childrensmentalhealth/symptoms.html

35 Hilt, R. J., & Nussbaum, A. M. (Eds.). (2016). *DSM-5 pocket guide for child and adolescent mental health.* https://doi.org/10.1176/appi.books.9781615370511

36 American Academy of Child & Adolescent Psychiatry. (2017, October). *Anxiety and children.* https://www.aacap.org/AACAP/Families_and_Youth/Facts_for_Families/FFF-Guide/The-Anxious-Child-047.aspx

37 American Academy of Child & Adolescent Psychiatry. (2019, January). *Oppositional defiant disorder.* https://www.aacap.org/aacap/families_and_youth/facts_for_families/fff-guide/Children-With-Oppositional-Defiant-Disorder-072.aspx

My Notes

Oppositional Defiant Disorder

All children are oppositional from time to time, particularly when they are feeling tired, hungry, stressed, or upset. They may argue, talk back, disobey, and defy parents, teachers, or other adults. Oppositional behavior is considered a normal part of development for children two to three years of age and early adolescents. However, uncooperative and hostile behavior becomes a serious concern when it is so frequent and consistent that it stands out when compared with other children of the same age or when it significantly affects the child's social, family, and academic life.[38]

When children act out persistently causing serious problems at home, in school, or with peers, they may be diagnosed with **oppositional defiant disorder (ODD)**. Up to 16 percent of all school-age children and adolescents have ODD. ODD usually starts before 8 years of age but no later than 12 years of age. Children with ODD are more likely to act oppositionally or defiantly around people they know well, such as family members, a regular care provider, or a teacher.[39]

Examples of ODD behaviors include the following[40]:

- Often being angry or losing one's temper
- Often arguing with adults or refusing to comply with adults' rules or requests
- Often being resentful or spiteful
- Deliberately annoying others or becoming annoyed with others
- Often blaming other people for one's own mistakes or misbehavior

Many children with ODD may have coexisting conditions such as anxiety, post-traumatic stress disorder (PTSD), ADHD, autism, learning disabilities, or substance abuse. See Figure 12.2[41] for an illustration of conditions that can be mistaken for ODD.

---

38 American Academy of Child & Adolescent Psychiatry. (2019, January). *Oppositional defiant disorder.* https://www.aacap.org/aacap/families_and_youth/facts_for_families/fff-guide/Children-With-Oppositional-Defiant-Disorder-072.aspx

39 Centers for Disease Control and Prevention. (2021, March 22). *Behavior or conduct problems in children.* https://www.cdc.gov/childrensmentalhealth/behavior.html#conduct

40 Centers for Disease Control and Prevention. (2021, March 22). *Behavior or conduct problems in children.* https://www.cdc.gov/childrensmentalhealth/behavior.html#conduct

41 "Instead_of_Oppositional_Defiant_Disorder_1_Wide.png" by MissLunaRose12 is licensed under CC BY-SA 4.0

My Notes

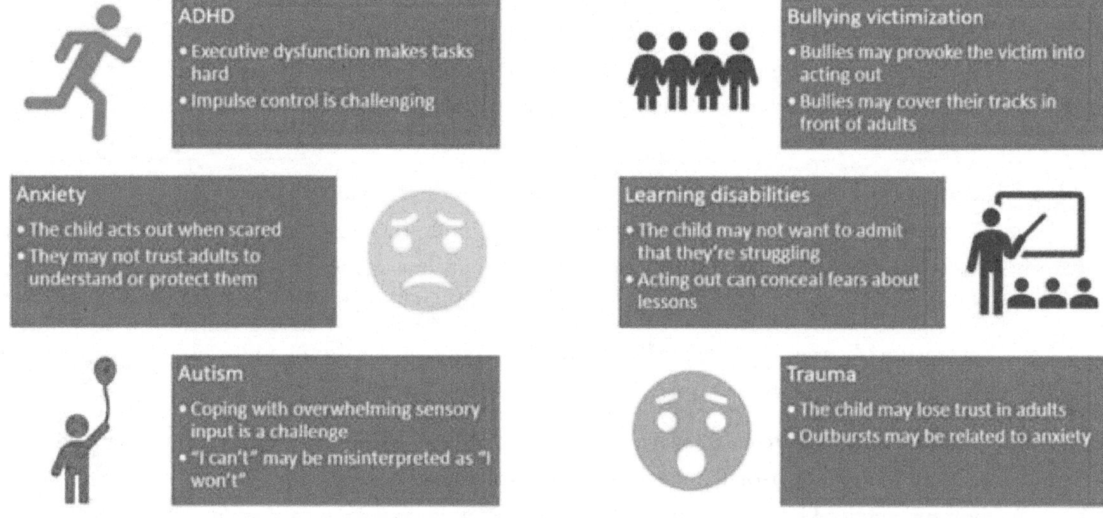

Figure 12.2 Conditions That Can Be Mistaken for Oppositional Defiant Disorder

Treatment of ODD

Treatment of ODD includes the following[42]:

- Parent behavioral management training to help parents manage the child's behavior
- Individual psychotherapy to develop more effective anger management skills
- Family psychotherapy to improve communication and mutual understanding
- Cognitive behavioral therapy and other psychotherapies to decrease negativity and enhance effective problem-solving
- Social skills training to increase flexibility and improve frustration tolerance with peers

Medications may be prescribed to control distressing symptoms of ODD, as well as symptoms related to coexisting conditions such as ADHD, anxiety, and mood disorders.[43]

---

42 American Academy of Child & Adolescent Psychiatry. (2019, January). *Oppositional defiant disorder.* https://www.aacap.org/aacap/families_and_youth/facts_for_families/fff-guide/Children-With-Oppositional-Defiant-Disorder-072.aspx

43 American Academy of Child & Adolescent Psychiatry. (2019, January). *Oppositional defiant disorder.* https://www.aacap.org/aacap/families_and_youth/facts_for_families/fff-guide/Children-With-Oppositional-Defiant-Disorder-072.aspx

My Notes

Parent Education

Parents of children diagnosed with ODD need support and understanding. Nurses can teach parents to help their child with ODD in the following ways[44]:

- **Build on the positives.** Give the child praise and positive reinforcement when they show flexibility or cooperation. Discipline will not work if there are no positive interactions.
- **Take a time-out or break.** If conflict with your child is progressively getting worse instead of better, take a time-out break. Demonstration of taking a break is also good modeling for the child. If the child decides to take a time-out to prevent overreacting, they should receive support for doing so.
- **Prioritize your battles.** Because the child with ODD has trouble avoiding power struggles, prioritize the things you want your child to do. For example, if you give your child a time-out in their room for misbehavior, don't add time to the time-out for arguing. Instead, calmly say, "Your time will start when you go to your room." Listen when they shout, but do not shout back.
- **Set reasonable, age-appropriate limits and consequences.** Set limits and establish consequences that can be enforced consistently.
- **Maintain other interests.** Manage your stress with healthy life choices such as exercise and relaxation. Maintain personal interests so that managing your child with ODD doesn't take all your time and energy. Use respite care and other breaks as needed.
- **Obtain support.** Collaborate and obtain support from other adults working with your child (e.g., teachers and coaches).

Conduct Disorder

Conduct disorder (CD) is diagnosed when a child shows an ongoing pattern of aggression toward others with serious violations of rules and social norms at home, school, and with peers. These rule violations may involve breaking the law and result in arrest.[45] Adults with antisocial conduct disorder typically show symptoms of CD before age 15.[46]

Examples of CD behaviors are as follows[47]:

- Breaking serious rules, such as running away, staying out all night, or skipping school
- Being aggressive in a way that causes harm, such as bullying, fighting, or being cruel to animals
- Lying, stealing, or purposefully damaging other people's property

---

44 American Academy of Child & Adolescent Psychiatry. (2019, January). *Oppositional defiant disorder*. https://www.aacap.org/aacap/families_and_youth/facts_for_families/fff-guide/Children-With-Oppositional-Defiant-Disorder-072.aspx

45 Centers for Disease Control and Prevention. (2021, March 22). *Behavior or conduct problems in children*. https://www.cdc.gov/childrensmentalhealth/behavior.html#conduct

46 Mayo Clinic. (2019, December 10.) *Antisocial personality disorder*. https://www.mayoclinic.org/diseases-conditions/antisocial-personality-disorder/symptoms-causes/syc-20353928#:~:text=Adults%20with%20antisocial%20personality%20disorder,Destruction%20of%20property

47 Centers for Disease Control and Prevention. (2021, March 22). *Behavior or conduct problems in children*. https://www.cdc.gov/childrensmentalhealth/behavior.html#conduct

My Notes

Children who exhibit these serious behaviors should receive a comprehensive evaluation and treatment by a mental health professional. Some signs of behavior problems, such as not following rules in school, can be related to learning disorders that require additional assessment and interventions. Without treatment, many youngsters with conduct disorder are likely to have ongoing problems resulting in the inability to adapt to the demands of adulthood.[48]

Treatment for CD

Starting treatment early for CD is important. For younger children, research indicates the most effective treatment is behavior therapy training for parents where a therapist helps the parent learn effective ways to strengthen the parent-child relationship and respond to the child's behavior. For school-age children and teens, a combination of behavior therapy training that includes the child, the family, and the school is most effective.[49] Read more about treatment in the "Psychological Therapies and Behavioral Interventions" section.

Developmental Disabilities

Developmental disabilities are a group of conditions with physical, learning, language, or behavioral impairments. These conditions begin during the developmental period, may impact day-to-day functioning, and usually last throughout a person's lifetime.[50] Research indicates about 17% of children are diagnosed with a developmental disability such as blindness, hearing loss, learning disability, intellectual disability, stuttering, attention deficit hyperactivity disorder (ADHD), or autism spectrum disorder.[51]

Keep in mind that having a developmental disability does not mean the person is not healthy. Being healthy means staying well so one can lead a full, active life.[52]

 Read more information about autism in the "Autism Spectrum Disorder" section and ADHD in the "Attention Disorder and Hyperactivity Disorder" subsection presented earlier in this section.

Causes and Risk Factors

Developmental disabilities begin anytime during the developmental period and usually last throughout a person's lifetime. Most developmental disabilities begin before a baby is born, but some can occur after birth because of injury, infection, or other factors. Many developmental disabilities are thought to be caused by a complex mix

---

48 American Academy of Child & Adolescent Psychiatry. (2018, June). *Conduct disorder.* https://www.aacap.org/aacap/families_and_youth/facts_for_families/fff-guide/conduct-disorder-033.aspx

49 American Academy of Child & Adolescent Psychiatry. (2018, June). *Conduct disorder.* https://www.aacap.org/aacap/families_and_youth/facts_for_families/fff-guide/conduct-disorder-033.aspx

50 Centers for Disease Control and Prevention. (2021, September 13). *Increase in developmental disabilities among children in the United States.* https://www.cdc.gov/ncbddd/developmentaldisabilities/features/increase-in-developmental-disabilities.html

51 Centers for Disease Control and Prevention. (2021, September 13). *Increase in developmental disabilities among children in the United States.* https://www.cdc.gov/ncbddd/developmentaldisabilities/features/increase-in-developmental-disabilities.html

52 Centers for Disease Control and Prevention. (2021, September 13). *Increase in developmental disabilities among children in the United States.* https://www.cdc.gov/ncbddd/developmentaldisabilities/features/increase-in-developmental-disabilities.html

My Notes

of factors including genetics, parental health and behaviors (such as maternal infections or substance use during pregnancy), complications during birth, infections the baby had very early in life, or exposure of the mother or child to high levels of environmental toxins, such as lead. However, there is no known cause for most developmental disabilities.[53]

Diagnosis of Developmental Disabilities

Developmental disabilities are diagnosed by developmental monitoring and developmental screening through a partnership between parents and health care professionals as a child's growth and development are monitored.

Every child should receive routine screenings for developmental delays at their well-child visits. During a well-child visit, the provider performs **developmental monitoring** by observing for signs of developmental delays and talking with parents about any concerns they might have about their child's growth and development. If any problems are noted during developmental monitoring, **developmental screening** is performed. Standardized tools used during developmental screening are formal questionnaires or checklists based on research that ask questions about a child's development, including language, movement, thinking, behavior, and emotions. Developmental screening can be done by a doctor or nurse but may also be performed by other professionals in health care, early childhood education, community, or school settings to determine if a child is learning as expected or if there are delays.[54]

View an image of developmental milestones in Figure 12.3.[55]

---

53 Centers for Disease Control and Prevention. (2021, September 13). *Facts about developmental disabilities.* https://www.cdc.gov/ncbddd/developmentaldisabilities/facts.html

54 Centers for Disease Control and Prevention. (2021, September 13). *Facts about developmental disabilities.* https://www.cdc.gov/ncbddd/developmentaldisabilities/facts.html

55 "Vroom-Poster_14x8.5_FNL-508" by National Center on Birth Defects and Developmental Disabilities, Centers for Disease Control and Prevention is in the Public Domain

My Notes

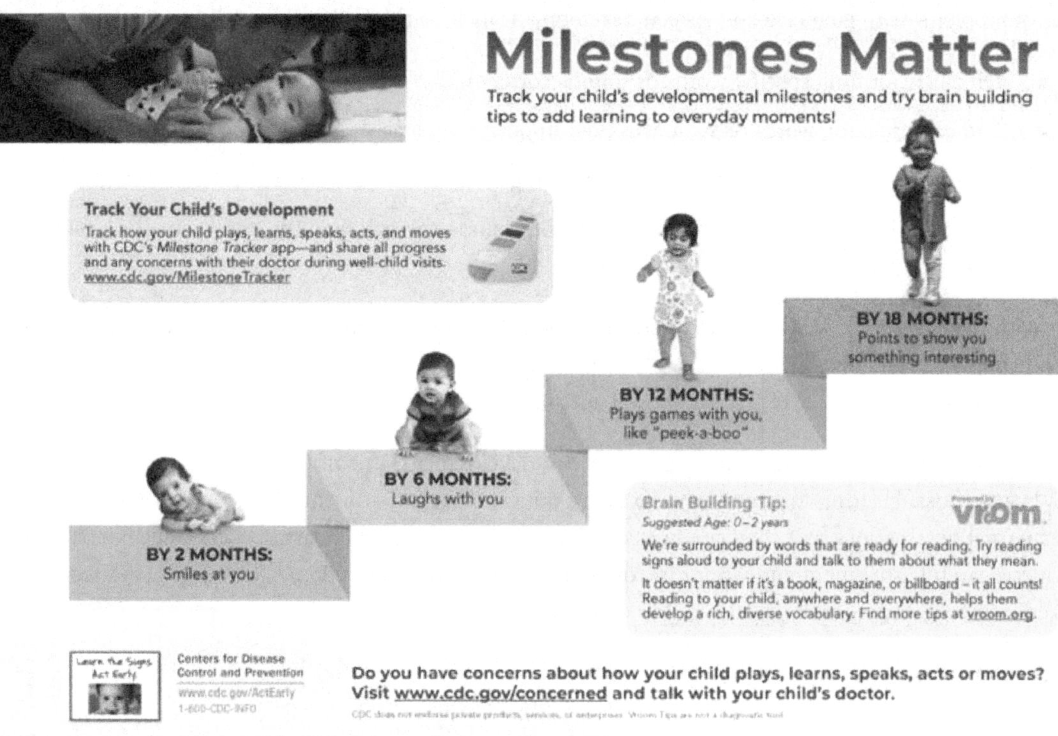

Figure 12.3 Developmental Milestones

View the CDC's Developmental Milestones and Milestone Checklists PDF.

Types of Disorders

Based on developmental screenings, children may require further evaluation for language and speech disorders, learning disorders, and intellectual disabilities.

Language and Speech Disorders

Some children struggle with understanding language and speaking. If they do not achieve the developmental milestones for language, it can be a sign of a language or speech disorder.[56]

Language development has many components. Children might have problems with one or more of the following[57]:

- **Receptive Language:** Difficulty understanding what others say due to not hearing the words (hearing loss) or not understanding the meaning of the words.
- **Expressive Language:** Difficulty communicating thoughts using language due to not knowing the words to use, not knowing how to put words together, or not being able to express the words.

---

56 Centers for Disease Control and Prevention. (2021, February 22). *Language and speech disorders in children.* https://www.cdc.gov/ncbddd/childdevelopment/language-disorders.html

57 Centers for Disease Control and Prevention. (2021, February 22). *Language and speech disorders in children.* https://www.cdc.gov/ncbddd/childdevelopment/language-disorders.html

My Notes

Examples of problems with language and speech development include the following conditions[58]:

- Difficulty forming specific words or sounds correctly
- Difficulty making words or sentences flow smoothly, such as stuttering
- Difficulty understanding language and speaking language
- Difficulty understanding the meaning of the sounds the ear sends to the brain (i.e., auditory processing disorder)

Children with language disorders may feel frustrated when they cannot understand others or make themselves understood and, as a result, may act out, act helpless, or withdraw. Language or speech disorders may also be present with other disorders such as ADHD, anxiety, or autism.[59]

If a child experiences difficulties with language or speech development, it is important to first determine if the child has hearing loss. Hearing loss may be difficult to notice, especially if a child has hearing loss in only one ear or has partial hearing loss (i.e., they can hear certain sounds but not others). A speech-language pathologist will conduct a careful assessment and work directly with the child and their parents, caregivers, and teachers for customized interventions according to the child's condition.[60]

Learning Disorders

Many children may struggle with learning certain topics or skills in school from time to time. However, when children struggle with learning specific skills over time, it can be a sign of a learning disorder. Having a **learning disorder** means that a child has difficulty in one or more areas of learning, even when their overall intelligence or motivation are not affected.[61]

Some symptoms of learning disorders are as follows[62]:

- Difficulty telling right from left
- Reversing letters, words, or numbers, after the first or second grade
- Difficulties recognizing patterns or sorting items by size or shape
- Difficulty understanding and following instructions or staying organized
- Difficulty remembering what was just said or what was just read
- Lacking coordination when moving around

---

58 Centers for Disease Control and Prevention. (2021, February 22). *Language and speech disorders in children.* https://www.cdc.gov/ncbddd/childdevelopment/language-disorders.html

59 Centers for Disease Control and Prevention. (2021, February 22). *Language and speech disorders in children.* https://www.cdc.gov/ncbddd/childdevelopment/language-disorders.html

60 Centers for Disease Control and Prevention. (2021, February 22). *Language and speech disorders in children.* https://www.cdc.gov/ncbddd/childdevelopment/language-disorders.html

61 Centers for Disease Control and Prevention. (2021, February 22). *Learning disorders in children.* https://www.cdc.gov/ncbddd/childdevelopment/learning-disorder.html

62 Centers for Disease Control and Prevention. (2021, February 22). *Learning disorders in children.* https://www.cdc.gov/ncbddd/childdevelopment/learning-disorder.html

My Notes

- Difficulty doing tasks with the hands, like writing, cutting, or drawing
- Difficulty understanding the concept of time

Examples of learning disorders include the following[63]:

- **Dyslexia:** Difficulty with reading
- **Dyscalculia:** Difficulty with math
- **Dysgraphia:** Difficulty with writing

Children with learning disorders may feel frustrated when they cannot learn a topic or skill (despite trying hard to do so) and may act out, act helpless, or withdraw. Learning disorders may also be present with other disorders, such as ADHD or anxiety, making it hard for a child to succeed in school. Children with learning disorders often require specialized instruction to meet their needs.[64]

Intellectual Disabilities

Intellectual disability is defined in the *Diagnostic and Statistical Manual of Mental Disorders (DSM5)* as a disorder with onset during the developmental period that includes both intellectual and adaptive functioning deficits in conceptual, social, and practical domains. The following criteria must be met for an individual to be diagnosed with an intellectual disability[65]:

- Deficits in intellectual functions, such as reasoning, problem-solving, planning, abstract thinking, judgment, academic learning, and learning from experience that is confirmed by both clinical assessment and individualized, standardized intelligence testing.
- Deficits in adaptive functioning that result in failure to meet developmental and sociocultural standards for personal independence and social responsibility. Without ongoing support, the adaptive deficits limit functioning in one or more activities of daily life, such as communication, social participation, and independent living, across multiple environments such as home, school, work, and the community.
- Onset of intellectual and adaptive deficits occurs during the developmental period.

Levels of intellectual disability vary greatly in children. Children with an intellectual disability might have a hard time communicating their needs, and an intellectual disability can cause them to develop more slowly than other children of the same age. Intellectual disability can be caused by a problem that starts any time before birth to when a child turns 18 years old. It can be caused by injury, disease, or other dysfunction in the brain. For many children, the cause of their intellectual disability is not known.[66]

---

63 Centers for Disease Control and Prevention. (2021, February 22). *Learning disorders in children.* https://www.cdc.gov/ncbddd/childdevelopment/learning-disorder.html

64 Centers for Disease Control and Prevention. (2021, February 22). *Learning disorders in children.* https://www.cdc.gov/ncbddd/childdevelopment/learning-disorder.html

65 American Psychiatric Association. (2013). *Desk reference to the diagnostic criteria from DSM-5.*

66 Centers for Disease Control and Prevention. (2021, August 24). *Facts about intellectual disabilities in children.* https://www.cdc.gov/ncbddd/childdevelopment/facts-about-intellectual-disability.html

My Notes

The more severe the degree of intellectual disability, the earlier the signs can be noticed during developmental monitoring, such as the following[67]:

- Sitting up, crawling, or walking later than other children
- Talking later than other children or having trouble speaking
- Difficulty remembering things
- Difficulty understanding social rules
- Difficulty seeing the results of their actions
- Difficulty solving problems

Children who are suspected to have an intellectual disability based on developmental screening are referred to a developmental pediatrician or other specialist for treatment.

Tics and Tourette Syndrome

Tourette syndrome (TS) and other tic disorders affect approximately 1% of school-aged children in the United States.[68] **Tics** are sudden twitches, movements, or sounds that people do repeatedly with the inability to stop their body from doing these actions. There are two types of tics: motor and vocal. **Motor tics** are movements of the body such as blinking, shrugging the shoulders, or jerking an arm. **Vocal tics** are sounds that a person makes with his or her voice such as grunting, humming, clearing the throat, or yelling out a word or phrase. Although the media often portray people with TS as involuntarily shouting out swear words (i.e., coprolalia) or constantly repeating the words of other people (i.e., echolalia), these symptoms are rare.[69]

The primary symptom of Tourette syndrome (TS) is tics that typically begin when a child is 5 to 10 years old. The first symptoms are often motor tics that occur in the head and neck area. Tics are often worse during times that are stressful or exciting and tend to improve when a person is calm or focused on an activity.[70]

In most cases, tics decrease during adolescence and early adulthood, and sometimes disappear entirely. However, many people with TS experience tics into adulthood and, in some cases, tics can become worse during adulthood.[71]

Tics are typically mild and do not require treatment, but it is essential to educate the individual and others about TS and provide appropriate support across all settings (e.g., school, work, and home). When tics become problematic or interfere with daily functioning, behavioral treatment or medication may be considered.[72]

---

67 Centers for Disease Control and Prevention. (2021, August 24). *Facts about intellectual disabilities in children.* https://www.cdc.gov/ncbddd/childdevelopment/facts-about-intellectual-disability.html

68 Tourette Association of American. (n.d.). *What is Tourette.* https://tourette.org/about-tourette/overview/what-is-tourette/#1461071628539-4f1f68e0-cd8d

69 Centers for Disease Control and Prevention. (2021, April 20). *What is Tourette syndrome?* https://www.cdc.gov/ncbddd/tourette/facts.html

70 Centers for Disease Control and Prevention. (2021, April 20). *What is Tourette syndrome?* https://www.cdc.gov/ncbddd/tourette/facts.html

71 Centers for Disease Control and Prevention. (2021, April 20). *What is Tourette syndrome?* https://www.cdc.gov/ncbddd/tourette/facts.html

72 Tourette Association of American. (n.d.). *What is Tourette.* https://tourette.org/about-tourette/overview/what-is-tourette/#1461071628539-4f1f68e0-cd8d

My Notes

View a video of individuals with tics: Tourette Syndrome Is . . . [73]

To read more about Tourette syndrome and tics, go to the Tourette Association of America.

Substance Use Disorders

Children and adolescents use alcohol and other substances for many reasons that may include maladaptive coping strategies. Alcohol is the most commonly used substance among young people in the United States. Data from several national surveys document frequent use of alcohol among young people. The 2019 Youth Risk Behavior Survey found these statistics among high school students during the past 30 days[74]:

- 29% drank alcohol.
- 14% binge drank.
- 5% of drivers drove after drinking alcohol.
- 17% rode with a driver who had been drinking alcohol.

Binge drinking is defined as a pattern of alcohol consumption that brings the blood alcohol concentration level to 0.08% or more. This pattern of drinking usually corresponds to five or more drinks on a single occasion for males or four or more drinks on a single occasion for females within about two hours.

Youth who binge drink alcohol are more likely to experience these issues[75]:

- School problems, such as higher rates of absences or lower grades
- Social problems, such as fighting or lack of participation in youth activities
- Legal problems, such as arrest for driving or physically hurting someone while drunk
- Physical problems, such as hangovers or illnesses
- Unwanted, unplanned, and unprotected sexual activity
- Disruption of normal growth or sexual development
- Physical and sexual violence
- Increased risk of suicide and homicide
- Alcohol-related motor vehicle crashes and other unintentional injuries, such as burns, falls, or drowning
- Memory problems
- Misuse of other substances

---

73 Tourette Association of American. (2018, January 24). *Tourette Syndrome is . . .* [Video]. YouTube. All rights reserved. https://youtu.be/M8clZP-PI2Y

74 Centers for Disease Control and Prevention. (2021, October 6). *Underage drinking.* https://www.cdc.gov/alcohol/fact-sheets/underage-drinking.htm

75 Centers for Disease Control and Prevention. (2021, October 6). *Underage drinking.* https://www.cdc.gov/alcohol/fact-sheets/underage-drinking.htm

My Notes

- Changes in brain development that may have lifelong effects
- Alcohol poisoning

Substance use disorders occur when the recurrent use of alcohol and/or drugs causes clinically significant impairment, including health problems, disability, and failure to meet major responsibilities at work, school, or home. The 2019 National Survey on Drug Use and Health reports that approximately 20.3 million people aged 12 or older had a substance use disorder in the past year.[76]

The Substance Abuse and Mental Health Services Administration (SAMHSA) has developed a national campaign called "Talk. They Hear You" to help parents and caregivers start talking with their children early about the dangers of alcohol and other drugs.[77] See Figure 12.4[78] for an example of a public service announcement from the "Talk. They Hear You" campaign.

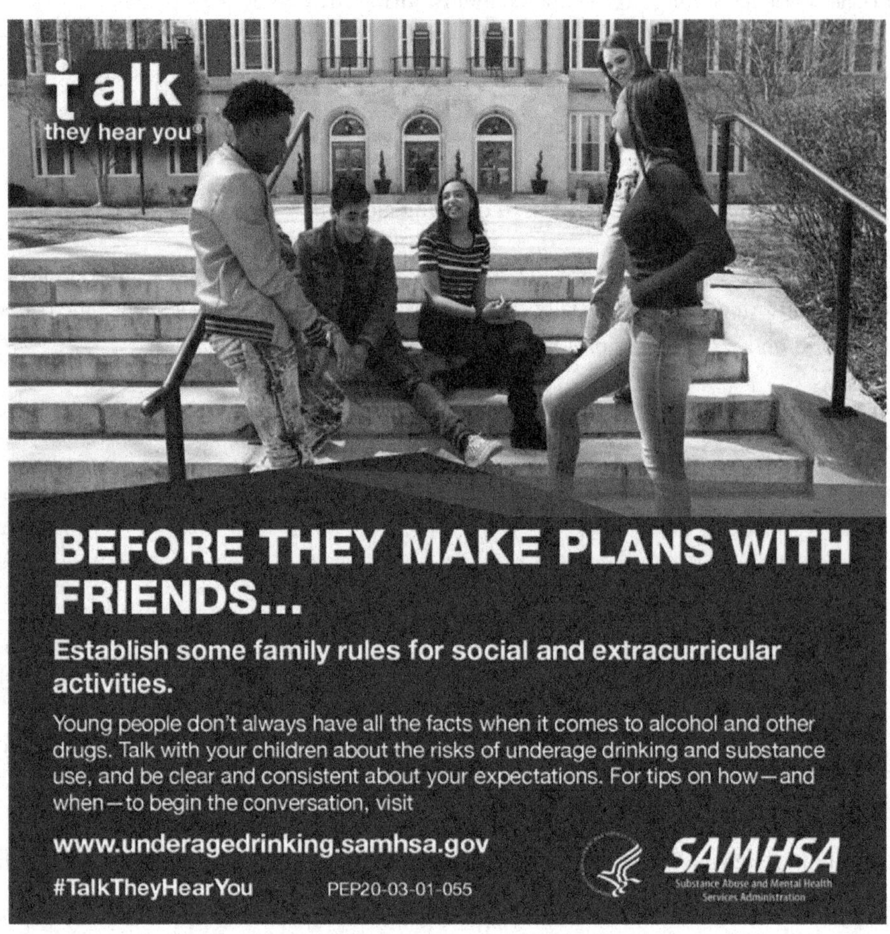

Figure 12.4 Image from "Talk. They Hear You" Campaign

---

76 Substance Abuse and Mental Health Services Administration. (2021, October 14). *Prevention of substance use and mental disorders.* https://www.samhsa.gov/find-help/prevention

77 Substance Abuse and Mental Health Services Administration. (2021, October 14). *Prevention of substance use and mental disorders.* https://www.samhsa.gov/find-help/prevention

78 "TTHY-friends-square-2020" by Substance Abuse and Mental Health Services Administration (SAMHSA) is in the Public Domain

Read more information in the "Substance Use Disorders" chapter.

My Notes

Gender Dysphoria

Distinctions between gender, sexual orientation, and sexual behavior are a critical concept in adolescent health and are greatly influenced by one's culture. Gender is assigned at birth based on the medical assessment of genitalia. Anatomical characteristics and chromosomes determine whether a person is biologically male or female. Gender identity, gender roles, and gender expression are psychological and cultural constructs referring to various aspects of maleness, femaleness, or other nonbinary designation.[79]

Gender identity is an individual's innate sense of being male, female, androgenous (i.e., of indeterminant sex), nonbinary (i.e., a blend of both genders or don't identify with either gender), or a preference to reject gender designation. An individual's gender identity is generally established during early childhood but may evolve across their life span. **Gender roles** are social constructs based on masculinity and femininity that embody one's culture's expectations, attitudes, behaviors, and personality traits based on one's biological sex. **Gender expression** refers to how an individual presents one's gender to the outside world, but it does not necessarily correlate with their gender identity.[80]

An individual's gender identity is influenced during early childhood by one's parents and immediate family members defining how a person expresses themselves as members of their gender. As children become adolescents, their influences broaden with peer, media, and community norms of gender and sexuality impacting their individual value systems.[81]

When a person's biological sex differs from their gender identity, they experience feelings of unease about their incongruent maleness or femaleness referred to as **gender dysphoria**. For example, a biologic male with an innate sense of being female may describe himself as "a woman trapped in a man's body."[82] People who are **transgender** have a gender identity or gender expression that differs from the sex they were assigned at birth. See Figure 12.5[83] for an image of a person displaying a sign at a rally for transgender equality.

---

79 Forcier, M. (2021, July 24). Adolescent sexuality. *UpToDate*. Retrieved February 22, 2022, from www.uptodate.com

80 Forcier, M. (2021, July 24). Adolescent sexuality. *UpToDate*. Retrieved February 22, 2022, from www.uptodate.com

81 Forcier, M. (2021, July 24). Adolescent sexuality. *UpToDate*. Retrieved February 22, 2022, from www.uptodate.com

82 Forcier, M. (2021, July 24). Adolescent sexuality. *UpToDate*. Retrieved February 22, 2022, from www.uptodate.com

83 "2013_Rally_for_Transgender_Equality_21175.jpg" by Ted Eytan is licensed under CC BY-SA 2.0

My Notes

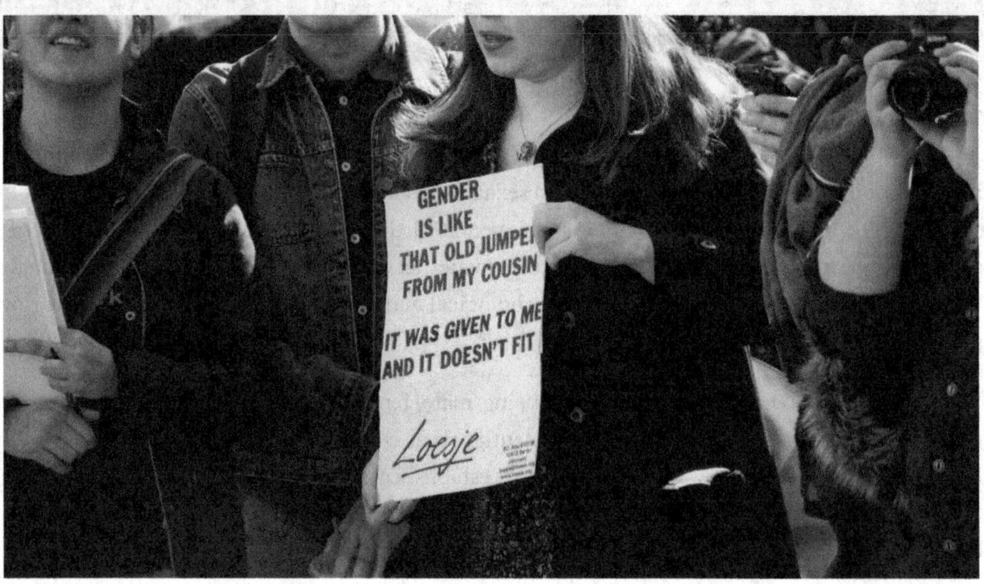

Figure 12.5 Transgender Equality Rally

Gender Dysphoria

According to the *DSM-5*, at least six of the following symptoms must be exhibited for at least six months and associated with distress or impaired functioning in order for a child to be diagnosed with gender dysphoria[84]:

- A strong desire to be of the other gender or an insistence they are another gender
- A strong preference for dressing in clothing stereotypical of the other gender
- A strong preference for playing with toys, games, or activities stereotypical of the other gender
- A strong rejection of the toys, games, and activities stereotypical of their assigned gender
- A strong preference for cross-gender roles when playing
- A strong preference for playmates of the other gender
- A strong dislike of one's sexual anatomy
- A strong desire to have the primary and/or secondary sex characteristics of the other gender

84 American Psychiatric Association. (2013). *Desk reference to the diagnostic criteria from DSM-5.*

My Notes

Only a small percentage of children who display gender dysphoria will continue to show these characteristics into adolescence or adulthood. Adolescents with gender dysphoria who dread the appearance of secondary sexual characteristics may seek hormones or surgery to alter their masculinity or femininity.[85]

Sexual orientation is different from gender identity and gender expression. Sexual orientation refers to an individual's pattern of physical, emotional, and romantic arousal (including fantasies, activities, and behaviors) and the gender(s) of persons to whom an individual is physically or sexually attracted. An individual's assessment of their sexual orientation is termed **sexual identity**. Formation of sexual identity may be fluid with experimentation with same-gender sexual contacts as part of adolescent development. Approximately 5 to 10 percent of teens identify as lesbian, gay, or bisexual.[86]

Adolescents and adults who are mature and healthy in their sexuality are able to do the following[87]:

- Take responsibility for one's own behavior
- Practice effective decision-making
- Affirm that human development includes sexual development, which may or may not include reproduction or sexual experience
- Seek further information about sexuality and reproduction as needed and make informed choices about family options and relationships
- Interact with all genders in respectful and appropriate ways
- Affirm one's own gender identity and sexual orientation and respect the gender identities and sexual orientations of others
- Appreciate one's body and enjoy one's sexuality throughout life, expressing one's sexuality in ways that are congruent with one's values
- Express love and intimacy in appropriate ways
- Develop and maintain meaningful relationships, avoiding exploitative or manipulative relationships
- Exhibit skills and communication that enhance personal relationships with family, peers, and romantic partners

Health risks and adverse outcomes can occur among youth who are gender-diverse or from sexual minorities. Risks and adverse outcomes can include child abuse, bullying, sexual harassment, teen dating violence, unprotected sex with risks for sexually transmitted infections and pregnancy, mental health problems (depression, anxiety, suicide, and disordered eating and body image), and substance use.[88]

Nurses should ask all clients, including adolescents, about their gender preferences and provide support if the client indicates a need for help. By promoting sexuality as healthy, respectful, and meaningful in the global context of adolescent development, nurses can encourage a positive model of empowerment for youth exploring their gender and sexual identities.[89]

---

85 American Psychiatric Association. (2013). *Desk reference to the diagnostic criteria from DSM-5.*

86 Forcier, M. (2021, July 24). Adolescent sexuality. *UpToDate*. Retrieved February 22, 2022, from www.uptodate.com

87 Forcier, M. (2021, July 24). Adolescent sexuality. *UpToDate*. Retrieved February 22, 2022, from www.uptodate.com

88 Forcier, M. (2021, July 24). Adolescent sexuality. *UpToDate*. Retrieved February 22, 2022, from www.uptodate.com

89 Forcier, M. (2021, July 24). Adolescent sexuality. *UpToDate*. Retrieved February 22, 2022, from www.uptodate.com

My Notes

12.3 PSYCHOLOGICAL THERAPIES AND BEHAVIORAL INTERVENTIONS

Mental, emotional, and behavioral disorders in childhood can cause long-term problems. Early treatment of a child's mental health or behavioral problems can reduce problems at home, in school, in forming friendships, and can promote healthy development into adulthood.[1] Treatments include psychological therapy, parent training in behavioral management, and behavioral interventions for the classroom.

Psychological Therapies

Depending on the type and severity of the mental health disorder, psychological therapy for children may be used in combination with prescribed medication. Psychological therapy helps a child manage their symptoms so that they can function well at home, in school, and in their community. For example, cognitive-behavioral therapy (CBT) works well for children with disruptive behavior disorders, depression, and anxiety.

Psychological therapy is conducted by trained mental health professionals for children and can be done individually or in groups. Psychological therapy with children can include talking, playing, or other activities to help the child express feelings and thoughts. Therapists may also observe parents and children together and make suggestions for different ways to respond to disruptive behaviors.[2] See Table 12.3 for a list of psychological therapies considered effective for common conditions in children and adolescents.[3]

Table 12.3 Psychological Therapies for Various Conditions in Children and Adolescents

Therapies	Description	Indications
Cognitive-Behavioral Therapy (CBT)	Teaches clients how to correct cognitive errors in thinking (such as, "nothing ever goes right for me") and coaches them to try different behaviors (i.e., behavioral activation) to lead to changes in how they feel. Exposure and response prevention (ERP) is a form of CBT for the treatment of obsessive-compulsive disorder (OCD).	Anxiety disorders Depressive disorders Oppositional defiant disorder Eating disorders Substance use disorder Post-traumatic stress disorder
Dialectical Behavior Therapy (DBT)	Specialized version of CBT with skills groups (to teach problem-solving, emotional regulation, distress tolerance, and interpersonal effectiveness skills), as well as individual therapy sessions. Mindfulness and meditation are often encouraged.	Chronic and significant suicide ideation and/or self-harm

1 Centers for Disease Control and Prevention. (2021, September 23). *Therapy to improve children's mental health.* https://www.cdc.gov/childrensmentalhealth/parent-behavior-therapy.html

2 Centers for Disease Control and Prevention. (2021, September 23). *Therapy to improve children's mental health.* https://www.cdc.gov/childrensmentalhealth/parent-behavior-therapy.html

3 Hilt, R. J., & Nussbaum, A. M. (Eds.). (2016). *DSM-5 pocket guide for child and adolescent mental health.* https://doi.org/10.1176/appi.books.9781615370511

My Notes

Therapies	Description	Indications
Family Therapy	Sessions that focus on the family relationship or interaction patterns that cause dysfunction and assist the family members to amend that pattern (rather than saying the problem resides within an individual).	Eating disorders Conduct disorder Depressive disorders Substance use disorders
Group Therapy	Addresses interaction pattern problems while also providing disorder-specific support within a group of strangers having similar challenges. Peer-based learning can be uniquely effective.	Anxiety disorders
Behavioral Management Training	Also known as parent management training, these programs teach and encourage skillful parent or caregiver responses to challenging child behaviors. Read more in the "Behavioral Interventions" subsection below.	Oppositional defiant disorder Conduct disorder
Social Skills Training	Variety of group and one-to-one techniques to teach basic behavioral and cognitive skills, reinforce prosocial behaviors, and teach social problem-solving. Group sessions are more beneficial than individual sessions because of peer learning influences.	Oppositional defiant disorder Attention deficit hyperactivity disorder (ADHD) Anxiety disorders Depressive disorders Autism spectrum disorder
Relaxation Training	Biofeedback, deep breathing, progressive muscle relaxation, and mindfulness are examples of strategies to increase mind-body awareness and enhance the ability to effectively calm emotional reactions. Read more about relaxation training in the "Stress" and "Coping" sections of the "Stress, Coping, and Crisis Intervention" chapter.	Anxiety disorders Depressive disorders
Motivational Interviewing (MI)	A specific type of therapeutic communication regarding health behaviors a client needs to change but has significant reluctance. It helps clients state their own reasons for changing behaviors, resolve their own ambivalence, and state actions they can take to change. Read more details in the "Motivational Interviewing" section of the "Therapeutic Communication and Nurse-Client Relationship" chapter.	Substance use disorders

Behavioral Interventions

Behavioral interventions reward desired behaviors and reduce maladaptive coping behaviors. Most child and adolescent treatment settings used structured programs to motivate and reward age-appropriate behaviors. For

My Notes

example, the point or star system may be used where the child receives points or stars for desired behaviors, and then specific privileges are awarded based on the points or stars earned each day.[4]

Parent Training in Behavior Management

Parent training in behavior management includes teaching skills and strategies such as positive reinforcement, structure, and consistent discipline to manage their child's behavior and help them succeed at school, at home, and in relationships.[5] See Figure 12.6[6] for an illustration of parent training in behavioral management.

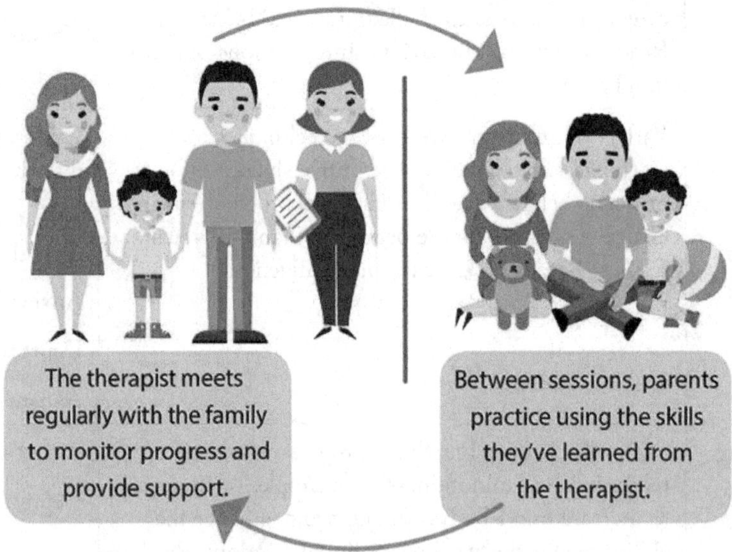

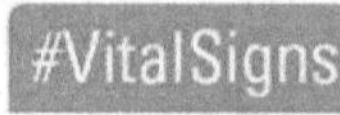

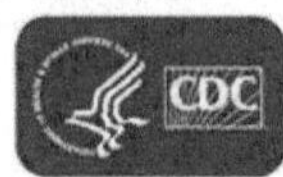

CDC Vitalsigns
www.cdc.gov/vitalsigns/adhd

Figure 12.6 Parent Training in Behavior Management

4 Halter, M. (2022). *Varcarolis' foundations of psychiatric-mental health nursing* (9th ed.). Saunders.

5 Centers for Disease Control and Prevention. (2021, September 23). *What is ADHD?* https://www.cdc.gov/ncbddd/adhd/facts.html

6 "adhd-behavior-therapy-parents-800px.png" by National Center on Birth Defects and Developmental Disabilities is in the Public Domain

My Notes

Behavioral Management Strategies

There are several evidence-based strategies that nurses can teach parents and caregivers to help manage behaviors of children and adolescents, such as Time-Out, Special Time, Functional Analysis of Behavior, Behavioral Activation, Sleep Hygiene, and Responding to Bullying.[7]

Time-Out

"Time-out" is a strategy for shaping a child's behavior through selective and temporary removal of the child's access to desired attention, activities, or other reinforcements following a behavioral transgression. This strategy works for children who experience regular positive praise and attention from their parents or caregivers because they feel motivated to maintain that positive regard. The length of time should be about one minute for each year of age, but adjustments need to be made based on the child's developmental level. For example, children with developmental delays should have shorter durations.[8]

Tips for caregivers implementing time-outs include the following[9]:

- Set consistent limits to avoid confusion.
- Focus on changing priority misbehaviors rather than everything at once.
- After setting a "time-out," decline further verbal engagement until a "time-in."
- Ensure time-outs occur immediately after misbehavior rather than being delayed.
- Follow through if using warnings (e.g., "I'm going to count to three . . .").
- State when the time-out is over. Setting a timer can be helpful.
- When the time-out finishes, congratulate the child on regaining personal control and then look for the next positive behavior to praise.
- Give far more positive attention than negative attention.

Special Time

"Special time" is a strategy for a caregiver and a young child to establish the enjoyment of each other's company. It is also referred to as "child-directed play" because it emphasizes that caregivers follow the child's lead. Tips for caregivers implementing special time include the following[10]:

- Commit to setting aside a regular time for "special time." Daily is best, but two to three times a week consistently also works.
- Select the time of day and label it as "our special time."

---

7 Hilt, R. J., & Nussbaum, A. M. (Eds.). (2016). *DSM-5 pocket guide for child and adolescent mental health.* https://doi.org/10.1176/appi.books.9781615370511

8 Hilt, R. J., & Nussbaum, A. M. (Eds.). (2016). *DSM-5 pocket guide for child and adolescent mental health.* https://doi.org/10.1176/appi.books.9781615370511

9 Hilt, R. J., & Nussbaum, A. M. (Eds.). (2016). *DSM-5 pocket guide for child and adolescent mental health.* https://doi.org/10.1176/appi.books.9781615370511

10 Hilt, R. J., & Nussbaum, A. M. (Eds.). (2016). *DSM-5 pocket guide for child and adolescent mental health.* https://doi.org/10.1176/appi.books.9781615370511

My Notes

- Choose a time short enough that it can happen reliably, usually 15-30 minutes. Ensure this time happens no matter how good or bad the day's behaviors were.
- Allow the child to select the activity, which must be something you do not actively dislike or does not involve spending money or completing a chore.
- Follow the child's lead during play, resisting the urge to tell them what to do.
- End of time; a timer may be helpful. Remind the child when the next special time will be.
- If the child refuses at first, explain you will just sit with them during the "special time."
- Expect greater success if you set your own special times for yourself, too.

Functional Analysis of Behavior

Functional analysis is a strategy for preventing a recurring problematic behavior by first identifying why a behavior keeps recurring and then devising a plan to prevent recurrences. For example, a parent reports their young child "throws temper tantrums every time we go to the store." As the mental health professional helps the parent analyze the behavior, the parent realizes they have been giving the child candy to halt the tantrums, which actually functions to reward the behavior and encourages it to happen again. If the parent were to stop delivering this unintentional reward, the tantrums would theoretically decrease. Alternatively, the parent may focus on avoiding reexposing the child to a recognized trigger for the behavior, such as the candy aisle.[11]

Behavioral Activation

Behavioral activation is a strategy to encourage a young person to reengage with other people and do things they find pleasurable. When an individual is sad or anxious, they are less likely to engage in activities they enjoy, and this withdrawal can cause isolation and worsen the mood. The following is a list of tips to provide clients for succeeding with behavioral activation[12]:

- Identify activities that you (not others) find motivating or rewarding. Develop a list with a variety of options because repetitively doing the same thing can become boring.
- Refine the list to things that can be measured as completed rather than vague goals.
- Rank the activities in order of those most easily completed to those more difficult to complete.
- Start by selecting something easy to accomplish to get started and then work up the list in increasing level of difficulty.
- Let others know your plans and enlist their help in motivating you.

---

11 Hilt, R. J., & Nussbaum, A. M. (Eds.). (2016). *DSM-5 pocket guide for child and adolescent mental health.* https://doi.org/10.1176/appi.books.9781615370511

12 Hilt, R. J., & Nussbaum, A. M. (Eds.). (2016). *DSM-5 pocket guide for child and adolescent mental health.* https://doi.org/10.1176/appi.books.9781615370511

My Notes

Sleep Hygiene

Insomnia is a common problem among children and adolescents. Most sleep problems can be resolved by changing habits and routines that affect sleep, commonly referred to as sleep hygiene. The following is a list of tips for caregivers for improving sleep hygiene[13]:

- Maintain consistent bedtimes and wake times every day of the week.
- Maintain a routine of pre-sleep activities (e.g., brush teeth, read a book).
- Avoid spending non-sleep time in or on one's bed. (i.e., "beds are for sleep").
- Ensure the bedroom is cool and quiet.
- Avoid highly stimulating activities just before bed (e.g., television, video games, social media, or exercise).
- Do not keep video games, televisions, computers, or phones in a child's bedroom.
- Exercise earlier in the day to help with sleeping later.
- Avoid caffeine in the afternoons and evenings. Caffeine causes shallow sleep and frequent awakenings.
- Encourage children and adolescents to discuss any worries with the caregiver before bed rather than ruminating on it during sleep time.
- Ensure that children go to bed drowsy but still awake. Falling asleep in places other than a bed forms habits that are difficult to break.
- Use security objects with young children who need a transitional object with which to feel safe and secure when their caregiver is not present (e.g., a special blanket or toy).
- When checking on a young child at night, briefly reassure the child you are present and they are OK.
- Avoid afternoon naps for all but very young children because they often interfere with nighttime sleep.
- If a child or adolescent is having sleep difficulties, keep a sleep diary to track sleep time, wake time, activities, and naps to identify patterns.

Responding to Bullying

Bullying occurs when a person seeks to harm, intimidate, or coerce someone perceived as vulnerable. If there is a sudden change in a child's mood, behavior, sleep, body symptoms, academic performance, or social functioning, there is a possibility they are experiencing bullying. Cyberbullying is a significant public health concern with rates of cyberbullying estimates ranging from 14 to 57%.[14]

---

13 Hilt, R. J., & Nussbaum, A. M. (Eds.). (2016). *DSM-5 pocket guide for child and adolescent mental health.* https://doi.org/10.1176/appi.books.9781615370511

14 Zhu, C., Huang, S., Evans, R., & Zhang, W. (2021). Cyberbullying among adolescents and children: A comprehensive review of the global situation, risk factors, and preventive measures. *Frontiers in Public Health,* 9. https://doi.org/10.3389/fpubh.2021.634909

My Notes

The following is a list of tips for assessing and responding to bullying[15]:

- **Detect:** Ask the child: "Sometimes kids get picked on or bullied. Have you ever seen this happen? Has it ever happened to you?" If the child responds "No" but bullying is suspected, suggest the caregivers speak with teachers and/or review the child's social media accounts.
- **Educate:** Let children know that bullying is unacceptable and if they experience bullying, you will help them respond.
- **Plan:** Plan ways with the child to avoid bullying.
    - Avoid places where bullying happens.
    - Teach them to walk away when bullying occurs and tell a trusted adult who can be quickly accessed.
    - Instruct the child to stay near adults where bullying occurs. Most bullying happens when adults are not around.
    - If a child feels they can confront the bully, teach them to say in a calm clear voice to stop the behavior and, "Bullying is not OK."
    - If the child is comfortable with deflating the situation with humor, they can use humor to challenge the bullying.
    - Encourage the child to ask their peers for support and ideas for dealing with the bully.
    - Encourage caregivers to communicate the bullying to the school and other families and jointly devise solutions.

Read more information about addressing bullying at www.stopbullying.gov.

Behavioral Interventions for the Classroom

Behavioral interventions for the classroom help children and adolescents succeed academically. Behavioral classroom management is a teacher-led approach that encourages a student's positive behaviors in the classroom through a reward system or a daily report card and discourages their negative behaviors. Organizational training teaches children and adolescents time management, planning skills, and ways to keep school materials organized to optimize student learning and reduce distractions.[16]

---

15 Hilt, R. J., & Nussbaum, A. M. (Eds.). (2016). *DSM-5 pocket guide for child and adolescent mental health.* https://doi.org/10.1176/appi.books.9781615370511

16 Centers for Disease Control and Prevention. (2021, September 23). *What is ADHD?* https://www.cdc.gov/ncbddd/adhd/facts.html

My Notes

12.4 AUTISM SPECTRUM DISORDER

Autism spectrum disorder (ASD) is a developmental disorder that affects an individual's communication and behavior. Although autism can be diagnosed at any age, it is classified as a developmental disorder because symptoms generally appear in the first two years of life.[1] An average of 2.3% of children in the United States have ASD.[2]

ASD is characterized by the following[3]:

- Difficulty with communication and interaction with other people
- Restricted interests and repetitive behaviors
- Symptoms that hurt the person's ability to function properly in school, work, and other areas of life

Autism is known as a "spectrum" disorder because there is wide variation in the type and severity of symptoms experienced by individuals. ASD occurs in all ethnic, racial, and economic groups. Although ASD is a lifelong disorder, treatments and services can improve a person's symptoms and ability to function.[4] See Figure 12.7[5] for an image depicting a child coping with the symptoms of autism.

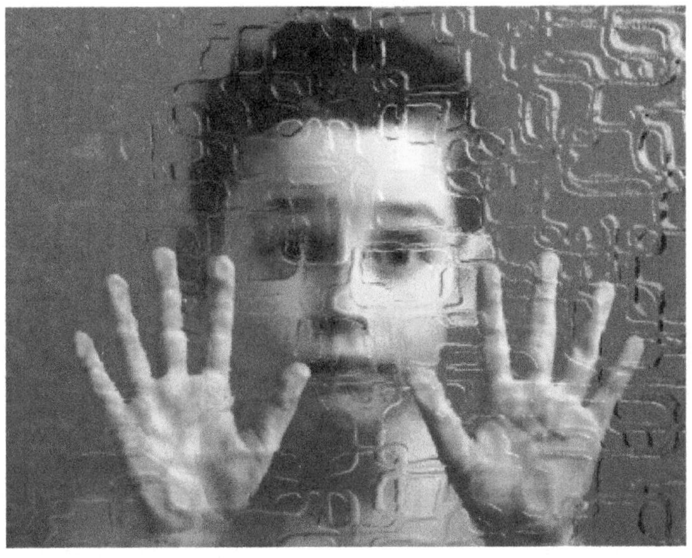

Figure 12.7 Child Coping With Autism Symptoms

1 National Institute of Mental Health. (2018, March 18). *Autism spectrum disorder.* U.S. Department of Health & Human Services. https://www.nimh.nih.gov/health/topics/autism-spectrum-disorders-asd

2 National Institute of Mental Health. (2022, January). *Autism spectrum disorder (ASD).* U.S. Department of Health & Human Services. https://www.nimh.nih.gov/health/statistics/autism-spectrum-disorder-asd#part_2547

3 National Institute of Mental Health. (2022, January). *Autism spectrum disorder (ASD).* U.S. Department of Health & Human Services. https://www.nimh.nih.gov/health/statistics/autism-spectrum-disorder-asd#part_2547

4 National Institute of Mental Health. (2022, January). *Autism spectrum disorder (ASD).* U.S. Department of Health & Human Services. https://www.nimh.nih.gov/health/statistics/autism-spectrum-disorder-asd#part_2547

5 "5299266366_0b6c8ae172_o" by hepingting is licensed under CC BY-SA 2.0

My Notes

Signs and Symptoms

People with ASD have difficulty with social communication and interaction, experience restricted interests, and exhibit repetitive behaviors. Here are some examples of behaviors in these categories:

Social Communication/Interaction Behaviors[6]:

- Making little or inconsistent eye contact
- Not looking at or listening to people
- Rarely sharing enjoyment of objects or activities by pointing or showing things to others
- Being slow to respond (or failing to respond) to someone calling one's name
- Having difficulties with the back-and-forth nature of a conversation
- Talking at length about a favorite subject without noticing that others are not interested or without giving others a chance to respond
- Exhibiting facial expressions, movements, and gestures that do not match what is being said
- Using a tone of voice that may sound flat and robot-like
- Having trouble understanding another person's point of view or being unable to understand other people's actions

Restricted Interests or Repetitive Behaviors[7]:

- Repeating certain behaviors or exhibiting unusual behaviors, such as repeating words or phrases (i.e., **echolalia**)
- Having a lasting intense interest in certain topics, such as numbers, details, or facts
- Having overly focused interests, such as with moving objects or parts of objects
- Getting upset by slight changes in a routine
- Being more or less sensitive than other people to sensory input, such as light, noise, clothing, or temperature
    - This sensitivity can present as physical touch, like a hug, actually being experienced as painful. Items such as seams on pants can be overwhelming and extremely agitating.

Although people with ASD experience many challenges, they also tend to have many strengths, including these strengths[8]:

- Being able to learn things in detail and remember information for long periods of time
- Being strong visual and auditory learners

---

6 National Institute of Mental Health. (2022, January). *Autism spectrum disorder (ASD)*. U.S. Department of Health & Human Services. https://www.nimh.nih.gov/health/statistics/autism-spectrum-disorder-asd#part_2547

7 National Institute of Mental Health. (2022, January). *Autism spectrum disorder (ASD)*. U.S. Department of Health & Human Services. https://www.nimh.nih.gov/health/statistics/autism-spectrum-disorder-asd#part_2547

8 National Institute of Mental Health. (2022, January). *Autism spectrum disorder (ASD)*. U.S. Department of Health & Human Services. https://www.nimh.nih.gov/health/statistics/autism-spectrum-disorder-asd#part_2547

- Excelling in math, science, music, or art

Causes and Risk Factors

Research suggests that genes can act together with influences from the environment to affect development in ways that can lead to ASD. Risk factors include the following[9]:

- A sibling with ASD
- Older parents at birth
- Genetic conditions such as Down syndrome and Fragile X syndrome
- Very low birth weight

Treatments

Current treatments for ASD seek to reduce symptoms that interfere with daily functioning and quality of life. ASD affects each person differently, meaning that people with ASD have unique strengths and challenges and thus different treatment needs. Treatment plans typically involve multiple professionals with interventions customized to the individual.[10]

As individuals with ASD exit high school and grow into adulthood, additional services can help improve their health and daily functioning and facilitate social engagement. Supports may be provided to complete job training, find employment, and secure housing and transportation.[11]

There are many categories of treatments available, and some treatments involve more than one approach. Treatment categories include the following[12]:

- Behavioral
- Developmental
- Educational
- Social-Relational
- Pharmacological
- Psychological
- Complementary and Alternative

---

9 National Institute of Mental Health. (2022, January). *Autism spectrum disorder (ASD).* U.S. Department of Health & Human Services. https://www.nimh.nih.gov/health/statistics/autism-spectrum-disorder-asd#part_2547

10 National Institute of Mental Health. (2022, January). *Autism spectrum disorder (ASD).* U.S. Department of Health & Human Services. https://www.nimh.nih.gov/health/statistics/autism-spectrum-disorder-asd#part_2547

11 National Institute of Mental Health. (2022, January). *Autism spectrum disorder (ASD).* U.S. Department of Health & Human Services. https://www.nimh.nih.gov/health/statistics/autism-spectrum-disorder-asd#part_2547

12 National Institute of Mental Health. (2022, January). *Autism spectrum disorder (ASD).* U.S. Department of Health & Human Services. https://www.nimh.nih.gov/health/statistics/autism-spectrum-disorder-asd#part_2547

My Notes

Behavioral Approaches

Behavioral approaches focus on changing an individual's behaviors by promoting understanding of what happens before and after the behavior. A notable behavioral treatment for people with ASD is called applied behavior analysis. Applied behavior analysis encourages desired behaviors and discourages undesired behaviors to improve a variety of skills, and progress is tracked and measured.[13]

Developmental Approaches

Developmental approaches focus on improving specific developmental skills, such as language skills or physical skills. Developmental approaches are often combined with behavioral approaches. The most common developmental therapy for people with ASD is speech and language therapy. Speech and language therapy helps improve the person's understanding and use of speech and language. Some people with ASD communicate verbally. Others with severe symptoms of ASD may communicate through the use of signs, gestures, pictures, or an electronic communication device.[14]

Occupational therapy teaches skills to help the person live as independently as possible. Skills may include dressing, eating, bathing, and relating to other people. Occupational therapy can also include sensory integration therapy to help improve responses to sensory input that may be restrictive or overwhelming.[15]

Physical therapy may be implemented to help improve physical skills, such as fine movements of the fingers or larger movements of the trunk and body.[16]

Educational Approaches

Educational treatments are provided in a classroom setting. One type of educational approach is the Treatment and Education of Autistic and Related Communication-Handicapped Children (TEACCH) approach. TEACCH is based on the idea that people with autism thrive on consistency and visual learning. It provides teachers with ways to adjust the classroom structure to improve academic and other outcomes. For example, daily routines can be written and placed in clear sight, boundaries can be set around learning stations, and verbal instructions can be complemented with visual instructions or physical demonstrations.[17]

Social-Relational Approaches

Social-relational treatments focus on improving social skills and building emotional bonds. For example, "social stories" provide simple descriptions of what to expect in a social situation. "Social skills groups" provide opportunities for people with ASD to practice social skills in a structured environment.

---

13 National Institute of Mental Health. (2022, January). *Autism spectrum disorder (ASD)*. U.S. Department of Health & Human Services. https://www.nimh.nih.gov/health/statistics/autism-spectrum-disorder-asd#part_2547

14 National Institute of Mental Health. (2022, January). *Autism spectrum disorder (ASD)*. U.S. Department of Health & Human Services. https://www.nimh.nih.gov/health/statistics/autism-spectrum-disorder-asd#part_2547

15 National Institute of Mental Health. (2022, January). *Autism spectrum disorder (ASD)*. U.S. Department of Health & Human Services. https://www.nimh.nih.gov/health/statistics/autism-spectrum-disorder-asd#part_2547

16 National Institute of Mental Health. (2022, January). *Autism spectrum disorder (ASD)*. U.S. Department of Health & Human Services. https://www.nimh.nih.gov/health/statistics/autism-spectrum-disorder-asd#part_2547

17 National Institute of Mental Health. (2022, January). *Autism spectrum disorder (ASD)*. U.S. Department of Health & Human Services. https://www.nimh.nih.gov/health/statistics/autism-spectrum-disorder-asd#part_2547

My Notes

Pharmacological Approaches

There are no medications used to treat ASD, but medications may be used to treat symptoms and improve functioning. For example, medication may be used to manage high energy levels, improve focus, or limit self-harming behavior, such as head banging or hand biting. Medication may also be used to treat concurrent psychological and medical conditions, such as anxiety, depression, seizures, or sleep problems.[18]

Psychological Approaches

Psychological approaches can help people with ASD cope with anxiety, depression, and other mental health issues. For example, cognitive behavioral therapy (CBT) helps individuals focus on the connections between their thoughts, feelings, and behaviors. During CBT a therapist and the individual work together to identify goals and change how the person thinks about a situation to change how they react to the situation.[19]

Complementary and Alternative Treatments

Some individuals with autism use special diets, herbal supplements, chiropractic care, animal therapy, art therapy, mindfulness, or relaxation therapies.[20] Treatment is most effective when tailored to the individual, and additional enriching therapies can help individuals with ASD to thrive.

To find resources related to caring for children with autism, go to the Autism Society.

18 National Institute of Mental Health. (2022, January). *Autism spectrum disorder (ASD)*. U.S. Department of Health & Human Services. https://www.nimh.nih.gov/health/statistics/autism-spectrum-disorder-asd#part_2547

19 National Institute of Mental Health. (2022, January). *Autism spectrum disorder (ASD)*. U.S. Department of Health & Human Services. https://www.nimh.nih.gov/health/statistics/autism-spectrum-disorder-asd#part_2547

20 National Institute of Mental Health. (2022, January). *Autism spectrum disorder (ASD)*. U.S. Department of Health & Human Services. https://www.nimh.nih.gov/health/statistics/autism-spectrum-disorder-asd#part_2547

My Notes

12.5 APPLYING THE NURSING PROCESS TO MENTAL HEALTH DISORDERS IN CHILDREN AND ADOLESCENTS

Working with children and adolescents is very different from working with adults. Young people are often reluctant participants who have been brought for care they did not seek on their own. Additionally, their communication skills are limited based on their developmental stage. In addition to gathering information from the child, information must also be obtained from the parent or caregiver.[1]

The first step to successful care is to create a therapeutic nurse-client relationship. A therapeutic alliance can typically be created if the young person feels noticed, heard, and appreciated. It is often helpful to start the conversation with a relatively neutral question like, "Your mom said that you go to ____ school. What is that school like?" School, friends, family, and favorite activities are low-stress conversation starters. For a very young child, a conversation starter could be a simple observation like what they are wearing. For example, "I see you are wearing blue tennis shoes; did you pick those out yourself?"[2]

For young people who seem reluctant to start talking, it may be helpful to describe something you saw that shows you have been paying attention to them. For example, "It looked as though it was hard for you to sit and do nothing while your dad and I were talking. Am I right about that?"[3]

When caring for adolescents, it is helpful to gather data from the parent or caregiver, and then ask to speak with the adolescent alone. Reinforce that the conversation is "conditionally confidential" and invite the adolescent to sit alone with you to talk. A 1:1 conversation with an adolescent typically creates a better therapeutic alliance with more honest answers obtained.[4]

A more subtle strategy to build a therapeutic-nurse relationship with children and adolescents is to shape how you speak so you are perceived as a responsive problem-solving partner rather than an authority figure who will judge them. Building a therapeutic nurse-client relationship with a young person should lead to learning their true chief complaint because the chief complaint of an adolescent may be different from their parents' complaints.[5] Furthermore, goal setting and treatment plans will be more effective when the adolescent's concerns are addressed.

Privacy, Confidentiality, and Mandatory Reporting

Confidentiality should be discussed with the adolescent client and their parent/guardian before beginning an assessment or related conversations, and circumstances should be defined for when confidentiality is "conditional" for children and adolescents. State laws determine what information is considered confidential and what requires reporting to law enforcement or Child Protective Services. Examples of what must be reported to law enforcement

---

1 Hilt, R. J., & Nussbaum, A. M. (Eds.). (2016). *DSM-5 pocket guide for child and adolescent mental health.* https://doi.org/10.1176/appi.books.9781615370511

2 Hilt, R. J., & Nussbaum, A. M. (Eds.). (2016). *DSM-5 pocket guide for child and adolescent mental health.* https://doi.org/10.1176/appi.books.9781615370511

3 Hilt, R. J., & Nussbaum, A. M. (Eds.). (2016). *DSM-5 pocket guide for child and adolescent mental health.* https://doi.org/10.1176/appi.books.9781615370511

4 Hilt, R. J., & Nussbaum, A. M. (Eds.). (2016). *DSM-5 pocket guide for child and adolescent mental health.* https://doi.org/10.1176/appi.books.9781615370511

5 Hilt, R. J., & Nussbaum, A. M. (Eds.). (2016). *DSM-5 pocket guide for child and adolescent mental health.* https://doi.org/10.1176/appi.books.9781615370511

My Notes

include child abuse, gunshot or stabbing wounds, sexually transmitted infections, abortions, suicidal ideation, and homicidal ideation. Some state laws make it optional for clinicians to inform parents/guardians if their child is seeking services related to sexual health care, substance abuse, or mental health care. Nurses should be aware of the state laws affecting the confidentiality of child and adolescent care in the state in which they are practicing.[6]

Although it is important for nurses to respect adolescent clients' privacy and confidentiality, it is also important to encourage the adolescent to talk with their parents/guardians about personal issues that affect their health even if they feel uncomfortable doing so. Parent/guardian support can help ensure the adolescent's health needs are met.[7]

Research your state's laws regarding adolescent clients' rights.

Visit the Wisconsin Department of Health Services' Client Rights for Minors.

Assessment

Parents and caregivers typically bring a child or adolescent in for mental health evaluation due to common concerns, such as the following:

- Poor academic performance
- Developmental delays
- Disruptive or aggressive behavior
- Withdrawn or sad mood
- Irritable or labile mood
- Anxious or avoidant behavior
- Recurrent and excessive physical complaints
- Sleep problems
- Self-harm and suicidality
- Substance abuse
- Disturbed eating

Poor academic performance is a common concern. Keep in mind that assessing a child's/adolescent's ability to function in school is like assessing an adult's ability to function at work. Many factors can affect a young person's performance at school, such as their ability and effort, the classroom environment, life distractions, or a mental health disorder.

Recall that ability may be impacted by hearing or visual impairments, learning disorders, or cognitive impairments. The nurse may assist with performing vision or hearing tests or providing a developmental rating scale. Signs of

---

6 Middleman, A. B., & Olson, K. A. (2021, August 10). Confidentiality in adolescent health care. *UpToDate.* Retrieved February 22, 2022, from www.uptodate.com

7 Middleman, A. B., & Olson, K. A. (2021, August 10). Confidentiality in adolescent health care. *UpToDate.* Retrieved February 22, 2022, from www.uptodate.com

My Notes

abuse, neglect, or bullying are important for the nurse to observe and report. Read more about abuse and neglect in the "Trauma, Abuse, and Violence" chapter.

Psychosocial Assessment and Mental Status Examination

Specific signs and symptoms of a mental health disorder should be assessed as part of the "health history" component of a comprehensive nursing assessment. While asking questions about specific symptoms and obtaining a health history, the nurse should also be simultaneously performing a mental status examination. The mental status examination includes these items:

- Appearance and General Behavior
- Speech
- Motor Activity
- Affect and Mood
- Thoughts and Perceptions
- Attitude and Insight
- Cognitive Abilities

Review details of a mental status examination in the "Application of the Nursing Process in Mental Health Care" chapter.

Family Dynamics

Family dynamics refers to the patterns of interactions among family members, their roles and relationships, and the various factors that shape their interactions. Because family members typically rely on each other for emotional, physical, and economic support, they are one of the primary sources of relationship security or stress. Secure and supportive family relationships provide love, advice, and care, whereas stressful family relationships may include frequent arguments, critical feedback, and unreasonable demands.[8]

Interpersonal interactions among family members have lasting impacts and influence the development and well-being of children. Unhealthy family dynamics can cause children to experience trauma and stress as they grow up, known as adverse childhood experiences (ACEs). Conflict between parents and adolescents is associated with adolescent aggression, whereas mutuality (cohesion and warmth) is shown to be a protective factor against aggressive behavior.[9]

Review information on adverse childhood experiences (ACEs) in the "Mental Health and Mental Illness" section of Chapter 1.

Effectively assessing and addressing a client's family dynamics and its role in a child's or adolescent's mental health disorder requires an interprofessional team of health professionals, including nurses, physicians, social workers, and therapists. Nurses are in a unique position to observe interaction patterns, assess family relationships, and attend to family concerns in clinical settings because they are in frequent contact with family members. Collaboration

8 This work is a derivative of *StatPearls* by Jabbari & Rouster and is licensed under CC BY 4.0

9 This work is a derivative of *StatPearls* by Jabbari & Rouster and is licensed under CC BY 4.0

My Notes

among interprofessional team members promotes family-centered care and provides clients and families with the necessary resources to develop and maintain healthy family dynamics.[10]

Life Span Considerations

Review theories of development across the life span in the "Application of the Nursing Process in Mental Health Care" chapter.

Adolescence is a time of exploration regarding gender identity, gender roles, and sexual orientation. As previously discussed, assuring conditional confidentiality is the first step in establishing basic trust and a therapeutic nurse-client relationship with an adolescent patient. Most adolescents require privacy to talk candidly about their gender identity and sexuality, so parents/guardians should be asked to leave the examination room at some point during the visit.[11]

Cultural Considerations

The Cultural Formulation Interview (CFI) is a structured tool in the *DSM-5* used to assess the influence oculture on a client's experience of distress. See the following box for an adapted version of the CFI tool for children and adolescents.[12]

Adapted Cultural Formulation Interview for Children and Adolescents[13]

- Suggested introduction to the child or adolescent: We have talked about the concerns of your family. Now I would like to know how you are feeling about being ____ years old.
- Feelings of age appropriateness in different settings: Do you feel you are like other people your age? In what way? Do you sometimes feel different from other people your age? In what way?
  - If they acknowledge sometimes feeling different: Does this feeling of being different happen more at home, at school, at work, and/or some other place? Do you feel your family is different from other families? Does your name have special meaning for you? Is there something special about you that you like or are proud of?
- Age-related stressors and supports: What do you like about being at home? At school? With friends? What don't you like at home? At school? With friends? Who is there to support you when you feel you need it? At home? At school? Among your friends?
- Age-related expectations: What do your parents or grandparents expect from a person your age in terms of chores, schoolwork, play, or religion? What do your teachers expect from a person

10 This work is a derivative of *StatPearls* by Jabbari & Rouster and is licensed under CC BY 4.0

11 Middleman, A. B., & Olson, K. A. (2021, August 10). Confidentiality in adolescent health care. *UpToDate.* Retrieved February 22, 2022, from www.uptodate.com

12 This work is a derivative of *StatPearls* by Jabbari & Rouster and is licensed under CC BY 4.0

13 This work is a derivative of *StatPearls* by Jabbari & Rouster and is licensed under CC BY 4.0

My Notes

your age? What do other people your age expect from a person your age? (If they have siblings, what do your siblings expect from a person your age?)

- Transition to adulthood (for adolescents): Are there any important celebrations or events in your community that recognize reaching a certain age or growing up? When is a youth considered ready to become an adult in your family or community? What is good about becoming an adult in your family? In school? In your community? How do you feel about "growing up"? In what ways are your life and responsibilities different from your parents' life and responsibilities?

Diagnoses

Health care professionals use the guidelines in the American Psychiatric Association's *Diagnostic and Statistical Manual (DSM-5)* to diagnose mental health disorders in children.[14]

Nurses customize nursing diagnoses based on the child's or adolescent's response to mental health disorders, their current signs and symptoms, and the effects on their and their family's functioning. Here are common nursing diagnoses related to childhood and adolescent disorders[15,16,17]:

- Anxiety
- Chronic Low Self-Esteem
- Disabled Family Coping
- Impaired Social Interactions
- Ineffective Impulse Control
- Risk for Delayed Development
- Risk-prone Health Behavior
- Risk for Impaired Parenting
- Risk for Spiritual Distress

Outcomes Identification

Broad goals focus on reducing symptoms of mental health disorders that interfere with the child's or adolescent's daily functioning and quality of life. SMART outcomes stand for outcomes that are specific, measurable, achievable, and realistic with a timeline indicated. They are customized according to each client's diagnoses and needs. Read more about SMART outcomes in the "Application of the Nursing Process in Mental Health Care" chapter.

14 American Psychiatric Association. (2013). *Desk reference to the diagnostic criteria from DSM-5.*

15 Halter, M. (2022). *Varcarolis' foundations of psychiatric-mental health nursing* (9th ed.). Saunders.

16 Ackley, B., Ladwig, G., Makic, M. B., Martinez-Kratz, M., & Zanotti, M. (2020). *Nursing diagnosis handbook: An evidence-based guide to planning care* (12th ed.). Elsevier.

17 Herdman, T. H., & Kamitsuru, S. (Eds.). (2018). *Nursing diagnoses: Definitions and classification, 2018-2020.* Thieme Publishers New York.

My Notes

For example, a SMART outcome for a child diagnosed with attention deficit disorder is, "The client will demonstrate reduced impulsive behaviors, as reported by parents and their teachers, within two weeks of initiating stimulant medication."

Planning Interventions

A public health approach to children's mental health includes promoting mental health for all children, providing preventative measures for children at risk, and implementing interventions.[18]

Prevention

It is not known why some children develop disruptive behavior disorders, but children are at greater risk if they are exposed to **adverse childhood experiences (ACEs)**. Toxic stress from ACEs can alter brain development and affect how the body responds to stress. ACEs are linked to chronic health problems, mental illness, and substance abuse. Children with three or more reported ACEs, compared to children with zero reported ACEs, had higher prevalence of one or more mental, emotional, or behavioral disorders (36.3% versus 11.0%).[19]

Review information on adverse childhood experiences (ACEs) in the "Mental Health and Mental Illness" section of Chapter 1.

Preventing ACEs can help children thrive into adulthood by lowering their risk for chronic health problems and substance abuse, improve their education and employment potential, and stop ACEs from being passed from one generation to the next.[20]

Raising awareness about ACEs can help reduce stigma around seeking help for parenting challenges, substance misuse, depression, or suicidal thoughts. Community solutions focus on promoting safe, stable, nurturing relationships and environments where children live, learn, and play. In addition to raising awareness and participating in community solutions, nurses should recognize ACE risk factors and refer clients and their families for effective services and support. See Figure 12.8[21] regarding strategies to prevent ACEs.

---

18 Centers for Disease Control and Prevention. (2021, September 23). *Therapy to improve children's mental health.* https://www.cdc.gov/childrensmentalhealth/parent-behavior-therapy.html

19 Centers for Disease Control and Prevention. (2022, February 24). *Data and statistics on children's mental health.* https://www.cdc.gov/childrensmentalhealth/data.html

20 Centers for Disease Control and Prevention. (2019, November 5). *Adverse childhood experiences (ACEs).* https://www.cdc.gov/vitalsigns/aces/index.html

21 This image is derived from "Preventing Adverse Childhood Experiences (ACEs): Leveraging the Best Available Evidence" by National Center for Injury Prevention and Control, Division of Violence Prevention and is in the Public Domain

My Notes

Strategy	Approach
Strengthen economic supports to families	• Strengthening household financial security • Family-friendly work policies
Promote social norms that protect against violence and adversity	• Public education campaigns • Legislative approaches to reduce corporal punishment • Bystander approaches • Men and boys as allies in prevention
Ensure a strong start for children	• Early childhood home visitation • High-quality child care • Preschool enrichment with family engagement
Teach skills	• Social-emotional learning • Safe dating and healthy relationship skill programs • Parenting skills and family relationship approaches
Connect youth to caring adults and activities	• Mentoring programs • After-school programs
Intervene to lessen immediate and long-term harms	• Enhanced primary care • Victim-centered services • Treatment to lessen the harms of ACEs • Treatment to prevent problem behavior and future involvement in violence • Family-centered treatment for substance use disorders

Figure 12.8 Strategies to Prevent ACEs

Read Preventing Adverse Childhood Experiences PDF by the CDC with evidence-supporting interventions.

Planned Interventions

The following interventions can be planned by nurses for children and adolescents in a variety of settings, including inpatient, outpatient, day treatment, outreach programs in schools, and home visits.[22]

Behavioral Interventions

Behavioral interventions reward desired behaviors to reduce maladaptive coping behaviors. Most child and adolescent treatment settings use structured programs to motivate and reward age-appropriate behaviors. For example, the point or star system may be used where the child receives points or stars for desired behaviors, and then specific privileges are awarded based on the points or stars earned each day.[23]

Read more about interprofessional behavioral interventions for the child, parents/caregivers, and teachers in the "Psychological Therapies and Behavioral Interventions" section.

22 Halter, M. (2022). *Varcarolis' foundations of psychiatric-mental health nursing* (9th ed.). Saunders.

23 Halter, M. (2022). *Varcarolis' foundations of psychiatric-mental health nursing* (9th ed.). Saunders.

My Notes

Play Therapy

Children develop physically, intellectually, emotionally, and socially through play. **Play therapy** encourages children to express feelings such as anxiety, self-doubt, and fear through their natural play. It also allows them to work through painful or traumatic memories. For example, nurses often use dolls or other toys to help children work through feelings of fear prior to a medical procedure.[24] See Figure 12.9[25] for an image of children with special needs playing at a school for autism.

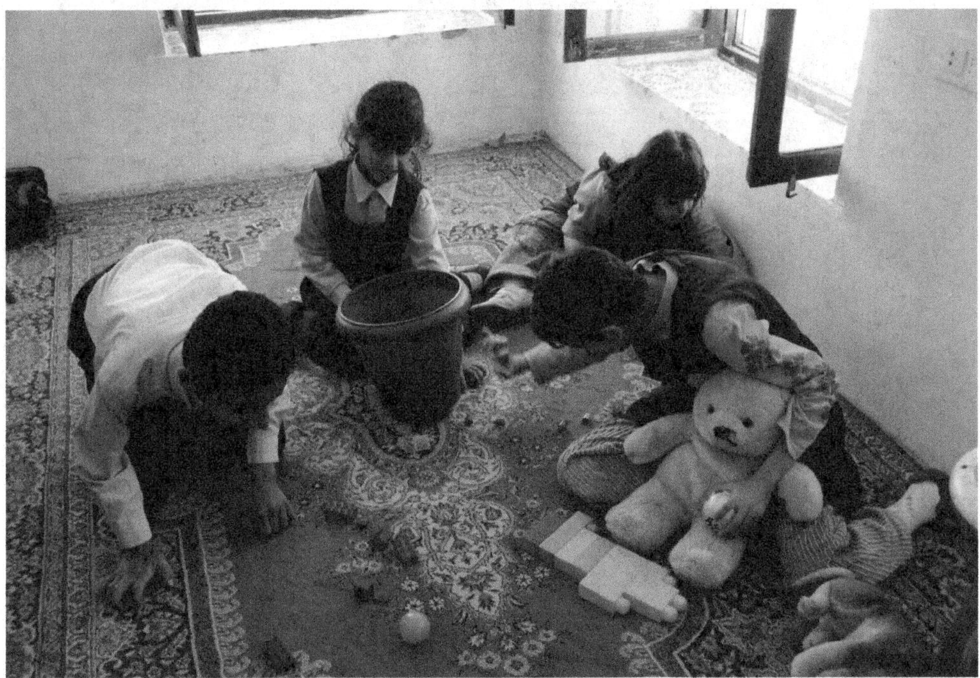

Figure 12.9 Children With Special Needs Playing at an Autism School

Bibliotherapy

Bibliotherapy uses books to help children express feelings in a supportive environment, gain insight into feelings and behavior, and learn new ways to cope with difficult situations. When children listen to or read a story, they identify with the characters and experience a catharsis of feelings. Stories and books should be selected based on the child's cognitive and developmental levels that reflect the situations or feelings the child is experiencing and their emotional readiness for the topic.[26] See Figure 12.10[27] for an image of bibliotherapy.

---

24 Halter, M. (2022). *Varcarolis' foundations of psychiatric-mental health nursing* (9th ed.). Saunders.

25 "4885680339_721cd1843e_k" by World Bank Photo Collection is licensed under CC BY-NC-ND 2.0

26 Halter, M. (2022). *Varcarolis' foundations of psychiatric-mental health nursing* (9th ed.). Saunders.

27 "Bibliotherapy.jpg" by Shelley Rodrigo is licensed under CC BY 2.0

My Notes

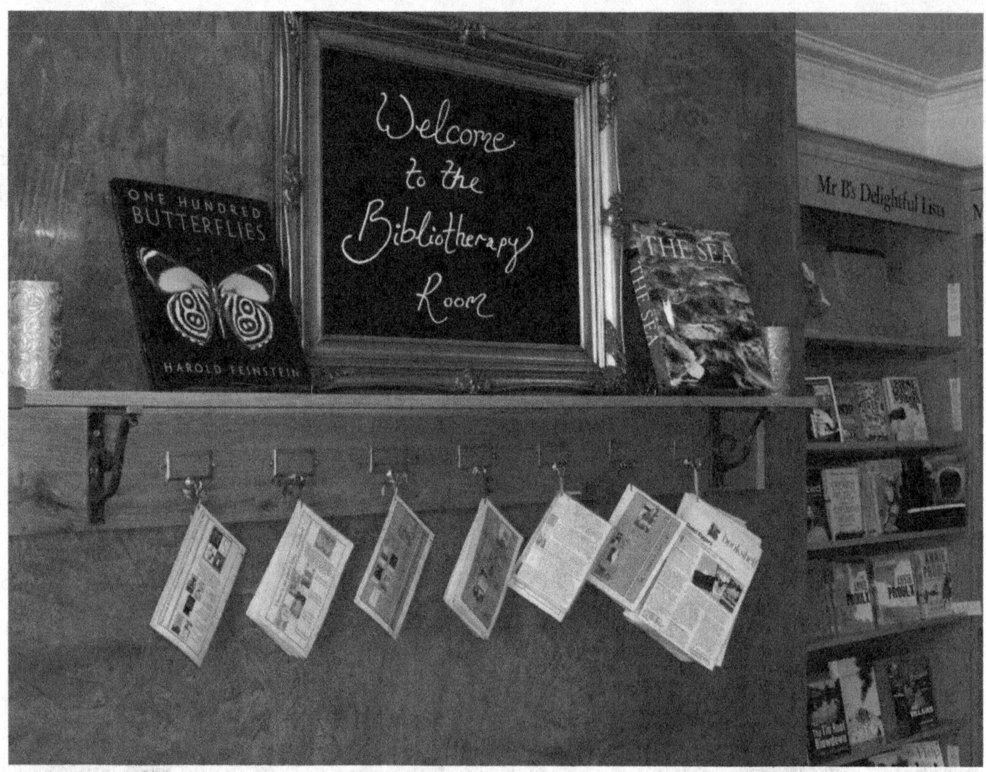

Figure 12.10 Bibliotherapy

Expressive Arts Therapy

Art provides a nonverbal method of expressing difficult or confusing emotions. Drawing, painting, and sculpting with clay are commonly used art therapies. Children who have experienced trauma often show the traumatic event in their drawing when asked to draw whatever they wish.[28]

Journaling

Journaling is an effective technique for older children and teenagers. Journaling is a tangible way to record emotions and begin dialogue with others. A daily journal is also helpful in setting goals and evaluating progress.[29]

Music Therapy

Music has been recognized for centuries as having healing power. **Music therapy** is an evidence-based approach to improve an individual's physical, psychological, cognitive, behavioral, and social functioning when listening to music, singing, or moving to music.[30] See Figure 12.11[31] for an image of music therapy.

---

28 Halter, M. (2022). *Varcarolis' foundations of psychiatric-mental health nursing* (9th ed.). Saunders.

29 Halter, M. (2022). *Varcarolis' foundations of psychiatric-mental health nursing* (9th ed.). Saunders.

30 Halter, M. (2022). *Varcarolis' foundations of psychiatric-mental health nursing* (9th ed.). Saunders.

31 "103909417_f36b60ceec_k" by midiman is licensed under CC BY 2.0

My Notes

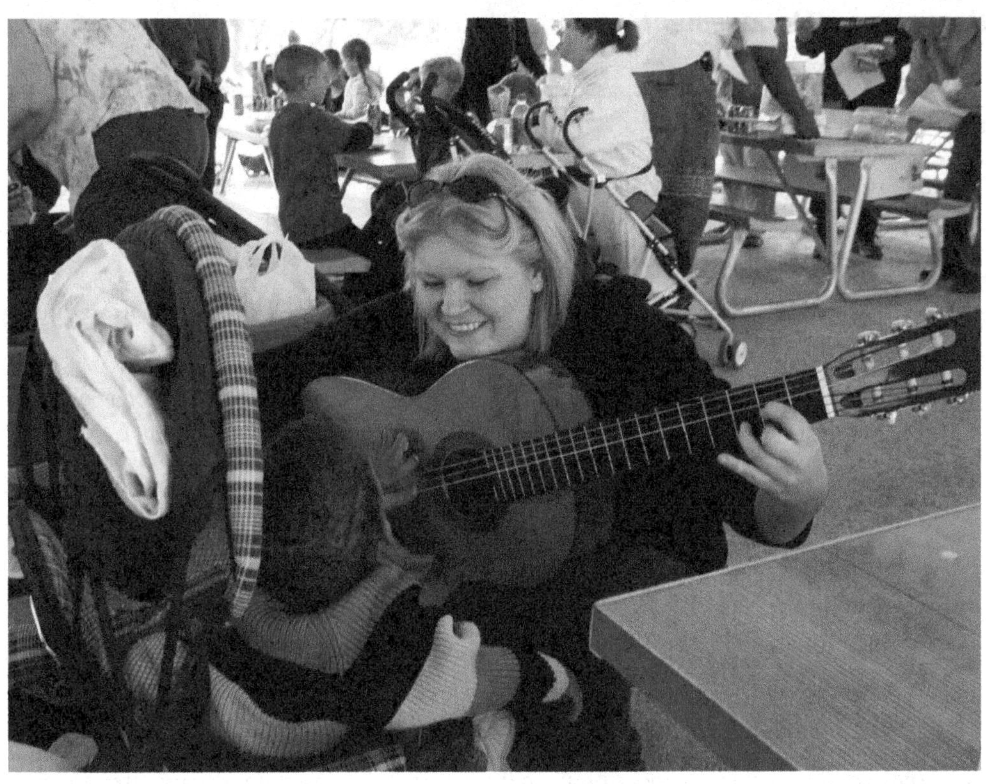

Figure 12.11 Music Therapy

Family Education and Support

Education of family members is a key component for treating child and adolescent mental health disorders. Read more about "Parent Training in Behavior Management" in the "Psychological Therapies and Behavioral Interventions" section. Nurses can help family members develop specific goals and identify interventions to achieve their family's goals.

Family members can also be encouraged to attend support groups or group education. Group education can be useful for learning how other families solve problems and build on strengths while developing insight and improved judgment about their own family.[32]

Find support groups for many disorders near you at Psychology Today's Support Groups.

Implementation

Treatment of mental health disorders in children and adolescents typically requires a combination of psychotherapy and pharmacotherapy. Read about specific multidisciplinary treatments for various disorders in the "Psychological Therapies and Behavioral Intervention," "Attention Deficit Hyperactivity Disorder," and "Autism Spectrum Disorder" areas of this chapter. Nurses should recognize and capitalize on the client's and family's strengths as they develop a nursing care plan and provide education and referral to resources as appropriate.

32 Halter, M. (2022). *Varcarolis' foundations of psychiatric-mental health nursing* (9th ed.). Saunders.

My Notes

Disruptive Behavior Management

Nurses can manage a child's or adolescent's disruptive behaviors by implementing many different types of interventions[33]:

- **Behavioral contract:** A verbal or written agreement is made between the client and other parties (e.g., nurses, parents, or teachers) about behaviors, expectations, and needs. The contract is periodically reviewed with positive and negative reinforcement provided.
- **Collaborative and proactive solutions:** The identification of problematic behaviors, their specific triggers, and mutually agreeable solutions.
- **Role playing:** The nurse or client acts out a specific role to practice new behaviors or skills in specific situations.
- **Planned ignoring:** When behaviors are determined to be attention-seeking and not dangerous, they may be ignored. Positive reinforcement is provided for on-task actions.
- **Signals or gestures:** An adult uses a word, gesture, or eye contact to remind the child to use self-control. For example, placing one's finger to one's lips and making eye contact may be used to remind a child to remain quiet during a quiet activity.
- **Physical distance:** It may be helpful to move closer to a child for a calming effect. However, some children may find this agitating and require more space and less physical closeness.
- **Redirection:** The engagement of an individual in an appropriate activity after an undesirable action.
- **Humor:** Appropriate joking can be used as a diversion to help relieve feelings of guilt or fear.
- **Restructuring:** The process of changing an activity to reduce stimulation or frustration.
- **Limit setting:** The process of giving direction, stating an expectation, or telling a child what to do or where to go. Caregivers and/or staff should do this firmly, calmly, and consistently without anger, preferably in advance of problem behavior occurring. For example, "I would like you to stop turning the light on and off."
- **Simple restitution:** The individual is expected to correct the adverse effects of their actions, such as apologizing to the people affected or returning upturned chairs to their proper position.

Restrictive Interventions

Restrictive interventions are only implemented after attempting less restrictive interventions that did not successfully manage the client's behavior. As a last resort, restrictive interventions, including seclusion or restraints, may be implemented to keep the client or others around them safe.[34]

The Centers for Medicare and Medicaid Services (CMS) and The Joint Commission (TJC) define seclusion as the involuntary confinement of a client alone in a room or area from which the client is physically prevented from leaving. Restraint is defined as any manual method, physical or mechanical device, material, or equipment that immobilizes or reduces the ability of a patient to move their arms, legs, body, or head freely. A drug is considered a

---

33 Halter, M. (2022). *Varcarolis' foundations of psychiatric-mental health nursing* (9th ed.). Saunders.

34 Halter, M. (2022). *Varcarolis' foundations of psychiatric-mental health nursing* (9th ed.). Saunders.

restraint when it is used as a restriction to manage the patient's behavior or restrict the patient's freedom of movement and is not a standard treatment or dosage for the patient's condition.[35]

Seclusion is viewed as less restrictive than restraints, but seclusion and restraint are psychologically harmful and can be physically dangerous. Nurses must vigilantly follow agency policy when implementing seclusion or restraints. Members of the health care team who assist with seclusion or restraint of children or adolescents must receive specific training to decrease the risk of injury to the youngster and themselves.[36]

Seclusion and restraints should be discontinued as soon as possible. Clients in seclusion or restraints must be continuously monitored. Hydration, elimination, comfort, and other psychological and physical needs must be monitored regularly and addressed per agency policy.[37]

After the child or adolescent is calm, staff should include the child in a debriefing session and discuss the events leading up to the restrictive interventions to explore ways it may have been prevented.[38]

Evaluation

Evaluation focuses on monitoring a child's and adolescent's progress towards meeting their individualized SMART goals and the revision of the nursing care plan as needed. Client progress monitoring may include symptom management, behavior management, academic performance, activities of daily living, and socialization. The nurse also monitors effectiveness of interprofessional treatments, support groups, and community resources for the client's families.

---

35 Knox, D. K., & Holloman, G. H., Jr. (2012). Use and avoidance of seclusion and restraint: Consensus statement of the American Association for Emergency Psychiatry Project BETA seclusion and restraint workgroup. *The Western Journal of Emergency Medicine, 13*(1), 35–40. https://doi.org/10.5811/westjem.2011.9.6867

36 Halter, M. (2022). *Varcarolis' foundations of psychiatric-mental health nursing* (9th ed.). Saunders.

37 Knox, D. K., & Holloman, G. H., Jr. (2012). Use and avoidance of seclusion and restraint: Consensus statement of the American Association for Emergency Psychiatry Project BETA Seclusion and Restraint Workgroup. *The Western Journal of Emergency Medicine, 13*(1), 35–40. https://doi.org/10.5811/westjem.2011.9.6867

38 Halter, M. (2022). *Varcarolis' foundations of psychiatric-mental health nursing* (9th ed.). Saunders.

My Notes

12.6 SPOTLIGHT APPLICATION

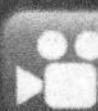

Dr. Temple Grandin was one of the first individuals to document the insights gained from her personal experience of autism. View a video of Dr. Temple Grandin describing her personal experience as, "Everything in my mind works like a search engine set for the image function": Temple Grandin on Her Search Engine | Blank on Blank.[1]

Reflective Questions:

1. What symptoms of autism does Dr. Temple Grandin illustrate?
2. What strengths does Dr. Temple Grandin illustrate and what has she achieved?

---

1 Blank on Blank. (2016, March 1). *Temple Grandin on her search engine | Blank on Blank.* [Video]. YouTube. All rights reserved. https://youtu.be/Ifsh6sojAvg

12.7 LEARNING ACTIVITIES

My Notes

Interactive Activities

An interactive H5P element has been excluded from this version of the text. You can view it online here: https://wtcs.pressbooks.pub/nursingmhcc/?p=640#h5p-41

An interactive H5P element has been excluded from this version of the text. You can view it online here: https://wtcs.pressbooks.pub/nursingmhcc/?p=640#h5p-42

An interactive H5P element has been excluded from this version of the text. You can view it online here: https://wtcs.pressbooks.pub/nursingmhcc/?p=640#h5p-44

My Notes

XII GLOSSARY

Adverse childhood experiences (ACEs): Potentially traumatic events that occur in childhood, such as violence, abuse, and growing up in a family with mental health or substance use problems.

Bibliotherapy: A behavioral intervention that uses books to help children express feelings in a supportive environment, gain insight into feelings and behavior, and learn new ways to cope with difficult situations.

Conduct disorder (CD): A behavioral disorder diagnosed when a child shows an ongoing pattern of aggression toward others with serious violations of rules and social norms at home, school, and with peers.

Developmental disabilities: A group of conditions with physical, learning, language, or behavioral impairments.

Developmental monitoring: Routine screenings for developmental delays during well-child visits based on observations of the child and discussion with parents.

Developmental screening: Formal questionnaires or checklists based on research that ask questions about a child's development, including language, movement, thinking, behavior, and emotions.

Dyscalculia: A learning disorder with difficulty with math.

Dysgraphia: A learning disorder with difficulty with writing.

Dyslexia: A learning disorder with difficulty with reading.

Echolalia: Repeating certain behaviors or exhibiting unusual behaviors, such as repeating words or phrases.

Expressive language disorder: Difficulty communicating thoughts using language due to not knowing the words to use, not knowing how to put words together, or not being able to express the words.

Intellectual disability: A person's ability to learn at an expected level and function in daily life is limited.

Learning disorder: Difficulty in one or more areas of learning, even when a child's overall intelligence or motivation are not affected.

Mental health disorders among children: Serious changes in the way children typically learn, behave, or handle their emotions, causing distress and problems getting through the day.

Music therapy: A behavioral intervention to improve an individual's physical, psychological, cognitive, behavioral, and social functioning by listening to music, singing, or moving to music.

Oppositional defiant disorder (ODD): A behavioral disorder diagnosed when children act out persistently, causing serious problems at home, in school, or with peers.

Play therapy: A behavioral intervention that encourages children to express feelings such as anxiety, self-doubt, and fear through their natural play. It also allows them to work through painful or traumatic memories.

Receptive language disorder: Difficulty understanding what others say due to not hearing the words (hearing loss) or not understanding the meaning of the words.

Restraint: Any manual method, physical or mechanical device, material, or equipment that immobilizes or reduces the ability of a patient to move their arms, legs, body, or head freely.

Seclusion: The involuntary confinement of a client alone in a room or area from which the client is physically prevented from leaving.

Separation anxiety: A condition of children being very afraid when away from parents or caregivers.

Tics: Sudden twitches, movements, or sounds that people do repeatedly with the inability to stop their body from doing these actions.

Chapter 13

Eating Disorders

13.1 INTRODUCTION

My Notes

- Apply the nursing process to clients with eating disorders
- Describe nursing assessments related to eating disorders
- Identify common nursing problems/diagnoses related to eating disorders
- Establish a safe environment
- Plan individualized goals and expected outcomes in collaboration with the client and their family members
- Apply evidence-based practice when planning and implementing nursing care
- Describe common treatments for eating disorders
- Identify appropriate referrals to community resources
- Evaluate the effectiveness of interventions
- Provide patient education to clients and their family members

Many people become concerned about their weight at some point in their lives. However, individuals with eating disorders have a distorted view of their weight and their body image and develop an unhealthy relationship with food. As a result of this psychological struggle, behaviors such as severe restriction of food intake, obsessive exercising, binging, and purging can occur. Eating disorders can affect anyone, regardless of gender, age, race, or economic status and often can also affect their family members and loved ones. The physiological consequences of eating disorders can be fatal if they are not identified and treated appropriately. This chapter will review different types of eating disorders and discuss common assessment findings, treatments, and related nursing interventions.

My Notes

13.2 BASIC CONCEPTS

Eating disorders are serious medical illnesses, and the way we talk about them with others matters.[1] See Figure 13.1[2] with facts nurses can use to help shape the conversation around eating disorders.

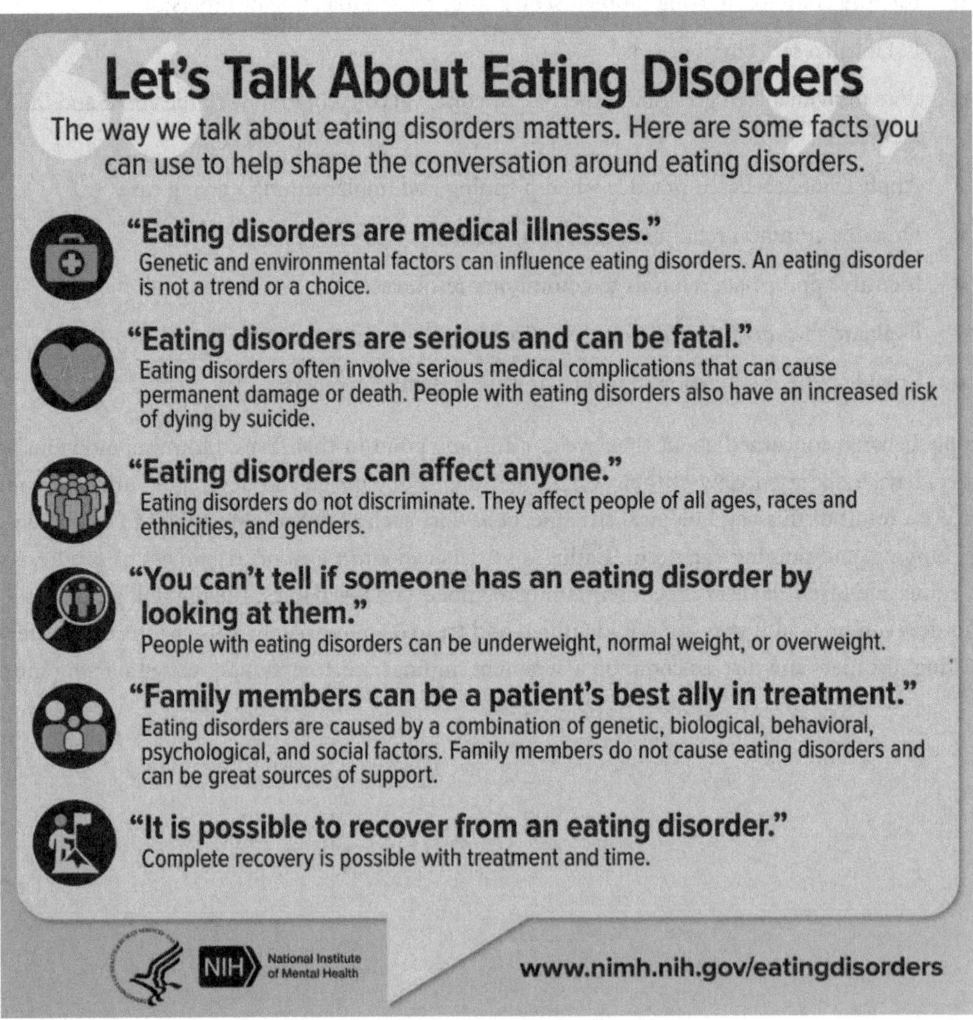

Figure 13.1 Facts About Eating Disorders

Common Eating Disorders

Common eating disorders include anorexia nervosa, bulimia nervosa, and binge eating disorder.[3]

1 National Institute of Mental Health. (2021, December). *Eating disorders.* U.S. Department of Health and Human Services. https://www.nimh.nih.gov/health/topics/eating-disorders

2 "2020_eatingdisorderinfographics_final.jpg" by U.S. Department of Health and Human Services, National Institutes of Health, National Institute of Mental Health is in the Public Domain

3 National Institute of Mental Health. (2021, December). *Eating disorders.* U.S. Department of Health and Human Services. https://www.nimh.nih.gov/health/topics/eating-disorders

Anorexia Nervosa

Anorexia nervosa is a condition where people avoid food, severely restrict food, or eat very small quantities of only certain foods. They have an intense fear of gaining weight or becoming fat, even if they are significantly underweight. People with anorexia nervosa often have distorted body image and view themselves as overweight.[4] See Figure 13.2[5] for an illustration of how a person with anorexia nervosa may perceive themselves.

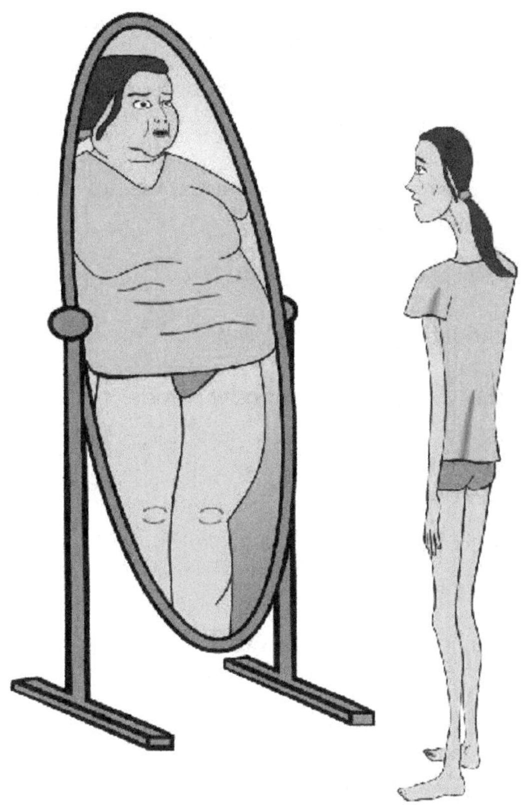

Figure 13.2 Body Perception of a Person With Anorexia Nervosa

There are two subtypes of anorexia nervosa: restricting type and a binge eating/purging type. People with the restrictive subtype of anorexia nervosa severely limit the amount and type of food they consume or engage in excessive exercise. People with the binge-purge subtype have binge eating and/or purging episodes. **Binge eating** episodes refer to eating large amounts of food in a short period of time with a feeling of a loss of control. **Purging episodes** refer to eating large amounts of food in a short time followed by self-induced vomiting or the misuse of laxatives, diuretics, or enemas to eliminate what was consumed.[6,7]

---

4 National Institute of Mental Health. (2021, December). *Eating disorders.* U.S. Department of Health and Human Services. https://www.nimh.nih.gov/health/topics/eating-disorders

5 "maxpixel.net/Bulimia-Anorexia-Nervosa-Skimmed-Delusional-4049661.png" by unknown author is licensed under CC0

6 National Institute of Mental Health. (2021, December). *Eating disorders.* U.S. Department of Health and Human Services. https://www.nimh.nih.gov/health/topics/eating-disorders

7 American Psychiatric Association. (2013). *Desk reference to the diagnostic criteria from DSM-5.*

My Notes

Anorexia nervosa can be fatal due to medical complications associated with starvation. It has an extremely high mortality (death) rate compared with other mental health disorders. Young people between the ages of 15 and 24 with anorexia have 10 times the risk of dying compared to their same-aged peers. Males represent 25% of individuals with anorexia nervosa and are at a higher risk of dying because they are often diagnosed later than females.[8,9]

Signs and symptoms of anorexia nervosa include the following[10]:

- Severely restricted eating
- Extreme thinness (also referred to as **emaciation**)
- A relentless pursuit of thinness and unwillingness to maintain a healthy weight
- Intense fear of gaining weight
- Distorted body image where a person's self-esteem is heavily influenced by their perception of their of body weight and shape
- Denial of the seriousness of low body weight

Other signs may develop over time, including these issues[11]:

- Thinning of the bones (i.e., osteopenia or osteoporosis)
- Anemia
- Muscle wasting and weakness
- Brittle hair and nails
- Dry and yellowish skin
- Growth of fine hair all over the body (**lanugo**)
- Severe constipation
- Low blood pressure
- Slowed breathing and pulse
- Drop in internal body temperature, causing the person to feel cold all the time
- Lethargy, sluggishness, or feeling tired all the time
- Infertility
- Damage to the structure and function of the heart
- Brain damage
- Multiorgan failure

---

8 National Institute of Mental Health. (2021, December). *Eating disorders.* U.S. Department of Health and Human Services. https://www.nimh.nih.gov/health/topics/eating-disorders

9 National Eating Disorders Association. (n.d.). *Statistics and research on eating disorders.* https://www.nationaleatingdisorders.org/statistics-research-eating-disorders

10 National Institute of Mental Health. (2021, December). *Eating disorders.* U.S. Department of Health and Human Services. https://www.nimh.nih.gov/health/topics/eating-disorders

11 National Institute of Mental Health. (2021, December). *Eating disorders.* U.S. Department of Health and Human Services. https://www.nimh.nih.gov/health/topics/eating-disorders

See the following box for criteria used to diagnose anorexia nervosa according to the *Diagnostic and Statistical Manual of Disorders (DSM-5)*.

DSM-5 Criteria for Anorexia Nervosa[12]

- Restrictions of energy intake relative to requirements, leading to significantly low body weight in the context of age, sex, developmental trajectory, and physical health. Significantly low weight is defined as weight less than minimally normal, or in children and adolescents, less than that minimally expected.
- Intense fear of gaining weight or becoming fat or persistent behavior that interferes with weight gain, even though already at a significantly low weight.
- Disturbance in the way in which one's body weight or shape is experienced, undue influence of body weight or shape on self-evaluation, or persistent lack of recognition of the seriousness of the current low body weight.

The type is specified as follows:

- Restricting type: Weight loss is accomplished primarily through dieting, fasting, or excessive exercise. During the last three months, the individual has not engaged in recurrent episodes of binge eating or purging behavior.
- Binge eating/purging type: During the last three months, the individual has engaged in recurrent episodes of binge eating or purging behavior (i.e., self-induced vomiting or the misuse of laxatives, diuretics, or enemas).

Bulimia Nervosa

Bulimia nervosa is a condition where people have recurrent and frequent episodes of binge eating (i.e., eating unusually large amounts of food in a short amount of time while also feeling a lack of control over these episodes). Binge eating is followed by behaviors used to eliminate the excess food such as forced vomiting, excessive use of laxatives or diuretics, fasting, excessive exercise, or a combination of these behaviors. People with bulimia nervosa may be slightly underweight, normal weight, or overweight.[13]

Signs and symptoms of bulimia nervosa include the following[14]:

- Chronically inflamed and sore throat
- Swollen salivary glands in the neck and jaw area

---

12 American Psychiatric Association. (2013). *Desk reference to the diagnostic criteria from DSM-5.*

13 National Institute of Mental Health. (2021, December). *Eating disorders.* U.S. Department of Health and Human Services. https://www.nimh.nih.gov/health/topics/eating-disorders

14 National Institute of Mental Health. (2021, December). *Eating disorders.* U.S. Department of Health and Human Services. https://www.nimh.nih.gov/health/topics/eating-disorders

My Notes

- Worn tooth enamel and increasingly sensitive and decaying teeth as a result of exposure to stomach acid
- Acid reflux disorder and other gastrointestinal problems
- Intestinal distress and irritation from laxative abuse
- Severe dehydration from purging of fluids
- Electrolyte imbalance (sodium, calcium, potassium, and other minerals) that can lead to dysrhythmias and cardiac arrest

See the following box for *DSM-5* criteria for diagnosing bulimia nervosa.

DSM-5 Criteria for Bulimia Nervosa[15]

- Recurrent episodes of binge eating. A binge eating episode is characterized by both of the following:
  - Eating in a discrete period of time (e.g., within any two-hour period) an amount of food that is definitely larger than what most individuals would eat in a similar period of time under similar circumstances.
  - A sense of lack of control overeating during the episode (i.e., feeling that one cannot stop eating or control what or how much one is eating).
- Recurrent inappropriate compensatory behavior to prevent weight gain, such as self-induced vomiting; misuse of laxatives, diuretics, or other medications; fasting; or excessive exercise.
- The binge eating and inappropriate compensatory behaviors both occur, on average, at least once a week for three months.
- Self-evaluation is unduly influenced by body shape and weight.
- The disturbance does not occur exclusively during episodes of anorexia nervosa.

Binge Eating Disorder

Binge eating disorder is the most common eating disorder in the United States.[16] **Binge eating disorder** is a condition where people lose control over their eating and have recurring episodes of eating unusually large amounts of food. However, unlike bulimia nervosa, periods of binge eating are not followed by purging, excessive exercise, or fasting. As a result, people with binge eating disorder often are overweight or obese.[17]

---

15 American Psychiatric Association. (2013). *Desk reference to the diagnostic criteria from DSM-5.*

16 National Institute of Mental Health. (2021, December). *Eating disorders.* U.S. Department of Health and Human Services. https://www.nimh.nih.gov/health/topics/eating-disorders

17 National Institute of Mental Health. (2021, December). *Eating disorders.* U.S. Department of Health and Human Services. https://www.nimh.nih.gov/health/topics/eating-disorders

My Notes

These are the signs and symptoms of a binge eating disorder[18]:

- Eating unusually large amounts of food in a specific amount of time, such as a two-hour period
- Eating even when feeling full or not hungry
- Eating at a fast pace
- Eating until uncomfortably full
- Eating alone or in secret to avoid embarrassment
- Feeling distressed, ashamed, or guilty about eating
- Frequent dieting, possibly without weight loss

See the *DSM-5* criteria for diagnosing binge eating disorder in the following box.

DSM-5 Criteria for Binge Eating Disorder[19]

- Recurrent episodes of binge eating.
- The binge eating episodes are associated with three (or more) of the following:
  - Eating much more rapidly than normal.
  - Eating until feeling uncomfortably full.
  - Eating large amounts of food when not feeling physically hungry.
  - Eating alone because of being embarrassed by how much one is eating.
  - Feeling disgusted with oneself, depressed, or very guilty afterward.
- Marked distress regarding binge eating is present.
- The binge eating occurs, on average, at least once a week for three months.
- The binge eating is not associated with the recurrent use of inappropriate compensatory behavior, such as in bulimia nervosa, and does not occur exclusively during the course of bulimia nervosa or anorexia nervosa.

Other Eating Disorders

Pica is another type of eating disorder in which an individual repeatedly eats things that are not considered food and have no nutritional value, such as paper, dirt, soap, hair, glue, or chalk. Individuals with pica do not usually have an aversion to food, and ingested items vary with age. The behavior is inappropriate to the developmental level of the individual and is not part of a culturally supported practice. A person diagnosed with pica is at risk for

---

18 National Institute of Mental Health. (2021, December). *Eating disorders.* U.S. Department of Health and Human Services. https://www.nimh.nih.gov/health/topics/eating-disorders

19 American Psychiatric Association. (2013). *Desk reference to the diagnostic criteria from DSM-5.*

My Notes

potential intestinal blockages or toxic effects of substances consumed (such as lead in paint chips). Treatment for pica involves testing for nutritional deficiencies and addressing them if needed. Behavioral interventions used to treat pica may include redirecting the individual from the nonfood items and rewarding them for setting aside or avoiding nonfood items.[20]

Avoidant restrictive food intake disorder (ARFID) is a condition where individuals limit the amount or type of food eaten. Unlike anorexia nervosa, people with ARFID do not have a distorted body image or extreme fear of gaining weight. ARFID is most common in middle childhood and usually has an earlier onset than other eating disorders. Many children go through phases of picky eating, but a child with ARFID does not eat enough calories to grow and develop properly, and an adult with ARFID does not eat enough calories to maintain basic body function.[21]

Signs and symptoms of ARFID include the following[22]:

- Dramatic restriction of types or amount of food eaten
- Lack of appetite or interest in food
- Dramatic weight loss
- Upset stomach, abdominal pain, or other gastrointestinal issues with no other known cause
- Limited range of preferred foods that becomes even more limited (i.e., "picky eating" that gets progressively worse)

ARFID does not include food restriction related to lack of availability of food; dieting; cultural practices, such as religious fasting; or developmentally normal behaviors, such as toddlers who are picky eaters. Food avoidance or restriction commonly develops in infancy or early childhood and may continue in adulthood, but it can start at any age. Regardless of the age of the person affected, ARFID can impact families, causing increased stress at mealtimes and in other social eating situations. Treatment for ARFID involves an individualized plan and may involve several specialists, including a mental health professional and a registered dietician.

Body Mass Index

Body mass index (BMI) is a person's weight in kilograms divided by the square of height in meters. BMI is an easy screening method to determine if an individual's weight is classified as underweight, healthy weight, overweight, or obese. However, it is important to remember that BMI is a screening method and does not take into account muscle mass, bone density, overall body composition, racial, and sex differences.[23] See Table 13.2a for adult weight status according to BMI ranges.

---

20 American Psychiatric Association. (2021, March). *What are eating disorders?* https://www.psychiatry.org/patients-families/eating-disorders/what-are-eating-disorders

21 National Institute of Mental Health. (2021, December). *Eating disorders.* U.S. Department of Health and Human Services. https://www.nimh.nih.gov/health/topics/eating-disorders

22 National Institute of Mental Health. (2021, December). *Eating disorders.* U.S. Department of Health and Human Services. https://www.nimh.nih.gov/health/topics/eating-disorders

23 Nordqvist, C. (2022, January 19). Why BMI is inaccurate and misleading. *Medical News Today.* https://www.medicalnewstoday.com/articles/265215

Table 13.2a Adult Weight Status by BMI[24]	
BMI	**Weight Status**
Below 18.5	Underweight
18.5 – 24.9	Healthy Weight
25.0 – 29.9	Overweight
30.0 or higher	Obese

For children and teens, the interpretation of BMI depends upon their age and sex. After BMI is calculated for children and teens, it is expressed as a percentile obtained from either a percentile calculator or growth chart. See categories of weight status based on BMI percentiles in Table 13.2b. Information pertaining to calculators and growth charts can be found in the following box.

Table 13.2b Child or Adolescent Weight Status by BMI Percentile[25]	
BMI Percentile	**Weight Status**
Less than 5th Percentile	Underweight
5th Percentile to Less Than 85th Percentile	Healthy Weight
85th Percentile to Less Than 95th Percentile	Overweight
95th Percentile or Higher	Obese

Calculating BMI

The CDC's Adult BMI Calculator conveniently calculates a person's BMI based on their height and weight. The following formulas can also be used to calculate a person's BMI[26]:

- weight (kg) / [height (m)]2 or
- weight (lb) / [height (in)]2 x 703

The CDC's BMI Percentile Calculator for Children and Adolescents conveniently calculates a child's or adolescent's BMI percentile based on their height, weight, gender, and age. Otherwise, gender

24 Centers for Disease Control and Prevention. (2021, August 27). *About adult BMI.* U.S. Department of Health & Human Services. https://www.cdc.gov/healthyweight/assessing/bmi/adult_bmi/index.html#Interpreted

25 Centers for Disease Control and Prevention. (2021, August 27). *About adult BMI.* U.S. Department of Health & Human Services. https://www.cdc.gov/healthyweight/assessing/bmi/adult_bmi/index.html#Interpreted

26 Centers for Disease Control and Prevention. (2021, August 27). *About adult BMI.* U.S. Department of Health & Human Services. https://www.cdc.gov/healthyweight/assessing/bmi/adult_bmi/index.html#Interpreted

My Notes

growth charts are used to determine BMI percentiles and then their weight status is determined using the appropriate table below:

- *BMI-for-Age Boys Growth Chart*
- *BMI-for-Age Girls Growth Chart*

Risk Factors

The exact cause of eating disorders is not fully understood, but research suggests that a combination of genetic, biological, behavioral, psychological, and cultural factors can increase a person's risk. Eating disorders are hereditary. Researchers are working to identify DNA variations that are linked to the increased risk of developing eating disorders. Brain imaging studies are also providing a better understanding of eating disorders. For example, researchers have found differences in patterns of brain activity in women with eating disorders in comparison to healthy women. This kind of research can help guide the development of new means of diagnosis and treatment of eating disorders.[27]

Although genetics increases the risk for developing eating disorders, the individual's environment plays a significant role. Onset can occur at nearly any point in the life span, but eating disorders commonly start in adolescence and young adulthood when there can be exceptional pressure from peers, social media, advertisements, etc., to diet or lose weight. For those genetically vulnerable to eating disorders, initial weight loss may reinforce a reward feedback mechanism and establish a maladaptive eating behavior pattern. Physiological and sensorial changes result in alterations in hunger and satiety, gastrointestinal motility, and decision-making around food and eating.

As you consider the genetic, environmental, and social influences of eating disorders, recognize that a combination of these factors can affect the severity and presenting characteristics for each client. Additionally, although eating disorders are commonly thought of as affecting young women, it can affect people of all genders, ages, races/ethnicities, body weights, and socioeconomic statuses. People with body weight or BMI within normal ranges can have eating disorder behaviors. See Figure 13.3[28] for an illustration of its diverse impact. Some individuals are mildly affected throughout their lives but then triggered by a significant physical or emotional life event that manifests clinical worsening.

---

27 National Institute of Mental Health. (2021, December). *Eating disorders.* U.S. Department of Health and Human Services. https://www.nimh.nih.gov/health/topics/eating-disorders

28 "eating-disorders-everyone-sm.jpg" by U.S. Department of Health and Human Services, National Institutes of Health, National Institute of Mental Health is in the Public Domain

My Notes

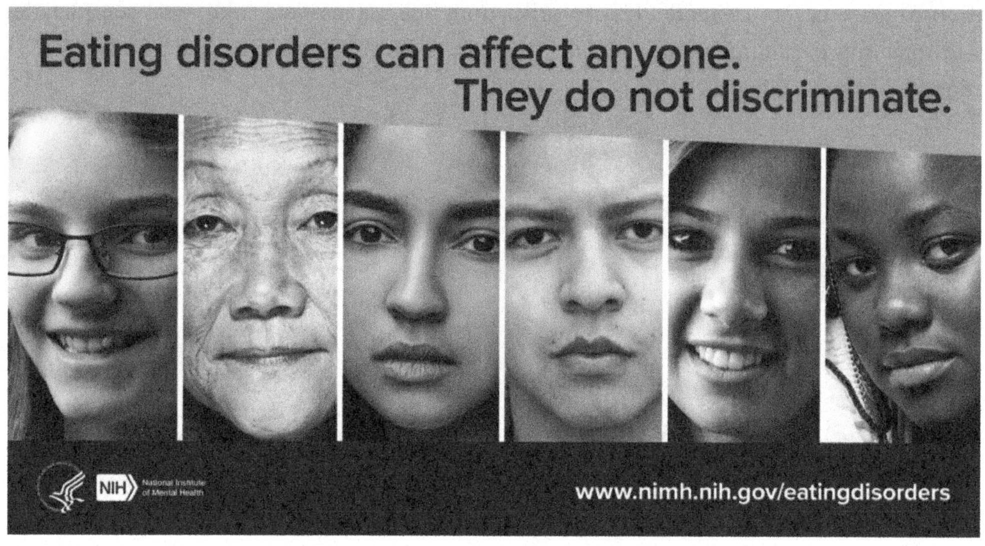

Figure 13.3 Eating Disorders Affect Anyone

Cultural Considerations

Cultural beliefs impact self-concept and satisfaction with body size. Anorexia nervosa is associated with cultures that value thinness. Furthermore, studies indicate that social media significantly influences these beliefs. For example, one study found that participants with higher use of social media had significantly greater odds of having eating concerns.[29] See Figure 13.4[30] for an image of an extremely underweight fashion model in a culture that values thinness.

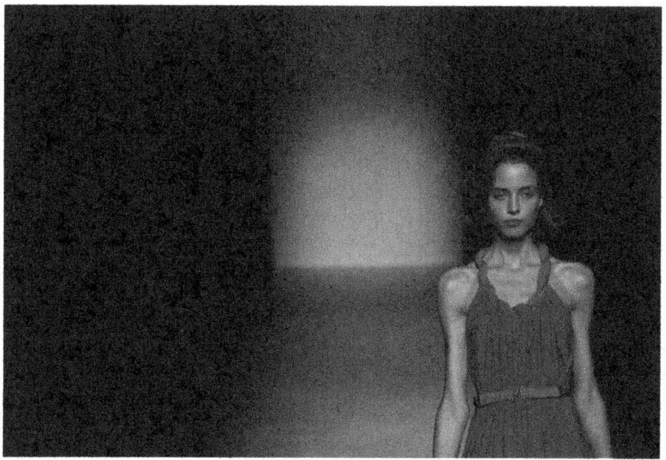

Figure 13.4 Underweight Model

---

29 Sidani, J. E., Shensa, A., Hoffman, B., Hanmer, J., & Primack, B. A. (2016). The association between social media use and eating concerns among us young adults. *Journal of the Academy of Nutrition and Dietetics, 116*(8), 1465-1472. https://doi.org/10.1016/j.jand.2016.03.021

30 "7991065935_8f05b38f46_k" by Farrukh is licensed under CC BY-NC 2.0

My Notes

Black and Hispanic teenagers are more likely to suffer from bulimia nervosa. Additional considerations are the influences of some sports' cultures on athletes where weight is a consideration, such as in wrestling, gymnastics, figure skating, and body building.[31]

31 National Eating Disorders Association. *Statistics and research on eating disorders.* https://www.nationaleatingdisorders.org/statistics-research-eating-disorders

13.3 TREATMENT FOR EATING DISORDERS

My Notes

Early treatment is important for individuals with eating disorders because of increased risk for suicide, self-injury behaviors, and medical complications. People with eating disorders may also have other mental health disorders (such as depression or anxiety) or problems with substance use. There are a variety of treatments that have been shown to be effective in treating eating disorders. Generally, treatment is more effective before the disorder becomes chronic, but even people with long-standing eating disorders can recover.[1]

Treatment plans are tailored to individual needs and may include one or more of the following:

- Individual, group, and/or family psychotherapy
- Medications
- Nutritional counseling
- Medical care and monitoring

Psychotherapy

Cognitive behavioral therapy (CBT) is used to reduce or eliminate binge eating and purging behaviors. Individuals learn how to identify distorted or unhelpful thinking patterns and recognize and change inaccurate beliefs.[2]

Read more about CBT in the "Treatments for Depression" section of the "Depressive Disorders" chapter.

Family-based therapy is a type of psychotherapy where parents of adolescents with anorexia nervosa assume responsibility for feeding their child. This therapy has been found to be very effective in helping adolescents gain weight and improve eating habits and moods.[3]

Medications

Evidence also suggests that medications such as antidepressants, antipsychotics, or mood stabilizers may also be helpful for treating eating disorders and other co-occurring mental illnesses such as anxiety or depression.[4]

Anorexia Nervosa

Standard treatment for clients with anorexia nervosa includes nutritional rehabilitation and psychotherapy. Acutely ill clients who do not gain weight despite this standard treatment may be prescribed olanzapine, a second-generation antipsychotic, or antidepressants for concurrent depressive disorders. Nurses should keep in mind that low weight clients are at increased risk for side effects. Additionally, medications such as antidepressants and

---

1 National Institute of Mental Health. (2021, December). *Eating disorders.* U.S. Department of Health and Human Services. https://www.nimh.nih.gov/health/topics/eating-disorders

2 National Institute of Mental Health. (2021, December). *Eating disorders.* U.S. Department of Health and Human Services. https://www.nimh.nih.gov/health/topics/eating-disorders

3 National Institute of Mental Health. (2021, December). *Eating disorders.* U.S. Department of Health and Human Services. https://www.nimh.nih.gov/health/topics/eating-disorders

4 National Institute of Mental Health. (2021, December). *Eating disorders.* U.S. Department of Health and Human Services. https://www.nimh.nih.gov/health/topics/eating-disorders

My Notes

antipsychotics can impact cardiac function. Bupropion is contraindicated in clients with eating disorders because of increased risk for seizures, and tricyclic antidepressants should not be used because of their cardiotoxicity.[5]

Bulimia Nervosa

Fluoxetine, an SSRI antidepressant, may be prescribed for adults with bulimia nervosa even in the absence of depressive symptoms. If fluoxetine is not tolerated, other selective serotonin reuptake inhibitors (SSRIs) may be used. However, bupropion is contraindicated in clients with bulimia because of increased risk of seizures.[6]

Binge Eating Disorder

Obese clients with binge eating disorder who do not respond to psychotherapy are encouraged to participate in behavioral weight loss therapy. SSRIs, anticonvulsants, or stimulants may be prescribed for clients with binge eating disorder.[7]

Read more about antidepressants in the "Treatments for Depression" section of the "Depressive Disorders" chapter.

Read more about antipsychotics in the "Schizophrenia" section of the "Psychosis and Schizophrenia" chapter.

Nutritional Counseling

Nutritional counseling by a dietician with specialized training is necessary for individuals with eating disorders. The counseling should incorporate education about nutritional needs, as well as planning and monitoring healthy food choices.[8]

Medical Care and Monitoring

Medical treatments for eating disorders can be delivered in a variety of settings. The following characteristics apply to the setting selected for an individual's treatment[9]:

- **Intensive Outpatient:** The client is medically and psychiatrically stable and does not need daily medical monitoring. Symptoms are under sufficient control for the individual to be able to function in normal social, educational, or vocational situations and continue to make progress in recovery.

---

5 Walsh, B. T. (2022). Anorexia nervosa in adults: Pharmacotherapy. *UpToDate.* Retrieved February 17, 2022, from www.uptodate.com

6 Halter, M. (2022). *Varcarolis' foundations of psychiatric-mental health nursing* (9th ed.). Saunders.

7 Sysko, R., & Devlin, M. (2022). Binge eating disorder in adults: Overview of treatment. *UpToDate.* Retrieved February 17, 2022, from www.uptodate.com

8 National Eating Disorders Association. (n.d.). *Treatment.* https://www.nationaleatingdisorders.org/treatment

9 National Eating Disorders Association. (n.d.). *Treatment.* https://www.nationaleatingdisorders.org/treatment

My Notes

- **Partial Hospitalization:**
  - The client is medically stable. The eating disorder impairs functioning but is without immediate risk. The client requires daily assessment of physiologic and mental status.
  - The client is psychiatrically stable but is unable to function in normal social, educational, or vocational situations. They engage in daily binge eating, purging, fasting, restricted food intake, or other pathogenic weight control techniques.
- **Residential:** The client is medically stable and requires no intensive medical intervention. They are psychiatrically impaired and unable to respond to partial hospital or outpatient treatment.
- **Inpatient:**
  - The client is medically unstable as determined by:
    - Unstable or depressed vital signs
    - Laboratory findings presenting acute health risk
    - Complications due to coexisting medical problems such as diabetes
  - The client is psychiatrically unstable as determined by:
    - Rapidly worsening symptoms
    - Suicidal ideation with a plan and unable to contract for safety

My Notes

13.4 APPLYING THE NURSING PROCESS TO EATING DISORDERS

People with eating disorders may appear healthy even when they are very ill. Additionally, individuals with anorexia nervosa often do not view their behavior as a problem. They are typically only seen in health care settings due to concerned family or friends who encourage them to seek treatment. Conversely, individuals with bulimia nervosa or binge eating disorder may feel shame and sensitivity to the perceptions of others regarding their illness. Therefore, it is vital for the nurse to build a therapeutic nurse-patient relationship with clients with eating disorders and empathize with possible feelings of low self-esteem and lack of control over eating.[1]

This section will apply the nursing process to anorexia and bulimia nervosa.

Assessment

When assessing an individual with a potential or diagnosed eating disorder, it is vital to obtain their perception of the problem while assessing for signs and symptoms. Care planning that does not address their perspective will not be effective. As previously mentioned, clients with anorexia nervosa often do not perceive their behaviors as a problem, so specialized therapeutic techniques may be required. Review signs and symptoms associated with various eating disorders in the "Basic Concepts" section.

Subjective Assessment

A complete nursing assessment includes health history, psychosocial assessment, and screening for risk of suicide or self-harm. Nutritional patterns, fluid intake, and daily exercise should also be assessed. If the client has a binging or purging pattern, the amount of food eaten and/or the frequency of these behaviors should be assessed.

Objective Assessment

Objective assessments include routine weight monitoring and orthostatic vital signs. Common objective assessment findings for individuals with anorexia nervosa and bulimia nervosa are compared in Table 13.4a. Clients with binge eating disorder may have obesity and gastrointestinal symptoms but do not typically have other associated abnormal assessment findings.

Table 13.4a Comparison of Assessment Findings in Anorexia Nervosa and Bulimia Nervosa[2]

Anorexia Nervosa	**Bulimia Nervosa**
Low weight	Normal to slightly low weight
Muscle weakening (from starvation and electrolyte imbalance)	Muscle weakening (from electrolyte imbalance)
Peripheral edema (from hypoalbuminemia)	Peripheral edema (from rebound fluids if diuretics are used)
Cardiovascular abnormalities (hypotension, bradycardia, heart failure from starvation, and dehydration)	Cardiovascular abnormalities (cardiomyopathy and cardiac dysrhythmias from electrolyte imbalances)

---

1 Halter, M. (2022). *Varcarolis' foundations of psychiatric-mental health nursing* (9th ed.). Saunders.

2 Halter, M. (2022). *Varcarolis' foundations of psychiatric-mental health nursing* (9th ed.). Saunders.

My Notes

Anorexia Nervosa	Bulimia Nervosa
Abnormal lab results (hypokalemia and anemia from starvation)	Electrolyte imbalances (hypokalemia and hyponatremia from diuretics, laxatives, or vomiting)
Other signs: Amenorrhea (lack of menstruation) Lanugo (growth of fine hair all over the body) Cold extremities Constipation Impaired renal function Decreased bone density	Other signs: Tooth erosion or dental caries (from vomiting reflux over enamel) Parotid swelling (due to increased serum amylase levels) Calluses or scars on hand (from self-induced vomiting) Seizures (purging via self-induced vomiting lowers seizure threshold)

Diagnostic and Lab Work

Laboratory and diagnostic testing are typically performed to rule out thyroid imbalances and to evaluate for potential physiological complications resulting from starvation, dehydration, and electrolyte imbalances. Laboratory testing may include the following[3]:

- Complete blood count
- Electrolyte levels
- Glucose level
- Thyroid function tests
- Erythrocyte sedimentation rate (ESR)
- Creatine phosphokinase (CPK)

Diagnostic testing may include these tests:

- Electrocardiogram (ECG)
- Dual energy X-ray absorptiometry (DEXA) to measure bone density

Diagnoses

Common nursing diagnoses for individuals diagnosed with anorexia nervosa or bulimia nervosa include these diagnoses[4]:

- *Imbalanced Nutrition: Less Than Body Requirements*
- *Risk for Electrolyte Imbalance*
- *Risk for Imbalanced Fluid Volume*
- *Impaired Body Image*

---

3 Halter, M. (2022). *Varcarolis' foundations of psychiatric-mental health nursing* (9th ed.). Saunders.

4 Halter, M. (2022). *Varcarolis' foundations of psychiatric-mental health nursing* (9th ed.). Saunders.

My Notes

- *Ineffective Coping*
- *Interrupted Family Processes*
- *Chronic Low Self-Esteem*
- *Powerlessness*
- *Risk for Spiritual Distress*

Outcomes Identification

These are the typical overall treatment goals for individuals with eating disorders[5]:

- Restoring adequate nutrition
- Bringing weight to a healthy level
- Reducing excessive exercise
- Stopping binge-purge and binge eating behaviors

SMART expected outcomes are individualized for each client based on their established nursing diagnoses and current status. (SMART is an acronym for Specific, Measurable, Attainable/Actionable, Relevant, and Timely.) An example of a SMART expected outcome for an individual hospitalized with anorexia nervosa who is experiencing electrolyte imbalances is:

The client will maintain a normal sinus heart rhythm with a regular rate during their hospitalization.[6]

Planning Interventions

Planning depends on the acuity of the client's situation. As previously discussed, clients are hospitalized for stabilization. Common criteria for hospitalization include extreme electrolyte imbalance, weight below 75% of healthy body weight, arrhythmias, hypotension, temperature less than 98 degrees Fahrenheit, or risk for suicide.[7] After a client is medically stable, the treatment plan includes a combination of psychotherapy, medications, and nutritional counseling. Review the "Treatment for Eating Disorders" section for more details.

Implementation

Nurses individualize interventions based on the client's current clinical status and their phase of treatment. Interventions can be categorized based on the American Psychiatric Nursing Association (APNA) standard for *Implementation* that includes the *Coordination of Care; Health Teaching and Health Promotion; Pharmacological, Biological, and Integrative Therapies; Milieu Therapy*; and *Therapeutic Relationship and Counseling*. (Review information about these subcategories in the "Application of the Nursing Process in Mental Health Care" chapter.) Read nursing interventions for clients with eating disorders categorized by APNA categories in Table 13.4b.

---

5 National Institute of Mental Health. (2021, December). *Eating disorders*. U.S. Department of Health and Human Services. https://www.nimh.nih.gov/health/topics/eating-disorders

6 Ackley, B., Ladwig, G., Makic, M. B., Martinez-Kratz, M., & Zanotti, M. (2020). *Nursing diagnosis handbook: An evidence-based guide to planning care* (12th ed.). Elsevier.

7 Halter, M. (2022). *Varcarolis' foundations of psychiatric-mental health nursing* (9th ed.). Saunders.

My Notes

Table 13.4b Examples of Nursing Interventions by APNA Subcategories[8,9]		
Subcategory of the APNA Standard of Implementation	**The nurse will . . .**	**Rationale**
Coordination of Care	Communicate client trends with interprofessional team members, such as risk for suicide and target weight. A target weight and daily caloric intake are set in collaboration with the dietician and the provider. Refer to community resources and outpatient treatment.	All team members providing care must be aware of the client's suicide risk to maintain a safe environment. A combination of treatments is used to achieve the client's goal weight and promote recovery. Discharge planning is a vital component of treatment and should include the client's family or loved ones.
Health Teaching and Health Promotion	Promote health by teaching adaptive coping strategies such as journaling. Support basic skills such as learning how to create meal plans, shopping at the grocery store, and navigating family or social eating situations.	Nurses encourage resilience by promoting healthy coping strategies, communication, and problem-solving skills.
Pharmacological, Biological, and Integrative Therapies	Deliver patient education about antidepressants or other medications with expected time frames for improvement.	Client understanding of their medications and potential side effects can increase medication adherence.
Milieu Therapy	Provide a pleasant, calm atmosphere at mealtimes. Emphasize the social nature of eating. Encourage conversations during mealtimes that do not involve the topics of eating or exercise. Observe clients during meals to prevent hiding or throwing away food and at least one hour after eating to prevent purging. Encourage the client to make their own menu choices as they approach their goal weight.	The milieu of an eating disorder specialty unit is purposefully organized to assist the client in establishing healthy eating patterns and normalization of eating. The highly structured environment provides precise mealtimes, adherence to the meal plan, close observation of bathroom trips, and monitoring potential access to laxatives or diuretics. Mealtimes can cause episodes of high anxiety. The client should feel accepted and safe from judgmental evaluations in the milieu with a focus on eating behaviors and underlying feelings of anxiety, dysphoria, low self-esteem, and a lack of control.[10]

8 Halter, M. (2022). *Varcarolis' foundations of psychiatric-mental health nursing* (9th ed.). Saunders.

9 American Nurses Association, American Psychiatric Nurses Association, and International Society of Psychiatric-Mental Health Nurses. (2014). *Psychiatric-mental health nursing: Scope and standards of practice* (2nd ed.).

10 Halter, M. (2022). *Varcarolis' foundations of psychiatric-mental health nursing* (9th ed.). Saunders.

My Notes

Subcategory of the APNA Standard of Implementation	The nurse will . . .	Rationale
Therapeutic Relationship and Counseling	Provide 1:1 therapeutic communication to encourage the client to develop adaptive coping strategies, use stress management techniques, develop supportive relationships, and seek spiritual resources. Acknowledge the emotional and physical difficulty the client is experiencing. Use motivational interviewing and contract with the client to increase their ownership of treatment goals. Weigh the client daily in their underwear for the first week and then three times a week. Do not allow oral intake before the morning weigh-in. It is permissible for the client to not view the scale during the weigh-in. Administer liquid supplements as prescribed. Be empathetic with the client's struggle to give up control of their eating and weight as they are expected to regain weight.	Effective therapeutic techniques for clients with depression can promote hope and positive self-esteem. The first priority is to establish a therapeutic relationship. The client's feelings of extreme fatigue can be used to engage cooperation in the treatment plan. Motivational interviewing is a collaborative, goal-oriented style of communication. It is designed to strengthen personal motivation and commitment to specific goals by eliciting and exploring the person's reasons for change within an atmosphere of acceptance and compassion.[11] Accurate weight taking and monitoring are vital. The client may try to control and sabotage the weight monitoring. The client is typically expected to gain 0.5 pound on a specific schedule. However, weight gain of more than five pounds in one week can cause pulmonary edema.

11 Miller, W. R., & Rollnick, S. (2013). *Motivational Interviewing: Helping people to change* (3rd ed.). Guilford Press.

My Notes

Subcategory of the APNA Standard of Implementation	The nurse will . . .	Rationale
	Encourage the clients to verbalize or use a journal to record their feelings surrounding eating disorder behaviors. Confront irrational thoughts and beliefs to promote healthy eating behaviors. Monitor physical activity and individualize the client's plans for exercise. Focus on the client's strengths, including their work on normalizing weight and eating behaviors. Reinforce the knowledge and skills gained from individual, family, and group therapy sessions.	The particulars of how patients should be weighed (i.e., open vs. blind weighed) is a point of debate in the field. Because viewing the scale can cause anxiety, blind weighing is typically used during the acute stage of treatment, whereas open weighing may be suitable at later stages of recovery.[12] Oral or enteral supplements may be prescribed based on the client's status. However, be alert for refeeding syndrome in severely malnourished clients. External control is required initially to promote good nutrition and a healthy weight. Cognitive and behavioral changes will occur gradually. The client often experiences a strong drive to exercise. Nurses can assist in planning a reasonable amount of exercise. Acknowledge milestones and encourage other sources of gratification other than eating.

Inpatient Care

If the client is exhibiting risk for suicide, a safety plan should be immediately implemented. Review nursing care for clients with risk for suicide in the "Application of the Nursing Process in Mental Health Care" chapter.

Severely malnourished clients may require therapeutic enteral nutrition. Any client with negligible food intake for more than five days is at risk of developing a potentially fatal complication called refeeding syndrome. The hallmark feature of **refeeding syndrome** is hypophosphatemia but may also involve serious sodium and fluid imbalances; changes in glucose, protein, and fat metabolism; thiamine deficiency; hypokalemia; and hypomagnesaemia. To avoid this syndrome, a thorough nutritional assessment must be performed followed by the slow reintroduction of nutrients and fluids according to evidence-based guidelines.[13]

After resolving acute symptoms, clients with anorexia begin a weight restoration program for incremental weight gain with a treatment goal set for 90% of ideal body weight. Specially trained dieticians assist in developing daily meal plans and caloric intake, and clients are generally weighed two or three times a week to gauge progress.[14]

---

12 Froreich, F. V., Ratcliffe, S. E., & Vartanian, L. R. (2020). Blind versus open weighing from an eating disorder patient perspective. *Journal of Eating Disorders 8*, 39. https://doi.org/10.1186/s40337-020-00316-1

13 Mehanna, H. M., Moledina, J., & Travis, J. (2008). Refeeding syndrome: What it is, and how to prevent and treat it. *BMJ, 336*, 1495–1498. https://doi.org/10.1136/bmj.a301

14 Halter, M. (2022). *Varcarolis' foundations of psychiatric-mental health nursing* (9th ed.). Saunders.

My Notes

Nurses should be aware that clients with bulimia nervosa typically establish a therapeutic nurse-client relationship more quickly than clients with anorexia nervosa. As previously discussed in this chapter, clients with anorexia nervosa often do not view their condition as a disorder and value their obsessive-compulsive behaviors with eating as a way to feel safe and secure and avoid negative feelings. Conversely, clients with bulimia nervosa view their behaviors as problematic and desire help.[15]

Outpatient Care

Outpatient partial hospitalization is an option for clients who have been medically stabilized. In this setting, clients are in a clinical setting during the day and then go home to practice skills in the afternoon. Outpatient treatment continues if the client maintains a contracted weight, vital signs are within a normal range, and there is an absence of disordered eating behaviors.[16]

A significant part of the recovery process includes rebuilding relationships with family. Family members or significant others often feel frustrated, powerless, and hopeless because the strategies they previously attempted, such as forcing the client to eat or begging the client to eat, were not successful. The nurse helps with this recovery process by providing education to the client and their loved ones about the illness, treatment, and meal planning. Adaptive coping skills to address disordered thoughts should be reinforced.[17]

Review information about coping strategies in the "Stress, Coping, and Crisis Intervention" chapter.

Resources

Nurses refer clients and their loved ones to resources as part of discharge planning. Review examples of community resources in the following box.

Resources for Individuals With Eating Disorders

- National Eating Disorders Association (NEDA): Support, resources, and treatment options
- Eating Disorders Resource Group: Resources including treatment apps
- ANAD: Eating disorder peer support groups

Evaluation

Evaluation is a continuous process of reviewing a client's progress towards their individualized goals and SMART outcomes. Interventions are continually evaluated and modified based on their success in meeting these short-term goals.

---

15 Halter, M. (2022). *Varcarolis' foundations of psychiatric-mental health nursing* (9th ed.). Saunders.

16 Halter, M. (2022). *Varcarolis' foundations of psychiatric-mental health nursing* (9th ed.). Saunders.

17 Halter, M. (2022). *Varcarolis' foundations of psychiatric-mental health nursing* (9th ed.). Saunders.

13.5 SPOTLIGHT APPLICATION

My Notes

Consider these real-life stories of people who have struggled with eating disorders.

1. Princess Diana raised public awareness about eating disorders after sharing her experience with bulimia nervosa in recordings featured in the documentary *Diana: In Her Own Words*. After the publication, there was a sudden spike in the number of reported cases of bulimia, and many people came forward to receive the treatment they needed. Because of Diana's openness and honesty about her struggles with her eating disorder, countless people were empowered to be open and admit their own similar struggles.

Read more about Princess Diana's experience in an NEDA blog titled 20 Years Later: How Princess Diana's Legacy Continues to Help People With Eating Disorders.

2. Mike Majama, a major league baseball player, experienced an eating disorder that impacted his sports career.

Read a *Good Morning America* interview with Mike Majama.

3. Karla Mosley, an actress on the television show *The Bold and the Beautiful.*

Read an NPR interview with Karla Mosley.

4. Veterans with eating disorders.

Read a Connecticut Health Team story about veterans with eating disorders.

Reflective Questions

1. Compare and contrast the experiences of these individuals.
2. What strikes you most about these real-life stories?

My Notes

13.6 LEARNING ACTIVITIES

Learning Activities

(Answers to "Learning Activities" can be found in the "Answer Key" at the end of the book. Answers to the interactive activities are provided as immediate feedback.)

Case Study:

Tiffany is a 24-year-old nursing student who works weekends as a certified nursing assistant. Her sister Sara brought Tiffany to a clinic appointment with a nurse practitioner because of their family's concerns about Tiffany's weight and eating habits. During the intake process, Tiffany states, "I don't think there is a problem; I just don't want to be fat." Tiffany is 5'7" and weighs 101 pounds in her street clothes, with a calculated BMI of 15.8. When asked to perform a 24-hour diet recall, Tiffany states, "I drink coffee for breakfast, eat a low-fat yogurt for lunch, and then eat a head of iceberg lettuce for dinner most days." She cannot recall the last time she had a menstrual cycle. Tiffany states, "I used to run five miles every day, but lately I have been too tired to run." She denies any purging episodes. Sara states, "Tiffany does not sit down and eat meals with the rest of us. We have tried everything and cannot get her to eat. My mom has tried talking to her, begging her, and even yelling at her. If Tiffany does eat something besides lettuce, she either goes in the bathroom and vomits or runs ten miles. We are very worried about her and don't know what to do."

Questions:

1. What symptoms of an eating disorder is Tiffany demonstrating?
2. What other assessments does the nurse plan for Tiffany?
3. What findings does the nurse anticipate as a result of a comprehensive assessment?
4. What laboratory tests will likely be ordered during this visit?
5. What is the goal of treatment for Tiffany?
6. What type of psychotherapy would be helpful for Tiffany?
7. What conditions would cause Tiffany to be hospitalized?
8. Tiffany is hospitalized. Create a brief nursing care plan for Tiffany including a nursing diagnosis, SMART goal, and 3-5 nursing interventions.

My Notes

Interactive Activities

An interactive H5P element has been excluded from this version of the text. You can view it online here: https://wtcs.pressbooks.pub/nursingmhcc/?p=672#h5p-45

An interactive H5P element has been excluded from this version of the text. You can view it online here: https://wtcs.pressbooks.pub/nursingmhcc/?p=672#h5p-46

My Notes

XIII GLOSSARY

Anorexia nervosa: A condition where people avoid food, severely restrict food, or eat very small quantities of only certain foods.

Avoidant restrictive food intake disorder (ARFID): A condition where individuals limit the amount or type of food eaten.

Binge eating disorder: A condition where people lose control over their eating and have recurring episodes of eating unusually large amounts of food. Unlike bulimia nervosa, periods of binge eating are not followed by purging, excessive exercise, or fasting.

Binge eating episode: An episode characterized by both eating in a discrete period of time (e.g., within any two-hour period) an amount of food that is definitely larger than what most individuals would eat and a sense of a lack of control over eating during the episode.

Body mass index (BMI): A person's weight in kilograms divided by the square of height in meters.

Bulimia nervosa: A condition where people have recurrent and frequent episodes of eating unusually large amounts of food and feeling a lack of control over these episodes.

Emaciation: A condition of extreme thinness.

Family-based therapy: A type of psychotherapy where parents of adolescents with anorexia nervosa assume responsibility for feeding their child.

Lanugo: Growth of fine hair all over the body.

Pica: An eating disorder in which an individual repeatedly eats things that are not considered food with no nutritional value, such as paper, dirt, soap, hair, glue, or chalk.

Purging: Behavior in eating disorders used to compensate for overeating, such as forced vomiting, excessive use of laxatives, or diuretics.

Refeeding syndrome: A potentially fatal complication for any client with negligible food intake for more than five days that involves hypophosphatemia; serious sodium and fluid imbalances; changes in glucose, protein, and fat metabolism; thiamine deficiency; hypokalemia; and hypomagnesaemia.

Chapter 14

Substance Use Disorders

14.1 INTRODUCTION

My Notes

Learning Objectives

- Assess clients for intoxication, dependency, withdrawal symptoms, and/or substance use disorders and intervene as appropriate
- Apply the nursing process to clients experiencing withdrawal or toxicity from substances
- Provide care and/or support clients with nonsubstance-related dependencies (e.g., gambling, sexual addiction)
- Describe the neurobiology and risk factors for substance use disorders
- Apply the nursing process to clients with substance use disorders
- Describe protective factors and prevention programs for substance use disorders
- Outline evidence-based treatments for clients with substance use disorders
- Discuss recovery services for clients with substance use disorders
- Evaluate client's response to a treatment plan and revise as needed
- Provide patient education to clients and their family members

Misuse of alcohol, drugs, and prescribed medications is estimated to cost the United States more than $400 billion in health care expenses, law enforcement and criminal justice costs (due to drug-related crimes), lost workplace productivity, and losses from motor vehicle crashes.[1] The Centers for Disease Control and Prevention (CDC) National Center for Health Statistics estimates 107,622 drug overdose deaths and 52,000 alcohol-induced deaths occurred in the United States in 2021.[2]

View a visualization of recent drug overdose death rates nationally and by state at the CDC National Center for Health Statistics' Vital Statistics Rapid Release web page: Provisional Drug Overdose Death Counts.

Chronic substance use disorders significantly impact individuals, families, communities, and our society. According to the 2020 National Survey on Drug Use and Health (NSDUH), 40.3 million people in the United States aged 12 or older (14.5 percent) have a substance use disorder (SUD).[3]

---

1 Substance Abuse and Mental Health Services Administration, & Office of the Surgeon General. (2016). *Facing addiction in America: The surgeon general's report on alcohol, drugs, and health.* United States Department of Health and Human Services. https://www.ncbi.nlm.nih.gov/books/NBK424857/

2 National Center for Health Statistics. (2022, May 11). *U.S. overdose deaths in 2021 increased half as much in 2020 - but are still up 15%* [Press release]. https://www.cdc.gov/nchs/pressroom/nchs_press_releases/2022/ 202205.htm

3 National Survey on Drug Use and Health. https://nsduhweb.rti.org/respweb/homepage.cfm

My Notes

This chapter will provide an overview of many topics related to substance use. It begins by reviewing signs of intoxication of various psychoactive substances and treatment for overdose and withdrawal symptoms. The neurobiology of substance use disorders and risk factors are explored, and then evidence-based treatment and prevention interventions are discussed based on the Surgeon General's Report on Alcohol, Drugs, and Health. Finally, the nursing process is applied to a hospitalized client receiving treatment for alcohol withdrawal.

14.2 SUBSTANCES: USE, INTOXICATION, AND OVERDOSE

My Notes

A **substance** is defined as a psychoactive compound with the potential to cause health and social problems, including substance use disorder. Substances can be divided into four major categories: alcohol, illicit drugs (including nonmedical use of prescription drugs), over-the-counter drugs, and other substances. See examples of substances known to have a significant public health impact in Table 14.2a. **Substance use** refers to the use of any of the psychoactive substances listed in Table 14.2a.

Table 14.2a Categories and Examples of Substances[1]

Substance Category	Examples
Alcohol	Beer, malt liquor, wine, and distilled spirits
Illicit drugs (including prescription drugs used nonmedically)	■ Opioids, including heroin ■ Cannabis ■ Sedatives, hypnotics, and anxiolytics ■ Hallucinogens ■ Stimulants, including methamphetamine-like substances, cocaine, and crack ■ Dextromethorphan and other cold medications
Over-the-counter drugs (used nonmedically)	Dextromethorphan, pseudoephedrine, and other cold medications
Other substances	Inhalants such as spray paint, gasoline, and cleaning solvents; Delta-8 THC

Millions of Americans misuse substances. See Figure 14.1[2] regarding the number of people aged 12 and older who reported using various substances in a one-month period of time.

1 Substance Abuse and Mental Health Services Administration, & Office of the Surgeon General. (2016). *Facing addiction in America: The surgeon general's report on alcohol, drugs, and health.* United States Department of Health and Human Services. https://www.ncbi.nlm.nih.gov/books/NBK424857/

2 This image is a derivative of "Past Month General Substance Use and Nicotine Vaping: Among People Aged 12 and Older; 2020" table by Substance Abuse and Mental Health Services Administration. (2021). Key substance use and mental health indicators in the United States: Results from the 2020 National Survey on Drug Use and Health (HHS Publication No. PEP21-07-01-003, NSDUH Series H-56). Rockville, MD: Center for Behavioral Health Statistics and Quality, Substance Abuse and Mental Health Services Administration. Used under Fair Use. Retrieved from https://www.samhsa.gov/data/report/2020-nsduh-annual-national-report

My Notes

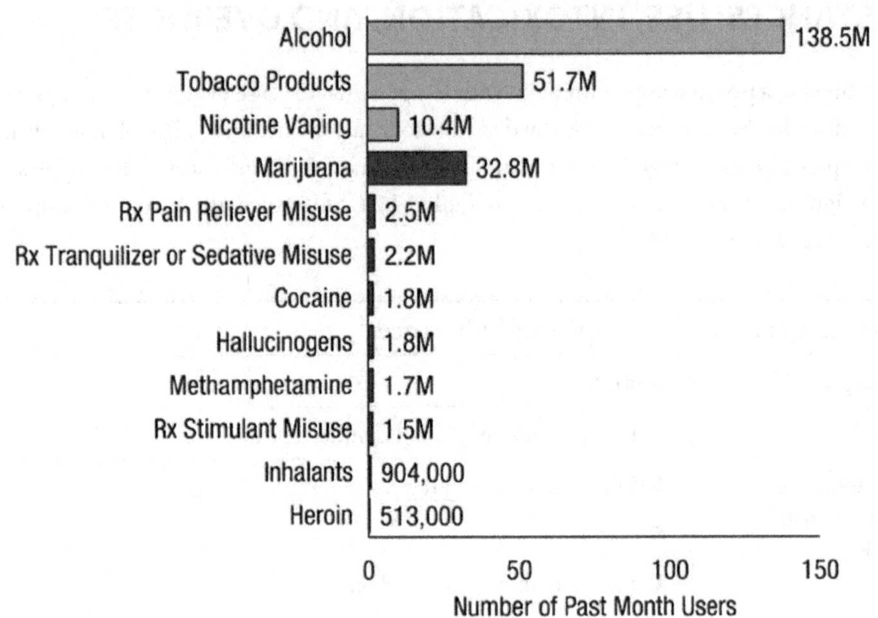

Figure 14.1 Number of People Aged 12 and OIder Who Reported Using Substances in the Past Month in 2020. Used under Fair Use.

Controlled Substances

The Controlled Substances Act is a federal law that places all **controlled substances** (i.e., substances regulated by the U.S. Drug Enforcement Agency) into one of five categories called schedules. This placement is based on the substance's medical use, its potential for abuse or dependency, and related safety issues. For example, Schedule I drugs have a high potential for abuse and potentially cause severe psychological and/or physical dependence, whereas Schedule V drugs represent the least potential for abuse.[3] **Dependence** means that when a person suddenly stops using a drug, their body goes through **withdrawal,** a group of physical and mental symptoms that can range from mild to life-threatening. See examples of controlled substances categorized by schedule in Table 14.2b.

Table 14.2b Examples of Substances by Schedule[4]

Schedule	Definition	Examples
Schedule I	No currently accepted medical use and a high potential for abuse.	Heroin, LSD, MDMA (Ecstasy), and cannabis (marijuana)
Schedule II	High potential for abuse, with use potentially leading to severe psychological or physical dependence. These drugs are also considered dangerous.	Hydrocodone, cocaine, methamphetamine, methadone, hydromorphone, meperidine, oxycodone, fentanyl, amphetamine/dextroamphetamine salts (Adderall), methylphenidate (Ritalin), and phencyclidine (PCP)

3 United States Drug Enforcement Administration. (n.d.). *The Controlled Substance Act.* U.S. Department of Justice. https://www.dea.gov/drug-information/csa

4 United States Drug Enforcement Administration. (n.d.). *The Controlled Substance Act.* U.S. Department of Justice. https://www.dea.gov/drug-information/csa

My Notes

Schedule	Definition	Examples
Schedule III	Moderate to low potential for physical and psychological dependence. Abuse potential is less than Schedule I and Schedule II drugs but more than Schedule IV.	Acetaminophen with codeine, ketamine, anabolic steroids, and testosterone
Schedule IV	Low potential for abuse and low risk of dependence.	Alprazolam (Xanax), diazepam (Valium), lorazepam (Ativan), zolpidem (Ambien), and tramadol (Ultram)
Schedule V	Lower potential for abuse than Schedule IV and consist of preparations containing limited quantities of certain narcotics. Generally used for antidiarrheal, antitussive, and analgesic purposes.	Cough medications with codeine, diphenoxylate/atropine (Lomotil), and pregabalin (Lyrica)

See the DEA alphabetized list of controlled substances PDF.

Substance Misuse

Substance misuse is defined as the use of alcohol or drugs in a manner, situation, amount, or frequency that could cause harm to the user or to those around them.[5] Misuse can be of low severity and temporary, but it can increase the risk for serious and costly consequences such as motor vehicle crashes; overdose death; suicide; various types of cancer; heart, liver, and pancreatic diseases; HIV/AIDS; and unintended pregnancies. Substance use during pregnancy can cause complications for the baby such as fetal alcohol spectrum disorders (FASDs) or neonatal abstinence syndrome (NAS). Substance misuse is also associated with intimate partner violence, child abuse, and neglect.[6] Substance abuse, an older diagnostic term, referred to unsafe substance use (e.g., drunk or drugged driving), use that caused legal problems, or use that continued despite failure to meet work and family responsibilities. However, the term "substance abuse" is now avoided by professionals because it does not accurately account for the neurobiological knowledge we now have about addictive disorders. Instead, the term "substance use disorder" is preferred and is further discussed in the "Substance Use Disorder" subsection of this chapter.[7]

Intoxication and Overdose

Intoxication refers to a disturbance in behavior or mental function during or after the consumption of a substance. **Overdose** is the biological response of the human body when too much of a substance is ingested. Signs of intoxication and overdose for categories of psychoactive substances are described in the following subsections.

5 Substance Abuse and Mental Health Services Administration, & Office of the Surgeon General. (2016). *Facing addiction in America: The surgeon general's report on alcohol, drugs, and health.* United States Department of Health and Human Services. https://www.ncbi.nlm.nih.gov/books/NBK424857/

6 Substance Abuse and Mental Health Services Administration, & Office of the Surgeon General. (2016). *Facing addiction in America: The surgeon general's report on alcohol, drugs, and health.* United States Department of Health and Human Services. https://www.ncbi.nlm.nih.gov/books/NBK424857/

7 Substance Abuse and Mental Health Services Administration, & Office of the Surgeon General. (2016). *Facing addiction in America: The surgeon general's report on alcohol, drugs, and health.* United States Department of Health and Human Services. https://www.ncbi.nlm.nih.gov/books/NBK424857/

My Notes

Anyone can call a regional poison control center at 1-800-222-1222 for consultation regarding toxic ingestion of substances and overdoses. Poison control centers are available at all times, every day of the year. Some hospitals also have toxicologists available for bedside consultation for overdoses.[8]

Alcohol Use and Intoxication

Based on the 2015-2020 Dietary Guidelines for Americans, a **standard drink** is defined as 14 grams (0.6 ounces) of pure alcohol. Examples of a standard drink are one 12-ounce beer, 8 – 9 ounces of malt liquor, 5 ounces of wine, or 1.5 ounces of distilled spirits. See Figure 14.2[9] for images of standard drinks.

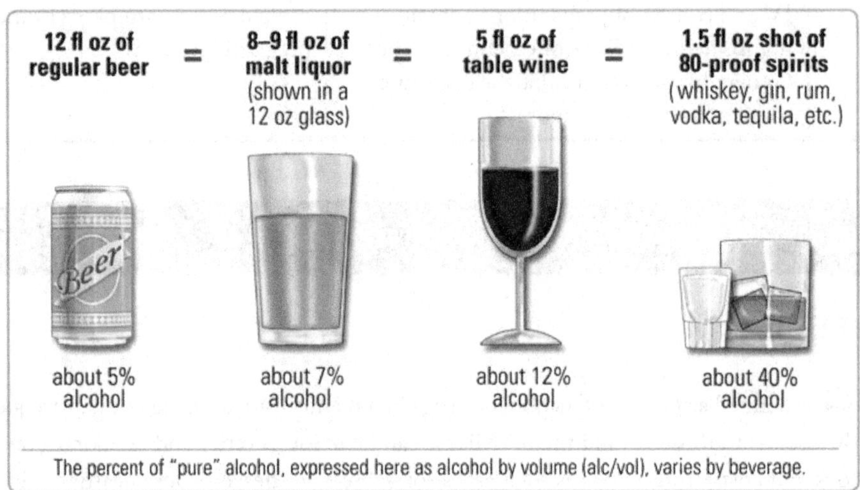

Figure 14.2 Standard Drink

The 2020 National Survey on Drug Use and Health reports that 50 percent (139.7 million) of Americans aged 12 or older use alcohol, 22.2 percent are binge drinkers, and 6.4 percent are heavy alcohol users.[10] **Heavy drinking** is defined as a female consuming 8 or more drinks per week or a male consuming 15 or more standard drinks per week, or either gender binge drinking on 5 or more days in the past 30 days. **Binge drinking** is defined as consuming several standard drinks on one occasion in the past 30 days; for men, this refers to drinking five or more standard alcoholic drinks on one occasion, and for women this refers to drinking four or more standard drinks on one occasion.[11] Alcohol intoxication refers to problematic behavioral or psychological changes (e.g., inappropriate sexual or aggressive behavior, mood lability, or impaired judgment) that develop during or shortly thereafter alcohol ingestion. Signs and symptoms of alcohol intoxication are as follows[12]:

- Slurred speech
- Incoordination

---

8 Rosenbaum, C., & Boyer, E. (2021, January 20). Dextromethorphan abuse and poisoning: Clinical features and diagnosis. *UpToDate*. Retrieved March 21, 2022, from www.uptodate.com

9 "NIH_standard_drink_comparison.jpg" by National Institutes of Health is in the Public Domain

10 National Survey on Drug Use and Health. https://nsduhweb.rti.org/respweb/homepage.cfm

11 National Survey on Drug Use and Health. https://nsduhweb.rti.org/respweb/homepage.cfm

12 American Psychiatric Association. (2013). *Desk reference to the diagnostic criteria from DSM-5*.

- Unsteady gait
- Nystagmus
- Impairment in attention or memory

Alcohol Overdose

An alcohol overdose occurs when there is so much alcohol in the bloodstream that areas of the brain controlling autonomic nervous system functions (e.g., breathing, heart rate, and temperature control) begin to shut down. Signs of alcohol overdose include mental confusion, difficulty remaining conscious, vomiting, seizures, trouble breathing, slow heart rate, clammy skin, dulled gag reflex, and extremely low body temperature. Alcohol intoxication while also taking opioids or sedative-hypnotics (such as benzodiazepines or sleep medications) increases the risk of an overdose. Alcohol overdose can cause permanent brain damage or death.[13] Anyone who consumes too much alcohol too quickly is in danger of an alcohol overdose, especially for individuals who engage in binge drinking. As blood alcohol concentration (BAC) increases, so does the risk of harm. When BAC reaches high levels, blackouts (gaps in memory), loss of consciousness (passing out), and death can occur. BAC can continue to rise even when a person stops drinking or is unconscious because alcohol in the stomach and intestine continues to enter the bloodstream and circulate throughout the body. See Figure 14.3[14] for the impairments related to rising BAC.

---

13 National Institute on Alcohol Abuse and Alcoholism, & National Institutes of Health. (2021, May). *Understanding the dangers of alcohol overdose.* https://www.niaaa.nih.gov/publications/brochures-and-fact-sheets/understanding-dangers-of-alcohol-overdose

14 "NIAAA_BAC_Increases_Graphic.jpg" by The National Institute on Alcohol Abuse and Alcoholism is in the Public Domain. Access for free at https://www.niaaa.nih.gov/publications/brochures-and-fact-sheets/understanding-dangers-of-alcohol-overdose

My Notes

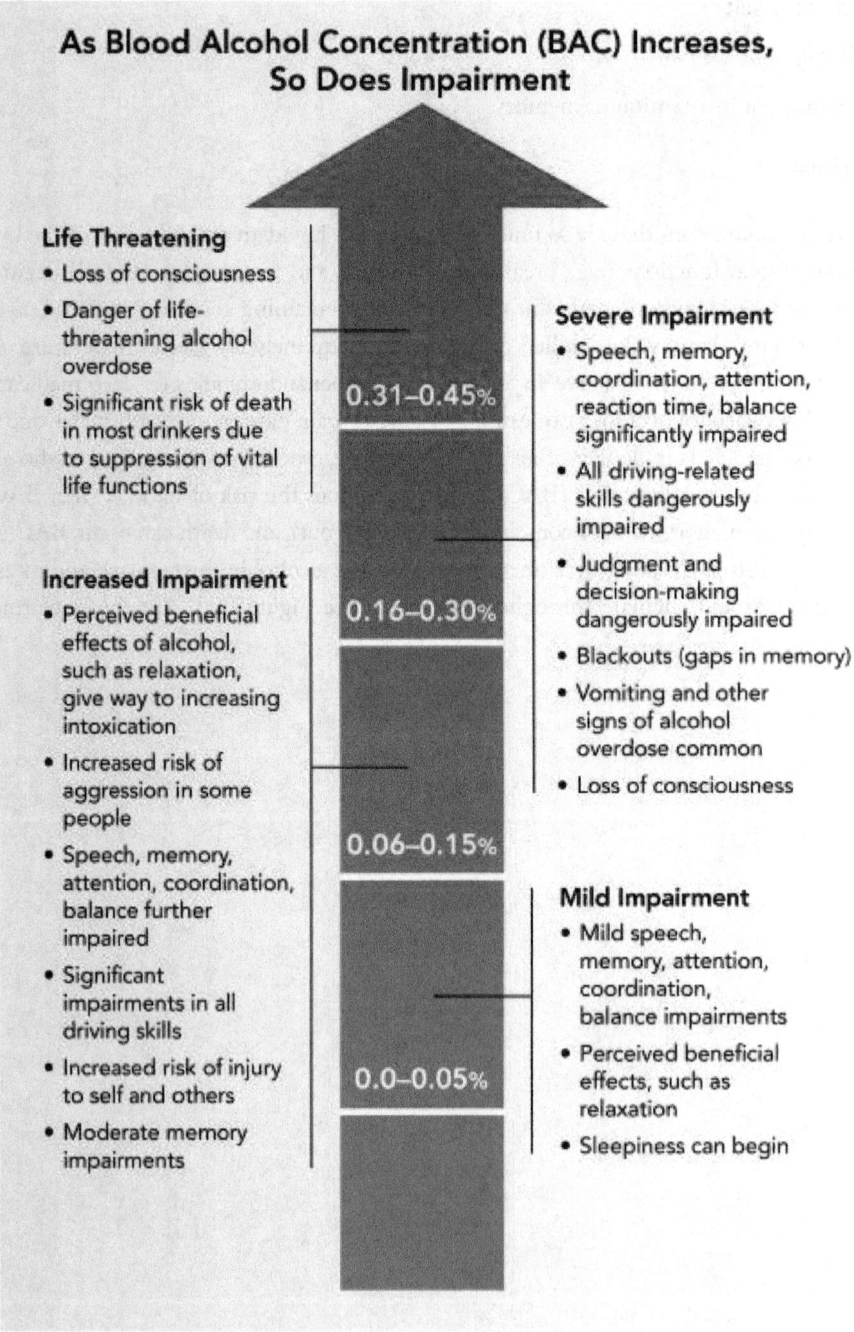

As Blood Alcohol Concentration (BAC) Increases, So Does Impairment

0.0–0.05%

Mild Impairment
- Mild speech, memory, attention, coordination, balance impairments
- Perceived beneficial effects, such as relaxation
- Sleepiness can begin

0.06–0.15%

Increased Impairment
- Perceived beneficial effects of alcohol, such as relaxation, give way to increasing intoxication
- Increased risk of aggression in some people
- Speech, memory, attention, coordination, balance further impaired
- Significant impairments in all driving skills
- Increased risk of injury to self and others
- Moderate memory impairments

0.16–0.30%

Severe Impairment
- Speech, memory, coordination, attention, reaction time, balance significantly impaired
- All driving-related skills dangerously impaired
- Judgment and decision-making dangerously impaired
- Blackouts (gaps in memory)
- Vomiting and other signs of alcohol overdose common
- Loss of consciousness

0.31–0.45%

Life Threatening
- Loss of consciousness
- Danger of life-threatening alcohol overdose
- Significant risk of death in most drinkers due to suppression of vital life functions

Figure 14.3 Impairments of Rising Blood Alcohol Concentrations

It is dangerous to assume that a person who drank an excessive amount of alcohol will "sleep it off." One potential danger of alcohol overdose is choking on one's vomit and dying from lack of oxygen because high levels of alcohol intake hinder the gag reflex, resulting in the inability to protect the airway. Asphyxiation can occur due to an obstructed airway or from aspiration of gastric contents into the lungs. For this reason, do not leave a person alone who has passed out due to alcohol misuse. Keep them in a partially upright position or roll them onto one

My Notes

side with an ear toward the ground to prevent choking if they begin vomiting.[15] Critical signs and symptoms of an alcohol overdose include the following[16]:

- Mental confusion or stupor
- Difficulty remaining conscious or inability to wake up
- Vomiting
- Seizures
- Slow respiratory rate (fewer than 8 breaths per minute)
- Irregular breathing (10 seconds or more between breaths)
- Slow heart rate
- Clammy skin
- No gag reflex
- Extremely low body temperature
- Bluish skin color or paleness

If you suspect someone has overdosed on alcohol, seek emergency assistance or call 911. While waiting for help to arrive, be prepared to provide information to the responders, such as the type and amount of alcohol the person drank and any other drugs they ingested, current medications, allergies to medications, and any existing health conditions.[17]

Medical Treatment of Acute Alcohol Intoxication

Acute alcohol intoxication can cause hypotension and tachycardia as a result of peripheral vasodilation or of the client's blood alcohol level (BAC). It is important to know if other drugs like opioids, benzodiazepines, or street drugs have been ingested because this increases the risk of overdose, and other treatments (such as naloxone) may be required. For clients with moderate to severe intoxication, routine lab work includes serum glucose and electrolytes to assess for hypoglycemia, hypokalemia, hypomagnesemia, hypocalcemia, hypophosphatemia, and hyperlactatemia. If hypoglycemia is present, a dextrose intravenous infusion is provided.[18] Severely intoxicated clients may receive intravenous thiamine, along with dextrose, to prevent Wernicke's encephalopathy. Wernicke's encephalopathy is an acute, life-threatening neurological condition characterized by nystagmus, ataxia, and confusion caused by thiamine (B1) deficiency associated with alcohol use disorder. Thiamine is required for cerebral

---

15 National Institute on Alcohol Abuse and Alcoholism, & National Institutes of Health. (2021, May). *Understanding the dangers of alcohol overdose.* https://www.niaaa.nih.gov/publications/brochures-and-fact-sheets/understanding-dangers-of-alcohol-overdose

16 National Institute on Alcohol Abuse and Alcoholism, & National Institutes of Health. (2021, May). *Understanding the dangers of alcohol overdose.* https://www.niaaa.nih.gov/publications/brochures-and-fact-sheets/understanding-dangers-of-alcohol-overdose

17 National Institute on Alcohol Abuse and Alcoholism, & National Institutes of Health. (2021, May). *Understanding the dangers of alcohol overdose.* https://www.niaaa.nih.gov/publications/brochures-and-fact-sheets/understanding-dangers-of-alcohol-overdose

18 Cowan, E., & Su, M. K. (2020, March 19). Ethanol intoxication in adults. *UpToDate.* Retrieved March 21, 2022, from www.uptodate.com

My Notes

energy utilization.[19] If untreated, Wernicke's encephalopathy can progress to Korsakoff's syndrome, a chronic, irreversible memory disorder resulting from thiamine deficiency.[20]

Some clients with acute alcohol intoxication can become agitated, violent, and uncooperative. Chemical sedation with administration of benzodiazepines may be required to prevent the client from harming themselves or others. However, benzodiazepines must be used with caution because they worsen the respiratory depression caused by alcohol.[21] Approximately one percent of clients with acute alcohol intoxication require critical care. Risk factors for admission to the intensive care unit (ICU) include abnormal vital signs (hypotension, tachycardia, fever, or hypothermia), hypoxia, hypoglycemia, and the need for parenteral sedation. If the client has inadequate respirations or airway maintenance, intubation and mechanical ventilation are required. Activated charcoal and gastric lavage are generally not helpful because of the rapid rate of absorption of alcohol from the gastrointestinal tract. Some acutely intoxicated clients experience head traumas due to severe intoxication from injuries sustained while intoxicated. If the client's mental status does not improve as their BAC level decreases, a CT scan of the head may be obtained.[22]

Opioid Use and Intoxication

In 2020, 9.5 million (3.4%) of Americans aged 12 and older reported using opioids in the past year. Among this population, 9.3 million people misused prescription pain relievers, and 902,000 people used heroin.[23] Opioids are substances that act on opioid receptors in the central nervous system. Medically, they are used for relief of moderate to severe pain and anesthesia. When misused, opioids cause a person to feel relaxed and euphoric (i.e., experience an intense feeling of happiness). Opioid prescription medications include Schedule II medications such as morphine, oxycodone, hydrocodone, fentanyl, and hydromorphone. Heroin, an illegal street drug, is also an opioid, but it is classified as a Schedule I drug.[24] Injected opioid misuse is a risk factor for contracting HIV, hepatitis B, hepatitis C, and bacterial endocarditis. The CDC reports that people who inject drugs accounted for 9 percent of HIV diagnoses in the United States in 2016.[25] Opioid intoxication causes problematic behavioral or psychological changes such as initial euphoria followed by apathy, dysphoria, psychomotor retardation or agitation, and impaired judgment. These are some signs of opioid intoxication[26]:

- Pupillary constriction (or dilation from severe overdose)
- Drowsiness or coma

---

19 This work is a derivative of *StatPearls* by Vasan and Kumar and is licensed under CC BY 4.0

20 National Institute of Neurological Disorders and Stroke. (n.d.). *Wernicke-Korsakoff syndrome.* https://www.ninds.nih.gov/health-information/disorders/wernicke-korsakoff-syndrome#:~:text=Korsakoff%20syndrome%20(also%20called%20Korsakoff's,the%20brain%20involved%20with%20memory

21 Cowan, E., & Su, M. K. (2020, March 19). Ethanol intoxication in adults. *UpToDate.* Retrieved March 21, 2022, from www.uptodate.com

22 Cowan, E., & Su, M. K. (2020, March 19). Ethanol intoxication in adults. *UpToDate.* Retrieved March 21, 2022, from www.uptodate.com

23 National Survey on Drug Use and Health. https://nsduhweb.rti.org/respweb/homepage.cfm

24 A.D.A.M. Medical Encyclopedia [Internet]. Atlanta (GA): A.D.A.M., Inc.; c1997-2022. Opioid intoxication; [updated 2022, February 18]. https://medlineplus.gov/ency/article/000948.htm

25 Substance Abuse and Mental Health Services Administration. (2022, March 2). *Alcohol, tobacco, and other drugs.* U.S. Department of Health & Human Services. https://www.samhsa.gov/find-help/atod

26 American Psychiatric Association. (2013). *Desk reference to the diagnostic criteria from DSM-5.*

My Notes

- Slurred speech
- Impairment in attention or memory

The typical signs of opioid overdose are referred to as the opioid overdose triad and include pinpoint pupils, respiratory depression, and decreased level of consciousness.[27]

Increasing Rates of Opioid Overdose Deaths

From 1999 to 2019, nearly 500,000 people died from an overdose involving prescription or illicit opioids. This rise in opioid overdose deaths can be outlined in three distinct waves. See Figure 14.4[28] for an illustration of these three waves of opioid overdose. The first wave of overdose deaths began with the increased prescription rate of opioids in the 1990s. The second wave began in 2010 with rapid increases in overdose deaths involving heroin. The third wave began in 2013 with significant increases in overdose deaths involving synthetic opioids, particularly illicitly manufactured fentanyl.[29]

There are two types of fentanyl: pharmaceutical fentanyl prescribed for severe pain, and illicitly manufactured fentanyl. Most recent cases of fentanyl-related overdose are associated with illicitly manufactured fentanyl that is added to other street drugs that make them more powerful, more addictive, and more dangerous.[30]

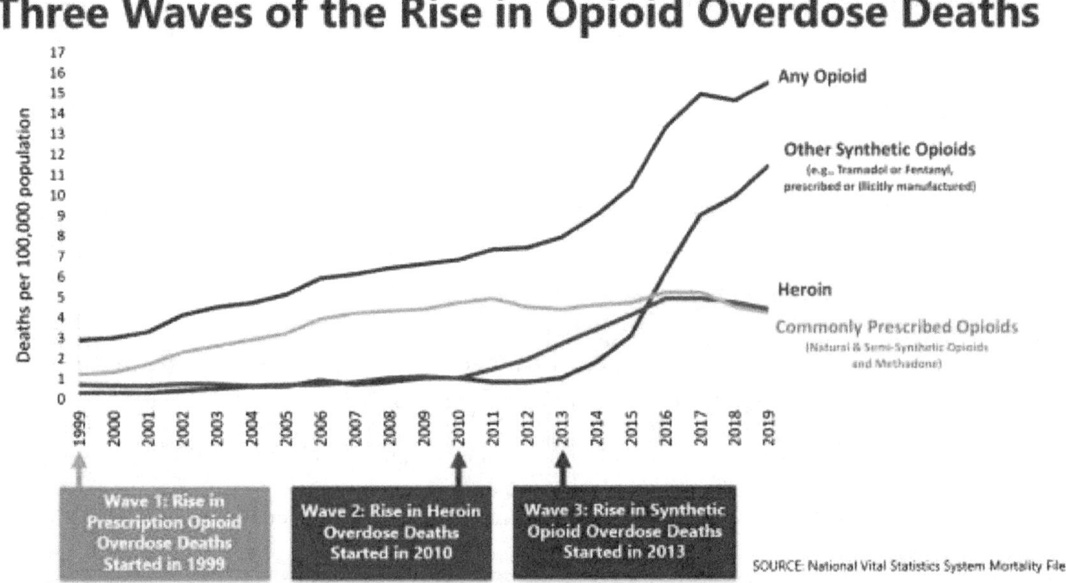

Figure 14.4 Three Waves of Opioid Overdose

---

27 *StatPearls* by Schiller, Goyal, & Mechanic is licensed under CC BY 4.0

28 "3-waves-2019-medium.PNG" by The Centers for Disease Control and Prevention is in the Public Domain. Access for free at https://www.cdc.gov/drugoverdose/epidemic/index.html

29 Centers for Disease Control and Prevention. (2021, March 17). *Understanding the epidemic.* U.S. Department of Health & Human Services. https://www.cdc.gov/drugoverdose/epidemic/index.html

30 Centers for Disease Control and Prevention. (n.d.). *The facts about fentanyl* [Handout]. https://www.cdc.gov/stopoverdose/fentanyl/pdf/fentanyl_fact_sheet_508c.pdf

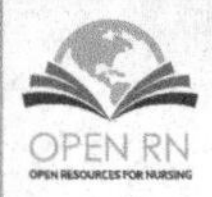

My Notes

Carfentanil is a new factor in opioid overdose rates. Carfentanil is synthetic opioid used to tranquilize large mammals like elephants. It is approximately 10,000 times more potent than morphine and 100 times more potent than fentanyl. A miniscule amount of powder containing two milligrams of carfentanil can be lethal. Carfentanil can be accidentally absorbed through the skin or inhaled by unsuspecting parties. If carfentanil or another fentanyl-related drug is suspected to be present on an individual, first responders and health care professionals must carefully follow safety protocols to avoid accidental lethal exposure.[31]

Read a U.S. Department of Justice Officer Safety Alert PDF: Carfentanil: A Dangerous New Factor in the U.S. Opioid Crisis.

Treating Opioid Overdose

Naloxone reverses the effects of an opioid overdose. A single-step nasal spray delivery of naloxone is the easiest and most successful route of administration for members of the community and first responders. Naloxone intramuscular injection is also available.[32]

Five basic steps are recommended for nurses, first responders, health professionals, and other bystanders to rapidly recognize and treat opioid overdose to prevent death.[33]

1. **Recognize Signs of Opioid Overdose**
    - Signs of opioid overdose include the following:
        - Unconsciousness or inability to awaken
        - Pinpoint pupils
        - Slow, shallow breathing; breathing difficulty manifested by choking sounds or a gurgling/snoring noise from a person who cannot be awakened; or respiratory arrest
        - Fingernails or lips turning blue or purple
    - If an opioid overdose is suspected, try to stimulate the person by calling their name or vigorously grinding one's knuckles into their sternum.
2. **Obtain Emergency Assistance:** If the person does not respond, call 911 or obtain emergency assistance.
3. **Provide Rescue Breathing, Chest Compressions, and Oxygen As Needed**[34]

---

31 Drug Enforcement Administration. (n.d.). *Officer safety alert.* U.S. Department of Justice. https://www.justice.gov/usao-edky/file/898991/download

32 Eggleston, W., Podolak, C., Sullivan, R.W., Pacelli, L., Keenan, M., & Wojcik, S. (2018). A randomized usability assessment of simulated naloxone administration by community members. *Addiction*, 113(12):2300-2304. https://doi.org/10.1111/add.14416

33 Substance Abuse and Mental Health Services Administration. (2018). *SAMHSA opioid overdose prevention toolkit: Five essential steps for first responders* [Manual]. U.S. Department of Health & Human Services. https://store.samhsa.gov/sites/default/files/d7/priv/five-essential-steps-for-first-responders.pdf

34 Substance Abuse and Mental Health Services Administration. (2018). *SAMHSA opioid overdose prevention toolkit: Five essential steps for first responders* [Manual]. U.S. Department of Health & Human Services. https://store.samhsa.gov/sites/default/files/d7/priv/five-essential-steps-for-first-responders.pdf

My Notes

- Provide rescue breathing if the person is not breathing on their own. A barrier device is recommended to reduce the risk of disease transmission. Rescue breathing for adults involves the following steps:
  - Be sure the person's airway is clear.
  - Place one hand on the person's chin, tilt the head back, and pinch the nose closed.
  - Place your mouth over the person's mouth to make a seal and give two slow breaths.
  - Watch for the person's chest (but not the stomach) to rise.
  - Follow up with one breath every five seconds.
- If the individual becomes pulseless, provide cardiopulmonary resuscitation (CPR).
- Administer oxygen as needed.

4. **Administer the First Dose of Naloxone**[35]

- Naloxone should be administered to anyone suspected of an opioid overdose.
- Research has shown that women, older adults, and those without obvious signs of opioid use disorder are undertreated with naloxone and, as a result, have a higher death rate. Therefore, naloxone should be considered for women and the elderly who are found unresponsive.
- Naloxone can be used in life-threatening opioid overdose circumstances in pregnant women.
- Naloxone can be given intranasally, intramuscularly, subcutaneously, or intravenously. The nasal spray is a prefilled device that requires no assembly and delivers a single dose into one nostril. An auto-injector is injected into the outer thigh to deliver naloxone intramuscularly or subcutaneously.
- All naloxone products are effective in reversing opioid overdose, including fentanyl-involved opioid overdoses, although overdoses involving potent or large quantities of opioids may require additional doses of naloxone.
- Withdrawal triggered by naloxone can feel unpleasant; some people may awaken confused, agitated, or aggressive. Provide safety, reassurance, and explain what is happening.

5. **Administer a Second Dose of Naloxone If the Person Does Not Respond**[36]:

- If the person overdosing does not respond within 2 to 3 minutes after administering a dose of naloxone, administer a second dose of naloxone.
- People who have taken long-acting or potent opioids (like fentanyl) may require additional intravenous bolus doses or an infusion of naloxone.
- The duration of effect of naloxone depends on dose, route of administration, and overdose symptoms. It is shorter than the effects of some opioids, so a second dose may be required.

---

35 Substance Abuse and Mental Health Services Administration. (2018). *SAMHSA opioid overdose prevention toolkit: Five essential steps for first responders* [Manual]. U.S. Department of Health & Human Services. https://store.samhsa.gov/sites/default/files/d7/priv/five-essential-steps-for-first-responders.pdf

36 Substance Abuse and Mental Health Services Administration. (2018). *SAMHSA opioid overdose prevention toolkit: Five essential steps for first responders* [Manual]. U.S. Department of Health & Human Services. https://store.samhsa.gov/sites/default/files/d7/priv/five-essential-steps-for-first-responders.pdf

My Notes

6. **Monitor the Person's Response**[37]:

- Most people respond to naloxone by returning to spontaneous breathing within 2 to 3 minutes. Continue resuscitation while waiting for the naloxone to take effect.
- The goal of naloxone therapy is to restore adequate spontaneous breathing but not necessarily achieve complete arousal.
- The individual should be monitored for recurrence of signs and symptoms of opioid toxicity for at least four hours from the last dose of naloxone. People who have overdosed on long-acting opioids like fentanyl require prolonged monitoring.
- Because naloxone has a relatively short duration of effect, overdose symptoms may return. Therefore, it is essential to get the person to an emergency department or other source of medical care as quickly as possible, even if the person revives after the initial dose of naloxone and seems to feel better.

Preventing Opioid Overdose

Nearly 85% of overdose deaths involve illicitly manufactured fentanyl, heroin, cocaine, or methamphetamine. Potential opportunities to link people to care or to implement life-saving actions have been identified for more than 3 in 5 people who died from drug overdose. Circumstances that represent a potential touchpoint for linkage to care are as follows[38]:

- **Bystander present:** Nearly 40% of opioid and stimulant overdose deaths occurred while a bystander was present.
- **Recent release from an institution:** Among the people who died from overdoses involving opioids, about 10% had recently been released from an institution (such as jail/prison, inpatient rehabilitation facilities, or psychiatric hospitals). Risk increased for this population because they were unaware of decreased tolerance to the drug due to abstinence from it while in the institution.
- **Previous overdose:** Among the people who died from overdoses involving opioids, about 10% had a previous overdose.
- **Mental health diagnosis:** Among all the people who died of a drug overdose, 25% had a documented mental health diagnosis.
- **Substance use disorder treatment:** Among the people who died from opioid overdose, nearly 20% had previously been treated for substance use disorder.

Opioid overdoses can be prevented by helping individuals struggling with opioid use disorder find the right treatment and recovery services, as well as providing public education about administering naloxone. See Figure 14.5.[39]

---

37 Substance Abuse and Mental Health Services Administration. (2018). *SAMHSA opioid overdose prevention toolkit: Five essential steps for first responders* [Manual]. U.S. Department of Health & Human Services. https://store.samhsa.gov/sites/default/files/d7/priv/five-essential-steps-for-first-responders.pdf

38 Centers for Disease Control and Prevention. (2020, September 4). *Overdose deaths and the involvement of illicit drugs.* U.S. Department of Health & Human Services. https://www.cdc.gov/drugoverdose/featured-topics/VS-overdose-deaths-illicit-drugs.html

39 "prevent-overdose-deaths-71k-large.jpg" by Centers for Disease Control and Prevention, National Center for Injury Prevention and Control is in the Public Domain. Access for free at https://www.cdc.gov/drugoverdose/resources/graphics/overdose.html

My Notes

for an image related to these strategies.[40] Read more about treatment and recovery in the "Treatment of Substance Use Disorders" section.

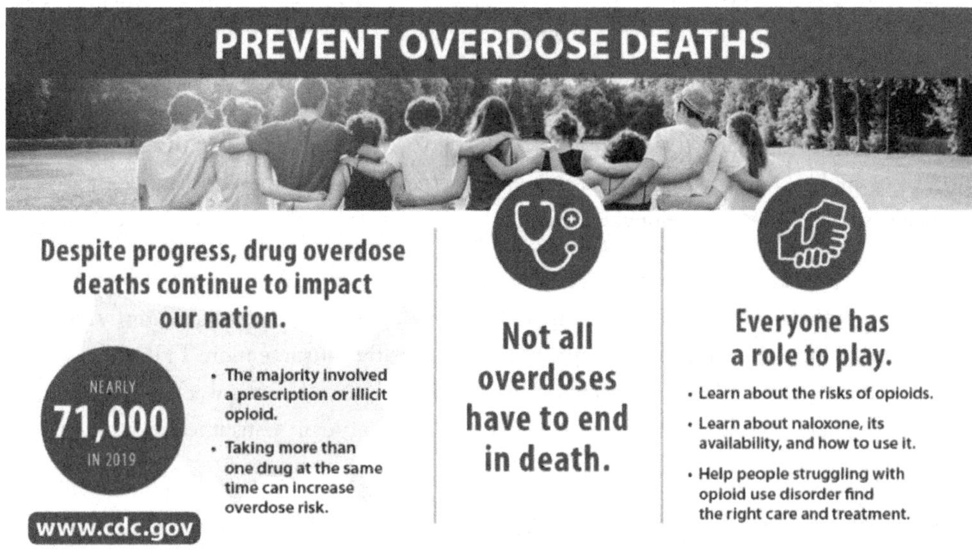

Figure 14.5 Preventing Overdose Deaths

Cannabis (Marijuana) Use and Intoxication

Approximately 48.2 million (17.5 percent) of Americans aged 12 or older used cannabis (marijuana) in the past year, and 14.2 million people (5.1%) have a cannabis use disorder.[41] Changes in marijuana policies across states have legalized marijuana for recreational and/or medicinal uses (e.g., pain control, increased appetite for individuals undergoing chemotherapy, etc.). Although many states now permit dispensing marijuana for medicinal purposes, the U.S. Food and Drug Administration has not approved "medical marijuana." Therefore, it is important for nurses to educate people about both the adverse health effects and the potential therapeutic benefits linked to marijuana.[42]

The main psychoactive chemical in marijuana is Delta-9-tetrahydrocannabinol (THC). THC alters the functioning of the hippocampus and other areas of the brain that enable a person to form new memories and shift their attentional focus. As a result, marijuana causes impaired thinking and interferes with a person's ability to learn and perform complicated tasks. THC also disrupts functioning of the cerebellum and basal ganglia that regulate

40 Centers for Disease Control and Prevention. (2020, September 4). *Overdose deaths and the involvement of illicit drugs.* U.S. Department of Health & Human Services. https://www.cdc.gov/drugoverdose/featured-topics/VS-overdose-deaths-illicit-drugs.html

41 National Institute on Drug Abuse. (2020). *Marijuana research report.* https://nida.nih.gov/publications/research-reports/marijuana/letter-director

42 National Institute on Drug Abuse. (2020). *Marijuana research report.* https://nida.nih.gov/publications/research-reports/marijuana/letter-director

My Notes

balance, posture, coordination, and reaction time. For this reason, people who have used marijuana may not drive safely and may have problems playing sports or engaging in other physical activities.[43]

When marijuana is smoked, THC and other chemicals pass from the lungs into the bloodstream and are rapidly carried to the brain. The person begins to experience effects such as euphoria and sense of relaxation almost immediately. Other common effects include heightened sensory perception (e.g., brighter colors), laughter, altered perception of time, and increased appetite. Other people experience anxiety, fear, distrust, or panic, especially if they take too much, the marijuana has high potency, or the person is inexperienced in using cannabis. People who have taken large or highly potent doses of marijuana may experience acute psychosis, including hallucinations, delusions, and a loss of the sense of personal identity.[44]

If marijuana is consumed in foods or beverages, the effects are delayed for 30 minutes to 1 hour because the drug must first pass through the digestive system. Eating or drinking marijuana delivers significantly less THC into the bloodstream. Because of the delayed effects, people may inadvertently consume more THC than they intend to.[45] Although detectable amounts of THC may remain in the body for days or even weeks after use, the noticeable effects of smoked marijuana generally last from 1 to 3 hours, and marijuana consumed in food or drink may last for many hours.[46]

Delta-8 THC products are manufactured from hemp-derived cannabidiol (CBD) and have psychoactive and intoxicating effects similar to Delta-9 THC. Some Delta-8 THC products are labeled as "hemp products," which can mislead consumers who associate "hemp" with being non-psychoactive. Delta-8 THC is available for purchase online and in stores but has not been approved by the U.S. Food and Drug Administration for safe use in any context. It should be kept out of reach of children and pets. Some manufacturers use unsafe chemicals to make Delta-8 THC through a chemical synthesis process that can contaminate the end product. As a result, there has been a recent increase in reports of adverse events with 8% of cases requiring admission to a critical care unit.[47]

THC affects brain systems that are still maturing through young adulthood, so regular use by teens may have negative and long-lasting effects on their cognitive development. Marijuana smoking is associated with large airway inflammation, increased airway resistance, lung hyperinflation, and chronic bronchitis. Vaping products that contain THC are associated with serious lung disease and death. Also, contrary to popular belief, marijuana can be addictive. THC stimulates neurons in the brain's reward system to release higher levels of dopamine and encourages the brain to repeat the rewarding behavior.[48]

The potential medicinal properties of marijuana and THC have been the subject of research and heated debate for decades. THC itself has proven medical benefits in particular formulations. For example, the U.S. Food and Drug

---

43 National Institute on Drug Abuse. (2020). *Marijuana research report.* https://nida.nih.gov/publications/research-reports/marijuana/letter-director

44 National Institute on Drug Abuse. (2020). *Marijuana research report.* https://nida.nih.gov/publications/research-reports/marijuana/letter-director

45 National Institute on Drug Abuse. (2020). *Marijuana research report.* https://nida.nih.gov/publications/research-reports/marijuana/letter-director

46 National Institute on Drug Abuse. (2020). *Marijuana research report.* https://nida.nih.gov/publications/research-reports/marijuana/letter-director

47 U.S. Food & Drug Administration. (2022, May 4). *5 things to know about Delta-8 tetrahydrocannabinol - Delta-8 THC.* https://www.fda.gov/consumers/consumer-updates/5-things-know-about-delta-8-tetrahydrocannabinol-delta-8-thc

48 National Institute on Drug Abuse. (2020). *Marijuana research report.* https://nida.nih.gov/publications/research-reports/marijuana/letter-director

My Notes

Administration (FDA) has approved the use of THC-based oral medications dronabinol (Marinol) and nabilone (Cesamet) for the treatment of nausea in clients undergoing cancer chemotherapy and to stimulate appetite in clients with wasting syndrome due to AIDS.[49] Marijuana is also used by individuals with certain illness such as multiple sclerosis for the management of spasticity, tics, convulsions, and dyskinesia.[50]

Cannabis intoxication is defined as problematic behavior or psychological changes (e.g., impaired motor coordination, euphoria, anxiety, sensation of slowed time, impaired judgment, social withdrawal) that developed during or shortly after cannabis use. Signs and symptoms of cannabis intoxication include the following[51]:

- Enlarged conjunctival vessels
- Increased appetite
- Dry mouth
- Tachycardia

According to the CDC, a fatal overdose caused solely by marijuana is unlikely. However, effects from marijuana can lead to unintentional injury, such as a motor vehicle crash, fall, or poisoning. Overconsumption of marijuana can occur when using marijuana-infused products like edibles and beverages because it can take up to two hours to feel the effects from the drug.[52] Additionally, marijuana purchased as a street drug may be laced with other substances like synthetic fentanyl that can cause overdose.

Sedative, Hypnotic, and Anxiolytic Use and Intoxication

Examples of medications in the sedative, hypnotic, or anxiolytic class include benzodiazepines, such as alprazolam (Xanax), diazepam (Valium), lorazepam (Ativan), chlordiazepoxide (Librium), and clonazepam (Klonopin). An example of a hypnotic is zolpidem (Ambien). Although these are prescription medications, they are commonly misused.

Chronic use of benzodiazepines causes changes in the gamma-aminobutyric acid (GABA) receptor, resulting in decreased GABA activity and the development of tolerance. When benzodiazepines are no longer present, or suddenly present at lower doses, withdrawal occurs.

Sedatives, hypnotics, and anxiolytic intoxication cause behavioral or psychological changes similar to alcohol intoxication, such as inappropriate sexual or aggressive behavior, mood lability, and impaired judgment. Symptoms of intoxication are as follows[53]:

- Slurred speech
- Incoordination

---

49 National Institute on Drug Abuse. (2020). *Marijuana research report.* https://nida.nih.gov/publications/research-reports/marijuana/letter-director

50 Shepard, S. (2021, December 6). *Can medical marijuana help your MS?* WebMD. https://www.webmd.com/multiple-sclerosis/multiple-sclerosis-medical-marijuana#:~:text=Surveys%20show%20that%20many%20people%20with%20MS%20already,that%20attacks%20your%20brain%2C%20spinal%20cord%2C%20and%20nerves

51 American Psychiatric Association. (2013). *Desk reference to the diagnostic criteria from DSM-5.*

52 Centers for Disease Control and Prevention. (2021, June 11). *Marijuana FAQs.* U.S. Department of Health & Human Services. https://www.cdc.gov/marijuana/faqs.htm

53 American Psychiatric Association. (2013). *Desk reference to the diagnostic criteria from DSM-5.*

My Notes

- Unsteady gait
- Nystagmus
- Impaired attention and memory
- Stupor or coma

Benzodiazepines are not detected by standard urine tests for drugs of abuse. However, specific benzodiazepine urine tests identify the metabolites of some benzodiazepines.[54]

Overdose

Benzodiazepines cause CNS depression and are commonly involved in drug overdose. They are often co-ingested with other drugs, such as alcohol or opioids that cause stupor, coma, and respiratory depression. When treating benzodiazepine overdose, end tidal CO2 (i.e., capnography) is used to monitor clients at risk for hypoventilation. Endotracheal intubation and mechanical ventilation may be required.[55,56] Flumazenil is an antidote to reverse benzodiazepine-induced sedation following general anesthesia and procedural sedation. However, it is used cautiously for benzodiazepine overdose because it is associated with withdrawal seizures in individuals who have developed a tolerance to benzodiazepines.

Hallucinogen Use and Intoxication

In 2020, 7.1 million (2.6 percent) people in America aged 12 or older used hallucinogens.[57] Hallucinogens are a diverse group of drugs that alter a person's awareness of their surroundings, as well as their own thoughts and feelings. They are commonly split into two categories: classic hallucinogens (such as LSD and peyote) and dissociative drugs (such as phencyclidine and ketamine). Dextromethorphan is an over-the-counter cough suppressant misused for its hallucinogenic and dissociative properties at high doses.

Hallucinogens cause hallucinations (sensations and images that seem real though they are not), and dissociative drugs can cause users to feel out of control or disconnected from their bodies and environments. Historically, some cultures have used hallucinogens like peyote as a part of religious or healing rituals.[58] Users of hallucinogens and dissociative drugs have increased risk for serious harm because of altered perceptions and moods. As a result, users might do things they would never do when not under the influence of a hallucinogen, like jump off a roof or act on suicidal thoughts.[59]

---

54 Greller, H., & Gupta, A. (2020, October 20). Benzodiazepine poisoning and withdrawal. *UpToDate.* Retrieved March 21, 2022, from www.uptodate.com

55 This work is a derivative of *StatPearls* by Kang, Galuska, & Ghassemzadeh and is licensed under CC BY 4.0

56 Greller, H., & Gupta, A. (2020, October 20). Benzodiazepine poisoning and withdrawal. *UpToDate.* Retrieved March 21, 2022, from www.uptodate.com

57 National Survey on Drug Use and Health. https://nsduhweb.rti.org/respweb/homepage.cfm

58 National Institute on Drug Abuse, & National Institutes of Health. (2021, November). *Hallucinogens drugfacts.* U.S. Department of Health & Human Services. https://nida.nih.gov/publications/drugfacts/hallucinogens

59 National Institute on Drug Abuse, & National Institutes of Health. (2021, November). *Hallucinogens drugfacts.* U.S. Department of Health & Human Services. https://nida.nih.gov/publications/drugfacts/hallucinogens

My Notes

Phencyclidine (PCP) is an example of a hallucinogen. It is an illegal street drug that usually comes as a white powder that can be inhaled through the nose, injected into a vein, smoked, or swallowed.[60] PCP intoxication causes problematic behavioral changes (e.g., belligerence, assaultiveness, impulsiveness, unpredictability, psychomotor agitation, impaired judgment) that occur during or shortly thereafter use.[61] Because of these symptoms, PCP is associated with violent and aggressive behavior including self-injury and violent criminal offenses (such as assaults, intimate partner violence, and homicide).[62] Within one hour of ingestion, two or more of the following signs or symptoms occur[63]:

- Vertical or horizontal nystagmus (an involuntary eye movement that causes the eye to rapidly move up and down or from side to side)
- Hypertension
- Tachycardia
- Numbness or diminished responsiveness to pain
- Ataxia (impaired balance or coordination)
- Slurred speech
- Muscle rigidity
- Seizures or coma
- Hyperacusis (sensitivity to noise)

Physical restraints may be necessary to control clients experiencing psychomotor agitation, followed by chemical sedation with intravenous benzodiazepines.[64]

Overdose

Overdose can occur with some dissociative drugs like PCP. High doses of PCP can cause seizures, coma, and death, especially if taken with depressants such as alcohol or benzodiazepines.[65]

Dextromethorphan is an over-the-counter medication that is misused due to its hallucinogenic effects and can cause overdose. Nonmedical use of dextromethorphan results in approximately 6,000 emergency department visits annually in the United States, often with co-ingestion of alcohol. Signs of toxic doses include neurobehavioral changes (e.g., hallucinations, inappropriate laughing, psychosis with dissociative features, agitation, and coma); tachycardia; dilated pupils; diaphoresis; and a "zombie-like" ataxic gait. Because acetaminophen is

---

60 A.D.A.M. Medical Encyclopedia [Internet]. Atlanta (GA): A.D.A.M., Inc.; c1997-2022. Substance use - phencyclidine (PCP); [updated 2022, February 18]. https://medlineplus.gov/ency/patientinstructions/000797.htm#:~:text=Phencyclidine%20(PCP)%20is%20an%20illegal,into%20a%20vein%20(shooting%20up)

61 American Psychiatric Association. (2013). *Desk reference to the diagnostic criteria from DSM-5.*

62 Crane, C. A., Easton, C. J., & Devine, S. (2013). The association between phencyclidine use and partner violence: An initial examination. *Journal of Addictive Diseases, 32*(2), 150–157. https://doi.org/10.1080/10550887.2013.797279.

63 American Psychiatric Association. (2013). *Desk reference to the diagnostic criteria from DSM-5.*

64 Heard, K., & Hoppe, J. (2020, March 19). Phencyclidine (PCP) intoxication in adults. *UpToDate.* Retrieved March 21, 2022, from www.uptodate.com

65 National Institute on Drug Abuse, & National Institutes of Health. (2021, November). *Hallucinogens drug facts.* U.S. Department of Health & Human Services. https://nida.nih.gov/publications/drugfacts/hallucinogens

My Notes

commonly present in cough and cold medications, toxic doses can cause severe delayed hepatotoxicity, hepatic failure, and death; serum acetaminophen levels should be obtained in all clients presenting with toxic levels of dextromethorphan.[66]

Stimulant Use and Intoxication

Stimulants include amphetamine-type substances, cocaine, and crack. Stimulants cause the release of dopamine in the brain and are highly addictive because the flood of dopamine in the brain's reward circuit strongly reinforces drug-taking behaviors. With continued drug use, the reward circuit adapts and becomes less sensitive to the drug. As a result, people take stronger and more frequent doses in an attempt to feel the same high and to obtain relief from withdrawal symptoms. Because the high from stimulants starts and fades quickly, people often take repeated doses in a form of binging, often giving up food and sleep while continuing to take the drug every few hours for several days. Both the use and withdrawal from amphetamines can cause psychosis with symptoms of hallucinations and paranoia.[67]

Approximately 2 million Americans used methamphetamine in the past year. The National Institute on Drug Abuse Data shows that overdose death rates involving methamphetamine quadrupled from 2011 to 2017.[68]

Methamphetamine comes in many forms and can be ingested by smoking, swallowing a pill, snorting, or injecting the powder that has been dissolved in water or alcohol. Methamphetamine can be easily made in small clandestine laboratories with relatively inexpensive over-the-counter ingredients such as pseudoephedrine, a common ingredient in cold medications. (To curb this illegal production, federal law requires pharmacies take steps to limit sales and obtain photo identification from purchasers.) Methamphetamine production also involves a number of other very dangerous chemicals. Toxic effects from these chemicals can remain in the environment long after the lab has been shut down, causing a wide range of health problems for people living in the area. These chemicals can also result in deadly lab explosions and house fires.[69]

Long-term use of methamphetamine has many negative consequences, including extreme weight loss, severe dental problems, intense itching leading to skin sores from scratching, involuntary movements (dyskinesia), anxiety, memory loss, and violent behavior.[70]

Cocaine is another powerfully addictive stimulant drug made from the leaves of the coca plant native to South America. It is estimated that 5.5 million people aged 12 or older have used cocaine, including about 778,000 users of crack.[71] Users may snort cocaine powder through the nose, rub it into their gums, or dissolve the powder and inject it into the bloodstream. Cocaine that has been processed to make a rock crystal is called "crack." The crystal

---

66 Rosenbaum, C., & Boyer, E. (2021, January 20). Dextromethorphan abuse and poisoning: Clinical features and diagnosis. *UpToDate.* Retrieved March 21, 2022, from www.uptodate.com

67 National Institute on Drug Abuse, & National Institutes of Health. (2019, May). *Methamphetamine drugfacts.* U.S. Department of Health & Human Services. https://nida.nih.gov/publications/drugfacts/methamphetamine

68 National Institute on Drug Abuse, & National Institutes of Health. (2019, May). *Methamphetamine drugfacts.* U.S. Department of Health & Human Services. https://nida.nih.gov/publications/drugfacts/methamphetamine

69 National Institute on Drug Abuse, & National Institutes of Health. (2019, May). *Methamphetamine drugfacts.* U.S. Department of Health & Human Services. https://nida.nih.gov/publications/drugfacts/methamphetamine

70 National Institute on Drug Abuse, & National Institutes of Health. (2019, May). *Methamphetamine drugfacts.* U.S. Department of Health & Human Services. https://nida.nih.gov/publications/drugfacts/methamphetamine

71 National Institute on Drug Abuse, & National Institutes of Health. (2019, May). *Methamphetamine drugfacts.* U.S. Department of Health & Human Services. https://nida.nih.gov/publications/drugfacts/methamphetamine

My Notes

is heated (making crackling sounds) to produce vapors that are inhaled into the lungs.[72,73] In the short-term, cocaine use can result in increased blood pressure, restlessness, and irritability. In the long-term, severe medical complications of cocaine use include heart attacks and seizures.[74]

Stimulant intoxication causes problematic behavioral or psychological changes such as euphoria or blunted affect; changes in sociability; hypervigilance; interpersonal sensitivity; anxiety, tension, or anger; and impaired judgment. These are some symptoms of stimulant intoxication:[75,76]

- Tachycardia
- Hypertension
- Pupillary dilation
- Elevated or decreased blood pressure
- Perspiration or chills
- Nausea or vomiting
- Weight loss
- Psychomotor agitation or retardation
- Muscular weakness
- Respiratory depression
- Chest pain or cardiac dysrhythmias
- Confusion, seizures, or coma
- Psychosis/hallucinations
- Dyskinesia (involuntary, erratic, writhing movements of the face, arms, legs, or trunk)
- Dystonia (involuntary muscle contractions that result in slow repetitive movements)

It is important for nurses to be aware that individuals with acute methamphetamine intoxication may, without provocation, develop severe agitation with extreme violence and place themselves, family members, medical staff, and other clients at risk of major injury. Control of agitation and hyperthermia (body temperature over 41 degrees Celsius) receive top priority for treatment with the following interventions[77]:

- Intravenous benzodiazepines are administered immediately for chemical sedation of severely agitated individuals.

---

72 American Psychiatric Association. (2013). *Desk reference to the diagnostic criteria from DSM-5.*

73 Boyer, E. W., & Hernon, C. (2019, December 24). Methamphetamine: Acute intoxication. *UpToDate.* Retrieved March 21, 2022, from www.uptodate.com

74 National Institute on Drug Abuse, & National Institutes of Health. (2019, May). *Methamphetamine drugfacts.* U.S. Department of Health & Human Services. https://nida.nih.gov/publications/drugfacts/methamphetamine

75 American Psychiatric Association. (2013). *Desk reference to the diagnostic criteria from DSM-5.*

76 Boyer, E. W., & Hernon, C. (2019, December 24). Methamphetamine: Acute intoxication. *UpToDate.* Retrieved March 21, 2022, from www.uptodate.com

77 Boyer, E. W., & Hernon, C. (2019, December 24). Methamphetamine: Acute intoxication. *UpToDate.* Retrieved March 21, 2022, from www.uptodate.com

My Notes

- Physical restraints should be avoided because clients who physically struggle against restraints undergo isometric muscle contractions that are associated with lactic acidosis, hyperthermia, sudden cardiac collapse, and death.
- Airway management with endotracheal intubation and mechanical ventilation may be required.
- Aggressive cooling is achieved through sedation, fluid resuscitation, external cooling blankets, or evaporative cooling techniques. Antipyretics are not used because the increased body temperature is caused by muscular activity, not an alteration in the hypothalamic temperature set point.

Read DrugFacts by the National Institute on Drug Abuse for more information about substances, intoxication, and overdose.

Inhalant Use and Intoxication

In 2020, 2.4 million (0.9 percent) of people aged 12 or older in America used inhalants. Unlike other illicit drugs, the percentage of inhalant use was highest among adolescents aged 12 to 17.[78] Inhalants are various products easily bought or found in the home, such as spray paints, markers, glue, gasoline, and cleaning fluids. People who use inhalants breathe in the fumes through their nose or mouth, usually by sniffing, snorting, bagging, or huffing. Although the high that inhalants produce usually lasts just a few minutes, people often try to make it last by continuing to inhale again and again over several hours.[79]

Prescription medications can also be misused as inhalants. For example, amyl nitrate is a prescription medication administered via inhalation to relieve chest pain. However, it is misused by individuals to cause a high. It is referred to by the street drug of "poppers."

Inhalant intoxication causes problematic behavioral or psychological changes such as belligerence, assaultiveness, apathy, and impaired judgment. Inhalant intoxication includes these symptoms[80]:

- Dizziness
- Nystagmus
- Incoordination
- Slurred speech
- Unsteady gait
- Lethargy
- Depressed reflexes
- Psychomotor retardation
- Tremor
- Generalized muscle weakness

---

78 National Institute on Drug Abuse, & National Institutes of Health. (2020, April). *Inhalants drugfacts.* U.S. Department of Health & Human Services. https://nida.nih.gov/publications/drugfacts/inhalants

79 National Institute on Drug Abuse, & National Institutes of Health. (2020, April). *Inhalants drugfacts.* U.S. Department of Health & Human Services. https://nida.nih.gov/publications/drugfacts/inhalants

80 American Psychiatric Association. (2013). *Desk reference to the diagnostic criteria from DSM-5.*

- Blurred or double vision
- Stupor or coma
- Euphoria

Long-term effects of inhalant use may include liver and kidney damage, hearing loss, bone marrow damage, loss of coordination and limb spasms (from nerve damage), delayed behavioral development (from brain problems), and brain damage (from cut-off oxygen flow to the brain).[81]

Acute intoxication with inhalants can cause life-threatening seizures and coma. Many solvents and aerosol sprays are highly concentrated with many other active ingredients; sniffing these products can cause the heart to stop within minutes. This condition, known as sudden sniffing death, can happen to otherwise healthy young people the first time they use an inhalant.[82] Treatment consists of maintaining cardiorespiratory function with 100 percent oxygen administration by rebreather mask and implementation of Pediatric Advanced Life Support (PALS) protocols that may require endotracheal intubation and mechanical ventilation.[83]

---

81 National Institute on Drug Abuse, & National Institutes of Health. (2020, April). *Inhalants drugfacts.* U.S. Department of Health & Human Services. https://nida.nih.gov/publications/drugfacts/inhalants

82 National Institute on Drug Abuse, & National Institutes of Health. (2020, April). *Inhalants drugfacts.* U.S. Department of Health & Human Services. https://nida.nih.gov/publications/drugfacts/inhalants

83 Boyer, E. W., & Hernon, C. (2019, December 24). Methamphetamine: Acute intoxication. *UpToDate.* Retrieved March 21, 2022, from www.uptodate.com

My Notes

14.3 WITHDRAWAL MANAGEMENT/DETOXIFICATION

Nurses working in medical-surgical hospital settings or emergency departments commonly provide care for clients receiving withdrawal treatment for alcohol, opioids, or other substances. Furthermore, clients frequently underreport alcohol and substance use, so nurses must be aware of signs of withdrawal in clients receiving medical care for other issues and notify the health care provider.[1]

Withdrawal management, also called detoxification, includes interventions aimed at managing the physical and emotional symptoms that occur after a person suddenly stops using a psychoactive substance. Withdrawal symptoms vary in intensity and duration based on the substance(s) used, the duration and amount of use, and the overall health of the individual. Some substances, such as opioids, sedatives, and tranquilizers, produce significant physical withdrawal effects, especially if they have been used in combination with heavy alcohol use. Rapid or unmanaged cessation from these substances can result in longer than expected course of withdrawal with seizures and other health complications.

Assessment and treatment of alcohol withdrawal and opioid withdrawal symptoms will be further discussed in the following sections.

Alcohol Withdrawal

The prevalence of alcohol use disorder is estimated to be as high as 40 percent among hospitalized clients. Approximately half of clients with alcohol use disorder experience alcohol withdrawal when they reduce or stop drinking, with as many as 20 percent experiencing serious manifestations such as hallucinations, seizures, and delirium tremens.[2] Severe alcohol withdrawal is considered a medical emergency that is best managed in an intensive care unit.

Symptoms of early or mild alcohol withdrawal include anxiety, minor agitation, restlessness, insomnia, tremor, diaphoresis, palpitations, headache, and alcohol craving. Clients often experience loss of appetite, nausea, vomiting, and diarrhea. Their risk for falls often increases when they try to go unassisted to the bathroom with these gastrointestinal symptoms. Physical signs include sinus tachycardia, systolic hypertension, hyperactive reflexes, and tremor. Without treatment, symptoms of mild alcohol withdrawal generally begin within 6 to 36 hours after the last drink and resolve within one to two days.[3]

Some clients develop moderate to severe withdrawal symptoms that can last up to six days, such as withdrawal hallucinations, seizures, or delirium tremens:

Hallucinations typically occur within 12 to 48 hours after the last drink. They are typically visual and commonly involve seeing insects or animals in the room, although auditory and tactile phenomena may also occur.[4]

---

1 Sellers, E. M. (n.d.). *CIWA-AR for alcohol withdrawal.* MDCalc. https://www.mdcalc.com/ciwa-ar-alcohol-withdrawal#why-use

2 Pace, C. (2022). Alcohol withdrawal: Epidemiology, clinical manifestations, course, assessment, and diagnosis. *UpToDate.* Retrieved March 19, 2022, from www.uptodate.com

3 Pace, C. (2022). Alcohol withdrawal: Epidemiology, clinical manifestations, course, assessment, and diagnosis. *UpToDate.* Retrieved March 19, 2022, from www.uptodate.com

4 Pace, C. (2022). Alcohol withdrawal: Epidemiology, clinical manifestations, course, assessment, and diagnosis. *UpToDate.* Retrieved March 19, 2022, from www.uptodate.com

My Notes

Alcohol withdrawal-related seizures can occur within 6 to 48 hours after the last drink. Risk factors for seizures include concurrent withdrawal from benzodiazepines or other sedative-hypnotic drugs.[5]

Delirium tremens (DTs) is a rapid-onset, fluctuating disturbance of attention and cognition that is sometimes associated with hallucinations. In its most severe manifestation, DTs are accompanied by agitation and signs of extreme autonomic hyperactivity, including fever, severe tachycardia, hypertension, and drenching sweats. DTs typically begin between 48 and 96 hours after the client's last drink. Mortality rates from withdrawal delirium have been historically as high as 20 percent, but with appropriate medical management, the mortality rate is between 1 and 4 percent. Death is attributed to cardiovascular complications, hyperthermia, aspiration, and severe fluid and electrolyte disorders.[6]

Clinical Institute Withdrawal Assessment for Alcohol Scale (CIWA-Ar)

The Clinical Institute Withdrawal Assessment for Alcohol Scale (CIWA-Ar) is the most widely used scale to determine the need for medically supervised withdrawal management. It is used in a wide variety of settings, including outpatient, emergency, psychiatric, and general medical-surgical units when there is a clinical concern regarding a client's alcohol withdrawal.

The CIWA-Ar scale is typically utilized in association with a protocol containing medications to guide symptom-triggered treatment. Clients with an alcohol use disorder who have a CIWA-Ar score of less than 10 do not typically require medical management.[7]

There are ten questions on the CIWA-Ar related to nausea/vomiting, tremor, paroxysmal sweats, anxiety, agitation, tactile disturbances, auditory disturbances, visual disturbances, headache, and level of orientation. The questions are rated from 0 to 7, except for orientation that is rated from 0 to 4. View the full CIWA-Ar scale in the following box.

 View the CIWA-Ar on the MDCalc medical reference website.

Treatment of Alcohol Withdrawal

Benzodiazepines are used to treat the psychomotor agitation most patients experience during alcohol withdrawal and prevent progression from minor symptoms to severe symptoms of seizures, hallucinations, or delirium tremens. Diazepam (Valium), lorazepam (Ativan), and chlordiazepoxide (Librium) are used most frequently to treat or prevent alcohol withdrawal symptoms.[8]

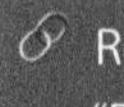 Review information about benzodiazepines in the "Antianxiety Medications" section of the "Psychotropic Medications" chapter.

---

5 Pace, C. (2022). Alcohol withdrawal: Epidemiology, clinical manifestations, course, assessment, and diagnosis. *UpToDate*. Retrieved March 19, 2022, from www.uptodate.com

6 Pace, C. (2022). Alcohol withdrawal: Epidemiology, clinical manifestations, course, assessment, and diagnosis. *UpToDate*. Retrieved March 19, 2022, from www.uptodate.com

7 Pace, C. (2022). Alcohol withdrawal: Epidemiology, clinical manifestations, course, assessment, and diagnosis. *UpToDate*. Retrieved March 19, 2022, from www.uptodate.com

8 Hoffman, R. (2022). Management of moderate and severe alcohol withdrawal symptoms. *UpToDate*. Retrieved May 5, 2022, from www.uptodate.com

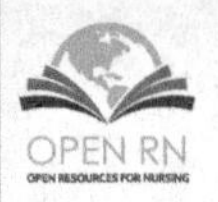

My Notes

Anticonvulsants may be used concurrently or instead of benzodiazepines. Anticonvulsants decrease the probability of withdrawal seizures.

Review information about anticonvulsants in the "Treatments for Bipolar Disorders" section of the "Bipolar Disorders" chapter.

Chronic alcohol use is associated with depletion of thiamine and magnesium. Clients receiving alcohol withdrawal treatment typically receive intravenous thiamine, along with dextrose, to prevent Wernicke's encephalopathy. Wernicke's encephalopathy is an acute, life-threatening neurological condition characterized by nystagmus, ataxia, and confusion caused by thiamine (B1) deficiency associated with alcohol use disorder.[9] If untreated, Wernicke's encephalopathy can progress to Korsakoff's syndrome, a chronic, irreversible memory disorder resulting from thiamine deficiency.[10] Treatment of other electrolyte deficiencies may be included during alcohol withdrawal treatment.

Opioid Withdrawal

Medically supervised opioid withdrawal, also known as detoxification, involves administering medication to reduce the severity of withdrawal symptoms that occur when an opioid-dependent client stops using opioids. However, supervised withdrawal alone does not generally result in sustained abstinence from opioids, nor does it address reasons the client became dependent on opioids.[11]

Clients may undergo detoxification for several reasons[12]:

- Initiating the process to "get clean and stay clean" from opioids. Some clients may follow up with inpatient or outpatient treatment after completing the detoxification process.
- Treating withdrawal symptoms when a client dependent on opioids or heroin becomes hospitalized and lacks access to the misused substance.
- Beginning the first step in treating opioid use disorder and transitioning to medication-assisted treatment like methadone or suboxone treatment.
- Establishing an abstinent state without withdrawal symptoms required for the client's setting or status (e.g., incarceration, probation, or a drug-free residential program).

---

9 This work is a derivative of *StatPearls* by Vasan and Kumar and is licensed under CC BY 4.0

10 National Institute of Neurological Disorders and Stroke. (n.d). *Wernicke-Korsakoff syndrome.* https://www.ninds.nih.gov/health-information/disorders/wernicke-korsakoff-syndrome#:~:text=Korsakoff%20syndrome%20(also%20called%20Korsakoff's,the%20brain%20involved%20with%20memory

11 Sevarino, K. A. (2022). Medically supervised opioid withdrawal during treatment for addiction. *UpToDate.* Retrieved March 19, 2022, from www.uptodate.com

12 Sevarino, K. A. (2022). Medically supervised opioid withdrawal during treatment for addiction. *UpToDate.* Retrieved March 19, 2022, from www.uptodate.com

My Notes

Clinical Opiate Withdrawal Scale

The Clinical Opiate Withdrawal Scale (COWS) is used in both inpatient and outpatient settings for the monitoring of withdrawal symptoms during opioid detoxification. It can be serially administered to track changes in the severity of withdrawal symptoms over time or in response to treatment.[13]

Symptoms of opioid withdrawal include drug craving, anxiety, restlessness, gastrointestinal distress, diaphoresis, and tachycardia. COWS rates the severity of 11 signs and symptoms of opioid withdrawal on a scale from 0 to 5, as described in the following box.

View the COWS on the MedCalc medical reference website.

Treatment of Opioid Withdrawal

A calm, quiet environment with supportive and reassuring staff is instrumental for helping clients overcome most symptoms of acute opioid withdrawal and can decrease the need for pharmacologic interventions. Clients who have associated diarrhea, vomiting, or sweating should be monitored for dehydration and have fluid levels maintained with oral and/or intravenous fluids.[14]

Medications used to treat withdrawal symptoms include opioid agonists such as buprenorphine and methadone, as well as Alpha-2 adrenergic agonists such as clonidine and lofexidine. Other medications may be prescribed to treat specific symptoms.[15]

Buprenorphine

Buprenorphine is an effective treatment for opioid withdrawal symptoms. A disadvantage of buprenorphine is it can worsen opioid withdrawal symptoms if not administered carefully. To avoid this situation, the client must be in a state of mild to moderate withdrawal before receiving their first dose of buprenorphine (i.e., have a COWS score greater than 10). The first dose of buprenorphine is typically 2 to 4 mg sublingually.[16]

Buprenorphine can cause respiratory depression. Common side effects include sedation, headache, nausea, constipation, and insomnia.[17]

---

13 Wesson, D. R. (n.d.). *COWS score for opiate withdrawal.* MDCalc. https://www.mdcalc.com/cows-score-opiate-withdrawal#why-use

14 Sevarino, K. A. (2022). Medically supervised opioid withdrawal during treatment for addiction. *UpToDate.* Retrieved March 19, 2022, from www.uptodate.com

15 Sevarino, K. A. (2022). Medically supervised opioid withdrawal during treatment for addiction. *UpToDate.* Retrieved March 19, 2022, from www.uptodate.com

16 Sevarino, K. A. (2022). Medically supervised opioid withdrawal during treatment for addiction. *UpToDate.* Retrieved March 19, 2022, from www.uptodate.com

17 Sevarino, K. A. (2022). Medically supervised opioid withdrawal during treatment for addiction. *UpToDate.* Retrieved March 19, 2022, from www.uptodate.com

My Notes

Buprenorphine/Naloxone

The combination medication buprenorphine/naloxone (Suboxone) is used for detoxification, as well as maintenance of abstinence from opioids. It may be used in outpatient settings as an opioid-blocker.[18]

Methadone

Methadone is a long-acting, synthetic opioid that reduces opioid craving and withdrawal symptoms by blocking the effect of opioids. It is typically prescribed in one of two ways[19]:

- Substitution Therapy: Methadone is prescribed to replace the use of an opioid and then is gradually tapered to prevent severe withdrawal symptoms.
- Maintenance Therapy: It is prescribed long-term as a one component of a comprehensive medication-assisted treatment plan for opioid use disorder. With counseling and other behavioral therapies, methadone helps individuals achieve and sustain recovery and lead active and meaningful lives.

In contrast to buprenorphine, methadone does not induce withdrawal symptoms when administered to a client with opioid in their system because it has an additive effect on opioids that are already present.[20]

A typical dose of methadone on Day 1 of withdrawal treatment varies from 10 – 20 mg orally. Injections are only recommended for clients unable to take oral medication. Dosing is titrated to control withdrawal symptoms while avoiding oversedation and motor impairment. Common side effects of methadone include constipation, mild drowsiness, excess sweating, peripheral edema, and erectile dysfunction.[21]

Due to its long half-life, clients are at risk for overdose if the dose is titrated up too quickly or their starting dose is too high for their tolerance level of opioids. Overdose with methadone can be lethal due to arrhythmia or respiratory depression. It is treated with naloxone with repeated doses as needed and rapid transfer to a medical unit.[22]

Alpha-2 Adrenergic Agonists

Alpha-2 adrenergic agonists, including clonidine and lofexidine, decrease many symptoms of opioid withdrawal and effectively relieve the autonomic symptoms of sweating, diarrhea, intestinal cramps, nausea, anxiety, and irritability. They are least effective for symptoms of myalgias, restlessness, insomnia, and craving.[23]

---

18 Substance Abuse and Mental Health Services Administration, & Office of the Surgeon General. (2016). *Facing addiction in America: The surgeon general's report on alcohol, drugs, and health.* United States Department of Health and Human Services. https://www.ncbi.nlm.nih.gov/books/NBK424857/

19 Substance Abuse and Mental Health Services Administration (SAMHSA). (2022, June 23). *Methadone.* https://www.samhsa.gov/medication-assisted-treatment/medications-counseling-related-conditions/methadone

20 Sevarino, K. A. (2022). Medically supervised opioid withdrawal during treatment for addiction. *UpToDate.* Retrieved March 19, 2022, from www.uptodate.com

21 Sevarino, K. A. (2022). Medically supervised opioid withdrawal during treatment for addiction. *UpToDate.* Retrieved March 19, 2022, from www.uptodate.com

22 Sevarino, K. A. (2022). Medically supervised opioid withdrawal during treatment for addiction. *UpToDate.* Retrieved March 19, 2022, from www.uptodate.com

23 Sevarino, K. A. (2022). Medically supervised opioid withdrawal during treatment for addiction. *UpToDate.* Retrieved March 19, 2022, from www.uptodate.com

My Notes

Clonidine can be taken orally or administered via a clonidine patch and changed weekly. Relief from withdrawal symptoms typically occurs within 30 minutes after a dose. However, common side effects of hypotension and sedation limit the use of these drugs. Contraindications to Alpha-2 adrenergic agonists include hypotension, renal insufficiency, cardiac instability, pregnancy, and psychosis. Tricyclic antidepressants should be stopped three weeks prior to use.[24]

Symptom-specific Medications

Various medications are prescribed to provide targeted relief for symptoms of opioid withdrawal[25]:

- Anxiety, irritability, restlessness: Diphenhydramine, hydroxyzine, lorazepam, and clonazepam
- Abdominal cramping: Dicyclomine
- Diarrhea: Bismuth and loperamide
- Nausea/vomiting: Ondansetron, prochlorperazine, and promethazine
- Insomnia: Trazodone, doxepin, mirtazapine, quetiapine, and zolpidem
- Muscle aches, joint pain, and headache: Ibuprofen, acetaminophen, ketorolac, and naproxen
- Muscle spasms and restless legs: Cyclobenzaprine, baclofen, diazepam, and methocarbamol

Warm baths, rehydration, and gentle stretching are also helpful for relieving muscle aches and cramps. Use of benzodiazepines and zolpidem is not recommended for clients receiving methadone or buprenorphine therapy unless they are under close medical supervision due to the risk of oversedation.[26]

Benzodiazepine Withdrawal

Rapid recognition and treatment of benzodiazepine withdrawal is critical because it can be life-threatening. Signs and symptoms of benzodiazepine withdrawal include tremors, anxiety, general malaise, perceptual disturbances, psychosis, seizures, and autonomic instability. Withdrawal is treated with a long-acting benzodiazepine (such as diazepam) and titrated to prevent withdrawal symptoms without causing excessive sedation or respiratory depression. The dose is then tapered gradually over a period of months.[27]

Treatment After Withdrawal Treatment

Withdrawal management is highly effective in preventing immediate and serious medical consequences associated with discontinuing substance use, but by itself, it is not an effective treatment for any substance use disorder. It is considered stabilization, meaning the client is assisted through a period of acute detoxification and withdrawal to be medically stable and substance-free. Stabilization often prepares the individual for treatment. It is considered a first step toward recovery, similar to the acute management of a diabetic coma as a first step toward managing the

---

24 Sevarino, K. A. (2022). Medically supervised opioid withdrawal during treatment for addiction. *UpToDate.* Retrieved March 19, 2022, from www.uptodate.com

25 Sevarino, K. A. (2022). Medically supervised opioid withdrawal during treatment for addiction. *UpToDate.* Retrieved March 19, 2022, from www.uptodate.com

26 Sevarino, K. A. (2022). Medically supervised opioid withdrawal during treatment for addiction. *UpToDate.* Retrieved March 19, 2022, from www.uptodate.com

27 Substance Abuse and Mental Health Services Administration. (2022, March 2). *Alcohol, tobacco, and other drugs.* U.S. Department of Health & Human Services. https://www.samhsa.gov/find-help/atod

My Notes

underlying illness of diabetes. Similarly, acute stabilization and withdrawal management are most effective when followed by evidence-based treatments and recovery services.[28]

Unfortunately, many individuals who receive withdrawal management do not become engaged in treatment. Studies have found that half to three quarters of individuals with substance use disorders who receive withdrawal management services do not enter treatment. One of the most serious consequences when individuals do not begin continuing care after withdrawal management is overdose. Because withdrawal management reduces acquired tolerance, those who attempt to reuse their former substance in the same amount or frequency may overdose, especially those with opioid use disorders.[29]

The remaining sections of this chapter will discuss substance abuse disorders and treatments, as well as prevention strategies.

---

28 Substance Abuse and Mental Health Services Administration, & Office of the Surgeon General. (2016). *Facing addiction in America: The surgeon general's report on alcohol, drugs, and health.* United States Department of Health and Human Services. https://www.ncbi.nlm.nih.gov/books/NBK424857/

29 Substance Abuse and Mental Health Services Administration, & Office of the Surgeon General. (2016). *Facing addiction in America: The surgeon general's report on alcohol, drugs, and health.* United States Department of Health and Human Services. https://www.ncbi.nlm.nih.gov/books/NBK424857/

14.4 SUBSTANCE-RELATED AND OTHER ADDICTIVE DISORDERS

My Notes

Substance-Related Disorders

Prolonged, repeated misuse of substances can produce changes to the brain that can lead to a substance use disorder. According to the *Diagnostic and Statistical Manual of Mental Disorders (DSM-5)*, **substance use disorder (SUD)** is an illness caused by repeated misuse of substances such as alcohol, caffeine, cannabis, hallucinogens, inhalants, opioids, sedatives, hypnotics, anxiolytics, stimulants (amphetamines, cocaine, and other stimulants), and tobacco. All of these substances taken in excess have a common effect of directly activating the brain reward system and producing such an intense activation of the reward system that normal life activities may be neglected. Nonsubstance related disorders such as gambling disorder activate the same reward system in the brain.[1]

Substance use disorders are diagnosed based on cognitive, behavioral, and psychological symptoms. See the *DSM-5* diagnostic criteria used for SUD in the following box. SUD can range from mild to severe and from temporary to chronic.[2]

DSM-5 Criteria for Substance Abuse Disorder

SUD diagnosis requires the presence of two or more of the following criteria in a 12-month period[3]:

- The substance is often taken in larger amounts or over a longer period than intended.
- There is a persistent desire or unsuccessful efforts to cut down or control substance use.
- A great deal of time is spent in activities necessary to obtain the substance, use the substance, or recover from its effects.
- There is a craving, or a strong desire or urge, to use the substance.
- There is recurrent substance use resulting in a failure to fulfill major role obligations at work, school, or home.
- There is continued substance use despite having persistent or recurrent social or interpersonal problems caused by or exacerbated by the effects of the substance.
- Important social, occupational, or recreational activities are given up or reduced because of substance use.
- There is recurrent substance use in situations in which it is physically hazardous.
- Substance use is continued despite knowledge of having a persistent or recurrent physical or psychological problem that is likely to have been caused or exacerbated by the substance.

---

1 American Psychiatric Association. (2013). *Desk reference to the diagnostic criteria from DSM-5.*

2 Substance Abuse and Mental Health Services Administration, & Office of the Surgeon General. (2016). *Facing addiction in America: The surgeon general's report on alcohol, drugs, and health.* United States Department of Health and Human Services. https://www.ncbi.nlm.nih.gov/books/NBK424857/

3 American Psychiatric Association. (2013). *Desk reference to the diagnostic criteria from DSM-5.*

My Notes

- Tolerance develops to the substance, as defined by:
    - A need for markedly increased amounts of the substance to achieve intoxication or the desired effect.
    - There is a markedly diminished effect with continued use of the same amount of the substance.
- Withdrawal symptoms occur when substance use is cut back or stopped following a period of prolonged use.

The disorder is classified as mild, moderate, or severe. Individuals exhibiting two or three symptoms are considered to have a "mild" disorder, four or five symptoms constitute a "moderate" disorder, and six or more symptoms are considered a "severe" substance use disorder.

Millions of Americans are diagnosed with SUD. See Figure 14.6[4] for a graphic of the number of people aged 12 and older with a substance use disorder in 2020.

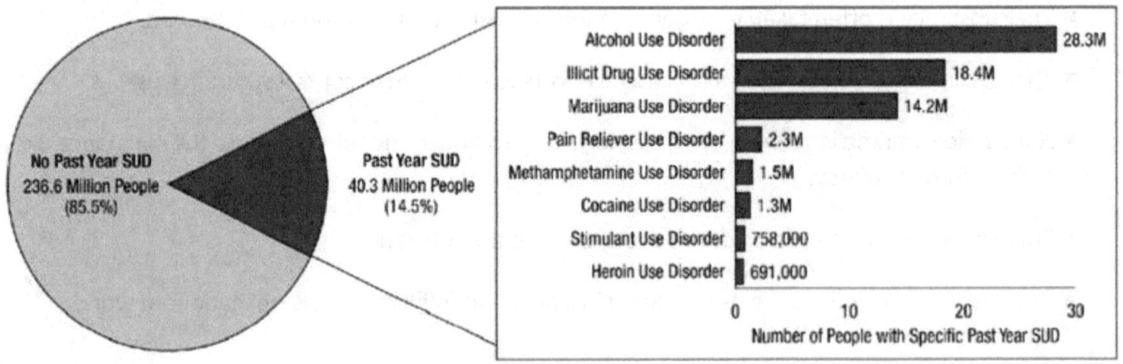

Figure 14.6 Number of People Aged 12 and Older With a Substance Use Disorder in 2020. Used under Fair Use.

SUD often develops gradually over time due to repeated misuse of a substance, causing changes in brain areas that control reward, stress, and executive functions like decision-making and self-control. Multiple factors influence whether a person will develop a substance use disorder such as the substance itself; the genetic vulnerability of the user; and the amount, frequency, and duration of the misuse.

4 This image is a derivative of "People Aged 12 or Older with a Past Year Substance Use Disorder (SUD); 2020" table by Substance Abuse and Mental Health Services Administration. (2021). Key substance use and mental health indicators in the United States: Results from the 2020 National Survey on Drug Use and Health (HHS Publication No. PEP21-07-01-003, NSDUH Series H-56). Rockville, MD: Center for Behavioral Health Statistics and Quality, Substance Abuse and Mental Health Services Administration. Used under Fair Use. Retrieved from https://www.samhsa.gov/data/report/2020-nsduh-annual-national-report

My Notes

Severe substance use disorders are commonly referred to as addictions. **Addiction** is associated with compulsive or uncontrolled use of one or more substances. Addiction is a chronic illness that has the potential for both relapse and recovery. **Relapse** refers to the return to substance use after a significant period of abstinence. **Recovery** is a process of change through which individuals improve their health and wellness, live a self-directed life, and strive to reach their full potential. Although abstinence from substance misuse is a primary feature of a recovery lifestyle, it is not the only healthy feature.[5] The chronic nature of addiction means that some individuals may relapse after an attempt at abstinence, which can be a normal part of the recovery process. Relapse does not mean treatment failure. Relapse rates for substance use are similar to rates for adherence to therapies for other chronic medical illnesses. There are a variety of medications that can be prescribed to assist with relapse prevention.[6]

Individuals with severe substance use disorders can overcome their disorder with effective treatment and regain health and social function, referred to as **remission**. When positive changes and values become part of a voluntarily adopted lifestyle, this is referred to as "being in recovery."[7] Among the 29.2 million adults in 2020 who have ever had a substance use problem, 72.5 percent considered themselves to be in recovery.[8]

Many individuals seeking care in health care settings, such as primary care, obstetrics and gynecology, emergency departments, and medical-surgical units, have undiagnosed substance use disorders. Recognition and early treatment of substance use disorders can improve their health outcomes and reduce overall health care costs.[9]

Substance Use Disorder in Nurses

Health care professionals are not immune to developing SUD. SUD is a chronic illness that can affect anyone regardless of age, occupation, economic circumstances, ethnic background, or gender. The National Council of State Boards of Nursing (NCSBN) created a brochure called *A Nurse's Guide to Substance Use Disorder in Nursing*. This brochure states that many nurses with substance use disorder (SUD) are unidentified, untreated, and may continue to practice when their impairment may endanger the lives of their clients. Because of the potential safety hazards to clients, it is a nurse's legal and ethical responsibility to report a colleague's suspected SUD to their manager or supervisor. It can be hard to differentiate between the subtle signs of SUD and stress-related behaviors, but three significant signs include behavioral changes, physical signs, and drug diversion.[10]

---

5 Substance Abuse and Mental Health Services Administration, & Office of the Surgeon General. (2016). *Facing addiction in America: The surgeon general's report on alcohol, drugs, and health.* United States Department of Health and Human Services. https://www.ncbi.nlm.nih.gov/books/NBK424857/

6 National Institute on Drug Abuse. (2022). *Drugs, brains, and behavior: The science of addiction treatment and recovery.* https://nida.nih.gov/publications/drugs-brains-behavior-science-addiction/treatment-recovery

7 Substance Abuse and Mental Health Services Administration, & Office of the Surgeon General. (2016). *Facing addiction in America: The surgeon general's report on alcohol, drugs, and health.* United States Department of Health and Human Services. https://www.ncbi.nlm.nih.gov/books/NBK424857/

8 Substance Abuse and Mental Health Services Administration. (2021). *Key substance use and mental health indicators in the United States: Results from the 2020 national survey on drug use and health.* Center for Behavioral Health Statistics and Quality, Substance Abuse, & Mental Health Services Administration. https://www.samhsa.gov/data/

9 Substance Abuse and Mental Health Services Administration, & Office of the Surgeon General. (2016). *Facing addiction in America: The surgeon general's report on alcohol, drugs, and health.* United States Department of Health and Human Services. https://www.ncbi.nlm.nih.gov/books/NBK424857/

10 NCSBSN. (2018). *A nurse's guide to substance use disorder in nursing* [Brochure]. https://www.ncsbn.org/SUD_Brochure_2014.pdf

My Notes

Behavioral changes include decreased job performance, absences from the unit for extended periods, frequent trips to the bathroom, arriving late or leaving early, and making an excessive number of mistakes including medication errors.[11]

Physical signs include subtle changes in appearance that may escalate over time; increasing isolation from colleagues; inappropriate verbal or emotional responses; and diminished alertness, confusion, or memory lapses. Signs of diversion include frequent discrepancies in opioid counts, unusual amounts of opioid wastage, numerous corrections of medication records, frequent reports of ineffective pain relief from clients, offers to medicate coworkers' patients for pain, and altered verbal or phone medication orders.[12]

Drug diversion occurs when medication is redirected from its intended destination for personal use, sale, or distribution to others. It includes drug theft, use, or tampering (adulteration or substitution). Drug diversion is a felony that can result in a nurse's criminal prosecution and loss of license.[13]

The earlier that a nurse is diagnosed with SUD and treatment is initiated, the sooner that client safety is protected and the better the chances for the nurse to recover and return to work. In most states, a nurse diagnosed with a SUD enters a nondisciplinary program designed by the Board of Nursing for treatment and recovery services. When a colleague treated for an SUD returns to work, nurses should create a supportive environment that encourages their continued recovery.[14]

View the NCSBN PDF pamphlet A Nurse's Guide to Substance Use Disorder in Nursing.

Nonsubstance-Related Disorders

Nonsubstance-related disorders are excessive behaviors related to gambling, viewing pornography, compulsive sexual activity, Internet gaming, overeating, shopping, overexercising, and overusing mobile phone technologies. These behaviors are thought to stimulate the same addiction centers of the brain as addictive substances. However, gambling disorder is the only nonsubstance use disorder with diagnostic criteria listed in the *DSM-5*. See the *DSM-5* criteria for the diagnosis of a gambling disorder in the following box. Additional research is being performed to determine the criteria for diagnosing other nonsubstance-related disorders.[15]

---

11 NCSBSN. (2018). *A nurse's guide to substance use disorder in nursing* [Brochure]. https://www.ncsbn.org/SUD_Brochure_2014.pdf

12 NCSBSN. (2018). *A nurse's guide to substance use disorder in nursing* [Brochure]. https://www.ncsbn.org/SUD_Brochure_2014.pdf

13 Nyhus, J. (2021). Drug diversion in healthcare. *American Nurse*. https://www.myamericannurse.com/drug- diversion-in-healthcare/

14 NCSBSN. (2018). *A nurse's guide to substance use disorder in nursing* [Brochure]. https://www.ncsbn.org/SUD_Brochure_2014.pdf

15 National Institute on Drug Abuse, & National Institutes of Health. (2019, May). *Methamphetamine drugfacts.* U.S. Department of Health & Human Services. https://nida.nih.gov/publications/drugfacts/methamphetamine

My Notes

DSM-5 Criteria for Gambling Disorder[16]

Gambling disorder is defined as persistent and recurrent problematic gambling behavior leading to clinically significant impairment or distress, as indicated by four or more of the following criteria in a 12-month period. Additionally, the gambling behavior is not better explained by a manic episode.

- Needs to gamble with increasing amounts of money to achieve the desired excitement
- Is restless or irritable when attempting to cut down or stop gambling
- Has made repeated unsuccessful efforts to control, cut back, or stop gambling
- Is often preoccupied with gambling (e.g., persistent thoughts of reliving past gambling experiences, planning the next venture, or thinking of ways to get money with which to gamble)
- Often gambles when feeling distressed (e.g., helpless, guilty, anxious, or depressed)
- After losing money gambling, often returns another day to get even (otherwise known as "chasing one's losses")
- Lies to conceal the extent of involvement with gambling
- Has jeopardized or lost a significant relationship, job, or educational or career opportunity because of gambling
- Relies on others to provide money to relieve desperate financial situation caused by gambling

16 American Psychiatric Association. (2013). *Desk reference to the diagnostic criteria from DSM-5.*

14.5 NEUROBIOLOGY OF SUBSTANCE USE DISORDERS

Severe substance use disorders, also called addictions, were once considered a moral failing or character flaw but are now known to be chronic illnesses. Scientific evidence shows that addiction to alcohol or drugs is a chronic brain disease that has potential for relapse and recovery.[1]

All addictive substances have powerful effects on the brain. These effects account for the euphoric or intensely pleasurable feelings that people experience during their initial use of alcohol or other substances. These feelings motivate people to use those substances again and again, despite the risks for significant harm. As individuals continue to misuse alcohol or other substances, progressive changes, called **neuroadaptations**, occur in the structure and function of the brain. These neuroadaptations drive the transition from controlled, occasional substance use to chronic misuse that can be difficult to control and can endure long after an individual stops using the substances. These changes can lead to the need for increased amounts of substances to achieve the same effect, referred to as tolerance. They may produce continued, periodic craving for the substance that can lead to relapse. More than 60 percent of people treated for a substance use disorder experience relapse within the first year after they are discharged from treatment, and a person can remain at increased risk of relapse for many years.[2]

For many people, initial substance use involves an element of impulsivity (i.e., acting without foresight or regard for the consequences). For example, an adolescent may impulsively take a first drink, smoke a cigarette, experiment with marijuana, or succumb to peer pressure and try a party drug like Ecstasy. If the experience is pleasurable, this feeling positively reinforces the substance use, making the person more likely to take the substance again. Another person may take a substance to relieve negative feelings such as stress, anxiety, or depression. In this case, the temporary relief the substance brings from the negative feelings reinforces substance use, increasing the likelihood that the person will use again.[3]

Many other environmental and social stimuli can reinforce a behavior. For example, peer approval positively reinforces substance use for some people. Likewise, if drinking or using drugs with others provides a feeling of relief from social isolation, substance use is reinforced.[4]

Eventually, in the absence of the substance, a person may experience negative emotions such as stress, anxiety, or depression or the individual may feel physically ill. This is called withdrawal, which often leads the person to use the substance again to relieve the withdrawal symptoms. As use becomes an ingrained behavior, impulsivity shifts to compulsivity, and the primary drivers of repeated substance use shift from positive reinforcement (feeling pleasure) to negative reinforcement (feeling relief) as the person seeks to stop the negative feelings and physical illness that accompany withdrawal. Eventually, the person begins taking the substance not to get "high," but rather

---

1 Substance Abuse and Mental Health Services Administration, & Office of the Surgeon General. (2016). *Facing addiction in America: The surgeon general's report on alcohol, drugs, and health.* United States Department of Health and Human Services. https://www.ncbi.nlm.nih.gov/books/NBK424857/

2 Substance Abuse and Mental Health Services Administration, & Office of the Surgeon General. (2016). *Facing addiction in America: The surgeon general's report on alcohol, drugs, and health.* United States Department of Health and Human Services. https://www.ncbi.nlm.nih.gov/books/NBK424857/

3 Substance Abuse and Mental Health Services Administration, & Office of the Surgeon General. (2016). *Facing addiction in America: The surgeon general's report on alcohol, drugs, and health.* United States Department of Health and Human Services. https://www.ncbi.nlm.nih.gov/books/NBK424857/

4 Substance Abuse and Mental Health Services Administration, & Office of the Surgeon General. (2016). *Facing addiction in America: The surgeon general's report on alcohol, drugs, and health.* United States Department of Health and Human Services. https://www.ncbi.nlm.nih.gov/books/NBK424857/

My Notes

to escape the "low" feelings from withdrawal. Compulsive substance seeking is a key characteristic of addiction, as well as loss of control over use. Compulsivity helps to explain why many people with addiction experience relapses after abstinence.[5]

Three regions of the brain are the key components in the development and persistence of substance use disorders: the basal ganglia, the extended amygdala, and the prefrontal cortex:

- The basal ganglia controls the rewarding, pleasurable effects of substance use and is responsible for the formation of habitual substance taking. Two subregions of the basal ganglia are particularly important in substance use disorders:
  - The nucleus accumbens, involved in motivation and the experience of reward.
  - The dorsal striatum, involved in forming habits and other routine behaviors.
- The extended amygdala is involved in the stress response and the feelings of unease, anxiety, and irritability that typically accompany substance withdrawal.
- The prefrontal cortex is involved in executive function (e.g., the ability to organize thoughts and activities, prioritize tasks, manage time, and make decisions), including exerting control over substance use.

These changes in the brain persist long after substance use stops and are associated with a high incidence of relapse with substance use disorders.

Addiction Cycle

The addiction process involves a three-stage cycle that becomes more severe as a person continues to misuse substances, causing neuroadaptions in brain function that reduce a person's ability to control their substance use. Each stage is associated with one of the brain regions previously described (i.e., basal ganglia, extended amygdala, and prefrontal cortex). See Figure 14.7[6] for an image of the brain regions associated with the three stages of addiction.

This three-stage model provides a useful way to understand the symptoms of addiction, the ways it can be prevented and treated, and the steps for recovery.[7]

These are the three stages of addiction:

- **Binge/Intoxication:** The stage at which an individual consumes an intoxicating substance and experiences its rewarding or pleasurable effects.

5 Substance Abuse and Mental Health Services Administration, & Office of the Surgeon General. (2016). *Facing addiction in America: The surgeon general's report on alcohol, drugs, and health.* United States Department of Health and Human Services. https://www.ncbi.nlm.nih.gov/books/NBK424857/

6 Substance Abuse and Mental Health Services Administration (US); Office of the Surgeon General (US). *Facing addiction in America: The surgeon general's report on alcohol, drugs, and health* [Internet]. Washington (DC): US Department of Health and Human Services; 2016 Nov. Figure 2.3, The Three Stages of the Addiction Cycle and the Brain Regions Associated with Them. Used under Fair Use. Available from https://www.ncbi.nlm.nih.gov/books/NBK424849/figure/ch2.f3/

7 Substance Abuse and Mental Health Services Administration, & Office of the Surgeon General. (2016). *Facing addiction in America: The surgeon general's report on alcohol, drugs, and health.* United States Department of Health and Human Services. https://www.ncbi.nlm.nih.gov/books/NBK424857/

My Notes

- **Withdrawal/Negative Affect:** The stage at which an individual experiences a negative emotional state in the absence of the substance.
- **Preoccupation/Anticipation:** The stage at which one seeks substances again after a period of abstinence.

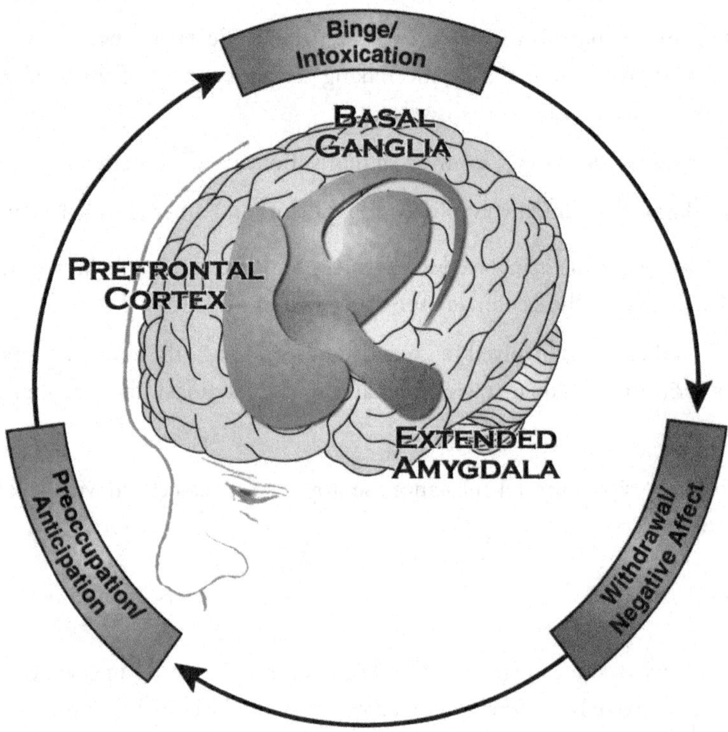

Figure 14.7 Brain Regions Associated With the Three Stages of Addiction. Used under Fair Use.

Binge/Intoxication

All addictive substances produce feelings of pleasure. These "rewarding effects" positively reinforce their use and increase the likelihood of repeated use. The rewarding effects of substances involve activity in the nucleus accumbens, including activation of the brain's dopamine and opioid signaling system. Studies show that antagonists, or inhibitors, of dopamine and opioidreceptors can block drug and alcohol-seeking behaviors.[8] See Figure 14.8[9] for an illustration of rewarding actions of addictive substances on the nucleus accumbens.

---

8 Substance Abuse and Mental Health Services Administration, & Office of the Surgeon General. (2016). *Facing addiction in America: The surgeon general's report on alcohol, drugs, and health.* United States Department of Health and Human Services. https://www.ncbi.nlm.nih.gov/books/NBK424857/

9 Substance Abuse and Mental Health Services Administration (US); Office of the Surgeon General (US). Facing Addiction in America: The Surgeon General's Report on Alcohol, Drugs, and Health [Internet]. Washington (DC): US Department of Health and Human Services; 2016 Nov. Figure 2.5, Actions of Addictive Substances on the Brain. Used under Fair Use. Available from: https://www.ncbi.nlm.nih.gov/books/NBK424849/figure/ch2.f5/

My Notes

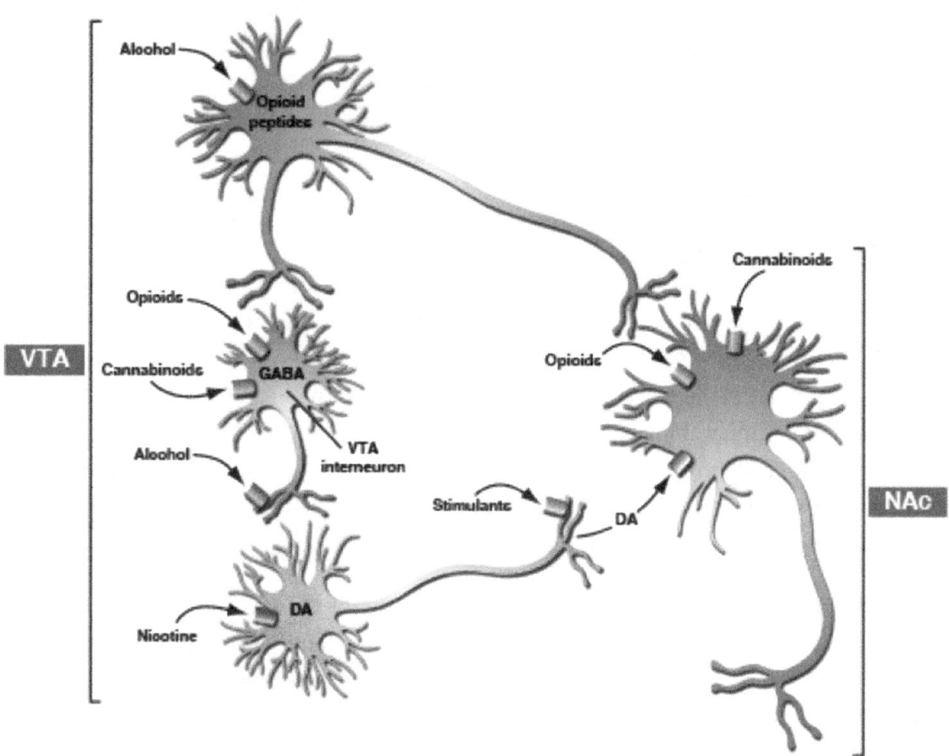

Figure 14.8 Rewarding Actions of Addictive Substances on the Nucleus Accumbens (NAc). Used under Fair Use.

Dopamine neurons (DA) are activated, either directly or indirectly, by all addictive substances, but particularly by stimulants and nicotine.[10]

The brain's opioid system includes naturally occurring opioid molecules (i.e., endorphins) and three types of opioid receptors (i.e., mu, delta, and kappa) and plays a key role in mediating the rewarding effects of opioids and alcohol. Activation of the opioid system stimulates the nucleus accumbens (NAc) directly or indirectly through the GABA and dopamine (DA) system.[11]

Tetrahydrocannabinol (THC), the primary psychoactive component of marijuana, targets GABA neurons that stimulate the dopamine (DA) system, as well as directly stimulating the nucleus accumbens (NAc).[12]

Activation of the brain's reward system by alcohol and drugs not only generates the pleasurable feelings associated with those substances, but also ultimately triggers changes in the way a person responds to stimuli associated with

---

10 Substance Abuse and Mental Health Services Administration, & Office of the Surgeon General. (2016). *Facing addiction in America: The surgeon general's report on alcohol, drugs, and health.* United States Department of Health and Human Services. https://www.ncbi.nlm.nih.gov/books/NBK424857/

11 Substance Abuse and Mental Health Services Administration, & Office of the Surgeon General. (2016). *Facing addiction in America: The surgeon general's report on alcohol, drugs, and health.* United States Department of Health and Human Services. https://www.ncbi.nlm.nih.gov/books/NBK424857/

12 Substance Abuse and Mental Health Services Administration, & Office of the Surgeon General. (2016). *Facing addiction in America: The surgeon general's report on alcohol, drugs, and health.* United States Department of Health and Human Services. https://www.ncbi.nlm.nih.gov/books/NBK424857/

the use of those substances. A person learns to associate the stimuli present while using a substance, including people, places, drug paraphernalia, and even internal states, such as mood, with the substance's rewarding effects. Over time, these stimuli can activate the dopamine system on their own and trigger powerful urges to take the substance. These "cravings" can persist even after the rewarding effects of the substance have diminished. As a result, exposure to people, places, or things previously associated with substance use can serve as triggers or cues that promote substance seeking and taking, even in people who are in recovery.[13]

Withdrawal/Negative Affect Stage

The withdrawal/negative affect stage of addiction follows the binge/intoxication stage, and, in turn, sets up future rounds of binge/intoxication. During this stage, a person who has been using alcohol or drugs experiences withdrawal symptoms, including negative emotions and symptoms of physical illness when they stop taking the substance. Symptoms of withdrawal may occur with all addictive substances, although they vary in intensity and duration depending on both the type of substance and the severity of use. The negative feelings associated with withdrawal are thought to come from two sources: diminished activation in the reward circuitry of the basal ganglia and activation of the brain's stress systems in the extended amygdala.[14]

When used long-term, all addictive substances cause dysfunction in the brain's dopamine reward system. For example, brain imaging studies in individuals with addictions show long-lasting decreases in dopamine receptors even after stopping substance abuse. See Figure 14.9[15] for an image of brain imaging studies comparing an individual with cocaine addiction to someone without addiction. Decreases in the activity of the dopamine system have also been observed during withdrawal from stimulants, opioids, nicotine, and alcohol. Other studies also show that when an addicted person is given a stimulant, it causes a smaller release of dopamine than when the same dose is given to a person who is not addicted.[16]

---

13 Substance Abuse and Mental Health Services Administration, & Office of the Surgeon General. (2016). *Facing addiction in America: The surgeon general's report on alcohol, drugs, and health.* United States Department of Health and Human Services. https://www.ncbi.nlm.nih.gov/books/NBK424857/

14 Substance Abuse and Mental Health Services Administration, & Office of the Surgeon General. (2016). *Facing addiction in America: The surgeon general's report on alcohol, drugs, and health.* United States Department of Health and Human Services. https://www.ncbi.nlm.nih.gov/books/NBK424857/

15 Substance Abuse and Mental Health Services Administration, & Office of the Surgeon General. (2016). *Facing addiction in America: The surgeon general's report on alcohol, drugs, and health.* United States Department of Health and Human Services. https://www.ncbi.nlm.nih.gov/books/NBK424857/

16 Substance Abuse and Mental Health Services Administration, & Office of the Surgeon General. (2016). *Facing addiction in America: The surgeon general's report on alcohol, drugs, and health.* United States Department of Health and Human Services. https://www.ncbi.nlm.nih.gov/books/NBK424857/

My Notes

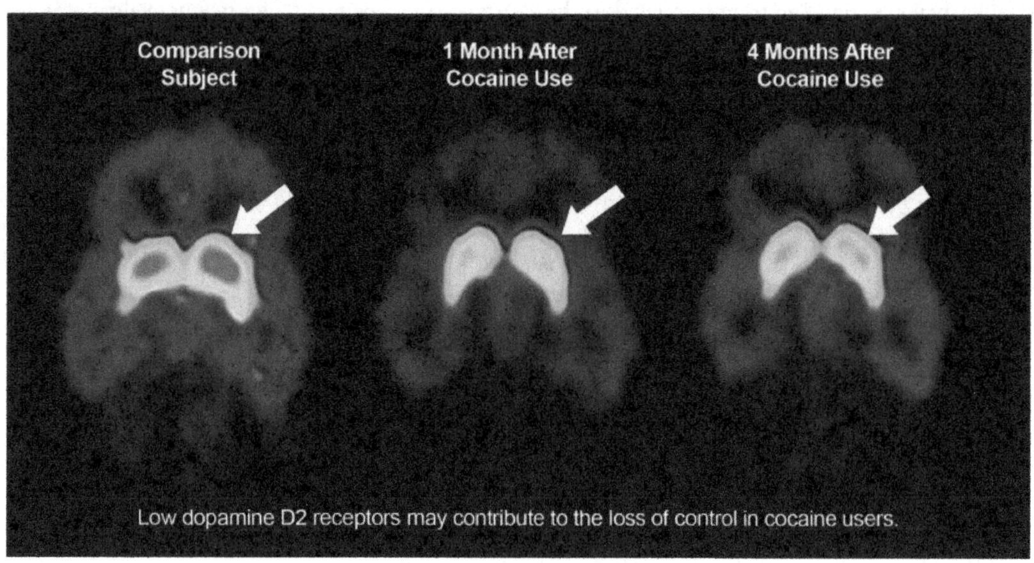

Figure 14.9 Decreased Dopamine Receptors in an Individual With a Cocaine Addiction. Used under Fair Use.

These findings suggest that people addicted to substances experience an overall reduction in the sensitivity of the brain's reward system (especially in the brain circuits involving dopamine), both to addictive substances and also to natural reinforcers, such as food and sex. This impairment explains why individuals who develop a substance abuse disorder often do not derive the same level of satisfaction or pleasure from once-pleasurable activities and may neglect eating. This loss of reward sensitivity may also account for the compulsive escalation of substance use as addicted individuals attempt to regain the pleasurable feelings the reward system once provided.[17]

At the same time, a second process occurs during the withdrawal stage related to the activation of stress neurotransmitters in the extended amygdala. These stress neurotransmitters include corticotropin releasing factor (CRF), norepinephrine, and dynorphin. These neurotransmitters play a key role in the negative feelings associated with withdrawal and in stress-triggered substance use. When researchers used antagonists to block activation of addicted individuals' stress neurotransmitter systems, it reduced their substance intake in response to withdrawal and stress.[18]

Preoccupation/Anticipation Stage: Prefrontal Cortex

The preoccupation/anticipation stage of the addiction cycle is the stage in which a person may begin to seek to use substances again after a period of abstinence. In this stage, an addicted person becomes preoccupied with using substances again, referred to as craving. This stage of addiction involves the brain's prefrontal cortex, the region that controls executive function (e.g., the ability to organize thoughts and activities; prioritize tasks; manage time; make decisions; and regulate one's own actions, emotions, and impulses). Executive function is essential for a person to make appropriate choices about whether or not to use a substance and to override strong urges to use

---

17 Substance Abuse and Mental Health Services Administration, & Office of the Surgeon General. (2016). *Facing addiction in America: The surgeon general's report on alcohol, drugs, and health.* United States Department of Health and Human Services. https://www.ncbi.nlm.nih.gov/books/NBK424857/

18 Substance Abuse and Mental Health Services Administration, & Office of the Surgeon General. (2016). *Facing addiction in America: The surgeon general's report on alcohol, drugs, and health.* United States Department of Health and Human Services. https://www.ncbi.nlm.nih.gov/books/NBK424857/

My Notes

it, especially when experiencing triggers related to the substance (e.g., being at a party where alcohol is served) or stressful experiences. People with alcohol, cocaine, or opioid use disorders show impairments in executive function, including disruption of decision-making and behavioral inhibition.[19]

19 Substance Abuse and Mental Health Services Administration, & Office of the Surgeon General. (2016). *Facing addiction in America: The surgeon general's report on alcohol, drugs, and health.* United States Department of Health and Human Services. https://www.ncbi.nlm.nih.gov/books/NBK424857/

14.6 RISK FACTORS

My Notes

Many factors influence the development of substance use disorders, including developmental, environmental, social, and genetic factors, and co-occurring mental health disorders. Other conditions called protective factors protect people from developing a substance use disorder or addiction. The relative influence of these factors varies across individuals and the life span.

Whether an individual ever uses alcohol or another substance and whether that initial use progresses to a substance use disorder of any severity depends on a number of factors including the following[1]:

- A person's genetic makeup and biological factors
- The age when substance use begins
- Psychological factors related to a person's unique history and personality
- Environmental factors, such as the availability of drugs, family and peer dynamics, financial resources, cultural norms, exposure to stress, and access to social support

Early Life Experiences

The experiences a person has early in childhood and in adolescence can set the stage for substance use and sometimes escalate to substance use disorder. Early life stressors (referred to as adverse childhood experiences) include physical, emotional, and sexual abuse; neglect; household instability (such as parental substance use and conflict, mental illness, or incarceration of household members); and poverty.[2]

Review information on adverse childhood experiences in the "Mental Health and Mental Illness" section of Chapter 1.

Adolescence is a critical vulnerable period for substance misuse and the development of substance use disorders because a characteristic of this developmental period is risk taking and experimentation. For some young people, this includes trying alcohol, marijuana, or other drugs. Additionally, the brain undergoes significant changes during this life stage, making it particularly vulnerable to substance exposure. For example, the frontal cortex, a region in the front part of the brain that includes the prefrontal cortex, does not fully develop until the early to mid-20s. Research shows that heavy drinking and drug use during adolescence affects development of this critical area of the brain.[3]

Approximately 74 percent of 18- to 30-year-olds admitted to treatment programs began using substances at the age of 17 or younger. Individuals who start using substances during adolescence often experience more chronic

1 Substance Abuse and Mental Health Services Administration, & Office of the Surgeon General. (2016). *Facing addiction in America: The surgeon general's report on alcohol, drugs, and health.* United States Department of Health and Human Services. https://www.ncbi.nlm.nih.gov/books/NBK424857/

2 Substance Abuse and Mental Health Services Administration, & Office of the Surgeon General. (2016). *Facing addiction in America: The surgeon general's report on alcohol, drugs, and health.* United States Department of Health and Human Services. https://www.ncbi.nlm.nih.gov/books/NBK424857/

3 Substance Abuse and Mental Health Services Administration, & Office of the Surgeon General. (2016). *Facing addiction in America: The surgeon general's report on alcohol, drugs, and health.* United States Department of Health and Human Services. https://www.ncbi.nlm.nih.gov/books/NBK424857/

My Notes

and intensive use, and they are at greater risk of developing a substance use disorder compared with those who begin use at an older age. In other words, the earlier the exposure, the greater the risk.[4]

Genetic and Molecular Factors

Genetic factors are thought to account for 40 to 70 percent of individual differences in risk for addiction. Although multiple genes are likely involved in the development of addiction, only a few specific gene variants have been identified that either predispose to or protect against addiction. Some of these variants have been associated with the metabolism of alcohol and nicotine, while others involve receptors and other proteins associated with key neurotransmitters and molecules involved in all parts of the addiction cycle. Genes involved in strengthening the connections between neurons and in forming drug memories have also been associated with addiction risk. Like other chronic health conditions, substance use disorders are influenced by the complex interplay between a person's genes and environment.[5]

Concurrent Mental Health Disorders

In 2020, 17 million adults (6.7%) had both a substance use disorder (SUD) and a mental health illness (AMI) as illustrated in Figure 14.10.[6] The relationship between SUDs and mental disorders is known to be bidirectional, meaning the presence of a mental health disorder may contribute to the development or exacerbation of an SUD, or an SUD may contribute to the development or exacerbation of a mental health disorder. The combined presence of SUDs and mental health disorders results in greater functional impairment; worse treatment outcomes; higher morbidity and mortality; increased treatment costs; and higher risk for homelessness, incarceration, and suicide.

---

4 Substance Abuse and Mental Health Services Administration, & Office of the Surgeon General. (2016). *Facing addiction in America: The surgeon general's report on alcohol, drugs, and health.* United States Department of Health and Human Services. https://www.ncbi.nlm.nih.gov/books/NBK424857/

5 Substance Abuse and Mental Health Services Administration, & Office of the Surgeon General. (2016). *Facing addiction in America: The surgeon general's report on alcohol, drugs, and health.* United States Department of Health and Human Services. https://www.ncbi.nlm.nih.gov/books/NBK424857/

6 Image is a derivative of "Past Year Substance Abuse Disorder (SUD) and Any Mental Illness (AMI): Among Adults Aged 18 or Older; 2020" table by Substance Abuse and Mental Health Services Administration. (2021). Key substance use and mental health indicators in the United States: Results from the 2020 National Survey on Drug Use and Health (HHS Publication No. PEP21-07-01-003, NSDUH Series H-56). Rockville, MD: Center for Behavioral Health Statistics and Quality, Substance Abuse and Mental Health Services Administration. Used under Fair Use. Retrieved from https://www.samhsa.gov/data/report/2020-nsduh-annual-national-report

My Notes

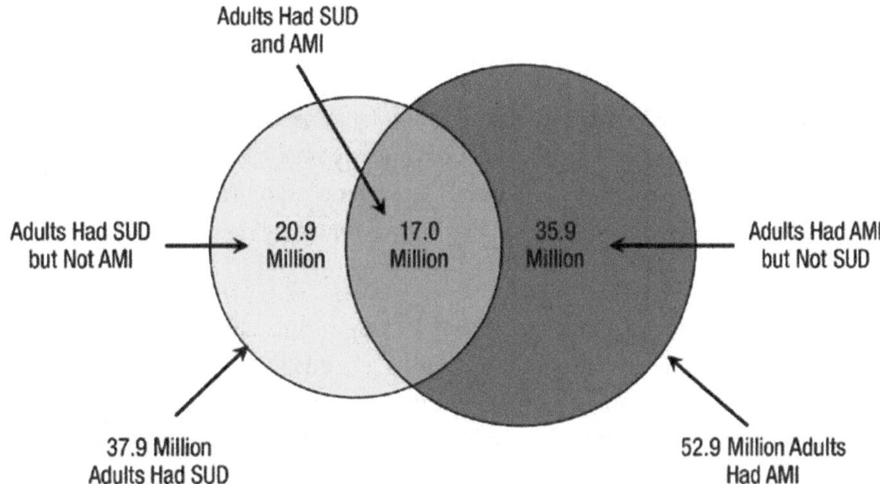

Figure 14.10 Concurrent Mental Illness (AMI) and Substance Use Disorder (SUD) in Adults in 2020. Used under Fair Use.

The reasons why substance use disorders and mental health disorders often occur together are not clear, but there are three possible explanations. One reason may be because certain substances may temporarily mask the symptoms of mental health disorders (such as anxiety or depression). A second reason may be that certain substances trigger a mental health disorder that otherwise would not have developed. For example, research suggests that alcohol use increases risk for PTSD by altering the brain's ability to recover from traumatic experiences. A third possible reason is that both substance use disorders and mental health disorders are caused by overlapping factors, such as particular genes, neurobiology, or exposure to traumatic or stressful life experiences.[7]

Mental health disorders and substance use disorders have overlapping symptoms, making diagnosis and treatment planning challenging. For example, people who use methamphetamine for a long period of time may experience paranoia, hallucinations, and delusions that can be mistaken for symptoms of schizophrenia.[8]

Gender

Some groups of people are more vulnerable to substance misuse and substance use disorders. For example, biological males tend to drink more than biological females and are at higher risk for alcohol use disorder. However, biological females who use cocaine, opioids, or alcohol may progress from initial use to a substance use disorder

7 Substance Abuse and Mental Health Services Administration, & Office of the Surgeon General. (2016). *Facing addiction in America: The surgeon general's report on alcohol, drugs, and health.* United States Department of Health and Human Services. https://www.ncbi.nlm.nih.gov/books/NBK424857/

8 Substance Abuse and Mental Health Services Administration, & Office of the Surgeon General. (2016). *Facing addiction in America: The surgeon general's report on alcohol, drugs, and health.* United States Department of Health and Human Services. https://www.ncbi.nlm.nih.gov/books/NBK424857/

My Notes

faster than males. Compared with biological males, biological females also exhibit greater withdrawal symptoms from some drugs such as nicotine and have higher levels of the stress hormone cortisol.[9]

Race and Ethnicity

Neurobiological factors contributing to differential rates of substance use disorders across racial and ethnic groups have been researched. A study using functional magnetic resonance imaging (fMRI) found that African American smokers showed greater activation of the prefrontal cortex upon exposure to smoking-related cues than did White smokers, an effect that may partly contribute to the lower smoking-cessation success rates among African Americans.[10]

Alcohol research on racial and ethnic groups has shown that approximately 36 percent of East Asians carry a gene variant that alters the rate of alcohol metabolism, causing a buildup of acetaldehyde, a toxic by-product that produces symptoms such as flushing, nausea, and rapid heartbeat. Although these effects may protect some individuals of East Asian descent from alcohol use disorder, those who drink despite the effects are at increased risk for esophageal and head and neck cancers.[11]

Individual, Family, and Community Level Risk Factors

An individual's risk factors for developing SUD include the following[12]:

- **Early initiation of substance use:** Engaging in alcohol or drug use at a young age
- **Early and persistent problem behavior:** Emotional distress, aggressiveness, and "difficult" temperaments in adolescents
- **Rebelliousness:** High tolerance for deviance and rebellious activities
- **Favorable attitudes toward substance use:** Positive feelings towards alcohol or drug use; low perception of risk
- **Peer substance use:** Friends and peers who engage in alcohol or drug use
- **Genetic predictors:** Genetic susceptibility to alcohol or drug use
- **Academic failure beginning in late elementary school:** Poor grades in school
- **Lack of commitment to school:** When a young person no longer considers the role of being a student as meaningful and rewarding or lacks investment or commitment to school

---

9 Substance Abuse and Mental Health Services Administration, & Office of the Surgeon General. (2016). *Facing addiction in America: The surgeon general's report on alcohol, drugs, and health.* United States Department of Health and Human Services. https://www.ncbi.nlm.nih.gov/books/NBK424857/

10 Substance Abuse and Mental Health Services Administration, & Office of the Surgeon General. (2016). *Facing addiction in America: The surgeon general's report on alcohol, drugs, and health.* United States Department of Health and Human Services. https://www.ncbi.nlm.nih.gov/books/NBK424857/

11 Substance Abuse and Mental Health Services Administration, & Office of the Surgeon General. (2016). *Facing addiction in America: The surgeon general's report on alcohol, drugs, and health.* United States Department of Health and Human Services. https://www.ncbi.nlm.nih.gov/books/NBK424857/

12 Substance Abuse and Mental Health Services Administration, & Office of the Surgeon General. (2016). *Facing addiction in America: The surgeon general's report on alcohol, drugs, and health.* United States Department of Health and Human Services. https://www.ncbi.nlm.nih.gov/books/NBK424857/

My Notes

Risk factors at the family level for an individual developing SUD are as follows[13]:

- **Family management problems:** Poor parental management practices, including failure to set clear expectations for children's behavior, failure to supervise and monitor children, and excessively harsh or inconsistent punishment
- **Family conflict:** Conflict between parents or between parents and children, including abuse or neglect
- **Favorable parental attitudes:** Parental attitudes that are favorable to drug use and parental approval of drinking and drug use
- **Family history of substance misuse:** Persistent or generalized substance misuse by family members

These are the risk factors at the community level for individuals developing SUD[14]:

- **Low cost of alcohol:** Low alcohol sales tax, happy hour specials, and other price discounting
- **High availability of substances:** High number of alcohol outlets in a defined geographical area or per a sector of the population
- **Community laws and norms favorable to substance use:** Community reinforcement of norms suggesting alcohol or drug use is acceptable for youth
- **Low neighborhood attachment:** Low level of bonding to the neighborhood
- **Community disorganization:** Living in neighborhoods with high population density, lack of public places, physical deterioration, or high rates of adult crime
- **Low socioeconomic status:** Parents' low socioeconomic status, as measured through a combination of education, income, and occupation
- **Transitions and mobility:** Communities with high rates of mobility within or between communities
- **Media portrayal of alcohol use:** Exposure to actors using alcohol or drugs in movies or television

13 Substance Abuse and Mental Health Services Administration, & Office of the Surgeon General. (2016). *Facing addiction in America: The surgeon general's report on alcohol, drugs, and health.* United States Department of Health and Human Services. https://www.ncbi.nlm.nih.gov/books/NBK424857/

14 Substance Abuse and Mental Health Services Administration, & Office of the Surgeon General. (2016). *Facing addiction in America: The surgeon general's report on alcohol, drugs, and health.* United States Department of Health and Human Services. https://www.ncbi.nlm.nih.gov/books/NBK424857/

My Notes

14.7 TREATMENT OF SUBSTANCE USE DISORDERS

Research has shown that substance use disorders are similar in course, management, and outcome to other chronic illnesses, such as hypertension, diabetes, and asthma. It is possible to adopt the same type of chronic care management approach to the treatment of substance use disorders as is used to manage chronic physical illnesses. Remission of substance use disorders and even full recovery can be achieved if evidence-based care is provided for adequate periods of time by properly trained health care professionals and augmented with supportive monitoring, recovery support services, and social services.[1]

There are a spectrum of effective strategies and services available to identify, treat, and manage substance use disorders. Research shows that the most effective way to help someone with a substance misuse problem who is at risk for developing a substance use disorder is to intervene early, before the condition can progress. Screening for substance misuse is increasingly being provided in general health care settings so that emerging problems can be detected and early intervention provided. The addition of services to address substance use problems and disorders in mainstream health care has extended the continuum of care and includes a range of effective, evidence-based medications; behavioral therapies; and supportive services. However, a number of barriers have limited the widespread adoption of these services, including common myths about addiction, lack of resources, insufficient training, and workforce shortages. This is particularly true for the treatment of individuals with co-occurring substance use and mental health disorders.[2]

There are several common myths about addiction that make it harder for people with substance use disorders to seek treatment to get well. Review these myths in the following box.

Common Myths About Addiction[3]

- Using drugs or alcohol is a choice, so if someone gets addicted, it's their fault.
  - **Reality:** Addiction is a consequence of many contributing factors, including genetics, neurobiology, adverse childhood effects (ACEs), trauma, and other influences.
- If someone just uses willpower, they should be able to stop using the substance.
  - **Reality:** For people who are genetically vulnerable to addiction, substance uses can cause profound changes in the brain that hijack the reward pathway of the brain. Addictive substances flood the brain with neurotransmitters than signal pleasure. These changes create intense impulses to continue using the substances despite negative consequences of doing so.

1 Substance Abuse and Mental Health Services Administration, & Office of the Surgeon General. (2016). *Facing addiction in America: The surgeon general's report on alcohol, drugs, and health.* United States Department of Health and Human Services. https://www.ncbi.nlm.nih.gov/books/NBK424857/

2 Substance Abuse and Mental Health Services Administration, & Office of the Surgeon General. (2016). *Facing addiction in America: The surgeon general's report on alcohol, drugs, and health.* United States Department of Health and Human Services. https://www.ncbi.nlm.nih.gov/books/NBK424857/

3 Face It Together. (n.d.) *Common myths about addiction.* https://www.wefaceittogether.org/learn/common-myths

My Notes

- Addiction affects certain types of people.
    - **Reality:** Addiction can affect anyone, no matter one's age, income, ethnicity, religion, family, or profession. Nationally, about one in eight people ages 12 and older are impacted.
- If someone has a stable job and family life, they can't be suffering from addiction.
    - **Reality:** Anyone is vulnerable to addiction. Many people hide the severity of their illness or don't get help because of stigma or shame.
- People have to become seriously ill before they can get well.
    - **Reality:** The longer a person waits to get help, the more changes happen to the brain, which can have deadly consequences like overdose. Studies show that people forced into treatment have an equal chance of successful recovery as people who initiate treatment on their own.
- Going to rehab will fix the problem.
    - **Reality:** Addiction is a chronic disease, similar to hypertension or diabetes, that can be controlled but not cured. Treatment is the first step towards wellness, but it is just the beginning. Staying well requires a lifelong commitment to managing the chronic disease.
- If someone relapses, they can never get better.
    - **Reality:** Relapse is no more likely with addiction than other chronic illnesses like diabetes. Getting well involves changing deeply embedded behaviors that are significantly rewarded in the brain. Behavioral change takes time and effort, and setbacks can occur. A relapse can signal that the treatment approach or other supports need to change or that other treatment methods are needed. There is hope that people who experience a relapse will return to recovery.

Substance use disorder treatment is designed to help individuals stop or reduce harmful substance misuse, improve their health and social function, and manage their risk for relapse. For example, mild substance use disorders can be identified quickly in many medical settings and often respond to brief motivational interventions and/or supportive monitoring, referred to as guided self-change. In contrast, severe and chronic substance use disorders often require specialty substance use disorder treatment and continued post-treatment support to achieve full remission and recovery. To address the spectrum of problems associated with substance use disorders, a continuum of care is planned and implemented based on an individual's needs, including early intervention, treatment, and recovery support services.[4]

4 Substance Abuse and Mental Health Services Administration, & Office of the Surgeon General. (2016). *Facing addiction in America: The surgeon general's report on alcohol, drugs, and health.* United States Department of Health and Human Services. https://www.ncbi.nlm.nih.gov/books/NBK424857/

My Notes

Early Intervention

Early intervention services can be provided in a variety of settings (e.g., school clinics, primary care offices, mental health clinics) to people who have substance misuse problems or mild substance use disorders. These services are usually provided when an individual presents for another medical condition or social service need and is not necessarily seeking treatment for a substance use disorder. The goals of early intervention are to reduce the harms associated with substance misuse, reduce risk behaviors before they lead to injury, improve health and social function, and prevent progression from misuse to a substance use disorder. Early intervention consists of providing education about risks of substance use, safe levels of alcohol and medication use, and strategies to quit substance use. Referral to treatment services is provided as needed.[5]

Populations Who Should Receive Early Intervention

Early intervention should be provided to children, adolescents, and adults who show signs of substance misuse or a mild substance use disorder. One group in need of early intervention is people who binge drink, particularly those aged 12 to 17, who are at higher risk for future substance use disorders because of their young age. Available research shows that brief, early interventions given by a respected care provider (such as a nurse, nurse educator, or physician) in the context of routine medical care can educate and motivate many individuals who are misusing substances to understand and acknowledge their risky behavior and reduce their substance use.[6]

Regardless of the substance, the first step of early intervention is using a screening tool to identify behaviors that put the individual at risk for harm or for developing a substance use disorder. Positive screening results should be followed by brief educational sessions tailored to the specific problems and interests of the individual. It should be delivered in a nonjudgmental manner, emphasizing both the importance of reducing substance use and the individual's ability to accomplish this goal. Follow-up evaluation should assess whether the screening and the brief intervention were effective in reducing the substance misuse or if formal treatment is required.[7]

Components of Early Intervention

One structured approach to delivering early intervention to people showing signs of substance misuse and/or early signs of a substance use disorder is through screening and brief intervention (SBI). Research has shown that several methods of SBI are effective in decreasing substance misuse for a variety of populations in a variety of health care settings.

Screening

Ideally, substance misuse screening should occur for all individuals who present to health care settings, including primary care, urgent care, mental health care, and emergency departments. Several validated screening instruments have been developed to help nonspecialty providers identify individuals who may have, or be at risk for, a

---

5 Substance Abuse and Mental Health Services Administration, & Office of the Surgeon General. (2016). *Facing addiction in America: The surgeon general's report on alcohol, drugs, and health.* United States Department of Health and Human Services. https://www.ncbi.nlm.nih.gov/books/NBK424857/

6 Substance Abuse and Mental Health Services Administration, & Office of the Surgeon General. (2016). *Facing addiction in America: The surgeon general's report on alcohol, drugs, and health.* United States Department of Health and Human Services. https://www.ncbi.nlm.nih.gov/books/NBK424857/

7 Substance Abuse and Mental Health Services Administration, & Office of the Surgeon General. (2016). *Facing addiction in America: The surgeon general's report on alcohol, drugs, and health.* United States Department of Health and Human Services. https://www.ncbi.nlm.nih.gov/books/NBK424857/

substance use disorder. An example of an evidence-based screening tool is the Alcohol Use Disorders Identification Test (AUDIT).[8] Based on a World Health Organization study, the AUDIT has become the world's most widely used alcohol screening instrument and is available in approximately 40 languages. It is a self-administered questionnaire consisting of ten questions pertaining to an individual's alcohol use. Read additional details about the AUDIT tool in the following box.

My Notes

AUDIT Screening Tool

Review the full AUDIT tool: Check Your Drinking: An Interactive Self-test.

The screening tool includes ten questions with answers ranging from 0 (Never) to 4 (4 or more times a week):

- How often do you have a drink containing alcohol?
- How many standard drinks containing alcohol do you have on a typical day when drinking?
- How often do you have six or more drinks on one occasion?
- During the past year, how often have you found that you were not able to stop drinking once you had started?
- During the past year, how often have you failed to do what was normally expected of you because of drinking?
- During the past year, how often have you needed a drink in the morning to get yourself going after a heavy drinking session?
- During the past year, how often have you had a feeling of guilt or remorse after drinking?
- During the past year, how often have you been unable to remember what happened the night before because you had been drinking?
- Have you or someone else been injured as a result of your drinking?
- Has a relative, friend, doctor, or other health worker been concerned about your drinking or suggested you cut down?

Brief Interventions

Brief interventions is a term used to describe quick therapeutic techniques used to initiate change in individuals with unhealthy behaviors. For example, motivational interviewing (MI) is a client-centered therapeutic technique that can be used to address a person's ambivalence to change their use of substances. It uses a conversational

8 Substance Abuse and Mental Health Services Administration, & Office of the Surgeon General. (2016). *Facing addiction in America: The surgeon general's report on alcohol, drugs, and health.* United States Department of Health and Human Services. https://www.ncbi.nlm.nih.gov/books/NBK424857/

My Notes

approach to help the client discover their interest in changing their behavior. The nurse asks the client to express their desire for change and any ambivalence they might have and then begins to work with the client on making a plan to change their behavior and a commitment to the change process. Individuals who receive MI are more likely to adhere to a treatment plan and subsequently achieve better outcomes.[9]

Referral

When an individual's substance use problem meets criteria for a substance use disorder or when brief interventions do not produce change, referral to specialized treatment should occur. This is called Screening, Brief Intervention, and Referral to Treatment (SBIRT). A referral for assessment and development of a clinical treatment plan is created with the client and tailored to meet their needs. Effective referral processes should incorporate strategies to motivate the client to accept the referral and assistance in navigating barriers for treatment.[10]

Compare the effectiveness of communication with a client being treated in the emergency department for injuries sustained when driving under the influence of alcohol in these YouTube videos:

 Video 1[11]: Anti-SBIRT (Doctor A)

 Video 2 (Using SBIRT)[12]: Using SBIRT Effectively (Doctor B)

Treatment

Treatment can occur in a variety of settings, but treatment for severe substance use disorders has traditionally been provided in specialty substance use disorder treatment programs. The National Institute on Drug Abuse (NIDA) outlines the following evidence-based principles for effective treatment of adults and adolescents with substance use disorders[13]:

---

9 Substance Abuse and Mental Health Services Administration, & Office of the Surgeon General. (2016). *Facing addiction in America: The surgeon general's report on alcohol, drugs, and health.* United States Department of Health and Human Services. https://www.ncbi.nlm.nih.gov/books/NBK424857/

10 Substance Abuse and Mental Health Services Administration, & Office of the Surgeon General. (2016). *Facing addiction in America: The surgeon general's report on alcohol, drugs, and health.* United States Department of Health and Human Services. https://www.ncbi.nlm.nih.gov/books/NBK424857/

11 SBIRTInsitute. (2011, March 2). *Anti-SBIRT (Doctor A).* [Video]. YouTube. All rights reserved. https://youtu.be/ZGETDcFcAbI

12 SBIRTInsitute. (2011, March 2). *Using SBIRT Effectively (Doctor B).* [Video]. YouTube. All rights reserved. https://youtu.be/uL8QyJF2wVw

13 Substance Abuse and Mental Health Services Administration, & Office of the Surgeon General. (2016). *Facing addiction in America: The surgeon general's report on alcohol, drugs, and health.* United States Department of Health and Human Services. https://www.ncbi.nlm.nih.gov/books/NBK424857/

My Notes

Addiction is a complex but treatable disease that affects brain function and behavior. Psychoactive substances alter the brain's structure and function, resulting in changes that persist long after substance use has ceased. This may explain why individuals with substance use disorder are at risk for relapse even after long periods of abstinence and despite the potentially devastating consequences of their behaviors.[14]

No single treatment is appropriate for everyone. Treatment varies depending on the type of drug and the characteristics of the individuals. Matching treatment settings, interventions, and services to an individual's particular problems and needs is critical to their ultimate success in returning to productive functioning in the family, workplace, and society.[15]

Treatment must be readily available. Because individuals may be uncertain about entering treatment, taking advantage of available services the moment people are ready for treatment is critical. Potential clients can be lost if treatment is not immediately available or readily accessible. As with other chronic diseases, the earlier treatment is offered in the disease process, the greater the likelihood of positive outcomes.[16]

Effective treatment attends to multiple needs of the individual, not just their substance abuse. To be effective, treatment must address the individual's substance abuse, as well as associated medical, psychological, social, vocational, and legal problems. It is also important that treatment is tailored to the individual's age, gender, ethnicity, and culture.[17]

Remaining in treatment for an adequate period of time is critical. The appropriate duration for an individual depends on the type and degree of the client's problems and needs. Research indicates that most addicted individuals need at least three months in treatment to significantly reduce or stop their substance use and that the best outcomes occur with longer durations of treatment. Recovery from substance use disorder is a long-term process and frequently requires multiple episodes of treatment. As with other chronic illnesses, relapses can occur and should signal a need for treatment to be reinstated or adjusted. Because individuals often leave treatment prematurely, programs should include strategies to engage and keep clients in treatment.[18]

Behavioral therapies, including individual, family, or group counseling, are the most common types of treatment. Behavioral therapies vary in focus and may address a client's motivation to change, provide incentives for abstinence, build skills to resist drug use, replace substance-using activities with constructive and rewarding

---

14 National Institute on Drug Abuse. (2018, January). *Principles of drug addiction treatment: A research-based guide* (3rd ed.). National Institutes of Health. https://nida.nih.gov/publications/principles-drug-addiction-treatment-research-based-guide-third-edition/principles-effective-treatment

15 National Institute on Drug Abuse. (2018, January). *Principles of drug addiction treatment: A research-based guide* (3rd ed.). National Institutes of Health. https://nida.nih.gov/publications/principles-drug-addiction-treatment-research-based-guide-third-edition/principles-effective-treatment

16 National Institute on Drug Abuse. (2018, January). *Principles of drug addiction treatment: A research-based guide* (3rd ed.). National Institutes of Health. https://nida.nih.gov/publications/principles-drug-addiction-treatment-research-based-guide-third-edition/principles-effective-treatment

17 National Institute on Drug Abuse. (2018, January). *Principles of drug addiction treatment: A research-based guide* (3rd ed.). National Institutes of Health. https://nida.nih.gov/publications/principles-drug-addiction-treatment-research-based-guide-third-edition/principles-effective-treatment

18 National Institute on Drug Abuse. (2018, January). *Principles of drug addiction treatment: A research-based guide* (3rd ed.). National Institutes of Health. https://nida.nih.gov/publications/principles-drug-addiction-treatment-research-based-guide-third-edition/principles-effective-treatment

My Notes

activities, improve problem-solving skills, and facilitate interpersonal relationships. Additionally, participation in group therapy and other peer support programs during and following treatment can help maintain abstinence.[19]

An individual's treatment plan must be continually evaluated and modified as needed to ensure it meets their changing needs. A client may require varying combinations of services and treatment components during the course of treatment and recovery. In addition to counseling or psychotherapy, clients may require medication, medical services, family therapy, parenting instruction, vocational rehabilitation, and/or social and legal services. For many clients, a recovery-oriented systems approach provides the best results, with the treatment intensity varying according to a person's changing needs.[20]

Many individuals with substance use disorders also have other mental health disorders. Treatment should address all conditions using appropriate medications.[21]

Treatment does not need to be voluntary to be effective. Sanctions or enticements from family, employment settings, and/or the criminal justice system can significantly increase treatment entry, retention rates, and the ultimate success of drug treatment interventions. Substance use during treatment must be monitored continuously because relapses during treatment do occur. Knowing their substance use is being monitored can be a powerful incentive for individuals to withstand urges to use substances. Monitoring also provides an early indication of a relapse, signaling an adjustment is needed in the individual's treatment plan to better meet their needs.[22]

Treatment programs should test clients for the presence of HIV/AIDS, hepatitis B and C, tuberculosis, and other infectious diseases, as well as provide targeted risk-reduction counseling. Many substance misuse-related behaviors put people at risk of infectious diseases. Targeted counseling reduces infectious disease. Counseling can also help those who are already infected to manage their illness. Moreover, engaging in substance abuse treatment can facilitate adherence to other medical treatments.[23]

Evidence-based treatment interventions include medications, behavioral therapies, and recovery services.[24]

---

19 National Institute on Drug Abuse. (2018, January). *Principles of drug addiction treatment: A research-based guide* (3rd ed.). National Institutes of Health. https://nida.nih.gov/publications/principles-drug-addiction-treatment-research-based-guide-third-edition/principles-effective-treatment

20 National Institute on Drug Abuse. (2018, January). *Principles of drug addiction treatment: A research-based guide* (3rd ed.). National Institutes of Health. https://nida.nih.gov/publications/principles-drug-addiction-treatment-research-based-guide-third-edition/principles-effective-treatment

21 National Institute on Drug Abuse. (2018, January). *Principles of drug addiction treatment: A research-based guide* (3rd ed.). National Institutes of Health. https://nida.nih.gov/publications/principles-drug-addiction-treatment-research-based-guide-third-edition/principles-effective-treatment

22 National Institute on Drug Abuse. (2018, January). *Principles of drug addiction treatment: A research-based guide* (3rd ed.). National Institutes of Health. https://nida.nih.gov/publications/principles-drug-addiction-treatment-research-based-guide-third-edition/principles-effective-treatment

23 National Institute on Drug Abuse. (2018, January). *Principles of drug addiction treatment: A research-based guide* (3rd ed.). National Institutes of Health. https://nida.nih.gov/publications/principles-drug-addiction-treatment-research-based-guide-third-edition/principles-effective-treatment

24 Substance Abuse and Mental Health Services Administration, & Office of the Surgeon General. (2016). *Facing addiction in America: The surgeon general's report on alcohol, drugs, and health.* United States Department of Health and Human Services. https://www.ncbi.nlm.nih.gov/books/NBK424857/

Medications

My Notes

Medications are an important element of treatment for many clients, especially when combined with counseling and other behavioral therapies. For example, methadone, buprenorphine, and naltrexone are effective in helping individuals addicted to heroin or other opioids stabilize their lives and reduce their substance misuse. Acamprosate, disulfiram, and naltrexone are medications approved for treating alcohol dependence. For persons addicted to nicotine, a nicotine replacement product (available as patches, gum, lozenges, or nasal spray) or an oral medication (such as bupropion or varenicline) can be an effective component of treatment when part of a comprehensive behavioral treatment program.[25] See Table 14.7 for a list of medications approved by the FDA to treat alcohol and opioid use disorders.

Table 14.7 Pharmacotherapy to Treat Alcohol and Opioid Use Disorders[26]

Medication	**Use**	**DEA Schedule**	**Application**
Buprenorphine-naloxone	Opioid use disorder	CIII	Used for detoxification or maintenance of abstinence.
Methadone	Opioid use disorder	CII	Used for withdrawal and long-term maintenance of abstinence of opioid addiction. Dispersed only at opioid treatment centers certified by SAMHSA and approved by state authority.
Naltrexone	Opioid use disorder and alcohol use disorder	Not scheduled under the Controlled Substances Act	Block opioid receptors, reduce cravings, and diminish rewarding effects of opioids and alcohol. Extended-release injections are recommended to prevent relapse.
Acamprosate	Alcohol use disorder	Not scheduled under the Controlled Substances Act	Used for maintenance of alcohol abstinence.
Disulfiram	Alcohol use disorder	Not scheduled under the Controlled Substances Act	Causes severe physical reactions when alcohol is ingested, such as nausea, flushing, and heart palpitations. The knowledge that the reaction will occur acts as a deterrent to drinking alcohol.

25 National Institute on Drug Abuse. (2018, January). *Principles of drug addiction treatment: A research-based guide* (3rd ed.). National Institutes of Health. https://nida.nih.gov/publications/principles-drug-addiction-treatment-research-based-guide-third-edition/principles-effective-treatment

26 Substance Abuse and Mental Health Services Administration, & Office of the Surgeon General. (2016). *Facing addiction in America: The surgeon general's report on alcohol, drugs, and health.* United States Department of Health and Human Services. https://www.ncbi.nlm.nih.gov/books/NBK424857/

My Notes

Medically assisted detoxification is only the first stage of treatment and by itself does little to change long-term substance misuse. Although medically assisted detoxification can safely manage the acute physical symptoms of withdrawal, detoxification alone is rarely sufficient to help individuals achieve long-term abstinence of substances. Clients should be encouraged to continue long-term treatment and recovery services following detoxification.[27]

Behavioral Therapies

In addition to medications, effective treatment of SUD includes behavioral therapies to help clients recognize the impact of substance misuse on their interpersonal relationships and ability to function in a healthy, safe, and productive manner. Behavioral therapies also teach and motivate clients to change their behaviors as a way to control their substance use disorders.[28]

Evidence-based behavioral therapies include cognitive-behavioral therapy, dialectical behavior therapy, family therapy, contingency management, community reinforcement approach, motivational enhancement therapy, matrix model, and twelve-step facilitation. These therapies are further described in the following subsections.

Cognitive-Behavioral Therapy

The theoretical foundation for cognitive-behavioral therapy (CBT) is that substance use disorders develop, in part, as a result of maladaptive behavior patterns and dysfunctional thoughts. As a result, CBT treatments involve techniques to modify such behaviors and improve coping skills by emphasizing the identification and modification of dysfunctional thinking. CBT is a short-term approach, usually involving 12 to 24 weekly individual sessions. These sessions typically explore the positive and negative consequences of substance use with self-monitoring as a mechanism to recognize cravings and other situations that may lead the individual to relapse. They also help the individual develop healthy coping strategies.

Dialectical Behavior Therapy

Dialectical behavior therapy (DBT) is an evidence-based therapy that teaches a skill called mindfulness. Multiple research studies have noted that mindfulness is potentially useful in helping people diagnosed with SUD gain mastery over substance cravings.[29]

Review information about cognitive-behavioral therapy and dialectical behavior therapy in the "Treatments for Depression" section of the "Depressive Disorders" chapter.

Family Therapy

Family behavior therapy (FBT) is a therapeutic approach used for both adolescents and adults that addresses not only substance use but also other issues the family may be experiencing, such as mental health disorders and family

---

27 National Institute on Drug Abuse. (2018, January). *Principles of drug addiction treatment: A research-based guide* (3rd ed.). National Institutes of Health. https://nida.nih.gov/publications/principles-drug-addiction-treatment-research-based-guide-third-edition/principles-effective-treatment

28 Substance Abuse and Mental Health Services Administration, & Office of the Surgeon General. (2016). *Facing addiction in America: The surgeon general's report on alcohol, drugs, and health.* United States Department of Health and Human Services. https://www.ncbi.nlm.nih.gov/books/NBK424857/

29 Substance Abuse and Mental Health Services Administration, & Office of the Surgeon General. (2016). *Facing addiction in America: The surgeon general's report on alcohol, drugs, and health.* United States Department of Health and Human Services. https://www.ncbi.nlm.nih.gov/books/NBK424857/

My Notes

conflict. FBT includes up to 20 treatment sessions that focus on developing skills and setting behavioral goals. Basic necessities are reviewed and inventoried with the client, and the family pursues resolution strategies and addresses activities of daily living, including violence prevention and HIV/AIDS prevention.[30]

Contingency Management

Behavior change involves learning new behaviors and changing old behaviors. Positive rewards or incentives for changing behavior can aid this process. Contingency management involves giving tangible rewards to individuals to support positive behavior change and has been found to effectively treat substance use disorders. In this therapy clients receive a voucher with monetary value that can be exchanged for food items, healthy recreational options (e.g., movies), or other sought-after goods or services when they exhibit desired behavior such as drug-free urine tests or participation in treatment activities. Clinical studies comparing voucher-based reinforcement to traditional treatment regimens have found that voucher-based reinforcement is associated with longer treatment engagement, longer periods of abstinence, and greater improvements in personal function. These positive findings, initially demonstrated with individuals with cocaine use disorders, have been reproduced in individuals with alcohol, opioid, and methamphetamine use disorders.[31]

Community Reinforcement Approach

Community reinforcement approach (CRA) plus vouchers is an intensive 24-week outpatient program that uses incentives and reinforcers to reward individuals who reduce their substance use. Individuals are required to attend one to two counseling sessions each week that emphasize improving relations, acquiring skills to minimize substance use, and reconstructing social activities and networks to support recovery. Individuals receiving this treatment are eligible to receive vouchers with monetary value if they provide drug-free urine tests several times per week. Research has demonstrated that CRA plus vouchers promotes treatment engagement and facilitates abstinence.[32]

Motivational Enhancement Therapy

Motivational enhancement therapy (MET) uses motivational interviewing techniques to help individuals resolve any uncertainties they have about stopping their substance use. MET works by promoting empathy, developing client awareness of the discrepancy between their goals and their unhealthy behavior, avoiding argument and confrontation, addressing resistance, and supporting self-efficacy to encourage motivation and change. The therapist supports the client in executing the behaviors necessary for change and monitors progress toward client-expressed goals.[33]

---

30 Substance Abuse and Mental Health Services Administration, & Office of the Surgeon General. (2016). *Facing addiction in America: The surgeon general's report on alcohol, drugs, and health.* United States Department of Health and Human Services. https://www.ncbi.nlm.nih.gov/books/NBK424857/

31 Substance Abuse and Mental Health Services Administration, & Office of the Surgeon General. (2016). *Facing addiction in America: The surgeon general's report on alcohol, drugs, and health.* United States Department of Health and Human Services. https://www.ncbi.nlm.nih.gov/books/NBK424857/

32 Substance Abuse and Mental Health Services Administration, & Office of the Surgeon General. (2016). *Facing addiction in America: The surgeon general's report on alcohol, drugs, and health.* United States Department of Health and Human Services. https://www.ncbi.nlm.nih.gov/books/NBK424857/

33 Substance Abuse and Mental Health Services Administration, & Office of the Surgeon General. (2016). *Facing addiction in America: The surgeon general's report on alcohol, drugs, and health.* United States Department of Health and Human Services. https://www.ncbi.nlm.nih.gov/books/NBK424857/

My Notes

Matrix Model

The matrix model is a structured, multi-component behavioral treatment that consists of evidence-based practices, including relapse prevention, family therapy, group therapy, drug education, and self-help, delivered in a sequential and clinically coordinated manner. The model consists of 16 weeks of group sessions held three times per week, which combine CBT, family education, social support, individual counseling, and urine drug testing.[34]

Twelve-Step Facilitation

Twelve-step facilitation (TSF), an individual therapy typically delivered in 12 weekly sessions, is designed to prepare individuals to understand, accept, and become engaged in Alcoholics Anonymous (AA), Narcotics Anonymous (NA), or similar 12-step programs.[35] Twelve-step programs are further discussed under the "Recovery Support Services" section below.

TSF focuses on three key ideas:

- Acceptance: Realizing that their substance use is part of a disorder, that life has become unmanageable because of alcohol or drugs, that willpower alone will not overcome the problem, and that abstinence is the best alternative
- Surrender: Giving oneself to a higher power, accepting the fellowship and support structure of other recovering individuals, and following the recovery activities laid out by a 12-step program
- Active involvement in a 12-step program

Recovery Support Services

In addition to medications and behavioral therapies, effective treatment of SUD includes recovery support services (RSS). Recovery support services provided by substance use disorder treatment programs and community organizations provide support to individuals receiving treatment for SUD, as well as ongoing support after treatment. These supportive services are typically delivered by trained case managers, recovery coaches, and/or peers. Specific RSS include assistance in navigating systems of care, removing barriers to recovery, staying engaged in the recovery process, and providing a social context for individuals to engage in community living without substance use. RSS can be effective in promoting healthy lifestyle techniques to increase resilience skills, reduce the risk of relapse, and help achieve and maintain recovery. Individuals who participate in RSS typically have better long-term recovery outcomes.[36]

---

34 Substance Abuse and Mental Health Services Administration, & Office of the Surgeon General. (2016). *Facing addiction in America: The surgeon general's report on alcohol, drugs, and health.* United States Department of Health and Human Services. https://www.ncbi.nlm.nih.gov/books/NBK424857/

35 Substance Abuse and Mental Health Services Administration, & Office of the Surgeon General. (2016). *Facing addiction in America: The surgeon general's report on alcohol, drugs, and health.* United States Department of Health and Human Services. https://www.ncbi.nlm.nih.gov/books/NBK424857/

36 Substance Abuse and Mental Health Services Administration, & Office of the Surgeon General. (2016). *Facing addiction in America: The surgeon general's report on alcohol, drugs, and health.* United States Department of Health and Human Services. https://www.ncbi.nlm.nih.gov/books/NBK424857/

My Notes

Recovery goes beyond abstinence and the remission of substance use disorder to include a positive change in the whole person. There are many paths to recovery. People choose their individual pathway based on their cultural values, socioeconomic status, psychological and behavioral needs, and the nature of their substance use disorder.[37]

A study of over 9,000 individuals with previous substance use disorders asked how they defined recovery. These three themes emerged[38]:

- **Abstinence:** 86 percent viewed abstinence as part of their recovery, but the remainder did not think abstinence was important for their recovery. However, abstinence was considered "essential" by those affiliated with 12-step mutual aid groups.
- **Personal growth:** "Being honest with myself" was endorsed as part of recovery by 98 percent of participants. Other almost universally endorsed elements included "handling negative feelings without using alcohol or drugs" and "being able to enjoy life without alcohol or drugs." Almost all study participants viewed their recovery as a process of growth and development, and about two thirds saw it as having a spiritual dimension.
- **Service to others:** Engaging in service to others was another prominent component of how study participants defined recovery. This is perhaps because during periods of heavy substance misuse, individuals may damage interpersonal relationships, which they later regret and attempt to resolve during recovery. Service to others has evidence of helping individuals maintain their own recovery.[39]

Recovery-Oriented Systems of Care (ROSC) embrace the idea that severe substance use disorders are most effectively addressed through a chronic care management model that includes long-term, outpatient care, recovery housing, and recovery coaching and management checkups. ROSC are designed to be easy to navigate for people seeking help, transparent in their operations, and responsive to the cultural diversity of the communities they serve. ROSC often use long-term recovery management protocols, such as recovery management checkups and telephone case monitoring.[40]

Even when remission is achieved after one or two years, it can take four to five more years before an individual's risk of relapse drops below 15 percent (the level of risk that people in the general population have of developing a substance use disorder in their lifetime). As a result, similar to other chronic illnesses, a person with a serious substance use disorder often requires ongoing monitoring and management to maintain remission and to provide early reintervention should relapse occur. Recovery support services (RSS) refer to the collection of community services that can provide emotional and practical support for continuing remission, as well as daily structure and

---

37 Substance Abuse and Mental Health Services Administration, & Office of the Surgeon General. (2016). *Facing addiction in America: The surgeon general's report on alcohol, drugs, and health.* United States Department of Health and Human Services. https://www.ncbi.nlm.nih.gov/books/NBK424857/

38 Substance Abuse and Mental Health Services Administration, & Office of the Surgeon General. (2016). *Facing addiction in America: The surgeon general's report on alcohol, drugs, and health.* United States Department of Health and Human Services. https://www.ncbi.nlm.nih.gov/books/NBK424857/

39 Substance Abuse and Mental Health Services Administration, & Office of the Surgeon General. (2016). *Facing addiction in America: The surgeon general's report on alcohol, drugs, and health.* United States Department of Health and Human Services. https://www.ncbi.nlm.nih.gov/books/NBK424857/

40 Substance Abuse and Mental Health Services Administration, & Office of the Surgeon General. (2016). *Facing addiction in America: The surgeon general's report on alcohol, drugs, and health.* United States Department of Health and Human Services. https://www.ncbi.nlm.nih.gov/books/NBK424857/

My Notes

rewarding alternatives to substance use. Recovery supports include services such as mutual aid groups, recovery coaches, recovery housing, community care, and education-based recovery support.

Mutual Aid Groups

Mutual aid groups, such as 12-step groups, are well-known recovery supports, and they share a number of features. Members share their substance use problem and value learning from each other's experiences as they focus on personal-change goals. The groups are voluntary associations that charge no fees and are member-led.

Alcoholics Anonymous

Alcoholics Anonymous (AA) has been in existence since 1935. Its philosophy, approach, and format have been adapted by groups focusing on recovery from other substances, such as Narcotic Anonymous, Cocaine Anonymous, Marijuana Anonymous, and Crystal Meth Anonymous. AA and derivative programs share two major components: social fellowship and a 12-step program of action that was formulated based on members' experiences of recovery from severe alcohol use disorders. These 12 steps are ordered in a logical progression, beginning with accepting that one cannot control one's substance use, followed by abstaining from substances permanently, and transforming one's spiritual outlook, character, and relationships with other people.[41]

Research studying 12-step mutual aid groups, specifically those focused on alcohol, has shown that participation in the groups promotes an individual's recovery by strengthening recovery-supportive social networks; increasing members' abilities to cope with risky social contexts and negative emotions; augmenting motivation to recover; reducing depression, craving, and impulsivity; and enhancing psychological and spiritual well-being.[42]

Find a local Alcoholics Anonymous group near you: Find A.A. Near You.

Al-Anon and Alateen

Friends and family members often suffer when a loved one has a substance use disorder. This can include worrying about their loved one experiencing accidents, injuries, legal consequences, diseases, or death or experiencing verbal or physical abuse. Mutual aid groups provide emotional support to concerned significant others to help them systematically and strategically cope with the problems related to the substance misuse of their loved one.[43]

Al-Anon is a mutual aid group for family members dealing with substance misuse in a loved one. Like AA, Al-Anon is based on a 12-step philosophy and provides support whether or not members' loved ones seek help or achieve remission or recovery. More than 80 percent of Al-Anon members are women. The principal goal of Al-Anon is to foster emotional stability and "loving detachment" from the loved one rather than coaching members to "get their loved one into treatment or recovery." Al-Anon includes Alateen that focuses on the specific needs of

---

41 Substance Abuse and Mental Health Services Administration, & Office of the Surgeon General. (2016). *Facing addiction in America: The surgeon general's report on alcohol, drugs, and health.* United States Department of Health and Human Services. https://www.ncbi.nlm.nih.gov/books/NBK424857/

42 Substance Abuse and Mental Health Services Administration, & Office of the Surgeon General. (2016). *Facing addiction in America: The surgeon general's report on alcohol, drugs, and health.* United States Department of Health and Human Services. https://www.ncbi.nlm.nih.gov/books/NBK424857/

43 Substance Abuse and Mental Health Services Administration, & Office of the Surgeon General. (2016). *Facing addiction in America: The surgeon general's report on alcohol, drugs, and health.* United States Department of Health and Human Services. https://www.ncbi.nlm.nih.gov/books/NBK424857/

My Notes

adolescents affected by a parent's or other family member's substance use. Research studies regarding the effectiveness of Al-Anon show that participating family members experience reduced depression, anger, and relationship unhappiness at rates comparable to those of individuals receiving psychological therapies.[44]

Find a local Al-Anon group near you: Al-Anon Meetings.

Recovery Coaches

Voluntary and paid recovery coaches help individuals discharging from treatment to connect to community services while addressing any barriers or problems that may hinder the recovery process. A recovery coach's responsibilities may include providing strategies to maintain abstinence, connecting people to recovery housing and social services, and helping people develop personal skills that maintain recovery.[45]

Recovery Housing

Recovery-supportive houses provide both a substance-free environment and mutual support from fellow recovering residents. Many residents stay in recovery housing during or after outpatient treatment, with self-determined residency lasting for several months to years. Residents often informally share resources and give advice based on their experience in accessing health care, finding employment, managing legal problems, and interacting with the social service system.[46]

Community Care

Recovery community centers may host mutual aid group meetings; offer recovery coaching, education, and social events; and provide access to other resources such as housing, education, and employment. Some recovery community centers encourage community members to engage in advocacy to combat negative public attitudes, educate the community, and improve supports for recovery in the community.[47]

Education-Based Recovery Support

Education-based recovery support services are designed to help individuals in early substance use disorder recovery achieve their educational goals while also focusing on the areas of their social, emotional, spiritual, and physical well-being needed to help sustain recovery. High school and college environments can be difficult for students in recovery because of high levels of substance misuse among other students, peer pressure to engage in substance

---

44 Substance Abuse and Mental Health Services Administration, & Office of the Surgeon General. (2016). *Facing addiction in America: The surgeon general's report on alcohol, drugs, and health.* United States Department of Health and Human Services. https://www.ncbi.nlm.nih.gov/books/NBK424857/

45 Substance Abuse and Mental Health Services Administration, & Office of the Surgeon General. (2016). *Facing addiction in America: The surgeon general's report on alcohol, drugs, and health.* United States Department of Health and Human Services. https://www.ncbi.nlm.nih.gov/books/NBK424857/

46 Substance Abuse and Mental Health Services Administration, & Office of the Surgeon General. (2016). *Facing addiction in America: The surgeon general's report on alcohol, drugs, and health.* United States Department of Health and Human Services. https://www.ncbi.nlm.nih.gov/books/NBK424857/

47 Substance Abuse and Mental Health Services Administration, & Office of the Surgeon General. (2016). *Facing addiction in America: The surgeon general's report on alcohol, drugs, and health.* United States Department of Health and Human Services. https://www.ncbi.nlm.nih.gov/books/NBK424857/

My Notes

use, and widespread availability of alcohol and drugs. High school and collegiate recovery support programs provide recovery-supportive environments and peer engagement with other students in recovery.[48]

Planning Individualized Treatment

After an individual is assessed and diagnosed with substance use disorder (SUD) by a trained professional based on criteria in the *Diagnostic and Statistical Manual of Mental Disorders (DSM-5)*, a collaborative, personalized treatment plan is designed with the client to meet their specific needs. The treatment plan and goals should be person-centered and include strength-based approaches that draw upon an individual's strengths and resources to keep them engaged in care. Individualized treatment plans should consider age, gender identity, race and ethnicity, language, health literacy, religion/spirituality, sexual orientation, culture, trauma history, and co-occurring physical and mental health problems. This increases the likelihood of successful treatment engagement and retention. Throughout treatment, individuals should be periodically reassessed to determine response to treatment and to make any needed adjustments to the treatment plan.[49]

Nurses can improve engagement and retention in treatment programs by building a strong therapeutic alliance with the client, effectively using evidence-based motivational strategies, acknowledging the client's individualized barriers, and creating a positive environment. Referring individuals to recovery support services, such as child care, housing, and transportation, can also improve retention in treatment.[50]

Treatment Settings and Continuum of Care

The treatment of severe substance use disorder is typically delivered in freestanding programs in various settings (e.g., hospital, residential, or outpatient settings) that vary in the frequency of care delivery (e.g., daily sessions to monthly visits), range of treatment components offered, and planned duration of care. As clients progress in treatment and begin to meet the goals of their individualized treatment plan, they transfer from clinical management in residential or intensive outpatient programs to less clinically intensive outpatient programs that promote client self-management.[51]

A typical progression for someone who has a severe substance use disorder might start with 3 to 7 days in a medically managed withdrawal program, followed by a 1- to 3-month period of intensive rehabilitative care in a residential treatment program, followed by intensive outpatient program (2 to 5 days per week for a few months) and later in a traditional outpatient program that meets 1 to 2 times per month. For many clients whose current living situations are not conducive to recovery, outpatient services should be provided in conjunction with recovery-supportive housing. In general, clients with serious substance use disorders are recommended to stay

48 Substance Abuse and Mental Health Services Administration, & Office of the Surgeon General. (2016). *Facing addiction in America: The surgeon general's report on alcohol, drugs, and health.* United States Department of Health and Human Services. https://www.ncbi.nlm.nih.gov/books/NBK424857/

49 Substance Abuse and Mental Health Services Administration, & Office of the Surgeon General. (2016). *Facing addiction in America: The surgeon general's report on alcohol, drugs, and health.* United States Department of Health and Human Services. https://www.ncbi.nlm.nih.gov/books/NBK424857/

50 Substance Abuse and Mental Health Services Administration, & Office of the Surgeon General. (2016). *Facing addiction in America: The surgeon general's report on alcohol, drugs, and health.* United States Department of Health and Human Services. https://www.ncbi.nlm.nih.gov/books/NBK424857/

51 Substance Abuse and Mental Health Services Administration, & Office of the Surgeon General. (2016). *Facing addiction in America: The surgeon general's report on alcohol, drugs, and health.* United States Department of Health and Human Services. https://www.ncbi.nlm.nih.gov/books/NBK424857/

My Notes

engaged for at least one year in the treatment process, which may involve participating in three to four different programs or services at reduced levels of intensity, all of which are ideally designed to help the client prepare for continued self-management after treatment ends.[52]

The levels of the treatment continuum include the following:

- **Medically monitored and managed inpatient care:** An intensive service delivered in an acute, inpatient hospital setting. These programs are typically necessary for individuals who require withdrawal management, primary medical and nursing care, and for those with co-occurring mental and physical health conditions. Treatment is available 24 hours a day and usually provided by an interdisciplinary team of health care professionals who can address serious mental and physical health needs.
- **Residential services:** Organized services, also in a 24-hour setting but outside of a hospital. These programs typically provide support, structure, and an array of evidence-based clinical services. Such programs are appropriate for physically and emotionally stabilized individuals who may not have a living situation that supports recovery, may have a history of relapse, or have co-occurring physical and/or mental health illnesses.
- **Partial hospitalization and intensive outpatient services:** Services range from counseling and education to clinically intensive programming. Partial hospitalization programs are used as a step-down treatment option after completing residential treatment and are usually available 6 to 8 hours a day during the work week. These services are considered to be approximately as intensive but less restrictive than residential programs and are appropriate for clients living in an environment that supports recovery but who need structure to avoid relapse.
- **Outpatient services:** Group and individual behavioral interventions and medications when appropriate. These components of care can be offered during the day, before or after work or school, or in the evenings and weekends. Typically, outpatient programs are appropriate as the initial level of care for individuals with a mild to moderate substance use disorder or as continuing care after completing more intensive treatment. Outpatient programs are also suitable for individuals with concurrent mental health conditions.

Helping Individuals in Need of Treatment

Despite the fact that substance use disorders are widespread, only a small percentage of people receive treatment because of the barriers previously discussed. Results from the 2020 National Survey of Drug Use and Health (NSDUH) indicate that among people aged 12 or older in 2020, 14.9 percent (or 41.1 million people) needed substance use treatment in the past year (defined if they had a SUD diagnosed in the past year or if they received substance use treatment at a specialty facility in the past year). There are many common reasons people do not seek treatment[53]:

- Not ready to stop using (40.7 percent)

52 Substance Abuse and Mental Health Services Administration, & Office of the Surgeon General. (2016). *Facing addiction in America: The surgeon general's report on alcohol, drugs, and health.* United States Department of Health and Human Services. https://www.ncbi.nlm.nih.gov/books/NBK424857/

53 Substance Abuse and Mental Health Services Administration, & Office of the Surgeon General. (2016). *Facing addiction in America: The surgeon general's report on alcohol, drugs, and health.* United States Department of Health and Human Services. https://www.ncbi.nlm.nih.gov/books/NBK424857/

My Notes

- Do not have health care coverage/could not afford (30.6 percent)
- Perceived negative effect on their job (16.4 percent) or cause neighbors/community to have a negative opinion (8.3 percent)
- Do not know where to go for treatment (12.6 percent) or no program has the type of treatment desired (11.0 percent)
- Do not have transportation, the programs are too far away, or hours are inconvenient (11.8 percent)

Nurses can use motivational interviewing strategies to explore clients' reasons for not seeking treatment and address their perceived barriers to treatment.

Strategies to Reduce Harm

Strategies to reduce the harm associated with substance use have been developed to engage people in treatment, as well as address the needs of individuals who are not yet ready to participate in treatment. Harm reduction programs provide public health services to prevent and reduce substance use-related risks among those actively using substances. Strategies include outreach and education programs, needle/syringe exchange programs, overdose prevention education, and improving public access to naloxone to reverse potentially lethal opioid overdose. These strategies are designed to reduce negative consequences for people with substance use disorders and those around them, such as overdose and the transmission of HIV and other infectious diseases. They also encourage individuals to seek treatment to reduce, manage, and stop their substance use.[54]

---

54 Substance Abuse and Mental Health Services Administration, & Office of the Surgeon General. (2016). *Facing addiction in America: The surgeon general's report on alcohol, drugs, and health.* United States Department of Health and Human Services. https://www.ncbi.nlm.nih.gov/books/NBK424857/

My Notes

14.8 PREVENTION OF SUBSTANCE USE DISORDERS

The misuse of alcohol and drugs and substance use disorders has a significant impact on public health in the United States. The Centers for Disease Control and Prevention (CDC) reports over 100,000 drug overdose deaths occurred in the United States in 2021, and overdose deaths in urban and rural populations have shown a significant upward trend over the past 20 years.[1] See Figure 14.11[2] for a graphic of overdose rates in urban and rural areas.

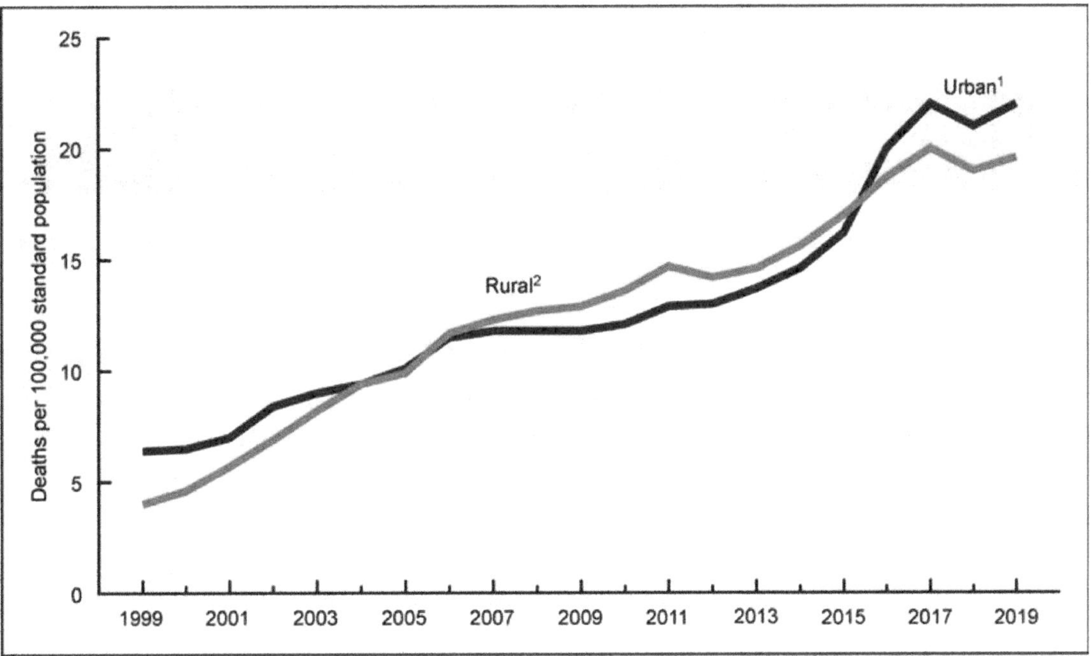

[1]Significant increasing trend from 1999 to 2017, with different rates of change over time; stable trend from 2017 through 2019, $p < 0.05$.
[2]Significant increasing trend from 1999 through 2019, with different rates of change over time, $p < 0.05$.
NOTES: Drug overdose deaths were identified using *International Classification of Diseases, 10th Revision* underlying cause-of-death codes X40–X44, X60–X64, X85, and Y10–Y14. Age-adjusted death rates were calculated using the direct method and the 2000 U.S. standard population. Decedent's county of residence was classified as urban or rural based on the 2013 NCHS Urban–Rural Classification Scheme for Counties. Access data table for Figure 1 at: https://www.cdc.gov/nchs/data/databriefs/db403-tables-508.pdf#1.
SOURCE: National Center for Health Statistics, National Vital Statistics System, Mortality.

Figure 14.11 Drug Overdose Rates in Urban and Rural Areas

Substance misuse is associated with a wide range of health and social problems, including heart disease, stroke, high blood pressure, various cancers (e.g., liver, lung, and colon cancer), mental health disorders, neonatal abstinence syndrome, driving under the influence (DUI) injuries and fatalities, incarcerations, sexual assaults and rapes, unintended pregnancies, sexually transmitted infections, and blood-borne pathogens like hepatitis and human

---

1 National Center for Health Statistics. (2021, November 21). *Drug overdose deaths in the U.S. top 100,000 annually* [Press Release]. Centers for Disease Control & Prevention. https://www.cdc.gov/nchs/pressroom/nchs_press_releases/2021/20211117.htm

2 "db403-fig1.png" from by Hedegaard, H., & Spencer, M. R. is in the Public Domain. Access the full report at https://www.cdc.gov/nchs/products/databriefs/db403.htm#fig1

My Notes

immunodeficiency virus (HIV).[3] Given the impact of substance misuse on public health, it is critical to implement preventative interventions to stop substance misuse from starting, as well as to identify and intervene early with individuals who have already begun to misuse substances.

Promoting Protective Factors

Experiencing a family member's substance use disorder is considered an adverse childhood event (ACE) that can impact a child's risk for developing behavioral problems, substance misuse, and chronic illness. Targeted prevention programs implemented at the family, school, and individual levels can complement broader population-level policies by promoting protective factors for children and adolescents.

Read more about ACEs in the "Adverse Childhood Experiences" section of the "Trauma, Abuse, and Violence" chapter.

Protective factors help prevent substance use disorders from developing despite the presence of risk factors. Protective factors exist at the individual, family, school, and community levels.

Examples of interventions to promote protective factors at the individual level include the following[4]:

- **Social, emotional, and behavioral competence:** Promoting interpersonal skills that help youth integrate feelings, thoughts, and actions to achieve specific social and interpersonal goals.
- **Self-efficacy:** Enhancing an individual's belief that they can modify, control, or abstain from substance use.
- **Spirituality:** Supporting beliefs in a higher being or involvement in spiritual practices or religious activities.
- **Resiliency:** Encouraging an individual's capacity for adapting to change and coping with stressful events in healthy and flexible ways.

Interventions to promote protective factors at the family, school, and community levels are as follows[5]:

- **Opportunities for positive social involvement:** Creating developmentally appropriate opportunities to be meaningfully involved with the family, school, or community.
- **Recognition for positive behavior:** Providing community and family recognition of individuals' efforts and accomplishments to encourage positive future behaviors.
- **Bonding:** Promoting attachment, commitment, and positive communication with family members, schools, and communities.

---

3 Substance Abuse and Mental Health Services Administration, & Office of the Surgeon General. (2016). *Facing addiction in America: The surgeon general's report on alcohol, drugs, and health.* United States Department of Health and Human Services. https://www.ncbi.nlm.nih.gov/books/NBK424857/

4 Substance Abuse and Mental Health Services Administration, & Office of the Surgeon General. (2016). *Facing addiction in America: The surgeon general's report on alcohol, drugs, and health.* United States Department of Health and Human Services. https://www.ncbi.nlm.nih.gov/books/NBK424857/

5 Substance Abuse and Mental Health Services Administration, & Office of the Surgeon General. (2016). *Facing addiction in America: The surgeon general's report on alcohol, drugs, and health.* United States Department of Health and Human Services. https://www.ncbi.nlm.nih.gov/books/NBK424857/

My Notes

- **Marriage or committed relationships:** Encouraging committed relationships with people who do not misuse alcohol or drugs.
- **Healthy beliefs and standards for behavior:** Establishing family, school, and community norms that communicate clear and consistent expectations about not misusing alcohol or drugs.

Prevention Interventions

The Institute of Medicine describes three categories of prevention interventions: universal, selective, and indicated. Universal interventions are aimed at all members of a given population, selective interventions are aimed at a subgroup determined to be at high-risk for substance use, and indicated interventions are targeted for individuals who are already misusing substances but have not developed a substance use disorder. Examples of evidence-based prevention interventions for each category are provided in the following subsections.

Universal Interventions

Universal interventions include policies that affect the entire population, such as the setting the minimum legal drinking age or reducing the availability of substances in a community. For example, laws targeting alcohol-impaired driving, such as license revocation for impaired driving and 0.08 legal blood alcohol (BAC) limits, have helped cut alcohol-related traffic deaths per 100,000 in half since the early 1980s.[6]

Several family-focused, universal prevention interventions show substantial preventive effects on substance use. Two examples are the Strengthening Families Program and the I Hear What You're Saying program[7]:

- **Strengthening Families Program (SFP):** A widely used seven-session, family-focused program that enhances parenting skills, such as nurturing, setting limits, and communicating, as well as promoting adolescents' skills in refusing substances. Across multiple studies conducted in rural United States communities, SFP showed reductions in tobacco, alcohol, and drug use up to nine years after the intervention (i.e., to age 21) compared with youth who were not assigned to the SFP. SFP also shows reductions in prescription drug misuse up to 13 years after the intervention (i.e., to age 25). Strong African American Families, a cultural adaptation of SFP, shows reductions in early initiation and rate of alcohol use for Black or African American rural youth.
- **I Hear What You're Saying:** An Internet-based program that involves nine 45-minute sessions to improve communication, establish family rules, and manage conflict. Specifically focused on mothers and daughters, follow-up results showed lower rates of substance use in an ethnically diverse sample.[8]

---

6 Substance Abuse and Mental Health Services Administration, & Office of the Surgeon General. (2016). *Facing addiction in America: The surgeon general's report on alcohol, drugs, and health.* United States Department of Health and Human Services. https://www.ncbi.nlm.nih.gov/books/NBK424857/

7 Substance Abuse and Mental Health Services Administration, & Office of the Surgeon General. (2016). *Facing addiction in America: The surgeon general's report on alcohol, drugs, and health.* United States Department of Health and Human Services. https://www.ncbi.nlm.nih.gov/books/NBK424857/

8 Substance Abuse and Mental Health Services Administration, & Office of the Surgeon General. (2016). *Facing addiction in America: The surgeon general's report on alcohol, drugs, and health.* United States Department of Health and Human Services. https://www.ncbi.nlm.nih.gov/books/NBK424857/

My Notes

Selective Interventions

Selective interventions are delivered to particular communities, families, or children who, due to exposure to risk factors, are at increased risk of substance misuse problems. Target audiences may include families living in poverty, the children of substance-misusing parents, or children who have difficulties with social skills. Selective interventions deliver specialized prevention services to individuals with the goal of reducing identified risk factors, increasing protective factors, or both. Examples of selective intervention programs are the Nurse-Family Partnership, Familias Unidas, and Brief Alcohol Screening and Intervention for College Students[9]:

Nurse-Family Partnership: A program focused on children younger than age 5 has shown significant reductions in the use of alcohol in the teen years compared with those who did not receive the intervention. Trained nurses provide an intensive home visitation intervention for at-risk, first-time mothers during pregnancy. This intervention provides ongoing education and support to improve pregnancy outcomes, infant health, and development of parenting skills.[10]

Familias Unidas: A family-based intervention for Hispanic or Latino youth that includes both multi-parent groups (eight weekly 2-hour sessions) and four to ten 1-hour individual family visits. It has been shown to lower substance use or delay the start of substance use among adolescents.[11]

Brief Alcohol Screening and Intervention for College Students (BASICS): A brief motivational intervention designed to help students reduce alcohol misuse and negative consequences of their drinking. It consists of two 1-hour interviews with a brief online assessment after the first session. The first interview gathers information about alcohol consumption patterns and personal beliefs about alcohol while providing instructions for self-monitoring drinking between sessions. The second interview uses data from the online assessment to develop personalized, normative feedback that reviews negative consequences and risk factors, clarifies perceived risks and benefits of drinking, and provides options for reducing alcohol use and its consequences. Follow-up studies of students who used BASICS have shown reductions in the quantity of drinking in the general college population, as well as fraternity members.

Indicated Prevention Interventions

Indicated prevention interventions are directed to those who are already involved in substance misuse but who have not yet developed a substance use disorder. An example of an indicated prevention intervention is Coping Power, a 16-month program for children in Grades 5 and 6. The program uses skills-based training to increase social competence, self-regulation, and positive parental involvement. Results include reduced substance use, delinquency, and aggressive behaviors.[12]

---

9 Substance Abuse and Mental Health Services Administration, & Office of the Surgeon General. (2016). *Facing addiction in America: The surgeon general's report on alcohol, drugs, and health.* United States Department of Health and Human Services. https://www.ncbi.nlm.nih.gov/books/NBK424857/

10 Substance Abuse and Mental Health Services Administration, & Office of the Surgeon General. (2016). *Facing addiction in America: The surgeon general's report on alcohol, drugs, and health.* United States Department of Health and Human Services. https://www.ncbi.nlm.nih.gov/books/NBK424857/

11 Substance Abuse and Mental Health Services Administration, & Office of the Surgeon General. (2016). *Facing addiction in America: The surgeon general's report on alcohol, drugs, and health.* United States Department of Health and Human Services. https://www.ncbi.nlm.nih.gov/books/NBK424857/

12 Substance Abuse and Mental Health Services Administration, & Office of the Surgeon General. (2016). *Facing addiction in America: The surgeon general's report on alcohol, drugs, and health.* United States Department of Health and Human Services. https://www.ncbi.nlm.nih.gov/books/NBK424857/

14.9 APPLYING THE NURSING PROCESS TO SUBSTANCE USE DISORDERS

My Notes

This section will apply the nursing process to caring for a hospitalized client diagnosed with a substance use disorder who is receiving withdrawal treatment.

Assessment

The following client history should be obtained from a client diagnosed with a substance use disorder[1]:

- **History of substance use:** Include names of the substances used, the time of last use, the duration of use, the quantity and frequency of use, and the method of use (e.g., oral, intravenous, inhaled, intranasal). A detailed substance use history helps determine the expected time frame for emergence of withdrawal symptoms and the potential for severe withdrawal syndromes.
- **Detailed history of previous withdrawal treatments:** For clients who have previously undergone withdrawal management, a history of these treatments should be obtained.
- **Treatment history:** The history of any previous treatment programs should be obtained. History should include previous treatments (such as inpatient or outpatient programs, 12-step programs such as Alcoholics Anonymous, or medications such as naltrexone or acamprosate), as well as what treatments have been helpful or not helpful.
- **Mental health history:** Concurrent mental health illness can impact the client's withdrawal symptoms. Clients should receive integrated post-withdrawal treatments for multiple diagnoses of mental health and substance use disorders.
- **Social history:** Identification of social supports (such as a supportive family member who can encourage abstinence and potentially dispense withdrawal medication), as well as barriers (such as poor transportation), can also help determine the most appropriate post-withdrawal treatment plan (e.g., residential, outpatient, and recovery programs).
- **Medical history and recent physical symptoms:** Medical problems can contribute to the client's symptoms and/or worsen withdrawal symptoms.

The client should receive a comprehensive physical examination to evaluate signs related to current withdrawal symptoms, as well as symptoms of concurrent medical and mental health diagnoses. If the client has been diagnosed with alcohol use disorder, signs of complications such as liver or pancreatic disease should be assessed.[2]

Screening Scales

Screening scales may be administered such as CIWA-aR (for alcohol withdrawal symptoms) and COWS (for opioid withdrawal symptoms). Read more information about these scales in the "Withdrawal Management/Detoxification" section of this chapter.

---

1 Pace, C. (2022). Alcohol withdrawal: Epidemiology, clinical manifestations, course, assessment, and diagnosis. *UpToDate.* Retrieved March 19, 2022, from www.uptodate.com

2 Pace, C. (2022). Alcohol withdrawal: Epidemiology, clinical manifestations, course, assessment, and diagnosis. *UpToDate.* Retrieved March 19, 2022, from www.uptodate.com

My Notes

Diagnostic and Lab Work

Laboratory testing for clients admitted for withdrawal treatment may include these items[3]:

- Complete blood count
- Serum electrolytes, including potassium, magnesium, and phosphate
- Glucose
- Creatinine
- Liver function tests
- Amylase and lipase
- Blood alcohol level
- Urine drug testing for benzodiazepines, cocaine, and opioids. (The opioid test may include testing for heroin, codeine, morphine, buprenorphine, oxycodone, methadone, and fentanyl.)
- Urine human chorionic gonadotropin (HCG) test for premenopausal women to check for pregnancy
- Electrocardiogram (ECG) for clients over 50 years of age or if there is a history of cardiac problems

Diagnoses

A nursing diagnosis related to the abrupt cessation of a psychoactive substance is a syndrome diagnosed as *Acute Substance Withdrawal Syndrome*. As a syndrome diagnosis, defining characteristics are the related nursing diagnoses, including *Acute Confusion, Anxiety, Disturbed Sleep Pattern, Nausea, Risk for Electrolyte Imbalance,* and *Risk for Injury*.[4]

Review information about syndrome nursing diagnosis in the "Diagnosis" section of the "Nursing Process" chapter of Open RN *Nursing Fundamentals*.

Outcomes Identification

An example of a broad goal related to withdrawal treatment is the following:

- The client will stabilize and remain free from injury.[5]

---

3 Pace, C. (2022). Alcohol withdrawal: Epidemiology, clinical manifestations, course, assessment, and diagnosis. *UpToDate.* Retrieved March 19, 2022, from www.uptodate.com

4 Ackley, B., Ladwig, G., Makic, M. B., Martinez-Kratz, M., & Zanotti, M. (2020). *Nursing diagnosis handbook: An evidence-based guide to planning care* (12th ed.). Elsevier

5 Ackley, B., Ladwig, G., Makic, M. B., Martinez-Kratz, M., & Zanotti, M. (2020). *Nursing diagnosis handbook: An evidence-based guide to planning care* (12th ed.). Elsevier

My Notes

These are some sample SMART outcomes[6]:

- The client's vital signs will remain within normal ranges during treatment.
- The client's electrolyte levels will remain within normal ranges during treatment.
- The client will participate in planning a post-withdrawal treatment program before discharge.

Planning Interventions

In addition to implementing the withdrawal treatment plan prescribed by the provider, the nurse collaboratively develops a post-withdrawal treatment plan with interprofessional health care team members. The plan should be client-centered and include their goals and readiness for change. Motivational interviewing is a helpful therapeutic technique when planning individualized treatment goals and programs.[7]

Implementation

Nursing interventions provide a supportive environment while the client undergoes withdrawal treatment. Vital signs are monitored closely because increases in temperature, pulse, and blood pressure are signs of withdrawal. After ensuring that an individual's physiological needs of airway, breathing, and circulation are met, safety measures receive top priority. Safety measures during withdrawal treatment may include interventions such as fall precautions, seizure precautions, or implementing restraints as needed to maintain the safety of the individual or those around them.[8]

Review information on fall precautions in the "Preventing Falls" section of the "Safety" chapter in Open RN *Nursing Fundamentals*.

Seizures can occur in clients experiencing alcohol withdrawal. Seizure precautions include keeping the bed in the lowest position with side rails padded. Suction and oxygen equipment must be available at all times at the patient's bedside.

Review information on safely implementing restraints in the "Workplace Violence" section of the "Trauma, Abuse, and Violence" chapter.

Medications are administered as prescribed to keep the client safe and comfortable, so they do not suffer.[9]

Review medications used during withdrawal treatment in the "Withdrawal Management/Detoxification" section of this chapter.

Clients with substance use disorders may exhibit a poor nutritional status due to long-term use of substances taking precedence over food and fluid intake. Nurses provide hydration and gradually reintroduce healthy foods while

---

6 Ackley, B., Ladwig, G., Makic, M. B., Martinez-Kratz, M., & Zanotti, M. (2020). *Nursing diagnosis handbook: An evidence-based guide to planning care* (12th ed.). Elsevier

7 Halter, M. (2022). *Varcarolis' foundations of psychiatric-mental health nursing* (9th ed.). Saunders.

8 Halter, M. (2022). *Varcarolis' foundations of psychiatric-mental health nursing* (9th ed.). Saunders.

9 Halter, M. (2022). *Varcarolis' foundations of psychiatric-mental health nursing* (9th ed.). Saunders.

My Notes

also promoting rest. Clients with alcohol use disorder are specifically at risk for thiamine (B1) and magnesium deficiencies that can lead to cardiac arrest. Thiamine and other electrolyte replacement are typically included during withdrawal treatment.[10]

Developing a therapeutic nurse-client relationship can encourage the client to explore harmful feelings of anxiety, hopelessness, and spiritual distress. Encouraging self-care and hygiene helps improve clients' self-esteem. Nurses educate clients about healthy coping skills and evidence-based treatment and recovery services available in the community.[11]

Review evidence-based treatments and recovery services in the "Treatment of Substance Use Disorders" section of this chapter.

Evaluation

Evaluation occurs on several levels by assessing the individualized SMART outcomes related to the effectiveness of the withdrawal treatment plan, symptom management, and the client's readiness and progress towards changes in their behavior.[12]

10 Halter, M. (2022). *Varcarolis' foundations of psychiatric-mental health nursing* (9th ed.). Saunders.

11 Halter, M. (2022). *Varcarolis' foundations of psychiatric-mental health nursing* (9th ed.). Saunders.

12 Halter, M. (2022). *Varcarolis' foundations of psychiatric-mental health nursing* (9th ed.). Saunders.

14.10 SPOTLIGHT APPLICATION

My Notes

> This case study is based on a sample client described in the "Assessment & Treatment of Substance Use Disorders" chapter of the *Foundations of Addiction Studies* book.

Jessica is a 26-year-old woman who recently received her second driving-under-the-influence (DUI) ticket and has been charged with a misdemeanor crime. She received her first DUI at age 21 and lost her license for one year. During that time, she completed a basic risk education DUI course and paid several thousand dollars in fines and attorney's fees.

Jessica continues to drink with her friends on weekends, usually having five or six drinks per night. In addition to alcohol, Jessica was recently prescribed Xanax to treat her anxiety disorder. Jessica often takes more than prescribed in the evening and sometimes mixes these pills with her alcohol consumption.

Jessica works from home full-time as a graphic designer. She says that she has little time to socialize during the week, so she looks forward to the weekend when she can see her friends and relax. Now that she has a second DUI, Jessica has lost her license again, although she is not overly concerned because she can continue working from home. She can walk or order a ride wherever she needs to go for groceries and other errands.

The court has ordered Jessica to have an evaluation done and to complete any treatment recommendations.

Reflective Questions

1. What were your initial feelings when you read this case study?
2. Can you identify any personal biases or assumptions you experienced while reading this scenario?
3. How many *DSM-5* criteria is Jessica displaying for a substance use disorder diagnosis?
4. List at least three issues to include in a treatment plan for Jessica.
5. How do Jessica's legal issues potentially impact her treatment plan?
6. How will you apply your new knowledge about substance use disorders to your nursing practice?

My Notes

14.11 LEARNING ACTIVITIES

Interactive Activities

An interactive H5P element has been excluded from this version of the text. You can view it online here: https://wtcs.pressbooks.pub/nursingmhcc/?p=875#h5p-47

An interactive H5P element has been excluded from this version of the text. You can view it online here: https://wtcs.pressbooks.pub/nursingmhcc/?p=875#h5p-48

An interactive H5P element has been excluded from this version of the text. You can view it online here: https://wtcs.pressbooks.pub/nursingmhcc/?p=875#h5p-49

XIV GLOSSARY

My Notes

Addiction: Severe substance use disorders are commonly referred to as addiction. Addiction is a chronic brain disease that has the potential for both recurrence (relapse) and recovery.[1]

Binge drinking: Consuming several standard drinks on one occasion in the past 30 days, defined for males as drinking five or more standard alcoholic drinks on one occasion, and for females as drinking four or more standard drinks on one occasion.[2]

Brief interventions: Therapeutic techniques used to initiate change in individuals with unhealthy behaviors.

Controlled substances: Substances regulated by the U.S. Drug Enforcement Agency into one of five categories called schedules. This placement is based on the substance's medical use, its potential for abuse or dependency, and related safety issues.

Delirium tremens (DTs): A rapid-onset, fluctuating disturbance of attention and cognition, sometimes associated with hallucinations, due to alcohol withdrawal. In its most severe manifestation, DTs are accompanied by agitation and signs of extreme autonomic hyperactivity, including fever, severe tachycardia, hypertension, and drenching sweats. DTs typically begin between 72 and 96 hours after the client's last drink.

Dependence: A condition that develops with chronic uses of a substance that causes a person to experience withdrawal symptoms if the substance is suddenly stopped.

Drug diversion: The act of redirecting medication from its intended destination for personal use, sale, or distribution to others. It includes drug theft, use, or tampering (adulteration or substitution). Drug diversion is a felony that can result in a nurse's criminal prosecution and loss of license.[3]

Heavy drinking: Excessive drinking defined as a female consuming 8 or more drinks per week and a male consuming 15 or more standard drinks per week, or either gender binge drinking on 5 or more days in the past 30 days.

Intoxication: A disturbance in behavior or mental function during or after the consumption of a substance.

Neuroadaptations: Progressive changes in the structure and function of the brain as a result of substance misuse. These neuroadaptations compromise brain function and also drive the transition from controlled, occasional substance use to chronic misuse that can be difficult to control.

Nonsubstance related disorders: Excessive behaviors such as gambling, viewing pornography, engaging in compulsive sexual activity, Internet gaming, overeating, shopping, overexercising, and overusing mobile phone technologies. These behaviors are thought to stimulate the same addiction centers of the brain as addictive substances. However, gambling disorder is the only nonsubstance use disorder with diagnostic criteria listed in the *DSM-5*.

Protective factors: Factors that help prevent substance use disorders from developing despite the risk factors that are present.

---

1 Substance Abuse and Mental Health Services Administration, & Office of the Surgeon General. (2016). *Facing addiction in America: The surgeon general's report on alcohol, drugs, and health.* United States Department of Health and Human Services. https://www.ncbi.nlm.nih.gov/books/NBK424857/

2 National Survey on Drug Use and Health. https://nsduhweb.rti.org/respweb/homepage.cfm

3 Nyhus, J. (2021). Drug diversion in healthcare. *American Nurse.* https://www.myamericannurse.com /drug- diversion-in-healthcare/

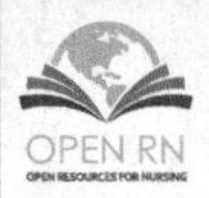

My Notes

Recovery: A process of change through which individuals improve their health and wellness, live a self-directed life, and strive to reach their full potential. Although abstinence from all substance misuse is a primary feature of a recovery lifestyle, it is not the only healthy feature.[4]

Relapse: The return to substance use after a significant period of abstinence.

Remission: The status of individuals with severe substance use disorders who overcome their disorder with effective treatment and regain health and social function.

Standard drink: 14 grams (0.6 ounces) of pure alcohol. Examples of a standard drink are one 12-ounce beer, 8 – 9 ounces of malt liquor, 5 ounces of wine, or 1.5 ounces distilled spirits.

Substance: A psychoactive compound with the potential to cause health and social problems, including substance use disorders. Substances can be divided into four major categories: alcohol, illicit drugs (including nonmedical use of prescription drugs), tobacco products, and over-the-counter drugs.

Substance misuse: The use of alcohol or drugs in a manner, situation, amount, or frequency that could cause harm to the user or to those around them.[5]

Substance use: The use (even one time) of any psychoactive substance.

Substance use disorder (SUD): A chronic illness caused by repeated misuse of psychoactive substances (e.g., alcohol, caffeine, cannabis, hallucinogens, inhalants, opioids, sedatives, hypnotics, anxiolytics, stimulants, and tobacco) that have a common effect of directly activating the brain's reward system.

Tolerance: A need for progressively increased amounts of a substance to achieve the desired effect or a diminished effect with continued use of the same amount of a substance.

Withdrawal: A group of physical and mental symptoms that can range from mild to life-threatening when a person suddenly stops using a substance.

Withdrawal management: Interventions that manage the physical and emotional symptoms that occur after a person stops using a psychoactive substance, also referred to as detoxification. Withdrawal symptoms vary in intensity and duration based on the substance(s) used, the duration and amount of use, and the overall health of the individual.

---

4 Substance Abuse and Mental Health Services Administration, & Office of the Surgeon General. (2016). *Facing addiction in America: The surgeon general's report on alcohol, drugs, and health.* United States Department of Health and Human Services. https://www.ncbi.nlm.nih.gov/books/NBK424857/

5 Substance Abuse and Mental Health Services Administration, & Office of the Surgeon General. (2016). *Facing addiction in America: The surgeon general's report on alcohol, drugs, and health.* United States Department of Health and Human Services. https://www.ncbi.nlm.nih.gov/books/NBK424857/

Chapter 15

Trauma, Abuse, and Violence

My Notes

15.1 INTRODUCTION

Learning Objectives

- Delineate adverse childhood experiences
- Incorporate trauma-informed care
- Assess clients for signs of abuse or neglect and intervene appropriately
- Promote safety for victims of abuse, neglect, or intimate partner violence
- Describe strategies to remain safe if workplace violence occurs

The health care system is composed of people who have experienced trauma, both those providing and those receiving care. Supporters of a trauma-informed approach recognize the prevalence of trauma survivors within health care settings and are aware that the service setting can also be a source of re-traumatization. As stated in the article "Trauma-Informed Nursing Practice," understanding how trauma has affected patients' lives and their interactions within the health care system is fundamental to responding to patients' needs and promotes better physical and mental health outcomes.[1]

Nurses provide care for clients who are experiencing or have experienced neglect, abuse, and intimate partner violence. In many settings, nurses may experience workplace violence while caring for clients who are agitated or combative. This chapter will discuss adverse childhood experiences and trauma-informed care, abuse and neglect of children and vulnerable adults, intimate partner violence, and workplace violence. Be aware that the content in this chapter may trigger powerful emotions, especially for survivors of similar traumatic experiences. Self-awareness and self-care practices should guide your engagement with this chapter.

Read the article "Trauma-Informed Nursing Practice" in the *Online Journal of Issues in Nursing* published by the American Nurses Association.

1 Fleishman, J., Kamsky, H., & Sundborg, S. (2019, May 31). Trauma-informed nursing practice. *OJIN: The Online Journal of Issues in Nursing, 24*(2). https://doi.org/10.3912/OJIN.Vol24No02Man03

My Notes

15.2 ADVERSE CHILDHOOD EXPERIENCES

In the late 1990s, a large research study evaluated the impact of adverse childhood experiences on adult health and health behaviors in over 17,000 participants. This research is referred to as the Adverse Childhood Experiences Study. **Adverse childhood experiences (ACE)** include neglect, abuse, witnessing violence, or experiencing substance abuse, mental illness, divorce, or imprisonment of a family member. The findings showed that the more negative events a child experienced, the higher the likelihood they had behavior problems and participated in adolescent risky behaviors, including substance abuse and unprotected sexual activity resulting in pregnancy. In addition, the findings showed that adults also struggled with substance abuse and had a higher likelihood of suffering with chronic illness, including alcoholism, chronic pulmonary disease, depression, liver disease, and many more.[1] Additionally, adults with the highest level of ACEs had a 20-year lower life expectancy than those without high levels of ACEs.[2] See Figure 15.1[3] for an infographic of ACEs.

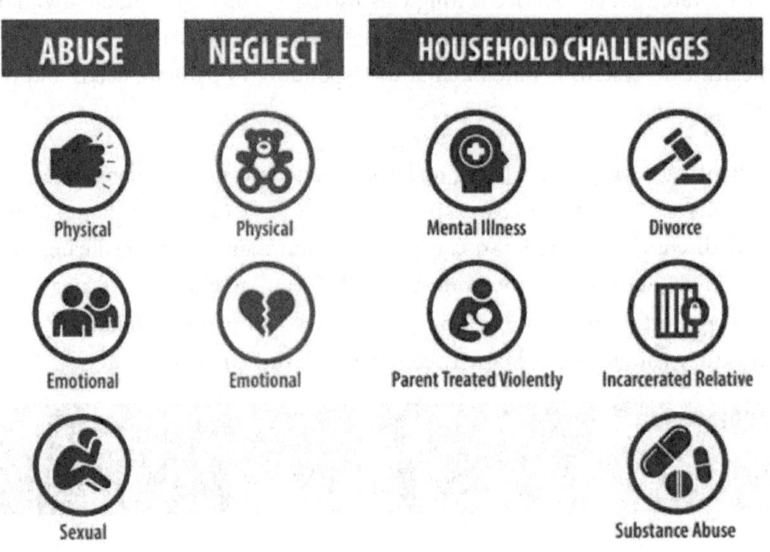

Figure 15.1 Adverse Childhood Events (ACEs)

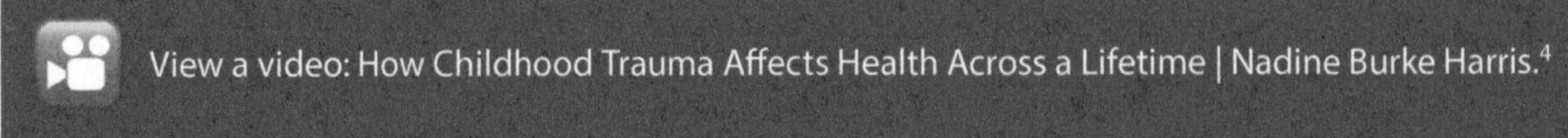

1 This work is a derivative of *Action steps using ACEs and trauma-informed care: A resilience model* by Laurie Leitch and is licensed under CC BY 4.0

2 This work is a derivative of *Action steps using ACEs and trauma-informed care: A resilience model* by Laurie Leitch and is licensed under CC BY 4.0

3 "ACEs.png" by unknown author for Centers for Disease Control and Prevention is licensed in the Public Domain. Access for free at https://www.cdc.gov/injury/pdfs/priority/ACEs-Strategic-Plan_Final_508.pdf

4 TED. (2015, February 17). *How childhood trauma affects health across a lifetime | Nadine Burke Harris.* [Video]. YouTube. All rights reserved. https://youtu.be/95ovIJ3dsNk

My Notes

Although many people who experience individual trauma continue to live their lives without lasting negative effects, others experience traumatic stress reactions causing lasting difficulties. Various biopsychosocial and cultural factors influence an individual's immediate response and long-term reactions to trauma. For most individuals, regardless of the severity of the trauma, the effects of trauma are met with resilience, defined as the ability to rise above circumstances or meet challenges with fortitude. Resilience includes the process of using available resources to negotiate hardship and/or the consequences of adverse events.[5]

The Centers for Disease Control and Prevention (CDC) created a resource titled *Preventing Adverse Childhood Experiences (ACEs): Leveraging the Best Available Evidence*. This resource contains these six strategies:

- Strengthen economic supports to families
- Promote social norms that protect against violence and adversity
- Ensure a strong start for children
- Teach skills
- Connect youth to caring adults and activities
- Intervene to lessen immediate and long-term harms

Read additional information about the CDC's prevention strategies in *Preventing Adverse Childhood Experiences (ACEs): Leveraging the Best Available Evidence* PDF.

View a video: We Can Prevent ACEs.[6]

Risk Factors, Protective Factors, and Prevention Strategies

By bringing attention to the powerful impact that negative childhood experiences have on future health and functioning, the ACE study demonstrates the importance of designing early intervention programs that target abuse, neglect, and violence.[7] Nurses can help prevent ACEs by educating parents, communities, and policymakers about how to help families provide safe and stable environments for children.

Risk Factors

Risk factors are conditions that increase the likelihood of experiencing ACEs. There are individual, family, and community risk factors for ACEs.

5 Center for Substance Abuse Treatment (US). (2014). *Trauma-informed care in behavioral health services.* Substance Abuse and Mental Health Services Administration. https://www.ncbi.nlm.nih.gov/books/NBK207201/

6 Centers for Disease Control and Prevention (CDC). (2018, April 5). *We can prevent ACEs.* [Video]. YouTube. All rights reserved. https://youtu.be/8gm-lNpzU4g

7 Center for Substance Abuse Treatment (US). (2014). *Trauma-informed care in behavioral health services.* Substance Abuse and Mental Health Services Administration. https://www.ncbi.nlm.nih.gov/books/NBK207201/

My Notes

Individual and Family Risk Factors

Individual and family risk factors include the following[8]:

- Families experiencing caregiving challenges related to children with special needs (for example, disabilities, mental health issues, and chronic physical illnesses)
- Children and adolescents who don't feel close to their parents/caregivers and feel as though they can't talk to them about their feelings
- Youth who start dating or engaging in sexual activity at an early age
- Children and youth with few or no friends or with friends who engage in aggressive or delinquent behavior
- Families with caregivers who have a limited understanding of children's needs or development
- Families with caregivers who were abused or neglected as children
- Families with young caregivers or single parents
- Families with low income
- Families with adults who have low levels of education
- Families experiencing high levels of stress from parenting or economic issues
- Families that have inconsistent discipline, use corporal punishment, and/or have low levels of parental supervision
- Families who are isolated from and not connected to other people (e.g., extended family, friends, neighbors)
- Families with high conflict and negative communication styles
- Families with attitudes accepting of or justifying violence or aggression

Community Risk Factors

Community risk factors include communities with these attributes[9]:

- High rates of violence and crime
- Limited educational and economic opportunities
- High rates of poverty, unemployment rates, and food insecurity
- Easy access to drugs and alcohol
- Low community involvement among residents
- Few community activities for youth
- Unstable housing where residents move frequently

---

8 Centers for Disease Control and Prevention. (2021, January 5). *Risk and protective factors.* https://www.cdc.gov/violenceprevention/aces/riskprotectivefactors.html

9 Centers for Disease Control and Prevention. (2021, January 5). *Risk and protective factors.* https://www.cdc.gov/violenceprevention/aces/riskprotectivefactors.html

Protective Factors

My Notes

Protective factors are conditions that protect people and decrease the possibility of experiencing ACEs.

Individual and Family Protective Factors

Individual and family protective factors against ACEs include the following[10]:

- Families where caregivers can meet basic needs of food, shelter, and health services for children
- Families that create a consistent family life where children feel safe, stable, and supported in nurturing relationships
- Children who have positive friendships and peer networks
- Children who experience academic success
- Children who have caring adults outside the family who serve as mentors/role models
- Families where caregivers have a college degree or higher education
- Families where caregivers have steady employment
- Families with strong social support networks and positive relationships with the people around them
- Families where caregivers engage in parental monitoring, supervision, and consistent enforcement of rules
- Families where caregivers/adults work through conflicts peacefully
- Families where caregivers help children work through problems
- Families that engage in fun, positive activities together
- Families that encourage the importance of school for children

Community Protective Factors

Communities can intervene to lessen the harms from ACEs and prevent future risks. Community protective factors include communities that demonstrate these qualities[11,12]:

- Families have access to education and support regarding positive parenting
- Families have access to economic and financial help
- Families have access to medical care and mental health services
- Individuals and families have access to safe, stable housing
- Families have access to nurturing and safe child care
- Families have access to high-quality preschool programs

---

10 Centers for Disease Control and Prevention. (2021, January 5). *Risk and protective factors.* https://www.cdc.gov/violenceprevention/aces/riskprotectivefactors.html

11 Centers for Disease Control and Prevention. (2021, January 5). *Risk and protective factors.* https://www.cdc.gov/violenceprevention/aces/riskprotectivefactors.html

12 Centers for Disease Control and Prevention (CDC). (2018, April 5). *We can prevent ACEs.* [Video]. YouTube. All rights reserved. https://youtu.be/8gm-lNpzU4g

My Notes

- Families have access to safe, engaging after-school programs and activities
- Adults have work opportunities with family-friendly policies
- There are strong partnerships among the community and business, health care, government, and other sectors
- Residents feel connected to each other and are involved in the community
- Violence is not tolerated or accepted in the community
- Positive parenting strategies are social norms in the community

Many factors contribute to ACEs, including personal traits and experiences, parents, the family environment, and the community itself. ACEs can have lasting negative effects on health and well-being, but these harms can be preventable. To prevent ACEs and protect children from neglect, abuse, and violence, nurses are involved in addressing these risk factors and protective factors with prevention strategies.[13]

Appropriately addressing traumatic experiences and promoting resilience are important parts of effective mental health care and integral for the healing and recovery process.[14]

---

13 Centers for Disease Control and Prevention. (2021, January 5). *Risk and protective factors.* https://www.cdc.gov/violenceprevention/aces/riskprotectivefactors.html

14 Substance Abuse and Mental Health Services Administration. (2022, March 22). *Trauma and violence.* https://www.samhsa.gov/trauma-violence

15.3 TRAUMA-INFORMED CARE

My Notes

Trauma has no age, gender, socioeconomic status, race, ethnicity, or sexual orientation boundaries. **Individual trauma** results from an event, series of events, or set of circumstances that is experienced by an individual as physically or emotionally harmful or life-threatening and can have lasting adverse effects on their functioning and mental, physical, social, emotional, or spiritual well-being. Adverse childhood experiences are examples of individual traumas.[1]

It is natural to feel afraid during and after a traumatic situation. The "fight, flight or freeze" reaction caused by the physiological stress response is intended to protect a person from harm. The sympathetic nervous system (SNS) automatically and unconsciously triggers this physiological stress response whenever there is a perception of threat.[2]

Review the physiology of the sympathetic nervous system and the parasympathetic nervous system in the "Psychotropic Medications" chapter.

Review activation of the stress response in the "Stress, Coping, and Crisis Intervention" chapter.

The SNS activates many organs during the stress response, resulting in symptoms like increased heart rate, increased blood pressure, rapid breathing, and tense muscles. Cumulative adverse childhood experiences can maintain this threat response in people's brains, which, over time, can "rewire" their level of physiological reactivity to stress and affect emotional regulation like depression, anxiety, and substance abuse. Trauma survivors are also susceptible to chronic physical and mental illnesses and suicide.[3] There also tends to be a decrease in positive social behaviors (such as collaboration and kindness) in individuals experiencing a chronic stress response because it requires their full cognitive capacity to respond by "fighting, fleeing, or freezing."

Arousal and reactivity symptoms include the following[4]:

- Being easily startled
- Feeling tense or "on edge"
- Having difficulty sleeping
- Having angry outbursts

---

1 This work is a derivative of *Action steps using ACEs and trauma-informed care: A resilience model* by Laurie Leitch and is licensed under CC BY 4.0

2 This work is a derivative of *Action steps using ACEs and trauma-informed care: A resilience model* by Laurie Leitch and is licensed under CC BY 4.0

3 Trauma-Informed Care Implementation Resource Center. (n.d.). *What is trauma-informed care?* Center for Health Care Strategies. https://www.traumainformedcare.chcs.org/what-is-trauma-informed-care/

4 National Institute of Mental Health. (2019, May). *Post-traumatic stress disorder.* U.S. Department of Health and Human Services. https://www.nimh.nih.gov/health/topics/post-traumatic-stress-disorder-ptsd

My Notes

These symptoms can make the person feel stressed and angry and can make it hard to do daily tasks, such as sleeping, eating, or concentrating[5].

Individuals who have a history of trauma may become triggered by engagement with the health care system. They may experience arousal and reactivity symptoms. As a result of the stimulation of the "fight, flight, or freeze" stress response, the parts of the brain involved in memory, planning, decision-making, and regulation are not engaged. This can impact the patient's involvement with health care services and affect their ability to adhere to treatment plans.[6] Nurses must understand this potential impact of previous trauma and incorporate patient-centered, trauma-informed care. Trauma-informed care is an approach that uses a lens of trauma to understand the range of cognitive, emotional, physical, and behavioral symptoms seen when individuals enter health care systems. **Trauma- informed care (TIC)** is a strengths-based framework that acknowledges the prevalence and impact of traumatic events in clinical practice, placing an emphasis on instilling in patients a sense of safety, control, and autonomy over their life and health care decisions. The basic goals of TIC are to avoid re-traumatization; emphasize survivor strengths and resilience; aid empowerment, healing, and recovery; and promote the development of survivorship skills.[7]

Two influential studies set the stage for the development of TIC[8]:

- The Adverse Childhood Experiences Study was an extensive study involving more than 17,000 individuals from the United States. It analyzed the long-term effects of childhood and adolescent traumatic experiences on adult health risks, mental health, health care costs, and life expectancy.[9]
- The Women, Co-Occurring Disorders, and Violence Study was a study focused on the role of interpersonal and other traumatic stressors among women. The researchers examined the interrelatedness of trauma, violence, and co-occurring substance use and mental health disorders and the incorporation of trauma-informed services.[10]

The Substance Abuse and Mental Health Services Administration (SAMHSA) as defined six core principles of TIC. See Figure 15.2[11] for an infographic related to these principles[12]:

---

5 National Institute of Mental Health. (2019, May). *Post-traumatic stress disorder.* U.S. Department of Health and Human Services. https://www.nimh.nih.gov/health/topics/post-traumatic-stress-disorder-ptsd

6 Fleishman, J., Kamsky, H., & Sundborg, S. (2019, May 31). Trauma-informed nursing practice. *OJIN: The Online Journal of Issues in Nursing, 24*(2). https://doi.org/10.3912/OJIN.Vol24No02Man03

7 Tracy, E. E., & Macias-Konstantopoulos, W. (2021, August 19). Human trafficking: Identification and evaluation in the health care setting. *UpToDate.* Retrieved April 4, 2022, from www.uptodate.com

8 Center for Substance Abuse Treatment (US). (2014). *Trauma-informed care in behavioral health services.* https://www.ncbi.nlm.nih.gov/books/NBK207201/

9 Felitti, V. J., Anda, R. F., Nordenberg, D., Edwards, V., Koss, M. P., & Marks, J. S. (1998). Relationship of childhood abuse and household dysfunction to many of the leading causes of death in adults: The adverse childhood experience (ACE) study. *American Journal of Preventive Medicine, 14*(3), 245-258. https://doi.org/10.1016/S0749-3797(98)00017-8

10 Clark, H. W., & Power, A. K. (2005). Women, co-occurring disorders, and violence study: A case for trauma-informed care. *Journal of Substance Abuse Treatment, 28*(2), 145-146. https://doi.org/10.1016/j.jsat.2005.01.002

11 This image is a derivative of "training_emergency_responders_final.jpg" by Centers for Disease Control and Prevention and in the Public Domain. Access for free at https://www.cdc.gov/cpr/infographics/6_principles_trauma_info.htm

12 Trauma-Informed Care Implementation Resource Center. (n.d.). *What is trauma-informed care?* Center for Health Care Strategies. https://www.traumainformedcare.chcs.org/what-is-trauma-informed-care/

My Notes

- **Safety:** Throughout the organization, patients and staff feel physically and psychologically safe.
- **Trustworthiness and Transparency:** Decisions are made with transparency and with the goal of building and maintaining trust.
- **Peer Support:** Individuals with shared experiences are integrated into the organization and viewed as integral to service delivery.
- **Collaboration and Mutuality:** Power differences between staff and clients and among organizational staff are leveled to support shared decision-making.
- **Empowerment Voice and Choice:** Patient and staff strengths are recognized, built on, and validated, including a belief in resilience and the ability to heal from trauma.
- **Cultural, Historical, and Gender Issues:** Biases and stereotypes (e.g., based on race, ethnicity, sexual orientation, age, geography) and historical trauma are recognized and addressed.

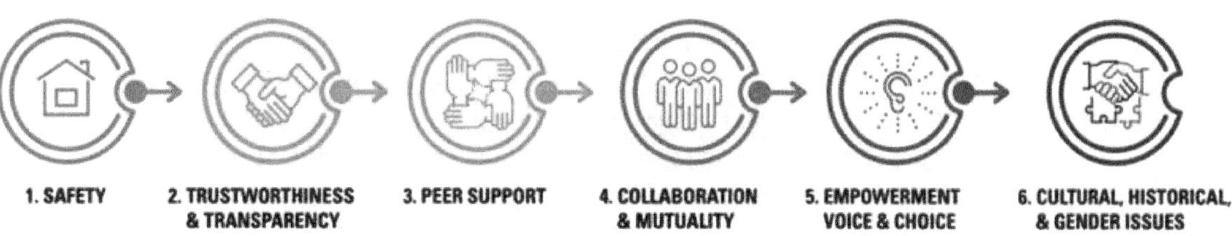

Figure 15.2 Core Principles of Trauma-Informed Care

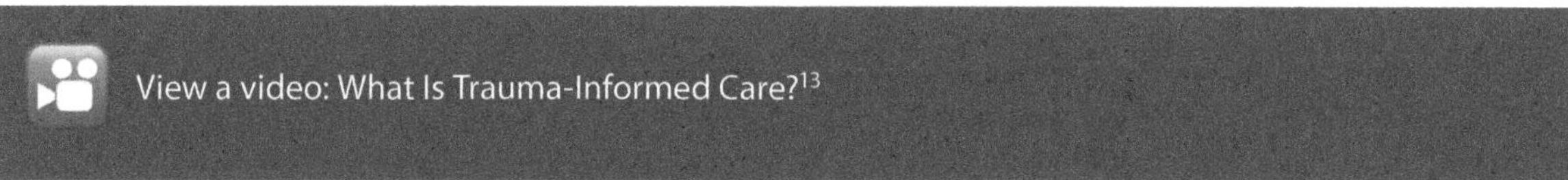

View a video: What Is Trauma-Informed Care?[13]

Trauma-Informed Nursing Practice

Nurses can incorporate trauma-informed care by routinely implementing the following practices with all clients[14]:

- **Introduce Yourself and Your Role in Every Patient Interaction:** Patients may recognize you, but they may not remember your role. This may lead to confusion and misunderstanding. When a patient understands who you are and your role in their care, they feel empowered to be actively engaged in their own care. They also feel less threatened because they know your name and why you are interacting with them. When one party is nameless, there can be an automatic power differential in the interaction.
- **Use Open and Nonthreatening Body Positioning:** Be aware of your body position when working with patients. Open body language conveys trust and a sense of value. Trauma survivors often feel powerless and trapped. Health care situations can trigger past experiences of lack of control or an inability to escape. Using nonthreatening body positioning helps prevent the threat detection

---

13 Center for Health Care Strategies. (2019, January 23). *What is trauma-informed care?* [Video]. YouTube. All rights reserved. https://youtu.be/fWken5DsJcw

14 Fleishman, J., Kamsky, H., & Sundborg, S. (2019, May 31). Trauma-informed nursing practice. *OJIN: The Online Journal of Issues in Nursing, 24*(2). https://doi.org/10.3912/OJIN.Vol24No02Man03

My Notes

areas of the patient's brain from taking over and helps patients stay regulated. A trauma-informed approach to body position includes attempting to have your body on the same level as the patient, often sitting at or below the patient. It could also include raising a hospital bed in order for the nurse and the patient to be on the same level, reducing the likelihood of creating a perceived power differential through positioning. Additionally, it is important to think about where you and the patient are positioned in the room in relation to the door or exit. Both nurse and patient should have access to the exit so that neither feels trapped.

- **Provide Anticipatory Guidance:** Verbalize what the patient can expect during a visit or procedure or what paperwork will cover. Knowing what to expect can reassure patients even if it is something that may cause discomfort. Past trauma is often associated with unexpected and unpredictable events. Knowing what to expect reduces the opportunity for surprises and activation of the SNS symptoms. It also helps patients feel more empowered in the care planning process.
- **Ask Before Touching:** For many trauma survivors, inappropriate or unpleasant touch was part of a traumatic experience. Touch, even when appropriate and necessary for providing care, can trigger a "fight, flight, or freeze" response and bring up difficult feelings or memories. This may lead to the individual experiencing increased anxiety and activation of the stress response, resulting in disruptive behaviors and possible dissociation. **Dissociation** is a break in how a person's mind handles information, causing disconnection from their thoughts, feelings, memories, and surroundings. Nurses are often required to touch patients, and sometimes this touch occurs in sensitive areas. Any touch can be interpreted as unwanted or threatening, so it is important to ask all clients permission to touch them. Asking permission before you touch patients gives them a choice and empowers them to have control over their body and physical space. Be alert to nonverbal signs such as eye tearing, flinching, shrinking away, or other body language indicating the person is feeling uncomfortable. If the client exhibits signs of discomfort when being touched, additional nursing interventions can be implemented such as a mindfulness or grounding practice.
- **Protect Patient Privacy:** Family members and other members of the medical team may be present when you care for a patient. Patients may not feel empowered or safe in asking others to step out. It is crucial that nurses do not put the responsibility on the patient to ask others to leave. It is the nurse's role to ask the patient (in private) whom they would like to be present during care and ask others to leave the room.
- **Provide Clear and Consistent Messaging About Services and Roles:** Trust is built when patients experience care providers who are forthright and honest. Dependability, reliability, and consistency are important when working with trauma survivors because previous trauma was often unexpected or unpredictable. Providing consistency from the nursing team regarding expectations and/or hospital rules can help patients feel secure and decrease opportunities for unmet expectations that might lead to triggering disruptive behavior.
- **Use Plain Language and Teach Back:** Avoid medical jargon and use clear, simple language. When patients are feeling triggered (i.e., their "fight, flight, or freeze" system is engaged), information processing and learning parts of the brain do not function optimally, and it is hard to remember new information. When providing education, information, or instructions, break information into small chunks and check for understanding. Offer to write important details down so they can accurately recall the information at a later time. Use clear language and "teach back" methods that empower patients with knowledge and understanding about their care.
- **Practice Universal Precaution:** Universal precaution means providing TIC to all patients regardless of a trauma history. Although ACE screening may be part of routine care, it can also

My Notes

have potential negative effects on patients. Unless a trauma-focused intervention is needed to amend the impact of trauma, many TIC experts propose universal precaution rather than direct screening.

Read a continuing education article titled "Trauma-Informed Nursing Practice" in the *American Journal of Nursing*.[15]

The Resilient Zone and Self-Regulation Skills

Individuals who have experienced repetitive or cumulative trauma may develop a dysregulated rhythm of their sympathetic nervous system (SNS) and parasympathetic nervous system (PNS), leaving them reactive and stuck in a state of hyperarousal, hypoarousal, or oscillating between the two extremes as their nervous system attempts to find balance. Simply put, the SNS "activates" the stress response, and the PNS "calms" the stress response. When out of balance, individuals may exhibit behaviors such as substance use disorders, self-harming, violence, poor school and work performance, bullying, and social disengagement.[16] Nurses can teach clients self-regulation skills by paying attention to their "fight, flight, or freeze" symptoms and learning how to balance their SNS and PNS systems.

Self-regulation skills teach clients how to return to a healthy balance of SNS and PNS stimulation called the resilient zone. See Figure 15.3[17] for an illustration of the **resilient zone** when the SNS and PNS are in balance. When in the resilient zone, the hormones released by the SNS during the "fight, flight, or freeze" stress response do not block conscious information processing by the brain. This balance promotes better capacity for flexibility and adaptability, prosocial behavior, improved problem-solving, and strategic thinking.[18]

---

15 Dowdell, E., & Speck, P.M. (2022). Trauma-informed care in nursing practice. *American Journal of Nursing, 122*(4), 30-38. https://journals.lww.com/ajnonline/Fulltext/2022/04000/CE__Trauma_Informed_Care_in_Nursing_Practice.22.aspx

16 This work is a derivative of *Action steps using ACEs and trauma-informed care: A resilience model* by Laurie Leitch and is licensed under CC BY 4.0

17 Leitch, L. (2017). Action steps using ACEs and trauma-informed care: A resilience model. *Health Justice 5*, 5. https://doi.org/10.1186/s40352-017-0050-5

18 This work is a derivative of *Action steps using ACEs and trauma-informed care: A resilience model* by Laurie Leitch and is licensed under CC BY 4.0

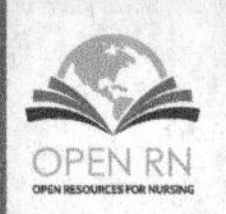

My Notes

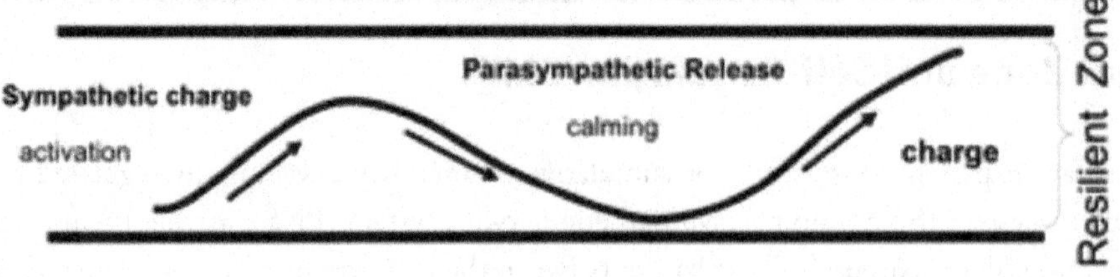

Figure 15.3 The Resilient Zone

Teaching self-regulation skills enables the individual to pay attention to symptoms of the stress response and use techniques to purposefully stimulate the PNS. They focus on quality of breath, heart rate, and muscle tension and then use relaxation breathing, progressive muscle relaxation, meditation, or other methods to stimulate the PNS. These skills can be used prior to and during challenging events, as well as practiced over time to build deeper nervous system balance.[19]

Read more about stress management, self-regulation skills, and grounding techniques in the "Stress, Coping, and Crisis Intervention" chapter.

Post-traumatic stress disorder (PTSD) is diagnosed in individuals who have been exposed to a traumatic event with chronic stress symptoms lasting more than one month that are so severe they interfere with relationships, school, or work. PTSD has been placed in a new diagnostic category in the *DSM-5* called "Trauma and Stressor-related Disorders." Read more about PTSD in the "Anxiety Disorders" chapter.

19 This work is a derivative of *Action steps using ACEs and trauma-informed care: A resilience model* by Laurie Leitch and is licensed under CC BY 4.0

15.4 ABUSE AND NEGLECT

My Notes

Child Neglect and Abuse

All 50 states and the District of Columbia have child abuse and neglect reporting laws that mandate certain professionals and institutions to refer suspected maltreatment to a Child Protective Services (CPS) agency. Each state has its own definitions of child abuse and neglect that are based on standards set by federal law. Federal legislation defines child abuse and neglect as, "Any recent act or failure to act on the part of a parent or caretaker which results in death, serious physical or emotional harm, sexual abuse or exploitation, or an act or failure to act, which presents an imminent risk of serious harm."[1] In 2019 there were 656,000 victims of child abuse and neglect, with a victim rate calculated as 9 victims per 1,000 children across the United States. In addition, 74.9 percent of victims were neglected, 17.5 percent were physically abused, and 9.3 percent were sexually abused. Child fatalities are the most tragic consequence of maltreatment. In 2019 it was estimated that 1,840 children died from abuse and neglect in the United States. The youngest children are the most vulnerable to maltreatment, with 45.4 percent of child fatalities younger than 1 year old. A perpetrator is the person who is responsible for the abuse or neglect of a child. Furthermore, 77.5% of perpetrators are a parent of the victim.[2]

An organization called A Safe Haven for Newborns is dedicated to preventing infant abuse and abandonment through education, prevention, and direct assistance (see Figure 15.4[3]).

Call the Helpline at 1-877-440-2229 or visit the A Safe Haven for Newborns website to find local resources.

---

1 Administration for Children & Families. (2021). *Child maltreatment 2019.* [Report]. U.S. Department of Health & Human Services. https://www.acf.hhs.gov/cb/report/child-maltreatment-2019

2 Administration for Children & Families. (2021). *Child maltreatment 2019.* [Report]. U.S. Department of Health & Human Services. https://www.acf.hhs.gov/cb/report/child-maltreatment-2019

3 "bc-english-ashfnb" by A Safe Haven for Newborns is used under Fair Use. Access for free at https://asafehavenfornewborns.com/international-safe-haven/

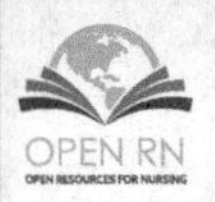

My Notes

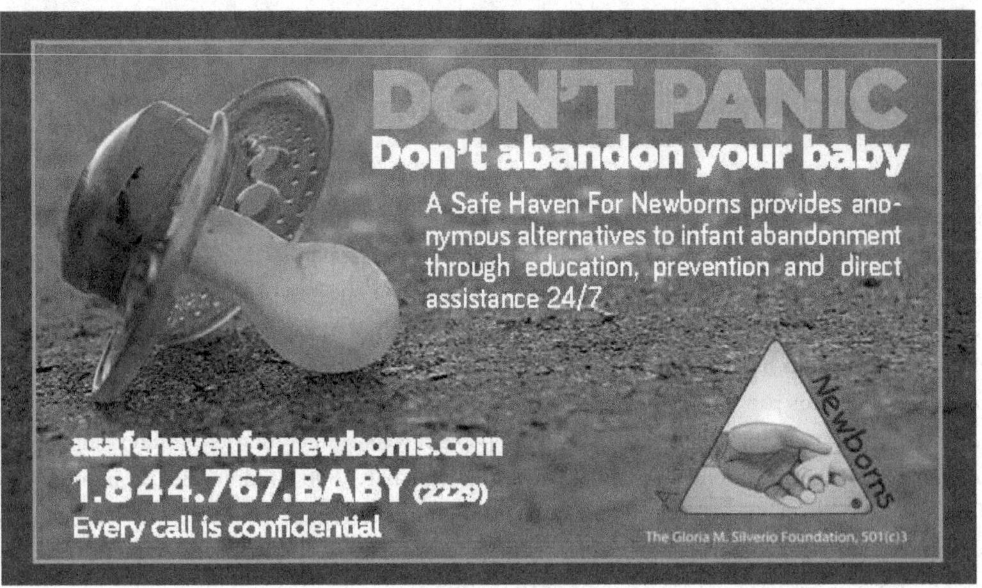

Figure 15.4 A Safe Haven For Newborns. Used under Fair Use.

Signs of Neglect and Abuse

Neglect

Neglect is a situation in which a parent or caretaker fails, refuses, or is unable, for reasons other than poverty, to provide the necessary care, food, clothing, or medical or dental care, which seriously endangers the physical, mental, or emotional health of the child. Signs of child neglect include the following[4]:

- Exhibits poor hygiene or body odor
- Is inappropriately dressed for weather
- Demonstrates needed medical or dental care
- Is left alone unsupervised for long periods of time
- Appears malnourished
- Is constantly hungry or begs for or steals food
- Demonstrates exhibits extreme willingness to please
- Is frequently absent from school
- Arrives early and stays late at school, play areas, or other people's home

4 Wisconsin Department of Children and Families. (n.d.). *Signs of child abuse and neglect.* https://dcf.wisconsin.gov/cps/signs

My Notes

Physical Abuse

Physical abuse is defined as injury inflicted on a child by other than accidental means. Physical injury includes, but is not limited to, lacerations, fractured bones, burns, internal injuries, severe or frequent bruising, or great bodily harm. Signs of physical abuse in children are as follows[5]:

- Bruises and/or welts on face, neck, chest, back, or soft muscle areas less prone to bruising by natural play or accidents (e.g., abdomen, breasts, under arm, inner thigh)
- Injuries in the shape of object (e.g., belt or cord)
- Unexplained burns on palms, soles of feet, or back; a line of demarcation from submerging in hot liquids (e.g., ankles, buttocks, wrists); burns in the shape of object (e.g., fork, cigarette)
- Fractures that do not fit the story of how an injury occurred
- Delay in seeking medical help
- Extremes in behavior (e.g., very aggressive or withdrawn and shy)
- Afraid to go home
- Frightened of parents
- Fearful of other adults
- Failure to thrive

However, some injuries are not visible to observation, such as shaken baby syndrome, a serious brain injury resulting from forcefully shaking an infant or toddler.

Sexual Abuse

Sexual abuse is defined as sexual intercourse or sexual touching of a child; sexual exploitation; human trafficking of a child; forced viewing of sexual activity; or permitting, allowing, or encouraging a child to engage in prostitution. Here are signs of sexual abuse in children[6]:

- Pain, swelling, or itching in genital area
- Bruises, bleeding, discharge in genital area
- Difficulty walking or sitting, frequent urination, or pain
- Stained or bloody underclothing
- Sexually transmitted diseases
- Refusal to take part in gym or other exercises
- Poor peer relationships
- Unusual interest in sex for age
- Drastic change in school achievement

---

5 Wisconsin Department of Children and Families. (n.d.). *Signs of child abuse and neglect.* https://dcf.wisconsin.gov/cps/signs

6 Wisconsin Department of Children and Families. (n.d.). *Signs of child abuse and neglect.* https://dcf.wisconsin.gov/cps/signs

My Notes

- Runaway or delinquent behavior
- Regressive to behaviors expected for a younger child

Read additional information about human trafficking in the "Vulnerable Populations" chapter.

Emotional Abuse

Emotional abuse is defined as harm to a child's psychological or intellectual functioning, which is exhibited by severe anxiety, depression, withdrawal, or aggression. Emotional damage may be demonstrated by substantial and observable changes in behavior, emotional response, or learning that are incompatible with the child's age or stage of development. Signs of emotional abuse in children include the following[7]:

- Low self-esteem
- Self-denigration
- Severe depression
- Unusual level of aggression
- Severe anxiety
- Extreme withdrawal
- Failure to learn

Child Protective Services

Child Protective Services (CPS) agencies provide services to children and their families, both in their homes and in foster care. Services are provided to prevent future instances of child maltreatment and remedy conditions that brought the children and their family to the attention of the agency.[8]

Elder Neglect and Abuse and Adults at Risk

Elder abuse is a common problem in the United States. Abuse, including neglect and exploitation, is experienced by about 1 in 10 people aged 60 and older who live at home. From 2002 to 2016, more than 643,000 older adults were treated in the emergency department for nonfatal assaults, and over 19,000 homicides occurred. This information is considered an underestimate of the problem because it is limited to those individuals treated in emergency departments and doesn't include those who do not seek treatment. Victims must decide whether to tell someone they are being hurt or continue being abused by someone they depend upon or care for deeply.[9]

---

7 Wisconsin Department of Children and Families. (n.d.). *Signs of child abuse and neglect.* https://dcf.wisconsin.gov/cps/signs

8 Administration for Children & Families. (2021). *Child maltreatment 2019.* [Report]. U.S. Department of Health & Human Services. https://www.acf.hhs.gov/cb/report/child-maltreatment-2019

9 Centers for Disease Control and Prevention. (2021, June 2). *Preventing elder abuse.* https://www.cdc.gov/violenceprevention/elderabuse/fastfact.html

My Notes

Elder abuse is defined as an intentional act or failure to act that causes or creates a risk of harm to an older adult. An older adult is defined as someone age 60 or older.[10] Adults at risk are also considered vulnerable adults at risk for abuse. **Adults at risk** are defined as adults who have a physical or mental condition that impairs their ability to care for their own needs.[11] Older adults and adults at risk are potentially susceptible for abuse, neglect, or financial exploitation by caregivers or a person they trust.[12] A **caregiver** is a person who has taken responsibility for all or part of an individual's care.

The following are types of elder abuse[13]:

- **Physical abuse:** Physical abuse refers to illness, pain, injury, functional impairment, distress, or death as a result of the intentional use of physical force and includes acts such as hitting, kicking, pushing, slapping, and burning. See Figure 15.5[14] for an infographic describing physical signs of elder abuse.
- **Sexual abuse:** Sexual abuse refers to forced or unwanted sexual interaction of any kind. This may include unwanted sexual contact or penetration or non-contact acts such as sexual harassment.
- **Emotional abuse:** Emotional abuse refers to verbal or nonverbal behaviors that inflict anguish, mental pain, fear, or distress, such as humiliation or disrespect, verbal and nonverbal threats, harassment, and geographic or interpersonal isolation.
- **Neglect:** Neglect is the failure to meet the person's basic needs, including food, water, shelter, clothing, hygiene, and essential medical care.
- **Financial abuse:** Financial abuse is the illegal, unauthorized, or improper use of money, benefits, belongings, property, or assets for the benefit of someone other than the individual.
- **Treatment without consent:** Treatment without consent refers to the administration of medication or the performance of psychosurgery, electroconvulsive therapy, or experimental research on an individual who has not provided informed consent.
- **Unreasonable confinement or restraint**: Unreasonable confinement or restraint refers to the intentional and unnecessary confinement of an individual in a locked room, involuntary separation from their living area, use of physical restraints, or the provision of unnecessary or excessive medication. (This does not include the use of these methods or devices if they conform with state and federal standards governing restraint or seclusion.)

---

10 Centers for Disease Control and Prevention. (2021, June 2). *Preventing elder abuse.* https://www.cdc.gov/violenceprevention/elderabuse/fastfact.html

11 Wisconsin Department of Health Services. (2018, November 13). *Adult protective services: Definitions.* https://www.dhs.wisconsin.gov/aps/definitions.htm#Abuse

12 Centers for Disease Control and Prevention. (2021, June 2). *Preventing elder abuse.* https://www.cdc.gov/ violenceprevention/elderabuse/fastfact.html

13 Centers for Disease Control and Prevention. (2021, June 2). *Preventing elder abuse.* https://www.cdc.gov/violenceprevention/elderabuse/fastfact.html

14 "Signs of Elder Abuse - Physical" by National Council on Aging is used under Fair Use. Access for free at https://www.ncoa.org/article/get-the-facts-on-elder-abuse

My Notes

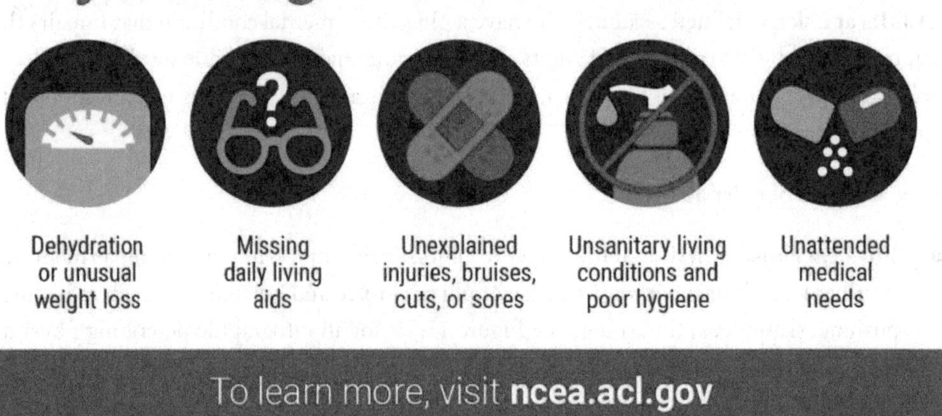

Figure 15.5 Physical Signs of Elder Abuse. Used under Fair Use.

Adult Protective Services

Adult Protective Services are available to provide aid to elder adults and adults at risk who have been abused, neglected, or exploited. Adult Protective Services are services provided to an individual with a developmental disability, degenerative brain disorder, serious mental illness, or other incapacity to keep them safe from abuse, neglect, or financial exploitation; prevent them from experiencing deterioration; or stop them from inflicting harm on themself or another person.

Protective services may include outreach, counseling, and referral for services; coordination of services for individuals; and tracking and follow-up. See Figure 15.6[15] for an illustration related to reporting concerns about vulnerable adults.

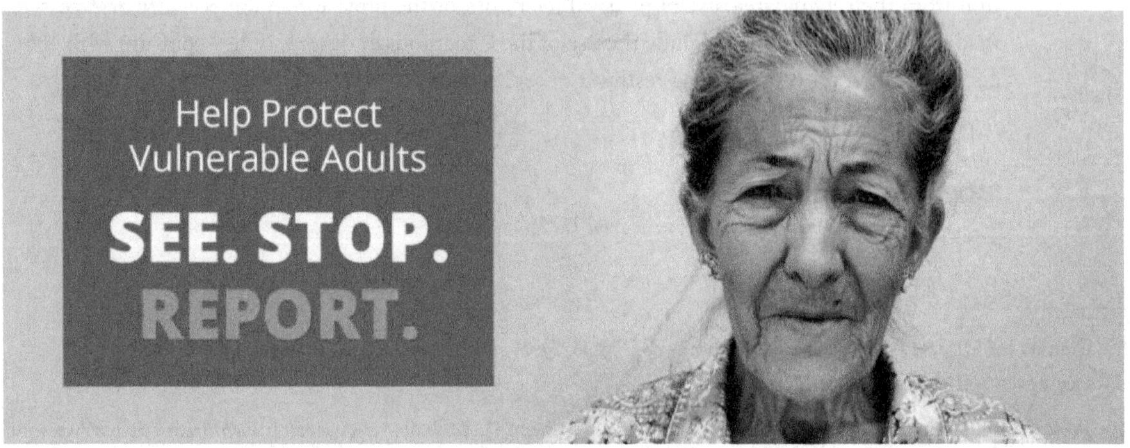

Figure 15.6 Reporting Concerns About Vulnerable Adults. Used under Fair Use.

15 "APS_header_3.jpg" by unknown author for Washington State Department of Social and Health Services is used under Fair Use.

My Notes

Find resources in your area for reporting elder abuse at the National Adult Protective Services Association website.

Read more about protective services in your state.

Find elder care resources in your community at Eldercare Locator.

Mandatory Reporting

Mandated reporters are required by law to report suspected abuse and neglect they see in the course of their professional duties. Nurses and other professionals are referred to as mandated reporters because they are required by state law to report suspected neglect or abuse of children, adults at risk, and the elderly. Nurses should be aware of the county or state agencies to whom they should report suspected abuse. For example, in Wisconsin, suspected neglect or abuse is reported to the Child Protective Services (CPS) or law enforcement. Persons required to report and who intentionally fail to report suspected child abuse or neglect may be fined up to $1,000 or imprisoned for up to six months or both.[16] See Figure 15.7[17] for an image related to reporting suspected abuse and neglect.

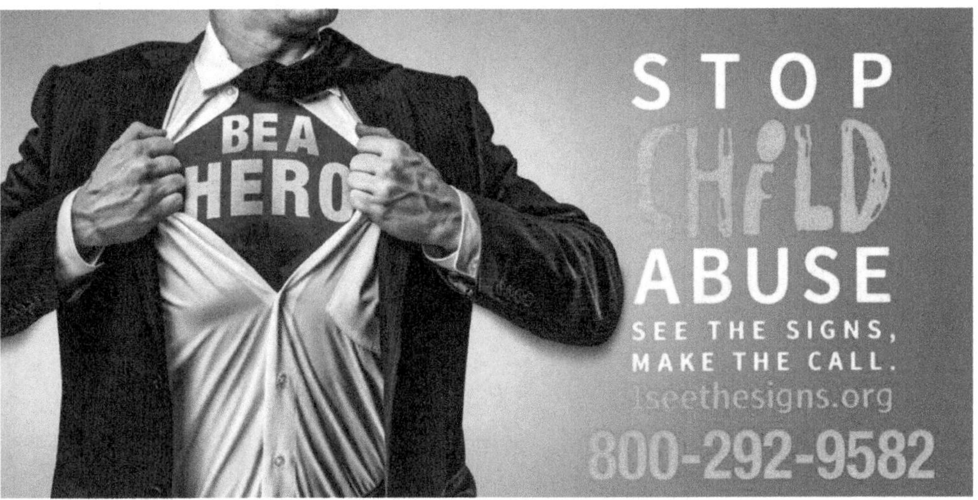

Figure 15.7 Report Suspected Child Abuse. Used under Fair Use.

What to Report

Mandatory reporters who suspect neglect or abuse should contact their county social/human services department, sheriff, or local police department immediately. When making a report, explain what happened or is happening to the child or vulnerable adult. Describe the nature of the abuse or neglect and be as specific as possible. Be

16 Wisconsin Department of Children and Families. (2019). *It shouldn't hurt to be a child . . . but sometimes it does.* [Brochure]. https://dcf.wisconsin.gov/files/publications/pdf/0101.pdf

17 "stop-child-abuse-see-the-signs-make-the-call-1536x748.jpg" by unknown author for Delaware Department of Services for Children, Youth & Their Families is used under Fair Use.

My Notes

prepared to give the name, DOB, address, and telephone number of the victim, as well as the name of their parent or caregiver. Include information on any known or reported Native American ancestry. If you do not know all of this information, report what you do know and explain all you know about the situation and family dynamics.[18]

When a report is filed, the receiving department will make a safety screening determination based on state statutes. If the report meets the criteria for alleged maltreatment, a social worker from the county department of social/human services will proceed with an investigation of the reported maltreatment and work with the parents to assess the situation to determine if any support or assistance is needed to protect the child or vulnerable adult and help the family.[19]

Find resources in your area for reporting suspected child abuse at the ChildHelp National Child Abuse Hotline.

Read more about protective services in your state. Access Wisconsin's information at Child Protective Services.

---

18 Wisconsin Department of Children and Families. (2019). *It shouldn't hurt to be a child . . . but sometimes it does.* [Brochure]. https://dcf.wisconsin.gov/files/publications/pdf/0101.pdf

19 Wisconsin Department of Children and Families. (2019). *It shouldn't hurt to be a child . . . but sometimes it does.* [Brochure]. https://dcf.wisconsin.gov/files/publications/pdf/0101.pdf

15.5 INTIMATE PARTNER VIOLENCE

My Notes

Intimate partner violence (IPV), sexual assault, and rape are crimes with long-lasting effects on victims and are a great cost to society. These crimes happen to both women and men and are often associated with substance use. A recent national survey found that 22 percent of women and 14 percent of men reported experiencing severe physical violence from an intimate partner in their lifetimes.[1] IPV is a significant public health issue that has many individual and societal costs. About 35% of female IPV survivors and more than 11% of male IPV survivors experience some form of physical injury related to IPV, and some deaths occur. About 1 in 5 homicide victims are killed by an intimate partner, and over half of female homicide victims in the US are killed by a current or former male intimate partner.[2] See Figure 15.8[3] for a CDC infographic related to IPV.

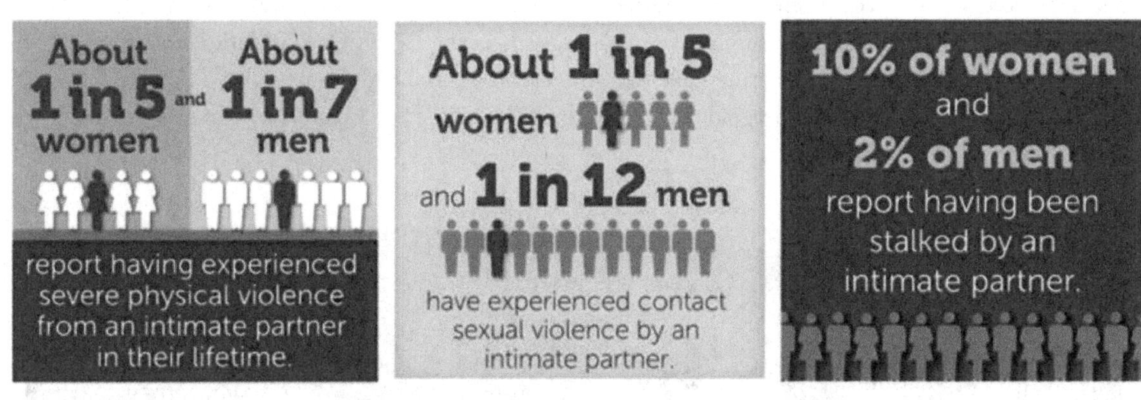

Figure 15.8 Intimate Partner Violence Statistics

Intimate partner violence (IPV) is abuse or aggression that occurs in a romantic relationship. "Intimate partner" refers to both current and former spouses and dating partners. IPV can vary in how often it happens and how severe it is. It can range from one episode of violence that could have lasting impact to chronic and severe episodes over multiple years. IPV can include any of the following types of behaviors[4]:

- **Physical violence:** When a person hurts or tries to hurt a partner by hitting, kicking, or using another type of physical force
- **Sexual violence:** Forcing or attempting to force a partner to take part in a sex act, sexual touching, or a nonphysical sexual event (e.g., sexting) when the partner does not or cannot consent

1 U.S. Department of Health and Human Services (HHS), Office of the Surgeon General. (2016). *Facing addiction in America: The surgeon general's report on alcohol, drugs, and health.* [Report]. https://addiction.surgeongeneral.gov/sites/default/files/surgeon-generals-report.pdf

2 U.S. Department of Health and Human Services (HHS), Office of the Surgeon General. (2016). *Facing addiction in America: The surgeon general's report on alcohol, drugs, and health.* [Report]. https://addiction.surgeongeneral.gov/sites/default/files/surgeon-generals-report.pdf

3 "how-big-is-the-problem-ipv-large" by Centers for Disease Control and Prevention is in the Public Domain. Access for free at https://www.cdc.gov/violenceprevention/intimatepartnerviolence/fastfact.html

4 Centers for Disease Control and Prevention. (2021, October 9). *Intimate partner violence.* https://www.cdc.gov/violenceprevention/intimatepartnerviolence/index.html

My Notes

- **Stalking:** A pattern of repeated, unwanted attention and contact by a partner that causes fear or concern for one's own safety or the safety of someone close to the victim
- **Psychological aggression:** The use of verbal and/or nonverbal communication with the intent to harm another partner mentally or emotionally and/or to exert control over another partner

View a video: What Is Intimate Partner Violence?[5]

Teen Dating Violence

When IPV occurs during adolescence, it is referred to as **teen dating violence (TDV)**. TDV affects millions of U.S. teens each year. Youth from marginalized groups, such as the LGBTQ+ population are at greatest risk of experiencing sexual and physical dating violence.[6] The use of alcohol and drugs is also a risk factor for non-consensual sexual contact among undergraduate and graduate students.[7] See Figure 15.9[8] for an infographic used to teach about healthy relationships.

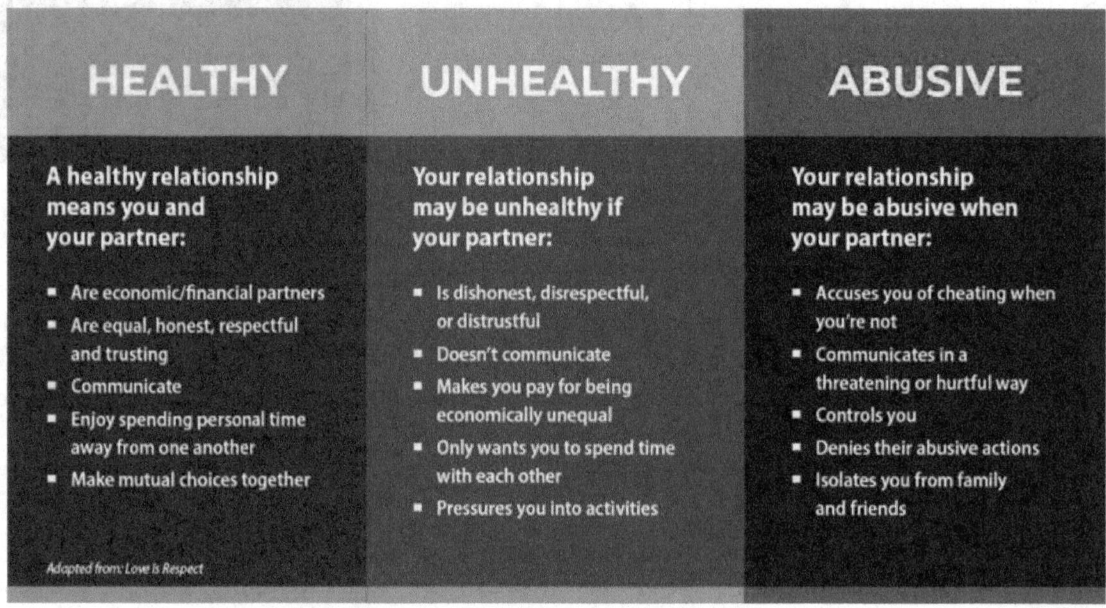

Figure 15.9 Healthy Versus Unhealthy and Abusive Relationships. Used under Fair Use.

---

5 Centers for Disease Control and Prevention. (2019, May 15). *What is intimate partner violence?* [Video]. YouTube. All rights reserved. https://youtu.be/VuMCzU54334

6 Weil, A. (2020, September 28). Intimate partner violence: Diagnosis and screening. *UpToDate.* Retrieved April 4, 2022, from www.uptodate.com

7 U.S. Department of Health and Human Services (HHS), Office of the Surgeon General. (2016). *Facing addiction in America: The surgeon general's report on alcohol, drugs, and health.* [Report]. https://addiction.surgeongeneral.gov/sites/default/files/surgeon-generals-report.pdf

8 "teen-dating-violence-relationship-range-chart-graphic.png" by unknown author for FairFax County Department of Family Services, Domestic and Violent Services is used under Fair Use. Access for free at https://www.fairfaxcounty.gov/familyservices/domestic-sexual-violence/teen-dating-violence

My Notes

Warning Signs of Intimate Partner Violence

These observations should heighten a nurse's suspicion of IPV[9]:

- Inconsistent explanation of injuries.
- Delay in seeking treatment for injuries.
- Frequent emergency department or urgent care visits. (Abusers typically do not want their victims to form an ongoing care relationship with one clinician. They may feel the victim will be less likely to find an ally in an emergency department where care may be more fragmented.)
- Missed appointments. The patient may not keep appointments because the abuser will not allow medical attention.
- Late initiation of prenatal care during pregnancy.
- Repeated abortions. Unplanned pregnancy may result from sexual assault and/or not being allowed to use birth control by the abuser.
- Medication nonadherence. Victims may not take medicines because the abuser has taken them away or not allowed the partner to fill prescriptions.
- Inappropriate affect. Victims may appear jumpy, fearful, or cry readily. They may avoid eye contact and seem evasive or hostile. Additionally, flat affect or dissociation may suggest post-traumatic stress disorder.
- Overly attentive or verbally abusive partner. The clinician should be suspicious if the partner answers questions for the patient. If the partner refuses to leave the examination room, the nurse should find a way to get the partner to leave before questioning the patient.
- Apparent social isolation.
- Reluctance to undress or have a genital, rectal, or oral examination or difficulty undergoing these or other examinations.

Assessment

The setting in which questioning occurs is important. The nurse must ensure that the patient feels safe and comfortable. Individuals are more likely to disclose their experiences of IPV when the nurse uses the following strategies[10]:

9 Weil, A. (2020, September 28). Intimate partner violence: Diagnosis and screening. *UpToDate.* Retrieved April 4, 2022, from www.uptodate.com

10 Weil, A. (2020, September 28). Intimate partner violence: Diagnosis and screening. *UpToDate.* Retrieved April 4, 2022, from www.uptodate.com

My Notes

- Provide privacy. Other people present in the room should be asked to leave for the interview and examination. Resistance of a partner to leave is a warning sign.
- Appear concerned with good eye contact.
- Be nonjudgmental and compassionate.
- Use open-ended questioning and ask only a few questions.
- Ask about "being hurt" or "treated badly" and avoid phrases like "domestic violence," "victim," "abused," or "battered."
- Assure confidentiality unless mandatory reporting is required or someone is in grave danger (i.e., duty to warn).
- Do not pressure to disclose, leave the relationship, or press charges.
- Encourage shared decision-making and respect for the patient's decisions.

The physical examination can provide warning signs that abuse may be occurring. The presence and location of injuries are important. Any injury without a good explanation, particularly involving the head and neck, teeth, or genital area, should raise suspicion. Typically, victims of domestic violence present with injuries on the central part of the body such as the breasts, abdomen, and genitals. Wounds on the head and neck, particularly neck bruising, may be caused by attempted strangulation. Wounds on the forearms often occur when a victim is in a defensive position. Bruises of different ages may be present due to repeated abuse. There may be other evidence of sexual assault, including sexually transmitted infections or unintended pregnancy.[11]

People experiencing abuse may deny the abuse for several reasons. They may not feel safe in disclosing information, especially if questions are not asked in a private environment or there is a fear of information not being kept confidential. They may not be emotionally ready to admit the reality of the situation, they may blame themselves, or they may feel like a failure if they admit to being abused. They may fear rejection, feel ashamed, believe that the abuse will not happen again, fear reprisal by the abuser, believe that they have no alternatives, or lack knowledge of resources that could help them. There may be language or cultural barriers between nurses and patients that interfere with communication or discomfort with using an interpreter to discuss sensitive issues.[12]

Patients for whom IPV is suspected but is not acknowledged should be asked again at subsequent visits. Research indicates patients are more likely to disclose information after they have been asked about IPV repeatedly in the health care setting and it is "normalized," meaning it happens frequently to many people.[13]

SAFE Survey

The Joint Commission recommends that hospitals use criteria to identify possible victims of abuse and neglect upon hospital entry and on an ongoingbasis, educate staff about how to recognize signs of abuse, assist with referrals of possible victims, and report abuse in accordance with law and regulation.

---

11 Weil, A. (2020, September 28). Intimate partner violence: Diagnosis and screening. *UpToDate.* Retrieved April 4, 2022, from www.uptodate.com

12 Weil, A. (2020, September 28). Intimate partner violence: Diagnosis and screening. *UpToDate.* Retrieved April 4, 2022, from www.uptodate.com

13 Weil, A. (2020, September 28). Intimate partner violence: Diagnosis and screening. *UpToDate.* Retrieved April 4, 2022, from www.uptodate.com

My Notes

Several IPV screening tools have been studied for use in emergency departments and clinics. SAFE is an example of a short survey tool that stands for the following assessments[14,15]:

- **S: Stress/Safety:** Do you feel safe in your relationship?
- **A: Afraid/Abused:** Have you ever been in a relationship where you were threatened, hurt, or afraid?
- **F: Friends/Family:** Are your friends or family aware you have been hurt?
- **E: Emergency Plan:** Do you have a safe place to go and the resources you need in an emergency?

Read the following PDF for additional information about Minnesota Department of Health's IPV screening tools: Family Home Visiting Intimate Partner Violence Screening & Referrals Toolkit.

Interventions and Safety Plans

Survivors of IPC are often afraid to leave their abusive partners because of the threats that have been made against them or their loved ones. The biggest threats for victims are strangulation (ten times more likely to be killed), the presence of a firearm (five times more likely), or if the abusive person is suicidal. It is not uncommon for an abusive person to threaten to kill themselves if they feel as if they're losing control over their partner, and they pose a serious risk to their victim if they have attempted suicide in the past, talk about a specific plan, or have access to a gun. Domestic violence is the single biggest indicator of murder-suicides in the United States, and this has escalated to include survivors' friends and family.[16]

Safety is a top priority when IPV is identified. Before the patient leaves the office, referrals to local resources should be made with a personalized safety plan in place. The most dangerous time in a relationship occurs when the abused person decides to leave. Nearly 77 percent of domestic violence-related homicides occur upon separation, and there is a 75 percent increase of violence upon separation for at least two years.[17] As the abuser realizes they are losing power and control over their partner, they often escalate tactics to increase fear in the individual leaving the relationship in an effort to make the individual stay. A **safety plan** is a set of actions that can help lower the risk of being hurt by an abusive partner. It includes specific information and resources that will increase one's safety at school, home, and other places visited regularly. View an infographic related to a safety plan in Figure 15.10.[18]

---

14 Weil, A. (2020, September 28). Intimate partner violence: Diagnosis and screening. *UpToDate.* Retrieved April 4, 2022, from www.uptodate.com

15 Rabin, R. F., Jennings, J. M., Campbell, J. C., & Bair-Merritt, M. H. (2009). Intimate partner violence screening tools. *American Journal of Preventive Medicine, 36*(5), 439-445.e4. https://doi.org/10.1016/j.amepre.2009.01.024

16 National Domestic Violence Hotline. (n.d.). *Plan for safety.* https://www.thehotline.org/plan-for-safety/

17 Battered Women's Support Services. (2020, June 11). *Eighteen months after leaving domestic violence is still the most dangerous time.* https://www.bwss.org/eighteen-months-after-leaving-domestic-violence-is-still-the-most-dangerous-time/

18 "vaw-covid-1.jpg" by unknown author for World Health Organization is licensed under CC BY-NC-SA 3.0 IGO. Access for free at https://www.who.int/multi-media/details/make-a-safety-plan-for-you-and-your-children

My Notes

Make a safety plan for you and your children:

If you are experiencing violence at home and need to leave in a hurry

Identify a friend, neighbour, relative, or shelter you can go to

Plan how to get there

Keep ready essential personal items to take with you

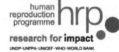

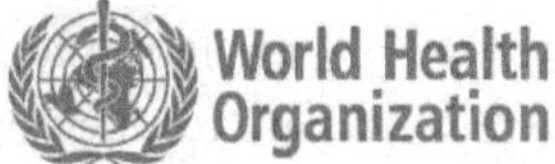

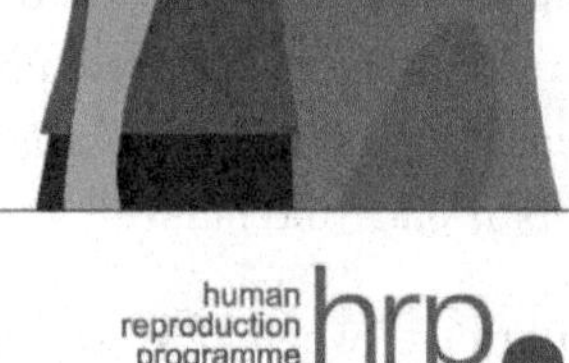

Figure 15.10 Safety Plan

Resources for Survivors of IPV

- Guide clients experiencing IPV to create a personalized online safety plan at the National Domestic Violence Hotline's Create a Safety Plan web page.
- If you need help or know someone who is experiencing IPV, visit the National Domestic Violence Hotline or call 1-800-799-7233. Online resources for developing a customized safety plan are available.
- Read about teen dating and healthy relationships at the Love is Respect website.

My Notes

Preventing IPV

There are many negative health outcomes associated with IPV, including chronic conditions affecting the heart, digestive, reproductive, musculoskeletal, and nervous systems. Survivors may experience mental health problems such as depression and post-traumatic stress disorder (PTSD) and are at higher risk for engaging in behaviors such as smoking, binge drinking, and risky sexual behaviors.[19]

Nurses and communities can promote healthy, respectful, and non-violent relationships to help reduce the occurrence of IPV.[20] See Figure 15.11[21] for an infographic related to IPV prevention strategies from the CDC.

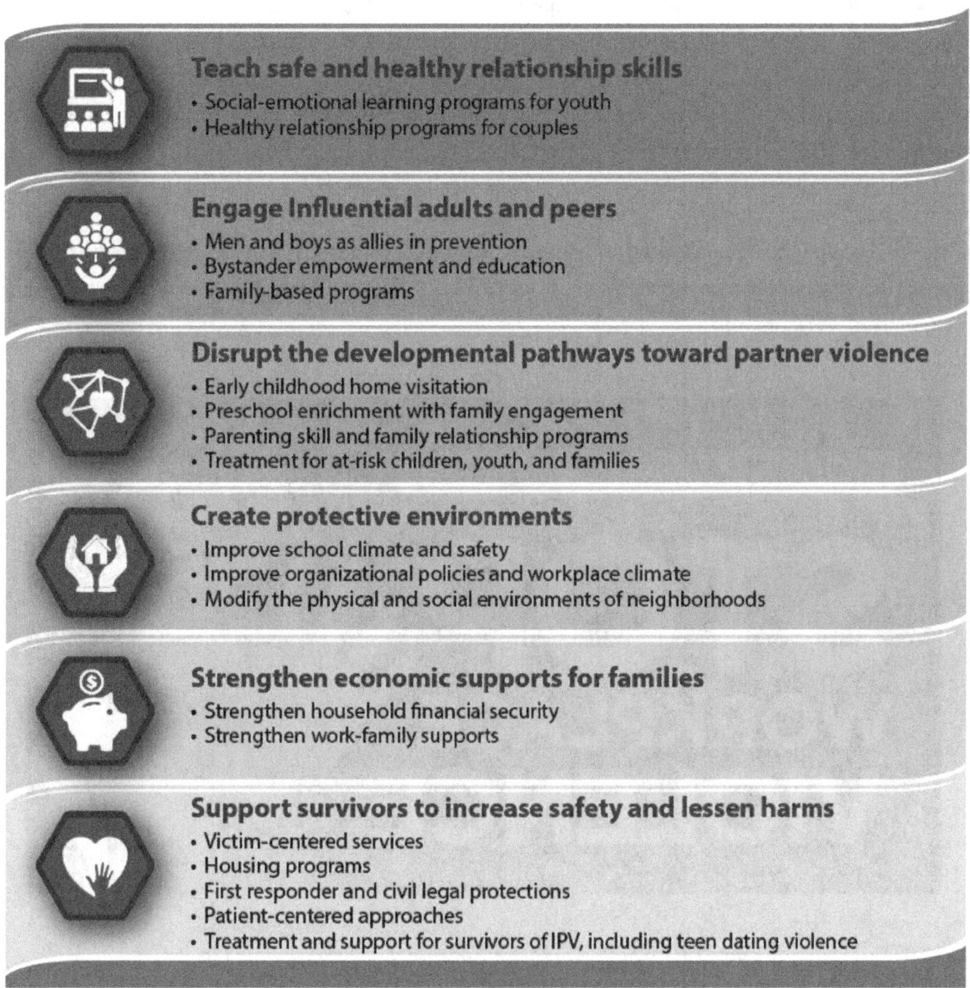

Figure 15.11 Preventing Intimate Partner Violence

---

19 Centers for Disease Control and Prevention. (2021, October 9). *Intimate partner violence.* https://www.cdc.gov/violenceprevention/intimatepartnerviolence/index.html

20 Centers for Disease Control and Prevention. (2021, October 9). *Intimate partner violence.* https://www.cdc.gov/violenceprevention/intimatepartnerviolence/index.html

21 "how-can-we-stop-ipv.PNG" by National Center for Injury Prevention and Control, Division of Violence Prevention is in the Public Domain. Access for free at https://www.cdc.gov/violenceprevention/intimatepartnerviolence/fastfact.html

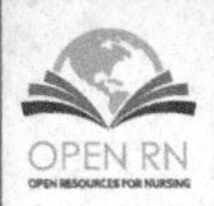

My Notes

15.6 WORKPLACE VIOLENCE

Workplace violence consists of physically and psychologically damaging actions that occur in the workplace or while on duty. Examples of workplace violence include direct physical assaults (with or without weapons), written or verbal threats, physical or verbal harassment, and homicide.[1]

Violence committed by patients or family members toward health care staff can occur in many health care settings, so nurses must be prepared to cope effectively with agitated patients to reduce the risk of serious injury to the patient, themselves, staff, and other clients. Up to 50 percent of health care professionals are victims of violence at some point during their careers. There is a wide range of risk factors for patient violence, including the environment, a patient's social and medical history, interpersonal relationships, genetics, neurochemistry and endocrine function, and substance abuse. In the emergency department (ED), substance intoxication or withdrawal is the most common diagnosis in combative patients. Known psychiatric illness is also a risk factor for violent behavior, with schizophrenia, personality disorders, mania, and psychotic depression most often associated with violence. Psychosis, delirium, and dementia can also lead to violent behavior.[2]

Some states are introducing legislation to increase the penalties for people who commit violence against nurses, making battery to a nurse a felony instead of a misdemeanor. A recent law passed in Wisconsin in 2022 makes it a felony to threaten a health care worker.[3] See Figure 51.12[4] for an illustration related to stopping workplace violence for nurses in Wisconsin.

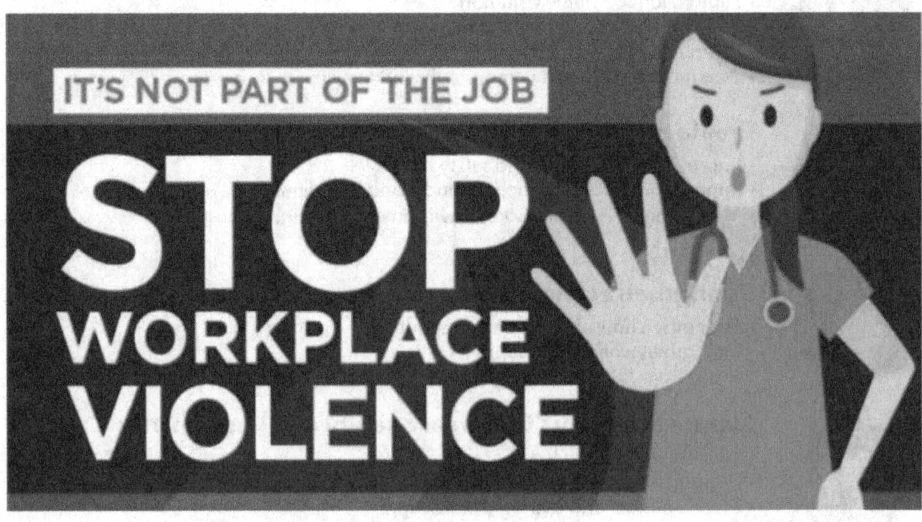

Figure 15.12 Stop Workplace Violence. Used under Fair Use.

---

1 Moore, G. P., & Pfaff, J. A. (2022, January 12). Assessment and emergency management of the acutely agitated or violent adult. *UpToDate.* Retrieved March 28, 2022, from www.uptodate.com

2 Moore, G. P., & Pfaff, J. A. (2022, January 12). Assessment and emergency management of the acutely agitated or violent adult. *UpToDate.* Retrieved March 28, 2022, from www.uptodate.com

3 Mensik, H. (2022, March 24). *Wisconsin passes law making threats against healthcare workers a felony.* HealthCareDive. https://www.healthcaredive.com/news/wisconsin-passes-law-threat-healthcare-workers-felony/620978/#:~:text=Wisconsin%20Governor%20Tony%20Evers%20signed,officers%20and%20other%20government%20workers

4 This image is a derivative of "WP-Violence-graphic-600x800.png" by Wisconsin Nurses Association is used under Fair Use. Access for free at https://www.wisconsinnurses.org/education/workplace-violence/

My Notes

Assessment of the combative patient begins with risk assessment and attention to safety measures. Violence typically erupts after a period of mounting tension. In a typical scenario, the patient first becomes angry, then resists authority, and finally becomes confrontational. However, violent behavior may erupt without warning, especially when caused by medical illness or dementia. A nurse may identify verbal and nonverbal cues of agitation and defuse the situation before violence happens. It is helpful to observe the nonverbal communication of a client's hands as an indicator of tension. Other signs of impending violence include the following[5]:

- Confrontational behavior
- Angry demeanor
- Loud, aggressive speech
- Tense posturing (e.g., gripping arm rails tightly or clenching fists)
- Frequently changing body position or pacing
- Aggressive acts (e.g., pounding walls, throwing objects, or hitting oneself)

Patients who are agitated but cooperative may be amenable to verbal de-escalation techniques. Actively violent patients and uncooperative, agitated patients, particularly those who exhibit signs of impending violence, require immediate physical restraint per an agency's policy. Assume that all violent patients are armed until proven otherwise, especially those presenting to an emergency department.[6]

Read about crisis intervention techniques in the "Stress, Coping, and Crisis Intervention" chapter.

Verbal De-Escalation Techniques

Verbal de-escalation techniques should be attempted before physical restraints or sedative medications are implemented. During initial interactions with the patient, it will rapidly become clear whether the patient will cooperate or continue to escalate. This interaction also enables the nurse to assess the patient's mental status. If the patient remains agitated or is incapable of interacting appropriately, then restraints become necessary.[7]

When attempting to de-escalate an individual, the nurse should adopt an honest and straightforward manner. Friendly gestures can be helpful. Offer a comfortable place to sit or something to eat or drink (but not a hot liquid that could be used as a weapon) to establish trust. Many individuals will decompress at this point because offering food or drink appeals to their most basic human needs and builds trust.[8]

The nurse should demonstrate a nonconfrontational, attentive, and receptive demeanor without conveying weakness or vulnerability. A calm and soothing tone of voice should be used. Avoid direct eye contact, do not approach

---

5 Moore, G. P., & Pfaff, J. A. (2022, January 12). Assessment and emergency management of the acutely agitated or violent adult. *UpToDate.* Retrieved March 28, 2022, from www.uptodate.com

6 Moore, G. P., & Pfaff, J. A. (2022, January 12). Assessment and emergency management of the acutely agitated or violent adult. *UpToDate.* Retrieved March 28, 2022, from www.uptodate.com

7 Moore, G. P., & Pfaff, J. A. (2022, January 12). Assessment and emergency management of the acutely agitated or violent adult. *UpToDate.* Retrieved March 28, 2022, from www.uptodate.com

8 Moore, G. P., & Pfaff, J. A. (2022, January 12). Assessment and emergency management of the acutely agitated or violent adult. *UpToDate.* Retrieved March 28, 2022, from www.uptodate.com

My Notes

the patient from behind or move suddenly, and stand at least two arm's lengths away.[9] The nurse should ensure a quick exit route to the door and never allow the individual to come between them and the door. Stethoscope and badge holders should not be worn around the neck to prevent strangulation risks.

In some cases, an agitated patient may be aware of their impulse control problem and may welcome limit-setting behavior by the nurse (e.g., "I can help you with your problem, but I cannot allow you to continue threatening me or the emergency department staff"). It is difficult to predict which patients will respond to this limit-setting approach. Some patients may interpret such statements as confrontational and escalate their behavior.[10]

A key mistake when interviewing an agitated or potentially violent individual is failing to address violence directly. They should be asked relevant questions, such as, "Do you feel like hurting yourself or someone else?" and "Do you carry a gun?" Stating the obvious (e.g., "You look angry") may help them to begin sharing their emotions. Speak in a conciliatory manner and offer supportive statements to diffuse the situation, such as, "You obviously have a lot of will power and are good at controlling your emotions."[11]

A consensus statement from the American Association for Emergency Psychiatry De-escalation Workgroup describes these ten key elements for verbal de-escalation[12]:

- **Respect personal space:** Maintain a distance of two arm's lengths and provide space for easy exit for either party.
- **Do not be provocative:** Keep your hands relaxed, maintain a open body posture, and do not stare at the patient.
- **Establish verbal contact:** The first person to contact the patient should take the lead in communicating.
- **Use concise, simple language:** Avoid elaborate and technical terms because they are hard for an impaired person to understand.
- **Identify feelings and desires:** "What are you hoping for?"
- **Listen closely to what the patient is saying:** After listening, restate what the patient said to improve mutual understanding (e.g., "Tell me if I have this right . . .").
- **Agree or agree to disagree:** Agree with clear specific truths or agree in general (e.g., "Yes, everyone should be treated respectfully.")
- **Set clear limits:** Inform the patient that violence or abuse cannot be tolerated.
- **Offer choices and optimism:** Patients feel empowered if they have some choice in matters.
- **Debrief the patient and staff.**

---

9 Moore, G. P., & Pfaff, J. A. (2022, January 12). Assessment and emergency management of the acutely agitated or violent adult. *UpToDate.* Retrieved March 28, 2022, from www.uptodate.com

10 Moore, G. P., & Pfaff, J. A. (2022, January 12). Assessment and emergency management of the acutely agitated or violent adult. *UpToDate.* Retrieved March 28, 2022, from www.uptodate.com

11 Moore, G. P., & Pfaff, J. A. (2022, January 12). Assessment and emergency management of the acutely agitated or violent adult. *UpToDate.* Retrieved March 28, 2022, from www.uptodate.com

12 Moore, G. P., & Pfaff, J. A. (2022, January 12). Assessment and emergency management of the acutely agitated or violent adult. *UpToDate.* Retrieved March 28, 2022, from www.uptodate.com

My Notes

The "philosophy of yes" is a de-escalation technique that encourages the nurse to respond affirmatively to an agitated individual. Examples of initial responses using this approach include "Yes, as soon as," "Okay, but first we need to," or "I absolutely understand why you want that done, but in my experience, there are better ways of getting what you need."[13]

However, some approaches to the combative patient are counterproductive and can lead to escalation. Arguing, condescension, or commanding the patient to calm down can have disastrous consequences. Patients often interpret such approaches as a challenge to "prove themselves." A threat to call security personnel can also invite aggression. Other potential mistakes include criticizing or interrupting the patient, responding defensively or taking the patient's comments personally, or not clarifying what the patient wants before responding.[14]

Never lie to a patient (e.g., stating "I am sure you will be out of here in no time" when this is not the case). After the lie becomes apparent, the patient may take out frustrations violently upon an unsuspecting nurse or colleague. Take all threats seriously. It is especially important not to deny or downplay threatening behavior. If verbal techniques are unsuccessful and escalation occurs, the nurse should excuse themselves and summon help.[15]

Applying Physical Restraints

Physical restraints may be used when verbal de-escalation techniques are unsuccessful despite a professional approach to the combative patient. Restraints should never be applied for convenience or punishment, and they should be removed as soon as possible, usually after adequate chemical sedation is achieved.

Restraints should be implemented systematically using an institutional protocol. The protocol typically begins after the examiner leaves the room when verbal de-escalation techniques have been unsuccessful, and assistance is summoned. It can be helpful to consider the application of restraints like a procedure, similar to running an advanced cardiac life support code.[16]

The restraint team should have at least five people, including a team leader. The leader is the only person giving orders and should be the person with the most experience implementing restraints, whether a clinician, nurse, or security officer. Before entering the room, the leader outlines the restraint protocol and warns the team of anticipated dangers (e.g., the presence of objects that may be used as weapons). All team members should remove personal effects (e.g., stethoscopes, pens, jewelry, etc.) the combative patient could use against them. If the patient to be restrained is female, at least one member of the restraint team should be female to diminish potential allegations of sexual assault.[17]

The restraint team should enter the room in force and display a professional, rather than threatening, attitude. Many violent individuals decompress at this point because the show of force protects their ego (e.g., "I would

---

13 Moore, G. P., & Pfaff, J. A. (2022, January 12). Assessment and emergency management of the acutely agitated or violent adult. *UpToDate.* Retrieved March 28, 2022, from www.uptodate.com

14 Moore, G. P., & Pfaff, J. A. (2022, January 12). Assessment and emergency management of the acutely agitated or violent adult. *UpToDate.* Retrieved March 28, 2022, from www.uptodate.com

15 Moore, G. P., & Pfaff, J. A. (2022, January 12). Assessment and emergency management of the acutely agitated or violent adult. *UpToDate.* Retrieved March 28, 2022, from www.uptodate.com

16 Moore, G. P., & Pfaff, J. A. (2022, January 12). Assessment and emergency management of the acutely agitated or violent adult. *UpToDate.* Retrieved March 28, 2022, from www.uptodate.com

17 Moore, G. P., & Pfaff, J. A. (2022, January 12). Assessment and emergency management of the acutely agitated or violent adult. *UpToDate.* Retrieved March 28, 2022, from www.uptodate.com

My Notes

have fought back, but there were too many against me"). The leader speaks to the patient in a calm and organized manner, explaining why restraints are needed and what the course of events will be (e.g., "You will receive a medical and psychiatric examination, as well as treatment"). The patient is instructed to cooperate and lie down to have restraints applied. Some patients will be relieved at the protection to self and others afforded by restraints when they feel themselves losing control. However, even if the patient suddenly appears less dangerous, physical restraints must be placed after the decision to use them has been made; do not negotiate with the patient at this point.[18]

If it becomes necessary to use force to control the patient, one team member restrains a preassigned extremity by controlling the major joint (e.g., knee or elbow). This can be accomplished by locking the major joint in extension. The team leader controls the head. If the patient is armed with a makeshift weapon, two mattresses can be used to charge and immobilize or sandwich the patient. Restraints are applied securely to each extremity and tied to the solid frame of the bed (not side rails because later repositioning of side rails also repositions the patient's extremity). To prevent their lower extremities from flailing independently, it may be best to cross the legs at the ankle and then attach the restraint to the bed frame on the opposite side.[19]

Leather is the optimal material for restraining a combative patient because it is strong, prevents escape, and is less constricting than typical soft restraints. Gauze should not be used. Soft restraints are helpful in restricting extremity use in a semi-cooperative patient but are less effective in a truly violent patient who continues to struggle. If chest restraints are used, it is vital to ensure adequate chest expansion for ventilation. Never apply pressure to the client's chest or back while they are immobilized due to asphyxiation risk. After the patient is immobilized, announcing "The crisis is over" can have a calming effect on the restraint team and the patient.[20]

After restraints have been applied, the patient should be monitored frequently and their position changed regularly to prevent circulatory obstruction, pressure injuries, and paresthesias, as well as to avoid rhabdomyolysis associated with continued combativeness. A standardized form based on agency policy is typically used for documentation. Documentation should include the specific indication for restraints and alternatives attempted. In addition to monitoring, nurses must ensure that basic needs (e.g., hydration, food, toileting) are met for any patient who is physically restrained or chemically sedated. Physical restraints should be removed as soon as possible.[21]

Chemical Sedation

Chemical sedation may be necessary, with or without physical restraints, in a combative patient who does not respond to verbal de-escalation techniques. The ideal sedative medication for an agitated or violent patient is rapid-acting with minimal side effects. The major classes of medications used to control the violent or agitated

18 Moore, G. P., & Pfaff, J. A. (2022, January 12). Assessment and emergency management of the acutely agitated or violent adult. *UpToDate.* Retrieved March 28, 2022, from www.uptodate.com

19 Moore, G. P., & Pfaff, J. A. (2022, January 12). Assessment and emergency management of the acutely agitated or violent adult. *UpToDate.* Retrieved March 28, 2022, from www.uptodate.com

20 Moore, G. P., & Pfaff, J. A. (2022, January 12). Assessment and emergency management of the acutely agitated or violent adult. *UpToDate.* Retrieved March 28, 2022, from www.uptodate.com

21 Moore, G. P., & Pfaff, J. A. (2022, January 12). Assessment and emergency management of the acutely agitated or violent adult. *UpToDate.* Retrieved March 28, 2022, from www.uptodate.com

patient include benzodiazepines, first-generation (typical) antipsychotics, second-generation (atypical) antipsychotics, and ketamine[22]:

- For severely violent patients requiring immediate sedation, a rapid-acting first-generation antipsychotic (e.g., haloperidol or droperidol), benzodiazepine (e.g., midazolam), or a combination of both may be prescribed. Second-generation antipsychotics, such as olanzapine, risperidone, and ziprasidone may also be prescribed.
- For patients with agitation from drug intoxication or withdrawal from an unknown cause, benzodiazepines are typically prescribed. Lorazepam and midazolam are used most often. Benzodiazepines may cause respiratory depression and excessive sedation, so close monitoring is essential after administration.
- Ketamine may be prescribed when initial treatments with benzodiazepines or antipsychotics have failed, especially in patients with excited delirium. However, clients receiving ketamine have increased risk for respiratory distress and may require endotracheal intubation and mechanical ventilation.

Post-Restraint Evaluation

After the patient is restrained, the cause of their agitation will be evaluated to determine if it is medical, psychiatric, or substance-use related. Patients over the age of 40 with new psychiatric symptoms are likely to have a medical cause. Elderly patients are at higher risk for delirium due to medical illness (such as a urinary tract infection) or adverse reactions to medications. Patients with a history of drug or alcohol use disorder may exhibit violent behavior as a manifestation of an intoxication or withdrawal syndrome. Violent behavior unrelated to medical illness, drug intoxication, or withdrawal should be followed by psychiatric consultation and evaluation.[23]

Defense Against Assault

Physical assault may occur despite appropriate precautions and interventions with a violent individual. If assaulted, immediately summon help. Maintain a sideward posture, keeping the arms ready for self-protection. If faced with an oncoming punch or a kick, deflect with an arm or a leg. If choking is attempted, tuck in the chin to protect the airway and carotid arteries. If bitten, do not pull away, but rather push toward the mouth and hold the nares shut to entice the opening of the mouth.[24] In a similar manner, don't pull away if your hair is pulled, but instead pull the client's hand toward your head and push up to bend their wrist backwards and increase the likelihood of them releasing their grip due to pain.

If threatened with a weapon, try to appear calm and comply with the individual's demands. Adopt a nonthreatening posture and avoid sudden movements. Do not attempt to reach for the weapon. Avoid arguing, despair, or whining. If taken hostage, attempt to establish a human connection with the hostage taker because there is less risk of violence if a relationship has been established. Do not bargain, make promises, or lie because the consequences could be disastrous. Reassure the hostage taker that an authorized person should arrive promptly to hear

---

22 Moore, G. P., & Pfaff, J. A. (2022, January 12). Assessment and emergency management of the acutely agitated or violent adult. *UpToDate.* Retrieved March 28, 2022, from www.uptodate.com

23 Moore, G. P., & Pfaff, J. A. (2022, January 12). Assessment and emergency management of the acutely agitated or violent adult. *UpToDate.* Retrieved March 28, 2022, from www.uptodate.com

24 Moore, G. P., & Pfaff, J. A. (2022, January 12). Assessment and emergency management of the acutely agitated or violent adult. *UpToDate.* Retrieved March 28, 2022, from www.uptodate.com

My Notes

their complaints or demands. If a weapon is put down, do not reach for it, but rather attempt to verbally resolve the crisis while awaiting arrival of law enforcement.[25]

Every hospital should have a written plan of action to implement in the case of extreme violence. The plan should include prevention and safety measures, a means for rapid notification of security and police personnel, evacuation plans, medical treatment, and crisis intervention. A novel approach uses a trained violence management team to provide a mechanism for dealing with aggressive patients and to protect the staff.[26]

Mandatory training for clinical and non-clinical staff must also be incorporated with written plans of action. This multifaceted approach improves nurses' self-perception and confidence against workplace violence.[27]

Interpersonal Conflict Among Health Care Team Members

Conflict is inevitable when working on a health care team composed of members with different personalities, roles, and responsibilities. Some conflicts among some team members can escalate to verbal threats or harassment. Common sources of interpersonal conflict in health care settings are passive-aggressiveness, horizontal aggression, defensiveness, peer informer behavior, and victimization behaviors. It is essential for all nurses to develop conflict resolution skills to effectively address these behaviors and maintain a safe work environment.

> Read more information about interpersonal conflict and conflict resolution skills in the "Conflict Resolution" section of the "Collaboration Within the Interprofessional Team" chapter of Open RN *Nursing Management and Professional Concepts.*

---

25 Moore, G. P., & Pfaff, J. A. (2022, January 12). Assessment and emergency management of the acutely agitated or violent adult. *UpToDate.* Retrieved March 28, 2022, from www.uptodate.com

26 Moore, G. P., & Pfaff, J. A. (2022, January 12). Assessment and emergency management of the acutely agitated or violent adult. *UpToDate.* Retrieved March 28, 2022, from www.uptodate.com

27 Ming, J. L., Huang, H. M., Hung, S. P., Chang, C. I., Hsu, Y. S., Tzeng, Y. M., Huang, H. Y., & Hsu, T. (2019). Using simulation training to promote nurses' effective handling of workplace violence: A quasi-experimental study. I*nternational Journal of Environmental Research and Public Health, 16(*19), 3648. http://dx.doi.org/10.3390/ijerph16193648

15.7 SPOTLIGHT ACTIVITY

My Notes

This Spotlight Activity is based on a real case originally presented in "Trauma-Informed Care in Nursing Practice" by Dowdell and Speck (2022). Identifying details have been changed or omitted to protect the anonymity of the client.[1]

Dana is a 34-year-old female who arrived at the Emergency Department with a neck injury she reports "happened this morning when I slipped and fell." The nurse notes that Dana's address given is in a different community about 50 miles away from the hospital. Initial physical examination revealed bruise patterns in various stages of healing all over Dana's body and three linear abrasions over the trapezius muscle on the right side of the neck consistent with attempted strangulation.

While awaiting diagnostic testing results, the nurse established a therapeutic nurse-client relationship and asked Dana a few follow-up questions about the events leading up to the injury and the relationship with the partner. Dana stated, "We fight a lot" and "My partner has a lot of angry outbursts." Upon the nurse's use of effective therapeutic communication, Dana shared that the injury resulted from "being choked and beaten," and the partner had done similar actions on "several previous occasions in front of the children." Dana then told the nurse, "My partner can't find out that I am here in this hospital."

A contrast computed tomography (CT) scan revealed swelling of Dana's right carotid artery and soft tissue in the neck. Laboratory tests also indicated that Dana had severely elevated blood sugars resulting in diabetic ketoacidosis (DKA). The health care team initiated a medication regimen to safely manage the DKA and also prevent a stroke from the injury.

The nurse noted that, over time, Dana became increasingly agitated in the ED with repetitive neurological assessments, fingersticks for bedside glucose levels, and the noises and high activity level of the ED. Establishing physical and psychological safety for both Dana and staff became a nursing priority during Dana's time in the ED.

Following trauma-informed care (TIC) guidelines to create a safe environment, the nurse asked Dana, "What do you need to feel safe here right now?" Dana immediately responded, "I can't have all these people coming at me. It's too much – too much noise, too many people touching me, it's just too much." The nurse moved Dana out of the trauma bay, which was near the ambulance entryway, and into a room where the nurse was able to close the door. The nurse also posted signage on the door asking all staff and visitors to contact the nurse before entering the room. Following agency protocol, the nurse swiftly gained Dana's consent for anonymity, meaning the client's name and room number(s) would not be shared with anyone outside of the hospital. Following these nursing actions, Dana's anxiety and agitation levels dropped noticeably in the ED. When an ICU bed became available, she was transferred there for medical management.

Dana was present during the handoff report from the ED nurse to the ICU nurse to validate information and it also improved Dana's sense of safety. Following the TIC cue given by the ED nurse, the ICU nurse asked Dana, "What else do you need to feel safe here right now?" Dana requested a private room, if available, to rest, listen to music, and "stay calm." The ICU nurses implemented a safety plan that included consistent staff and coordinated, clustered care. This plan minimized disturbances, thereby providing dedicated periods for rest between timed blood glucose monitoring and nursing monitoring of Dana's neurologic state and neck swelling.

---

1 Dowdell, E., & Speck, P. (2022). Trauma-informed care in nursing practice. *American Journal of Nursing, 122*(4), 30-38. https://journals.lww.com/ajnonline/Fulltext/2022/04000/CE__Trauma_Informed_Care_in_Nursing_Practice.22.aspx

My Notes

While in the ICU, the nurses taught Dana evidence-based methods for reducing anxiety, including deep breathing, grounding techniques, and moderating anxiety-provoking stimuli such as social media and electronics. In addition, the nurses noted the vocal and nonverbal cues that indicated Dana was feeling anxious, such as speaking in a raised voice or using rapid hand movements while speaking. Noticing these behaviors allowed nurses to ask follow-up questions such as "Do you feel safe at this moment?" and then review anxiety-reducing techniques by asking Dana, "Which technique would you like to use now?" By offering person-centered choices and creating a predictable structure around clustered nursing actions, the nurses promoted a feeling of safety for Dana, as well as techniques to self-regulate anxiety.

The health care team identified Dana's priority health concerns as DKA management and decreasing the risk for a stroke following nonfatal carotid trauma. The nursing team added Dana's increased risk for subsequent fatal strangulation as a priority concern that must be addressed before discharge. However, when asked by the nurses, "What is important to you to include in your discharge plan?" Dana identified the priorities of finding safe housing and employment with fair pay. Therefore, the nursing team recommended that upon discharge, Dana would transfer directly to community wraparound services for a variety of assistance, including transitional housing, job training, day care, medical care, and cognitive behavioral therapy.

Reflective Questions

1. What actions did the nurses perform with Dana to implement Trauma-Informed Care (TIC)?
2. What other actions do you plan to implement with your patients regarding TIC?
3. "Dana" could be a male or a female, and Dana's "partner" could be a male or a female. Do gender differences or sexual orientation affect your attitudes toward Dana's risks and follow-up care?
4. How might Dana's children be affected by Dana's ongoing abuse?
5. What if Dana's partner showed up at the hospital with a gun threatening to kill Dana? How would you respond as a nurse to keep yourself, other patients, and staff safe?

15.8 LEARNING ACTIVITIES

My Notes

Interactive Activities

An interactive H5P element has been excluded from this version of the text. You can view it online here: https://wtcs.pressbooks.pub/nursingmhcc/?p=1042#h5p-51

An interactive H5P element has been excluded from this version of the text. You can view it online here: https://wtcs.pressbooks.pub/nursingmhcc/?p=1042#h5p-50

An interactive H5P element has been excluded from this version of the text. You can view it online here: https://wtcs.pressbooks.pub/nursingmhcc/?p=1042#h5p-52

My Notes

XV GLOSSARY

Adults at risk: Adults who have a physical or mental condition that impairs their ability to care for their own needs.

Adverse childhood experiences (ACE): Traumatic experiences during childhood such as neglect, abuse, or witnessing violence, substance abuse, mental illness, divorce, or imprisonment of a family member.

Caregiver: A person who has taken responsibility for all or part of an individual's care.

Dissociation: A break in how the mind handles information, causing a person's disconnection from their thoughts, feelings, memories, and surroundings.

Elder abuse: An intentional act or failure to act that causes or creates a risk of harm to an older adult aged 60 or older.

Emotional abuse: Verbal or nonverbal behaviors that inflict anguish, mental pain, fear, or distress, such as humiliation or disrespect, verbal and nonverbal threats, harassment, and geographic or interpersonal isolation.

Financial abuse: The illegal, unauthorized, or improper use of money, benefits, belongings, property, or assets for the benefit of someone other than the individual.

Individual trauma: Trauma resulting from an event, series of events, or set of circumstances that is experienced by an individual as physically or emotionally harmful or life-threatening and can have lasting adverse effects on their functioning and mental, physical, social, emotional, or spiritual well-being. Adverse childhood experiences are examples of individual traumas.

Intimate partner violence (IPV): Abuse or aggression that occurs in a romantic relationship. IPV can include physical violence, sexual violence, stalking, or psychological aggression.

Mandated reporters: Nurses and other professionals required by state law to report suspected neglect or abuse of children, adults at risk, and the elderly they see in the course of their professional duties.

Neglect: When a parent or caregiver fails, refuses, or is unable, for reasons other than poverty, to provide the necessary care, food, clothing, or medical or dental care, which seriously endangers the physical health of a child or vulnerable adult.

Physical abuse: Injury inflicted on a child or vulnerable adult by other than accidental means. Physical injury includes, but is not limited to, lacerations, fractured bones, burns, internal injuries, severe or frequent bruising, or great bodily harm.

Resilience: The ability to rise above circumstances or meet challenges with fortitude. Resilience includes the process of using available resources to negotiate hardship and/or the consequences of adverse events.

Resilient zone: A healthy balance of stimulation by the sympathetic nervous system (SNS) and parasympathetic nervous system (PNS).

Safety plan: A set of actions that can help lower the risk of a person being hurt by an abusive partner that includes specific information and resources that increases their safety at school, home, and other places visited regularly.

Sexual abuse: Sexual intercourse or sexual touching; sexual exploitation; human trafficking; forced viewing of sexual activity; or permitting, allowing, or encouraging prostitution with a child or vulnerable adult.

Teen dating violence: Intimate partner violence that occurs during adolescence.

Trauma-informed care (TIC): A strengths-based framework that acknowledges the prevalence and impact of traumatic events in clinical practice, placing an emphasis on instilling in patients a sense of safety, control, and autonomy over their life and health care decisions. The basic goals of TIC are to avoid retraumatization; emphasize survivor strengths and resilience; aid empowerment, healing, and recovery; and promote the development of survivorship skills.

My Notes

Workplace violence: Physically and psychologically damaging actions that occur in the workplace or while on duty. Examples of workplace violence include direct physical assaults (with or without weapons), written or verbal threats, physical or verbal harassment, and homicide.

Chapter 16

Community Assessment

16.1 INTRODUCTION

My Notes

Learning Objectives

- Describe the characteristics of a healthy community
- Outline the roles of community health nurses and key community settings where they have an interprofessional role in health care services
- Explain resources and tools to use for community health needs assessments
- Apply the nursing process to community health nursing
- Define categories of preventative nursing interventions
- Explain how community resources help support the health needs of the members of the community

Most of your nursing education journey has likely focused on caring for clients in hospitals and long-term care settings. However, nurses also serve important roles in promoting the health and wellness of communities. Throughout history, nurses have served in public health roles and collaborated with community organizations to support health services. Florence Nightingale, the founder of modern nursing, advocated for two foundational components of community health nursing: health promotion and disease prevention.[1] Examples of current community health initiatives include public educational health sessions, blood pressure screenings, immunization clinics, and crisis intervention related to mental health care. See Figure 16.1[2] for an image of a community blood pressure screening.

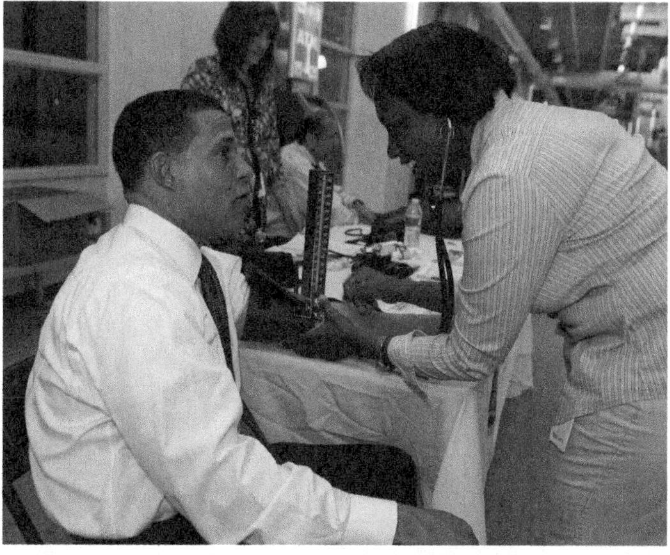

Figure 16.1 Community Health Screening

---

1 McDonald, L. (2006). *Florence Nightingale and public health policy: Theory, activism and public administration.* University of Guelph. https://cwfn.uoguelph.ca/nursing-health-care/fn-and-public-health-policy/

2 "7315182496_0cd3e18ed6_k" by Maryland GovPics is licensed under CC BY 2.0

My Notes

In recent years community health nursing has become increasingly important for several reasons:

- There are currently shorter hospital stays and decreasing hospital readmission rates.
- As the average age of the United States population increases, the need for community health services in members' homes increases.
- As the ability to successfully manage chronic conditions (including both physical and mental illness) improves, the need for outpatient health services also increases.
- As the usage of telehealth and virtual medical care expands, so does the need for community member support and patient education.

This chapter will introduce the roles of community health nurses, explore community health needs assessments, and discuss how nurses collaborate with community resources to support clients' physical and mental health care needs.

16.2 COMMUNITY HEALTH CONCEPTS

My Notes

Community Health Nursing

Nurses working in a community setting include public health nurses, school nurses, and parish nurses to name a few.

Public health nurses work across various settings in the community such as government agencies, community-based centers, shelters, and vaccine distribution sites. They provide disease prevention and health promotion services, such as working with mothers and children to improve nutrition, operating immunization clinics, and leading public health education initiatives such as smoking cessation campaigns. Public health nurses also prepare to respond quickly to public health emergencies such as natural disasters or epidemics.[1,2] Emergency preparedness is further discussed in the "Environmental Health and Emergency Preparedness" chapter. See Figure 16.2[3] for an image of a community health nurse providing health screenings in a maternal and child health clinic.

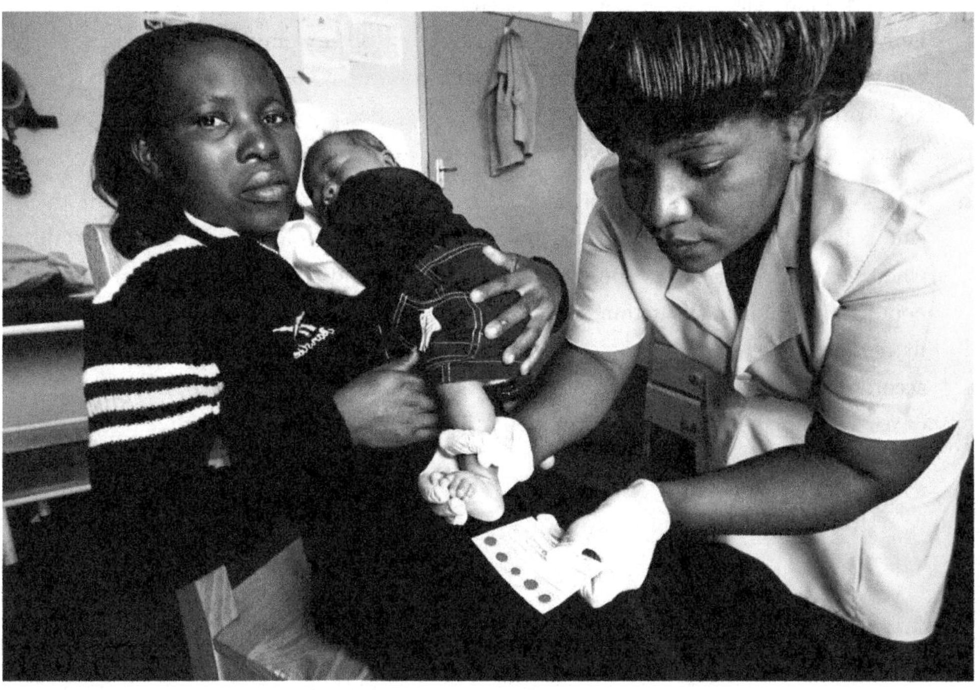

Figure 16.2 Health Screenings

School nurses work with over 56 million school-age children and adolescents. They provide direct care for chronic health problems and administer medications prescribed during school hours. They also provide mental health care, a need that has grown during the COVID-pandemic. Their work also affects the larger community. For

1 Greenwood, B. (2018, June 29). *What are the primary roles of the community nurse?* CHRON. https://work.chron.com/primary-roles-community-nurse-15144.html

2 National Academy of Medicine. (2021, May). *The future of nursing 2020-2030: Charting a path to achieve health equity* [Report]. https://www.phnurse.org/assets/docs/FON%20Valuing%20Community%20and%20Public%20Health%20Nursing.pdf

3 "PIXNIO-45563-3000x2000" by USAID on Pixnio is licensed under CC0

My Notes

example, school nurses may help develop disaster plans that coordinate activities in the school with the larger neighborhood.[4,5]

Parish nurses use their nursing skills for church or parish members in paid or volunteer positions. They provide health education, screening, advocacy, and referrals to other services in the community.[6]

Barriers for Community Health Nurses

Community health nurses serve important roles in identifying priority health needs of a community, as well as planning and implementing preventative health initiatives. However, community health nurses may face unique barriers when providing care to individuals, families, and community members. Three barriers are referred to as gaining entry, role negotiation, and confidentiality:

- **Gaining Entry:** Community health nurses may be considered "outsiders" as representatives of the established health care system and may not necessarily be trusted by community members. It is vital for community health nurses to build trust and supportive relationships. When working with individuals and families, nurses should assess specific community issues affecting that individual's health or their access to health care and then address those issues in their nursing care plan. Nurses can also investigate if there are community resources available to refer the client and/or their family members for additional services. See Figure 16.3[7] for an image of Red Cross volunteers working with caregivers of clients receiving palliative care.
- **Role Negotiation and Confidentiality:** Community health nurses must separate their roles as data collectors, health professionals, and neighbors. These roles can be difficult to differentiate when the nurse is assessing community health needs and providing nursing interventions for a population of individuals within their own home community. These individuals may include family members, friends, neighbors, or peers. Trust must be established and confidentiality assured according to legal and ethical parameters of nursing practice. Nurses should also establish a sense of partnership and encourage clients to participate in planning preventative health strategies for themselves and their families.

---

4 Greenwood, B. (2018, June 29). *What are the primary roles of the community nurse?* CHRON. https://work.chron.com/primary-roles-community-nurse-15144.html

5 National Academy of Medicine. (2021, May). *The future of nursing 2020-2030: Charting a path to achieve health equity* [Report]. https://www.phnurse.org/assets/docs/FON%20Valuing%20Community%20and%20Public%20Health%20Nursing.pdf

6 Greenwood, B. (2018, June 29). *What are the primary roles of the community nurse?* CHRON. https://work.chron.com/primary-roles-community-nurse-15144.html

7 "10716898813_74292ef548_k" by Department of Foreign Affairs and Trade is licensed under CC BY 2.0

My Notes

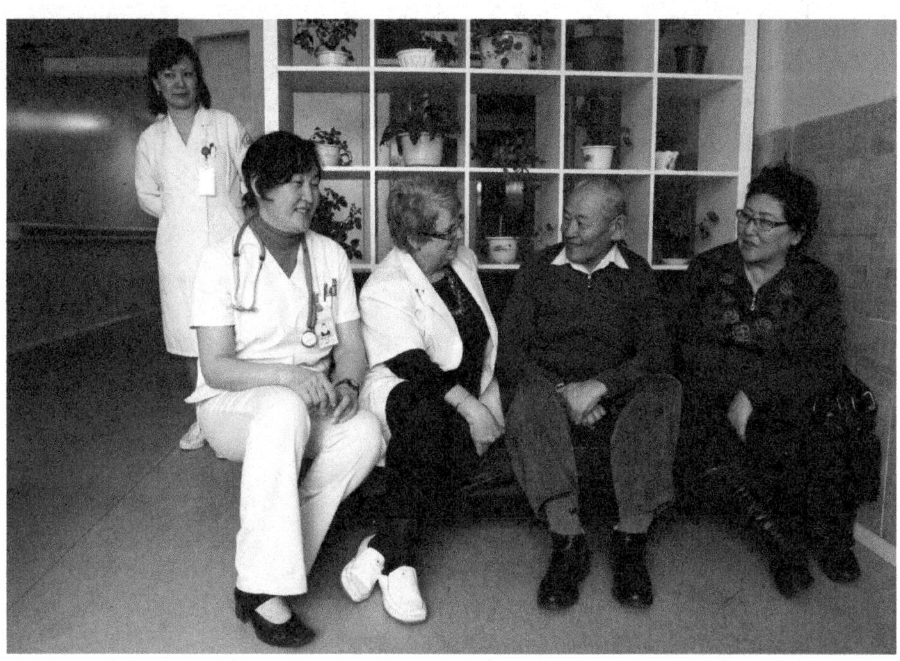

Figure 16.3 Setting Up Support Groups for Caregivers

Community Health

Community health nursing is based on several underlying concepts such as encouraging healthy living, preventing illness, promoting rehabilitation, evaluating the effectiveness of community resources, and advocating for improved overall community health.[8][9] In this manner, community health nurses pursue health equity. **Health equity** means that everyone has a fair and just opportunity to be as healthy as possible. This requires removing potential obstacles to obtaining and maintaining optimal health such as lack of access to health care services, good jobs with fair pay, quality education and housing, and safe environments.[10] Community health nurses address these conditions that are also known as social determinants of health.

Social determinants of health (SDOH) are the conditions in which people are born, grow, work, live, and age. Research shows that the SDOH can be more important than health care or lifestyle choices in influencing health and account for 30-55% of health outcomes.[11] See an illustration of SDOH in Figure 16.4.[12] SDOH can contrib-

---

8 Greenwood, B. (2018, June 29). *What are the primary roles of the community nurse?* CHRON. https://work.chron.com/primary-roles-community-nurse-15144.html

9 National Academy of Medicine. (2021, May). *The future of nursing 2020-2030: Charting a path to achieve health equity* [Report]. https://www.phnurse.org/assets/docs/FON%20Valuing%20Community%20and%20Public%20Health%20Nursing.pdf

10 Braveman, P., Arkin, E., Orleans, T., Proctor, D., & Plough, A. (2017, May 1). *What is health equity?* Robert Wood Johnson Foundation. https://www.rwjf.org/en/library/research/2017/05/what-is-health-equity-.html

11 World Health Organization. (n.d.). *Social determinants of health.* https://www.who.int/health-topics/social-determinants-of-health#tab=tab_1

12 "Healthy People 2030 SDOH Graphic.png" by U.S. Department of Health and Human Services, Office of Disease Prevention and Health Promotion is in the Public Domain. Access for free at https://health.gov/healthypeople/objectives-and-data/social-determinants-health

My Notes

ute to **health inequities**, defined as avoidable differences in health status seen within and between communities. In countries at all levels of income, health and illness follow a social gradient: the lower the socioeconomic position, the worse the health. According to the World Health Organization, SDOH can influence health equity in positive and negative ways[13]:

- Income and social protection
- Education
- Unemployment and job insecurity
- Working life conditions
- Food insecurity
- Housing, basic amenities, and the environment
- Early childhood development
- Social inclusion and nondiscrimination
- Structural conflict
- Access to affordable health services of decent quality

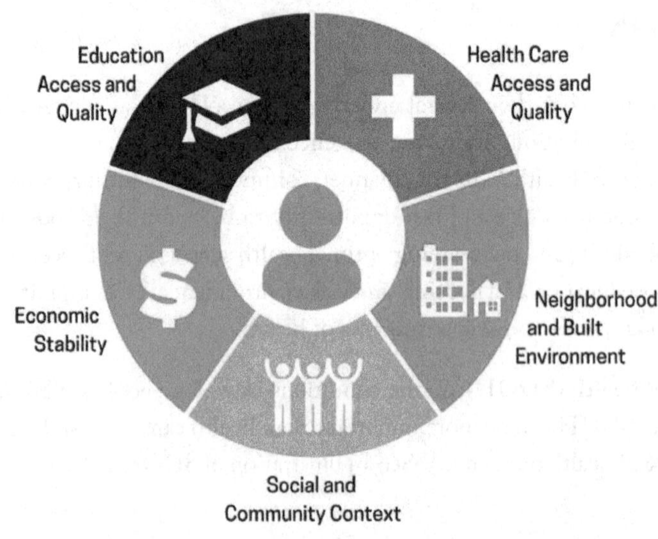

Figure 16.4 Social Determinants of Health

Health disparities are health differences that are linked with social, economic, and/or environmental disadvantages. Health disparities adversely affect groups of people who often experience greater obstacles to health based

---

13 World Health Organization. (n.d.). *Social determinants of health.* https://www.who.int/health-topics/social-determinants-of-health#tab=tab_1

on individual characteristics such as socioeconomic status, age, gender, culture, religion, mental illness, disability, sexual orientation, or gender identity.[14] These groups are often referred to as "vulnerable groups," and their care is further discussed in the "Vulnerable Populations" chapter.

As community health nurses strive to promote health equity, they assess SDOH, health disparities, and health inequities that are present in communities. They often begin by analyzing the context of the community because these characteristics can affect how community members respond to public health initiatives. The context of a community includes the following factors:

- **Physical aspects:** What geographical and man-made structures exist within the community? How do they shape the community's access to health care and other institutions within the community? How do they shape the community health nurse's access to the community members?
    - For example, is this a rural community that requires long-distance transportation to health care services?
- **Infrastructure:** In what condition are the local roads, bridges, and highways? Is there public transportation available for community members to use to access health care services, grocery stores, schools, and other institutions providing basic needs? Do members of the community have access to the Internet, electricity, landline phones, cellular phone towers, and other technology?
    - For example, are there buses or ride share services available for members to reach health care services?
- **Patterns of settlement, commerce, and industry:** How are residential and commercial areas located in the community? Are some residential areas located next to heavy industry? Are there areas of the community with higher crime rates? Are there areas defined by economic status within the community?
    - For example, is there an area of the community located next to a factory contributing to air pollution?
- **Demographics:** What are the ages, gender, sexual orientation, race, ethnicity, marital status, education, and first language of the members of the community? What is the average number of people living in a household in the community?
    - For example, is there an area where it is common for several multi-generation family members to live together in one residence?
- **History:** What local long- and short-term history affects the population of the community? What makes the community proud? What events in the community have helped shape the identity of the community members?
    - For example, do public parks commemorate war veterans?
- **Community leaders, both informal and formal:** Who are the elected officials in the community, and what are their roles and relationships to the members of the community? Are there other informal leaders, such as church leaders, academic leaders, corporate CEOs, community activists,

---

14 HealthyPeople.gov. (2022, February 6). *Disparities.* Office of Disease Prevention and Health Promotion, U.S. Department of Health and Human Services. https://www.healthypeople.gov/2020/about/foundation-health-measures/Disparities

My Notes

medical professionals, or others who serve an important role in the community? What are their roles and relationships to those in the community?

- For example, what relationships do the school board members have with community members?

- **Community culture, both informal and formal:** What are the spoken and unspoken rules and traditions of the community?
  - For example, does the community have a tradition of celebrating Memorial Day with a parade and public tributes at a local cemetery?
- **Existing groups and organizations:** What adult, youth, and community groups and organizations exist that can be used to help build alliances and collaboration within the community?
  - For example, is there a YMCA or other services in the community that promote physical activities for youth and other members of the community?
- **Existing institutions:** Where are the hospitals, medical care facilities, educational institutions, libraries, and religious institutions that serve the community? Are they accessible by public transportation? Who are the leaders in these institutions?
  - For example, is there an urgent care clinic in this community that can be accessed by bus service?
- **Economics:** Where do most of the community members work? Do any businesses or industries form a base industry in the community? How is wealth distributed? What is the community's average economic status: wealthy, upper middle class, working class, or poor?
  - For example, is this a working class community whose members primarily work in a few local factories?
- **Government/Politics:** Are political leaders highly influential in the community? How do they serve their role in relationship to the members of the community? Does political power lie with others in the community?
  - For example, how does the mayor of this city communicate with members of the community?
- **Social structure:** How do community members relate to one another on a routine basis? How are problems solved (or not solved) within the community? What symbols of respect and social relationships are evident?
  - For example, is there a town board that meets regularly and collaboratively makes decisions affecting planning and zoning of the community?
- **Attitudes and values:** What does the community care about? What issues does it ignore? What assumptions can be observed about how community members believe people should relate to one another, dress, communicate, do business, or treat one another? Is there evidence of discrimination of a particular group of individuals within the community? What norms exist for interacting with members of the community who look or behave "differently" than others?
  - For example, is it assumed in this community that neighbors will help clean up the neighborhood after storm damage occurs to several homes?

My Notes

According to the CDC, a **healthy community** is one in which local groups from all parts of the community work together to prevent disease and make healthy living options accessible. Working at the community level to promote healthy living brings the greatest health benefits to the greatest number of people. It also helps to reduce health gaps caused by differences in income, education, race and ethnicity, location, and other factors that can affect health.[15]

Community Health Needs Assessment

Community health needs assessment is a systematic process to identify and analyze community health needs and assets in order to prioritize these needs, plan, and act upon significant unmet community health needs.[16] A community health assessment gives nurses and community organizations comprehensive information about the community's current health status, needs, and issues. This information can be used to develop a community health improvement plan by justifying how and where resources should be allocated to best meet community needs.[17] Community health needs assessments are performed and reported at national, state, county, and local levels.

National Health Needs Assessments

Healthy People 2030 addresses the most current national public health priorities. It is published by the United States Department of Health and Human Services Office of Disease Prevention and Promotion. See Figure 16.5[18] for an illustration related to using Healthy People 2030 objectives and leading health indicators to assess community needs data, plan, and evaluate community health interventions.

---

15 Centers for Disease Control and Prevention. (2015, September 18). *A healthy community is a prepared community.* [Blog]. https://blogs.cdc.gov/publichealthmatters/2015/09/a-healthy-community-is-a-prepared-community/

16 Vigna, A. J. (2020). *The 2019 behavioral health gaps report for the state of Wisconsin.* University of Wisconsin Population Health Institute. https://uwphi.pophealth.wisc.edu/publications-2/evaluation-reports-2/

17 VHA Inc., & Healthy Communities Institute. (2013). *Assessing & addressing community health needs.* Catholic Heart Association of the United States. https://www.chausa.org/docs/default-source/general-files/cb_assessingaddressing-pdf.pdf?sfvrsn=4

18 "HP2030_HowtoUse_Screen1_2020-03-24.png" by unknown author for U.S. Department of Health and HumanServices is in the Public Domain. Access for free at https://health.gov/our-work/national-health-initiatives/healthy-people/healthy-people-2030/promoting-healthy-people-2030

My Notes

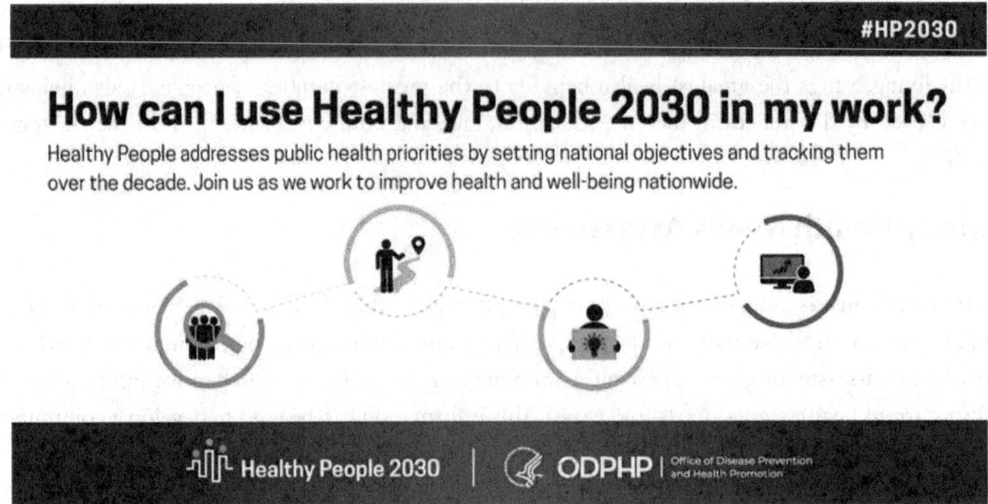

Figure 16.5 Healthy People 2030

A set of evidence-based Healthy People objectives is published every ten years based on current national data. Objectives are classified by categories[19]:

- Health Conditions
- Health Behaviors
- Populations
- Settings and Systems
- Social Determinants of Health

Examples of Healthy People 2030 community objectives include the following[20]:

- Increase the number of community organizations that provide preventative services
- Increase the rate of bystander CPR and AED use for nontraumatic cardiac arrests in public places
- Increase the proportion of adult stroke survivors who participate in rehabilitation services

Leading Health Indicators (LHIs) are a subset of high-priority Healthy People 2030 objectives to drive action toward improving health and well-being. Most LHIs address important factors that impact major causes of death and disease in the United States. They help organizations, communities, and community health nurses focus their resources and efforts to improve the health and well-being of all people. There are 23 LHIs that cover the life span from infants, children, adolescents, adults, and older adults. See a list of LHIs in Table 16.2.

19 Office of Disease Prevention and Health Promotion. *Healthy People 2030: Building a healthier future for all.* U.S. Department of Health and Human Services. https://health.gov/healthypeople

20 Office of Disease Prevention and Health Promotion. *Healthy People 2030: Building a healthier future for all.* U.S. Department of Health and Human Services. https://health.gov/healthypeople

My Notes

Table 16.2 Leading Health Indicators Across the Life Span

Life Stage	Leading Health Indicator
Infant	■ Infant Death
Children and Adolescents	■ 4th grade students whose reading skills are at or above the proficient achievement level for their grade ■ Adolescents with major depressive episodes (MDEs) who receive treatment ■ Children and adolescents with obesity ■ Current use of any tobacco products among adolescents
Adults and Older Adults	■ Adults engaging in binge drinking of alcoholic beverages during the past 30 days ■ Adults who meet current minimum guidelines for aerobic physical activity and muscle-strengthening activity ■ Adults who receive a colorectal cancer screening based on the most recent guidelines ■ Adults with hypertension whose blood pressure is under control ■ Cigarette smoking in adults ■ Employment among the working-age population ■ Maternal deaths ■ New cases of diagnosed diabetes in the population
All Ages	■ Children, adolescents, and adults who use the oral health care system (2+ years) ■ Consumption of calories from added sugars by persons aged 2 years and over ■ Drug overdose deaths ■ Exposure to unhealthy air ■ Homicides ■ Household food insecurity and hunger ■ Persons who are vaccinated annually against seasonal influenza ■ Persons who know their HIV status (13+ years) ■ Persons with medical insurance (<65 years) ■ Suicides

My Notes

Healthy People 2030 Resources

View Healthy People 2030 Objectives, Community Objectives, and Leading Health Indicators.

State Needs Assessments

States perform health needs assessments to develop state funding and program priorities for community health. For example, the Wisconsin Department of Health Services (DHS) performs a mental health and substance abuse needs assessment every other year. Data in this report include the following:

- **Prevalence of Needs:** The prevalence of disorders, conditions, and associated problems for the entire population and subpopulations
- **Access to Services:** Determination of which and how many services are received by individuals and exploration of barriers to access
- **Service Workforce and Capacity:** Examination of the mental health and substance use services workforce, including the number of providers of these services and the geographic dispersion of the workforce across the state

Another example of a state needs assessment related to mental health is the Behavioral Health Gaps Study funded by the Wisconsin DHS to assess gaps and needs in the behavioral health service system for individuals with mental health and substance use disorders. Key gaps documented in this study included shortages in child and geriatric psychiatrists; shortages in mental health inpatient beds and residential facilities for treating substance use; inadequacies of the medical transportation system; a need for improving crisis stabilization services in the community that focus on reducing contact with police officers; shortages in medication-assisted treatment providers and clinics; long waitlists across the service array; shortages in competent translation services; and the need to provide wraparound services, particularly for consumers with families.[21]

Explore your state's health needs assessments. Examples of health needs assessments in the state of Wisconsin are as follows:

Department of Health Service's Mental Health and Substance Abuse Needs Assessment PDF

The Behavioral Health Gaps Report for the State of Wisconsin PDF completed by University of Wisconsin-Madison Population Health Institute

County Health Rankings

County health rankings are created annually by the University of Wisconsin Population Health Institute for counties across the country.[22] These rankings provide a snapshot of a community's health and can be used as

---

21 Vigna, A. J. (2020). *The 2019 behavioral health gaps report for the state of Wisconsin.* University of Wisconsin Population Health Institute. https://uwphi.pophealth.wisc.edu/publications-2/evaluation-reports-2/

22 Vigna, A. J. (2020). *The 2019 behavioral health gaps report for the state of Wisconsin.* University of Wisconsin Population Health Institute. https://uwphi.pophealth.wisc.edu/publications-2/evaluation-reports-2/

My Notes

a starting point for implementing change to promote health equity in communities. See the following box to explore the health ranking for your community.

> Visit the Explore Health Rankings web page from the University of Wisconsin Population Health Institute to view the health ranking of your community.

Local Needs Assessments

Local communities perform health needs assessments and develop specific health initiatives for their community members. For example, the Eau Claire County Health Department Needs Assessment was used to create a county health plan. In 2021 the top health priorities were documented as drug use, mental health, alcohol misuse, obesity, and healthy nutrition. See Figure 16.6[23] with an image related to data from a county mental health needs assessment.

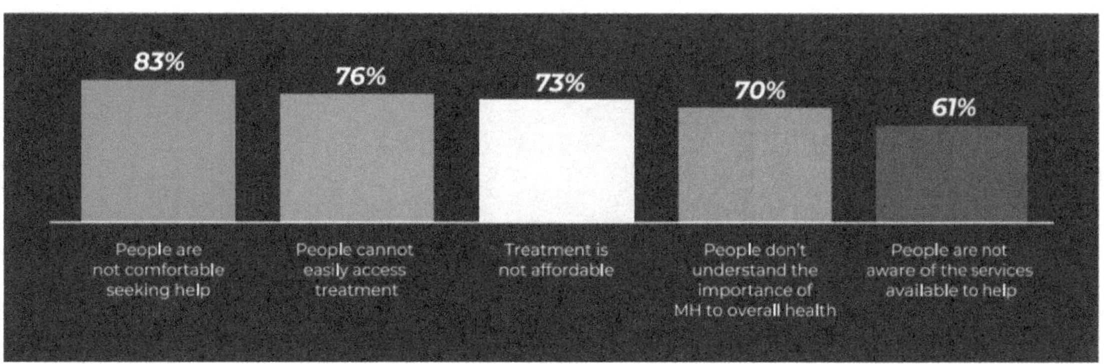

Figure 16.6 Mental Health Assessment

> Explore your community's health initiatives. View the example of Eau Claire City-County Health Department Needs Assessment.

Hospitals' Community Health Needs Assessments

Tax-exempt hospitals are required to conduct community health needs assessments according to the Patient Protection and Affordable Care Act (i.e., the Affordable Care Act). Hospitals are required to adopt implementation strategies to meet the community health needs identified through their needs assessment. This collaboration among hospitals and community partners expands the community's capacity to address health needs through a shared vision and creates a foundation for coordinated efforts to improve community health.[24]

---

23 This image is derived from 2021 Eau Claire County Community Health Assessment by Community Health Assessment Planning Partnership Committee and is in the Public Domain

24 VHA Inc., & Healthy Communities Institute. (2013). *Assessing & addressing community health needs.* Catholic Heart Association of the United States. https://www.chausa.org/docs/default-source/general-files/cb_assessingaddressing-pdf .pdf?sfvrsn=4

My Notes

View examples of hospitals' community health needs assessments:

- Mayo Clinic's Community Health Needs Assessment PDF
- Community Health Needs Assessments by HSHS Affiliated Hospitals in Wisconsin and Illinois

16.3 APPLYING THE NURSING PROCESS TO COMMUNITY HEALTH

My Notes

Community health nurses apply the nursing process to address needs of individuals, families, vulnerable populations, and entire communities. See Figure 16.7[1] for an illustration of the nursing process in community health nursing.

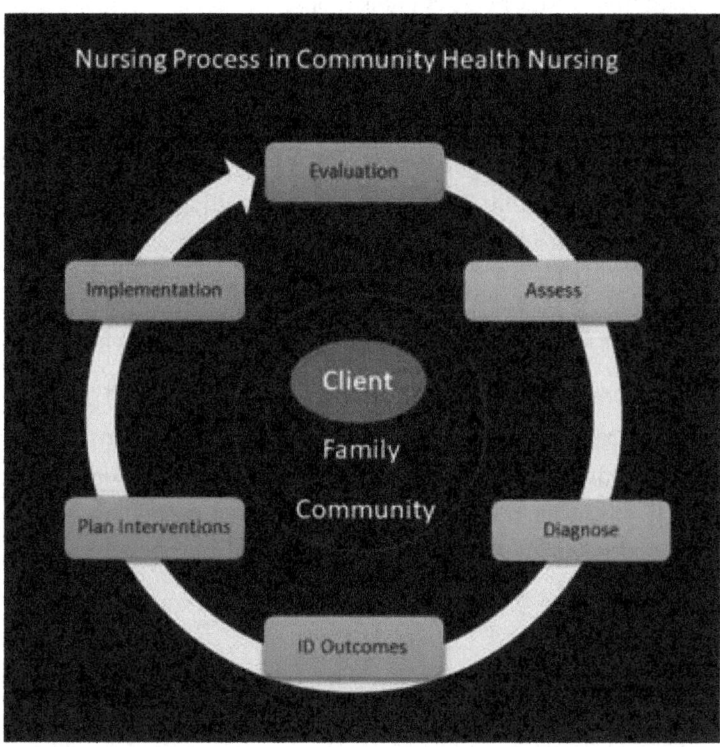

Figure 16.7 Nursing Process in Community Health Nursing

Assessment

The community health nurse typically begins a community health needs assessment by determining what data is already available.[2] As previously discussed in the "Community Health Concepts" section, national, state, county, and local health needs assessments are widely available. **Secondary analysis** refers to analyzing previously collected data to determine community needs.

Community health nurses may also engage in primary data collection to better understand the community needs and/or study who may be affected by actions taken as a result of the assessment.[3] **Primary data collection** includes tools such as public forums, focus groups, interviews, windshield surveys, surveys, and participant observation.

---

1 "Nursing Process in Community Health Nursing" by Open RN project is licensed under CC BY 4.0

2 *Community Tool Box* by Center for Community Health and Development at the University of Kansas is licensed under CC BY NC SA 3.0

3 *Community Tool Box* by Center for Community Health and Development at the University of Kansas is licensed under CC BY NC SA 3.0

My Notes

Public Forums

Public forums are gatherings where large groups of citizens discuss important issues at well-publicized locations and times. Forums give people of diverse backgrounds a chance to express their views and enhance understanding of the community's specific needs and resources. Forums should be planned in a convenient location with accessibility to public transportation and child care. They should also be scheduled at convenient times for working families to gain participation from a wide range of populations.

Focus Groups

Focus groups are a systematic method of data collection through small-group discussions led by a facilitator. Participants in focus groups are selected to represent a larger group of people. Groups of 6-10 people with similar backgrounds or interests are interviewed in an informal or formal setting. Focus groups should be scheduled at several dates and times to ensure a broad participation from members of the community. Here are advantages of focus groups:

- Community member involvement in assessing and planning community initiatives is encouraged.
- Different perceptions, values, and beliefs by community members are explored.
- Input can be obtained from specific subpopulations of the community. Example of subpopulations include young mothers caring for infants, individuals receiving home hospice care, individuals struggling to find housing, residents of the prison system, individuals coping with mental health disorders, or residents in group homes.

Interviews

Interviews are structured conversations with individuals who have experience, knowledge, or understanding about a particular topic or issue. **Key informant interviews** are conducted with people in key positions in the community and have specific areas of knowledge and experience. These interviews can be useful for exploring specific community problems and/or assessing a community's readiness to address those problems.[4]

Advantages of interviews include the following[5]:

- They can be conducted in a variety of settings (e.g., homes, schools, churches, stores, or community centers).
- They are low cost and generally have low dropout rates.
- Respondents define what is important from their perspective.
- It is possible to explore issues in depth, and there is an opportunity to clarify responses.
- They can provide leads to other data sources and key informants.
- They provide an opportunity to build partnerships with community members.
- Data can be compared among local government officials, citizens, and non-government leaders.

---

4 *A Guide to SAMHSA's Strategic Prevention Framework* by Substance Abuse and Mental Health Services Administration is available in the Public Domain

5 *A Guide to SAMHSA's Strategic Prevention Framework* by Substance Abuse and Mental Health Services Administration is available in the Public Domain

My Notes

Interviews can have these disadvantages:

- Interviews can be time-consuming to schedule and perform.
- They require trained interviewers.
- There is a potential for interviewer bias to affect the data collected during the interview.
- Rapport must be established before sensitive information is shared.
- It is more time-consuming to summarize and analyze findings.

Windshield Surveys

A **windshield survey** is a type of direct observation of community needs while driving and literally looking through the windshield. It can be used to observe characteristics of a community that impact health needs such as housing, pollution, parks and recreation areas, transportation, health and social services agencies, industries, grocery stores, schools, and religious institutions.

View a video: Windshield Survey Nursing.[6]

Surveys

Surveys use standardized questions that are relatively easy to analyze. They are beneficial for collecting information across a large geographic area, obtaining input from as many people as possible, and exploring sensitive topics.[7] Surveys can be conducted face to face, via the telephone, mailed, or shared on a website. Responses are typically anonymous but demographic information is often collected to focus on the needs of specific populations. Disadvantages of surveys can include the following[8]:

- Surveys can be time-consuming to design, implement, and analyze the results.
- The accuracy of survey results depends on who is surveyed and the size of the sample.
- Mailed surveys may have low response rates with higher costs due to postage.
- They offer little opportunity to explore issues in depth, and questions cannot be clarified.
- There is no opportunity to build rapport with respondents.

Participant Observation

Participant observation refers to nurses informally collecting data as a member of the community in which they live and work. This is considered a subjective observation because it is from the nurse's perspective. Informal observations are made, or discussions are elicited among peers and neighbors within the community.

---

6 Medrea, R. (2014, July 20). *Windshield survey nursing* [Video]. YouTube. All rights reserved. https://youtu.be/aAzW1bW_Dbw

7 McDonald, L. (2006). *Florence Nightingale and public health policy: Theory, activism and public administration.* University of Guelph. https://cwfn.uoguelph.ca/nursing-health-care/fn-and-public-health-policy/

8 *A Guide to SAMHSA's Strategic Prevention Framework* by Substance Abuse and Mental Health Services Administration is available in the Public Domain

My Notes

Sociocultural Considerations

When analyzing community health needs, it is essential to do so through a sociocultural lens. Just as an individual's health can be influenced by a wide variety of causes, community health problems are affected by various factors in the community. For example, a high rate of cancer in one community could be related to environmental factors such as pollution from local industry, but in another community, it may be related to the overall aging of the population. Both communities have a high rate of cancer, but the public health response would be very different. Another example related to mental health is related to various situational factors affecting depression. A high rate of depression in one community may be related to socioeconomic factors such as low-paying jobs, lack of support systems, and poor access to basic needs like grocery stores, whereas in another community it may be related to lack of community resources during frequent weather disasters. The public health response would be different for these two communities.

Nurses must also recognize and value cultural differences such as health beliefs, practices, and linguistic needs of diverse populations. They must take steps to identify subpopulations who are vulnerable to health disparities and further investigate the causes and potential interventions for these disparities. For example, mental health disparities pose a significant threat to vulnerable populations in our society, such as high rates of suicide among LGBTQ+ youth, reduced access to prevention services among people living in rural areas, and elevated rates of substance misuse among Native Americans. These disparities threaten the health and wellness of these populations.[9]

Key points to consider when assessing a community using a sociocultural lens include the following:

1. Have the trends of assessment data changed over time? What are the potential causes for these changes in this community?
2. How does the community's needs assessment data compare to similar communities at local, county, state, and national levels? What target goals and health initiatives have been successfully implemented in other communities?
3. What vulnerable subpopulations are part of this community, and what health disparities are they experiencing? What are potential causes and solutions for these health disparities?
4. Input from members of vulnerable subpopulations must be solicited regarding their perspectives on health disparities, as well as barriers they are experiencing in accessing health care.

Diagnosis

Similar to how nurses individualize nursing diagnoses for clients based on priority nursing problems identified during a head-to-toe assessment, community health nurses use community health needs assessment data to develop community health diagnoses. These diagnoses are broad, apply to larger groups of individuals, and address the priority health needs of the community. Resources such as Healthy People 2030 can be used to determine current public health priorities.

---

9 *A Guide to SAMHSA's Strategic Prevention Framework* by Substance Abuse and Mental Health Services Administration is available in the Public Domain

My Notes

A **community diagnosis** is a summary statement resulting from analysis of the data collected from a community health needs assessment.[10] A clear statement of the problem, as well as causes of the problem, should be included. A detailed community diagnosis helps guide community health initiatives that include nursing interventions.

A community diagnosis can address health deficits or services that support health in the community. A community diagnosis may also address a need for increased wellness in the community. Community diagnoses should include these four parts:

- The problem
- The population or vulnerable group
- The effects of the problem on the population/vulnerable group
- The indicators of the problem in this community

Here are some examples of community health diagnoses based on community health needs assessments:

- **Community Scenario A**
  - **Assessment data:** The local high school has had a 50% increase in the number of teen pregnancies in the past year, causing high school graduation rates to decrease due to pregnant students dropping out of high school.
  - **Community diagnosis:** Increased need for additional birth control and resources for prevention of pregnancy due to lack of current resources, as evidenced by 50% increase in teen pregnancies in the last year and a decrease in graduation rates.
- **Community Scenario B**
  - **Assessment data:** Fifty percent of residents of an assisted living facility were found to have blood pressure readings higher than 130/80 mmHg during a health fair last week at the facility.
  - **Community diagnosis:** Increased need for education about exercise and diet and referrals to primary care doctors for residents of an assisted living facility due to increased risk for mortality related to high blood pressure, as evidenced by a high number of residents with high blood pressure during a health fair.
- **Community Scenario C**
  - **Assessment data:** The local high school has had two cases of suicide in the past year.
  - **Diagnosis:** Increased need for community education regarding suicide prevention and crisis hotlines, as evidenced by an increase in adolescent suicide over the past twelve months.

Outcomes Identification

Outcomes refer to the changes in communities that nursing interventions and prevention strategies are intended to produce. Outcomes include broad overall goals for the community, as well as specific outcomes referred to as "SMART" outcomes that are specific, measurable, achievable, realistic, and with a timeline established.

---

10 Office of Disease Prevention and Health Promotion. *Healthy People 2030: Building a healthier future for all.* U.S. Department of Health and Human Services. https://health.gov/healthypeople

My Notes

Broad goals for communities can be tied to national objectives established by Healthy People 2030, as previously discussed in the "Community Health Concepts" section.

Healthy People objectives are classified by these five categories[11]:

- Health Conditions
- Health Behaviors
- Populations
- Settings and Systems
- Social Determinants of Health

SMART outcomes can be created based on the objectives listed under each category. For example, if an overall community goal is related to "Drug and Alcohol Use" under the "Health Behaviors" category, a SMART outcome could be based on the Healthy People objective, "Increase the proportion of people with a substance use disorder who got treatment in the past year."[12] Based on this Healthy People objective, an example of a SMART outcome could be the following:

- The proportion of people treated for a substance disorder in Smith County will increase to 14% within the next year.

View the Healthy People 2030 Objectives and Community Objectives.

Planning Interventions

Nursing interventions for the community can be planned based on the related Healthy People category and objective. For example, based on the sample SMART outcome previously discussed, a planned nursing intervention could be the following:

- The nurse will provide education and materials regarding evidence-based screening practices for substance use disorder in local clinics.

Community health nursing interventions typically focus on prevention of illness with health promotion interventions. After performing a community health needs assessment, identifying priority problems, and establishing health goals and SMART outcomes, the nurse integrates knowledge of health disorders (e.g., diabetes, cancer, obesity, or mental health disorders) and current health risks in a community to plan prevention interventions.

There are two common public health frameworks used to plan prevention interventions. A traditional preventive framework is based on primary, secondary, or tertiary prevention interventions. A second framework, often referred to as the Continuum of Care Prevention Model, was established by the Institute of Medicine (IOM) and

---

11 Office of Disease Prevention and Health Promotion. *Healthy People 2030: Building a healthier future for all.* U.S. Department of Health and Human Services. https://health.gov/healthypeople

12 Office of Disease Prevention and Health Promotion. *Healthy People 2030: Building a healthier future for all.* U.S. Department of Health and Human Services. https://health.gov/healthypeople

My Notes

includes universal, selected, and indicated prevention interventions. Both frameworks are further discussed in the following sections.[13]

Primordial, Primary, Secondary, Tertiary, and Quaternary Interventions

Preventive health interventions may include primordial, primary, secondary, tertiary, and quaternary prevention interventions. These strategies attempt to prevent the onset of disease, reduce complications of disease that develops, and promote quality of life.[14]

Primordial Prevention

Primordial prevention consists of risk factor reduction strategies focused on social and environmental conditions that affect vulnerable populations. In other words, primordial prevention interventions target underlying social determinants of health that can cause disease. These measures are typically promoted through laws and national policy. An example of a primordial prevention strategy is improving access to urban neighborhood playgrounds to promote physical activity in children and reduce their risk for developing obesity, diabetes, and cardiovascular disease.[15] See Figure 16.8[16] for an image of a neighborhood playground.

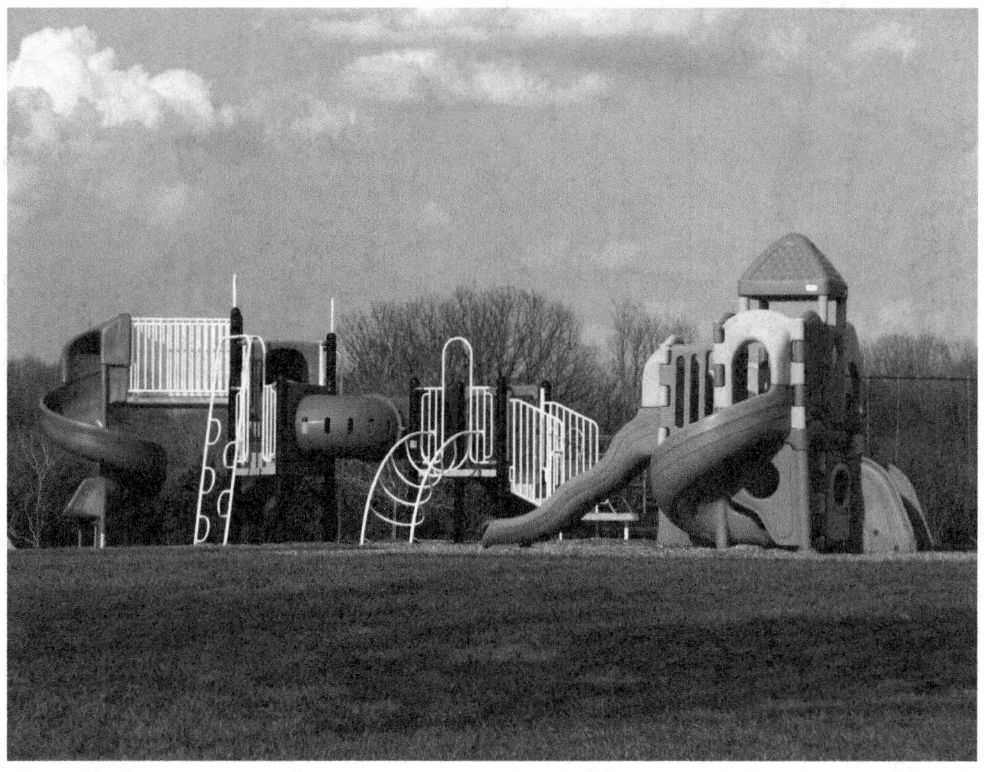

Figure 16.8 Primordial Prevention: Neighborhood Playgrounds

13 Savage, C. L. (2020). *Public/community health and nursing practice: Caring for populations* (2nd ed.). FA Davis.

14 This work is a derivative of *StatPearls* by Kisling and Das and is licensed under CC BY 4.0

15 This work is a derivative of *StatPearls* by Kisling and Das and is licensed under CC BY 4.0

16 "Playground_at_Hudson_Springs_Park.jpg" by Kevin Payravi is licensed under CC BY-SA 3.0

My Notes

Primary Prevention

Primary prevention consists of interventions aimed at susceptible populations or individuals to prevent disease from occurring. An example of primary prevention is immunizations.[17] Nursing primary prevention interventions also include public education and promotion of healthy behaviors.[18] See Figure 16.9[19] for an image of an immunization clinic sponsored by a student nurses' association.

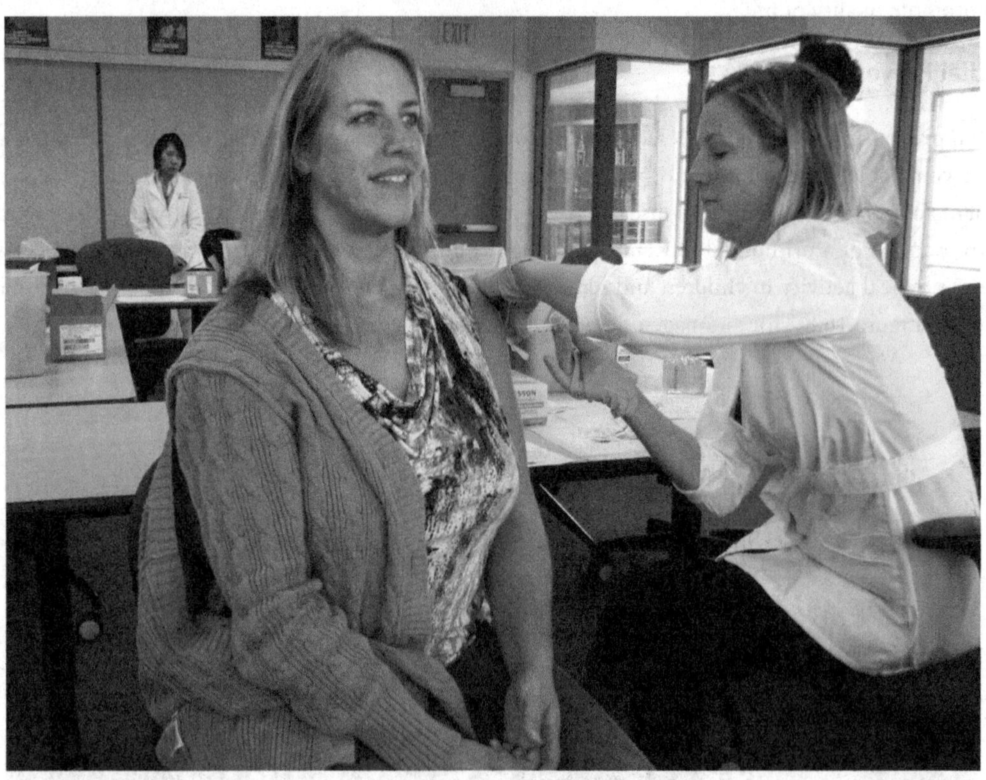

Figure 16.9 Primary Prevention: An Immunization Clinic

Secondary Prevention

Secondary prevention emphasizes early detection of disease and targets healthy-appearing individuals with subclinical forms of disease. Subclinical disease refers to pathologic changes with no observable signs or symptoms. Secondary prevention includes screenings such as annual mammograms, routine colonoscopies, Papanicolaou (Pap) smears, as well as screening for depression and substance use disorders[20]. Nurses provide education to community members about the importance of these screenings. See Figure 16.10[21] for an image of a mammogram.

---

17 This work is a derivative of *StatPearls* by Kisling and Das and is licensed under CC BY 4.0

18 Savage, C. L. (2020). *Public/community health and nursing practice: Caring for populations* (2nd ed.). FA Davis.

19 "10442934136_1f910af332_b" by Lower Columbia College (LCC) is licensed under CC BY_NC-ND 2.0

20 This work is a derivative of *StatPearls* by Kisling and Das and is licensed under CC BY 4.0

21 "US_Navy_021025-N-6498N-001_Mammogram_technician,_aids_a_patient_in_completing_her_annual_mam mogram_evaluation.jpg" by U.S. Navy photo by Ensign Ann-Marie Al Noad is in the Public Domain

My Notes

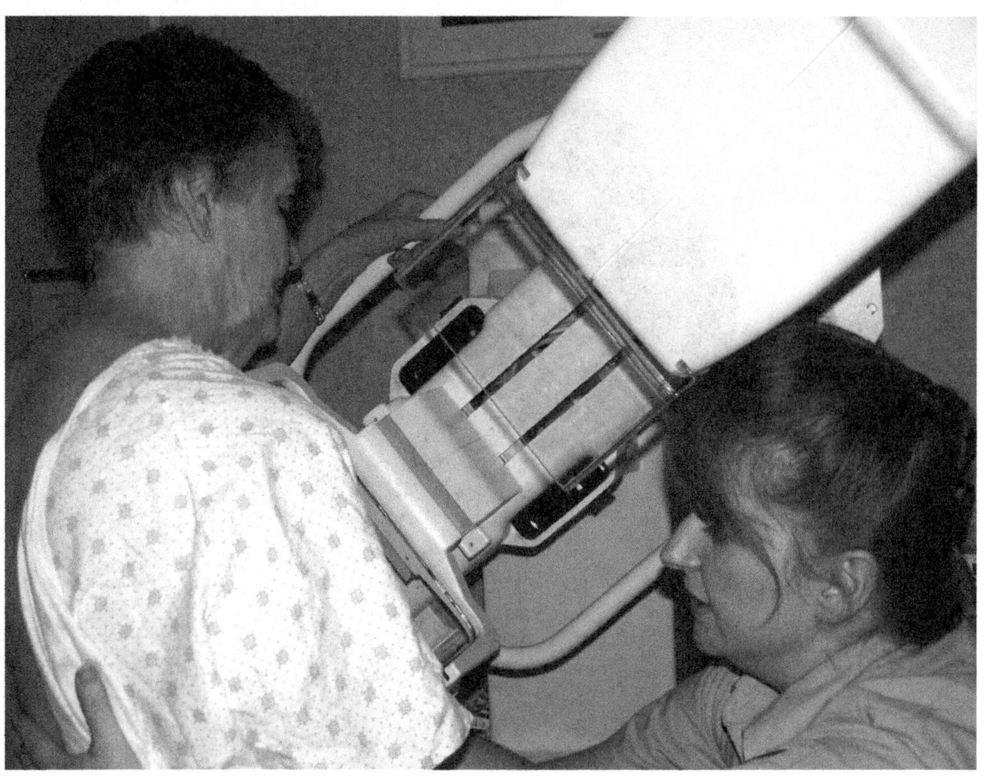

Figure 16.10 Secondary Prevention: Mammograms

Tertiary Prevention

Tertiary prevention is implemented for symptomatic clients to reduce the severity of the disease and potential long-term complications. While secondary prevention seeks to prevent the onset of illness, tertiary prevention aims to reduce the effects of the disease after it is diagnosed in an individual.[22] For example, rehabilitation therapy after an individual experiences a cerebrovascular accident (i.e., stroke) is an example of tertiary prevention. See Figure 16.11[23] for an image of a client receiving rehabilitation after experiencing a stroke.

The goals of tertiary prevention interventions are to reduce disability, promote curative therapy for a disease or injury, and prevent death. Nurses may be involved in providing ongoing home health services in clients' homes as a component of interprofessional tertiary prevention efforts. Health education to prevent the worsening or recurrence of disease is also provided by nurses.

22 This work is a derivative of *StatPearls* by Kisling and Das and is licensed under CC BY 4.0

23 "tech_zerog.jpg" by unknown author at Gaylord.org is included on the basis of Fair Use

My Notes

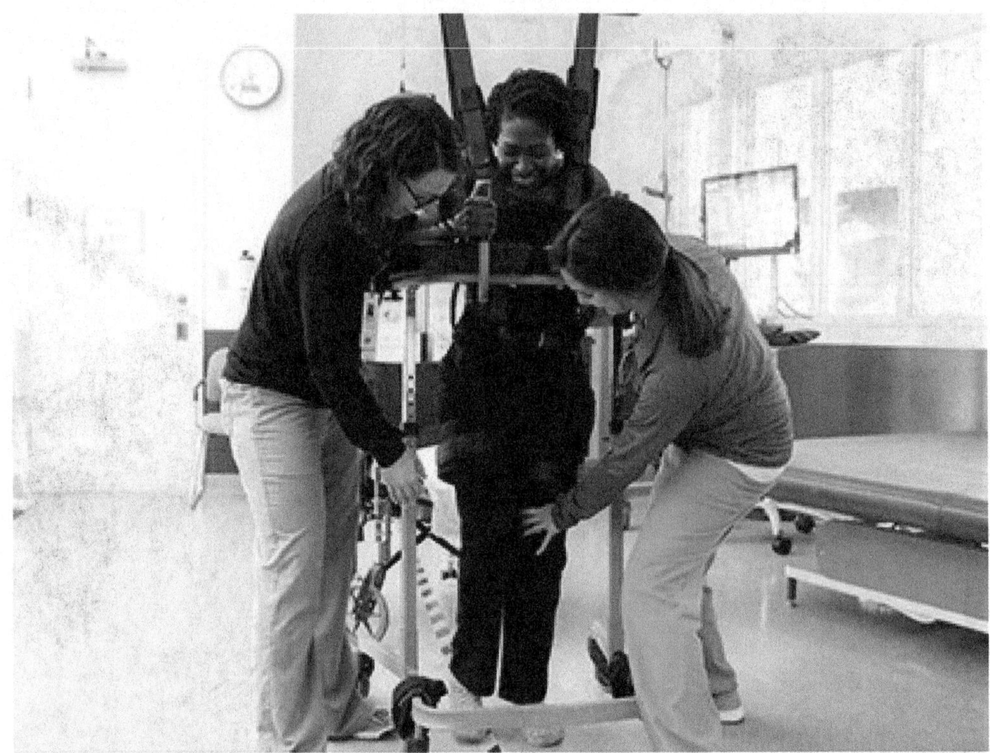

Figure 16.11 Tertiary Prevention: Post-Stroke Rehabilitation. Used under Fair Use.

Quaternary Prevention

Quaternary prevention refers to actions taken to protect individuals from medical interventions that are likely to cause more harm than good and to suggest interventions that are ethically acceptable. Targeted populations are those at risk of overmedicalization.[24] An example of quaternary prevention is encouraging clients with terminal illness who are approaching end of life to seek focus on comfort and quality of life and consider hospice care rather than undergo invasive procedures that will likely have no impact on recovery from disease.

See additional examples of primordial, primary, secondary, tertiary, and quaternary prevention strategies in Table 16.3a.

Table 16.3a Examples of Prevention Interventions[25,26]

Prevention Intervention Strategy	Examples
Primordial Prevention	■ Increased tax on cigarettes ■ Increased access to public walking paths and public parks

24 This work is a derivative of *StatPearls* by Kisling and Das and is licensed under CC BY 4.0

25 Savage, C. L. (2020). *Public/community health and nursing practice: Caring for populations* (2nd ed.). FA Davis.

26 This work is a derivative of *StatPearls* by Kisling and Das and is licensed under CC BY 4.0

My Notes

Prevention Intervention Strategy	Examples
Primary Prevention	■ Birthing and newborn classes for new parents at the local hospital ■ Television commercials regarding the importance of the influenza vaccines ■ Psychosocial health fairs in local malls or other public facilities ■ Tobacco cessation public education sessions ■ Television commercials about mindfulness classes at the community center
Secondary Prevention	■ Blood pressure screening events ■ Sexually transmitted disease screening in college students ■ Mammograms for early detection of breast cancer ■ Colonoscopies for early detection of colon cancer ■ Free testing for people exposed to another individual diagnosed with COVID-19 ■ Screening for substance abuse disorders in high schools ■ Screening for depression during annual physicals
Tertiary Prevention	■ Cardiac rehabilitation for individuals who have experienced a myocardial infarction ■ Occupational and physical therapy for individuals who experienced a cerebrovascular accident ■ Diabetic foot care provided at the local community center ■ Support groups for substance disorders in local churches
Quaternary Prevention	■ Routine education provided about advance directives and "Do Not Resuscitate" orders during clinic visits, hospital admissions, and long-term care admissions ■ Education provided about hospice care to clients diagnosed with terminal illness who are approaching end of life

In the United States, several governing bodies make prevention recommendations. For example, the United States Preventive Services Task Force (USPSTF) makes recommendations for primary and secondary prevention strategies, and the Women's Preventive Services Initiative (WPSI) makes recommendations specifically for females. The Advisory Committee on Immunizations Practices (ACIP) makes recommendations for vaccinations, and various specialty organizations such as the American College of Obstetrics and Gynecology (ACOG) and the American Cancer Society (ACS) make preventative care recommendations. Preventive services have been proven to be an essential aspect of health care but are consistently underutilized in the United States.[27] Nurses can help advocate for the adoption of evidence-based prevention strategies in their communities and places of employment.

Continuum of Care Prevention Model

A second framework for prevention interventions, referred to as the "Continuum of Care Prevention Model," was originally proposed by the Institute of Medicine (IOM) in 1994 and has been adopted by the Substance Abuse

27 This work is a derivative of *StatPearls* by Kisling and Das and is licensed under CC BY 4.0

My Notes

and Mental Health Services Administration (SAMHSA).[28] See Figure 16.12[29] for an illustration of the Continuum of Care Prevention Model.

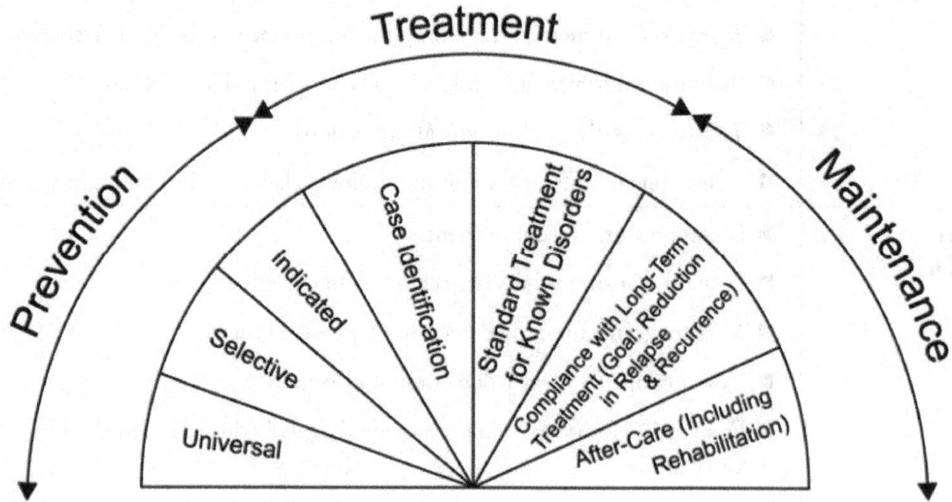

Figure 16.12 Continuum of Care Prevention Model. Used under Fair Use.

The Continuum of Care Prevention Model can be used to illustrate a continuum of mental health services for community members that includes prevention, treatment, and maintenance care:

- Prevention includes three types of strategies including universal, selective, and indicated interventions.
    - **Universal prevention:** Interventions designed to reach entire groups, such as those in schools, workplaces, or entire communities.[30,31] For example, wellness sessions regarding substance misuse can be planned and implemented at a local high school.

---

28 National Research Council (US); Institute of Medicine (US) Committee on the Prevention of Mental Disorders and Substance Abuse Among Children, Youth, and Young Adults; and Research Advances and Promising Interventions. Defining the scope of prevention. (2009). In M. E. O'Connell & Warner B. T. (Eds). *Preventing mental, emotional, and behavioral disorders among young people: Progress and possibilities. In Research advances and promising interventions.* National Academies Press. https://www.ncbi.nlm.nih.gov/books/ NBK32789/

29 This image is a derivative of the "IOM protractor" by unknown author and is included on the basis of Fair Use. Access for free at http://www.ca-sdfsc.org/docs/resources/SDFSC_IOM_Policy.pdf

30 National Research Council (US); Institute of Medicine (US) Committee on the Prevention of Mental Disorders and Substance Abuse Among Children, Youth, and Young Adults; and Research Advances and Promising Interventions. Defining the scope of prevention. (2009). In M. E. O'Connell & Warner B. T. (Eds). Preventing mental, emotional, and behavioral disorders among young people: Progress and possibilities. In Research advances and promising interventions. National Academies Press. https://www.ncbi.nlm.nih.gov/books/ NBK32789/

31 *A Guide to SAMHSA's Strategic Prevention Framework* by Substance Abuse and Mental Health Services Administration is available in the Public Domain

My Notes

- **Selected prevention:** Interventions that target individuals or groups with greater risk factors (and perhaps fewer protective factors) than the broader population.[32,33] For example, a research study showed that wellness programs implemented for adolescents who were already using alcohol or drugs reduced the quantity and frequency of their alcohol use and reduced episodes of binge drinking.[34]
- **Indicated prevention:** Interventions that target individuals who have a high probability of developing disease.[35] For example, interventions may be planned for adolescents who show early signs of substance misuse but have not yet been diagnosed with a substance use disorder. Interventions may include referrals to community support services for adolescents who have violated school alcohol or drug policies.[36]

- Treatment refers to identification of a mental health disorder and standard treatment for the known disorder. Treatment also includes interventions to reduce the likelihood of future co-occurring disorders.[37]
- Maintenance refers to long-term treatment to reduce relapse and recurrence, as well as provision of after-care services such as rehabilitation.[38]

See additional examples of prevention strategies using the Continuum of Care Prevention Model in Table 16.3b.

---

32 National Research Council (US); Institute of Medicine (US) Committee on the Prevention of Mental Disorders and Substance Abuse Among Children, Youth, and Young Adults; and Research Advances and Promising Interventions. Defining the scope of prevention. (2009). In M. E. O'Connell & Warner B. T. (Eds). *Preventing mental, emotional, and behavioral disorders among young people: Progress and possibilities. In Research advances and promising interventions.* National Academies Press. https://www.ncbi.nlm.nih.gov/books/NBK32789/

33 *A Guide to SAMHSA's Strategic Prevention Framework* by Substance Abuse and Mental Health Services Administration is available in the Public Domain

34 Werch, C., Moore, M. J., DiClemente, C. C., Bledsoe, R., & Jobli, E. (2005). A multihealth behavior intervention integrating physical activity and substance use prevention for adolescents. *Prevention Science, 6*(213). https://doi.org/10.1007/s11121-005-0012-3

35 National Research Council (US); Institute of Medicine (US) Committee on the Prevention of Mental Disorders and Substance Abuse Among Children, Youth, and Young Adults; and Research Advances and Promising Interventions. Defining the scope of prevention. (2009). In M. E. O'Connell & Warner B. T. (Eds). *Preventing mental, emotional, and behavioral disorders among young people: Progress and possibilities. In Research advances and promising interventions.* National Academies Press. https://www.ncbi.nlm.nih.gov/books/NBK32789/

36 *A Guide to SAMHSA's Strategic Prevention Framework* by Substance Abuse and Mental Health Services Administration is available in the Public Domain

37 National Research Council (US); Institute of Medicine (US) Committee on the Prevention of Mental Disorders and Substance Abuse Among Children, Youth, and Young Adults; and Research Advances and Promising Interventions. Defining the scope of prevention. (2009). In M. E. O'Connell & Warner B. T. (Eds). *Preventing mental, emotional, and behavioral disorders among young people: Progress and possibilities. In Research advances and promising interventions.* National Academies Press. https://www.ncbi.nlm.nih.gov/books/NBK32789/

38 National Research Council (US); Institute of Medicine (US) Committee on the Prevention of Mental Disorders and Substance Abuse Among Children, Youth, and Young Adults; and Research Advances and Promising Interventions. Defining the scope of prevention. (2009). In M. E. O'Connell & Warner B. T. (Eds). *Preventing mental, emotional, and behavioral disorders among young people: Progress and possibilities. In Research advances and promising interventions.* National Academies Press. https://www.ncbi.nlm.nih.gov/books/NBK32789/

My Notes

Table 16.3b Examples of Continuum of Care Prevention Strategies

Prevention Strategies	Examples
Universal Prevention	■ Handwashing education and posters in bathrooms of community gas stations ■ Parenting classes for new parents ■ Flu vaccine clinics at a local church
Selective Prevention	■ Backpack-buddy programs that provide food from schools to low-income families on weekends ■ Concussion training programs for youth athletes and their parents ■ Contact tracing procedures for individuals diagnosed with COVID-19
Indicated Prevention	■ Exercise programs at the local senior center targeted for individuals with diabetes ■ Food or clothing pantries established in a homeless shelter ■ Screening and consultation for the families of individuals who are admitted to hospitals with alcohol-related injuries

Read A Guide to SAMHSA's Strategic Prevention Framework PDF for more about planning prevention strategies for substance misuse and related mental health problems.

Culturally Competent Interventions

To overcome systemic barriers that can contribute to health disparities, nurses must recognize and value cultural differences of diverse populations and develop prevention programs and interventions in ways that ensure members of these populations benefit from their efforts.[39]

SAMHSA identified the following cultural competence principles for planning prevention interventions[40]:

- Include the targeted population in needs assessments and prevention planning
- Use a population-based definition of community (i.e., let the community define itself)
- Stress the importance of relevant, culturally appropriate prevention approaches
- Promote cultural competence among program staff

Review additional concepts related to culturally responsive care in the "Diverse Patients" chapter of Open RN *Nursing Fundamentals*.

39 *A Guide to SAMHSA's Strategic Prevention Framework* by Substance Abuse and Mental Health Services Administration is available in the Public Domain

40 *A Guide to SAMHSA's Strategic Prevention Framework* by Substance Abuse and Mental Health Services Administration is available in the Public Domain

My Notes

Evidence-Based Practice

It is essential to incorporate evidence-based practice when planning community health interventions. SAMHSA provides an evidence-based practice resource center for preventive practices related to mental health and substance abuse. See these resources, as well as examples of evidence-based programs and practices, in the following box.

Examples of Evidence-Based Prevention Practices Related to Mental Health and Substance Misuse[41]

- Blueprints for Healthy Youth Development: Youth violence, delinquency, and drug prevention and intervention programs that meet a strict scientific standard of program effectiveness
- Evidence-Based Behavioral Practice (EBBP): A project that creates training resources to help bridge the gap between behavioral health research and practice
- SAMHSA's Suicide Prevention Research Center (SPRC): A best practices registry that identifies, reviews, and disseminates information about best practices that address specific objectives of the National Strategy for Suicide Prevention
- The Athena Forum: Prevention 101: Substance misuse prevention programs and strategies with evidence of success from the Washington State Department of Social and Health Services
- National Institute on Drug Abuse: Preventing Drug Use Among Children and Adolescents: Research-based drug abuse prevention principles and an overview of program planning, including universal, selected, and indicated interventions
- View the SAMHSA Evidence-Based Practice Resource Center.

Implementation

Community health nurses collaborate with individuals, community organizations, health facilities, and local governments for successful implementation of community health initiatives. Depending on the established community health needs, goals, outcomes, and target group, the implementation of nursing interventions can be categorized as clinical, behavioral, or environmental prevention:

- **Clinical prevention:** Interventions are delivered one-on-one to individuals in a direct care setting. Examples of clinical prevention interventions include vaccine clinics, blood pressure monitoring, and screening for disease.
- **Behavioral prevention:** Interventions are implemented to encourage individuals to change habits or behaviors by using health promotion strategies. Examples of behavioral prevention

---

41 Substance Abuse and Mental Health Services Administration. (2019, July 19). *Finding evidence-based programs and practices.* https://www.samhsa.gov/sites/default/files/20190719-samhsa-finding_evidence-based-programs-practices.pdf

My Notes

interventions include community exercise programs, smoking cessation campaigns, or promotion of responsible alcohol drinking by adults.

- **Environmental prevention:** Interventions are implemented for the entire community when laws, policies, physical environments, or community structures influence a community's health. Examples of environmental prevention strategies include improving clean water systems, establishing no-smoking ordinances, or developing community parks and green spaces.

Evaluation

When evaluating the effectiveness of community health initiatives, nurses refer to the established goals and SMART outcomes to determine if they were met by the timeline indicated. In general, the following questions are asked during the evaluation stage:

- Did the health of the community improve through the interventions put into place?
- Are additional adaptations or changes to the interventions needed to improve outcomes in the community?
- What additional changes are needed to improve the health of the community?
- Have additional priority problems been identified?

16.4 LEARNING ACTIVITIES

My Notes

Interactive Activities

An interactive H5P element has been excluded from this version of the text. You can view it online here: https://wtcs.pressbooks.pub/nursingmhcc/?p=733#h5p-53

An interactive H5P element has been excluded from this version of the text. You can view it online here: https://wtcs.pressbooks.pub/nursingmhcc/?p=733#h5p-54

An interactive H5P element has been excluded from this version of the text. You can view it online here: https://wtcs.pressbooks.pub/nursingmhcc/?p=733#h5p-55

My Notes

XVI GLOSSARY

Community diagnosis: A summary statement resulting from analysis of the data collected from a community health needs assessment.

Community health needs assessment: A systematic process to identify and analyze community health needs and assets in order to prioritize these needs, plan, and act upon significant unmet community health needs.

Focus groups: A systematic way of collecting data through small group discussion. Focus group participants are chosen to represent a larger group of people.

Health disparities: Health differences that are linked with social, economic, and/or environmental disadvantages.

Health equity: A goal of everyone having a fair and just opportunity to be as healthy as possible.

Health inequities: Avoidable differences in health status seen within and between communities.

Healthy community: A community in which local groups from all parts of the community work together to prevent disease and make healthy living options accessible.

Indicated prevention: Interventions that target individuals who have a high probability of developing disease.

Interviews: Structured conversations with specific individuals who have experience, knowledge, or understanding about a topic or issue.

Key informant interviews: Interviews are conducted with select people who are in key positions and have specific areas of knowledge and experience.

Leading health indicators (LHIs): A subset of high-priority Healthy People 2030 objectives to drive action toward improving health and well-being.

Primary data collection: Data collected to better understand the community's needs and/or study who may be affected by actions taken for the community. Primary data collection includes tools such as public forums, focus groups, interviews, windshield surveys, surveys, and participant observation.[1]

Primary prevention: Interventions aimed at susceptible populations or individuals to prevent disease from occurring. Immunizations are an example of primary prevention.

Primordial prevention: Risk factor reduction strategies focused on social and environmental conditions targeted for vulnerable populations.

Public forms: Public gatherings where citizens discuss important issues at well-publicized locations and times.

Public health nurses: Public health nurses work across various settings in the community such as government agencies, community-based centers, shelters, and vaccine distribution sites.[2]

Quaternary prevention: Actions taken to protect individuals from medical interventions that are likely to cause more harm than good and to suggest interventions that are ethically acceptable.

Secondary analysis: Analyzing previously collected data and research about the community to determine community needs.

Secondary prevention: Interventions that emphasize early detection of disease and target healthy-appearing individuals with subclinical forms of disease.

---

1 *Community Tool Box* by Center for Community Health and Development at the University of Kansas is licensed under CC BY NC SA 3.0

2 Greenwood, B. (2018, June 29). *What are the primary roles of the community nurse?* CHRON. https://work.chron.com/primary-roles-community-nurse-15144.html

Selected prevention: Interventions that target individuals or groups with greater risk factors for illness (and perhaps fewer protective factors) than the broader population.

Social determinants of health (SDOH): The conditions in which people are born, grow, work, live, and age.

Surveys: Standardized questions that are relatively easy to analyze and are beneficial for collecting information across a large geographic area, hearing from as many people as possible, and exploring sensitive topics.

Tertiary prevention: Interventions implemented for symptomatic clients to reduce the severity of the disease and potential long-term complications.

Universal prevention: Interventions designed to reach entire groups or populations such as schools, whole communities, or workplaces.

Windshield survey: A form of direct observation of community needs while driving and literally looking through the windshield.

My Notes

Chapter 17

Vulnerable Populations

17.1 INTRODUCTION

My Notes

Learning Objectives

- Describe vulnerable populations
- Outline factors that may impact health-seeking behaviors of vulnerable populations
- Discuss support systems and organizations available for vulnerable populations
- Describe the role of the nurse as an advocate for vulnerable populations
- Apply the nursing process to caring for vulnerable populations using evidence-based practice
- Discuss interprofessional collaboration in providing care for vulnerable populations

The "Community Assessment" chapter describes how to assess community health needs and apply the nursing process to community health nursing. This chapter provides an overview of vulnerable populations and information for the nurse generalist to support their needs. The nursing process is applied to providing care for a vulnerable population in the "Spotlight Application" section.

My Notes

17.2 VULNERABLE POPULATIONS

A **vulnerable population** is a group of individuals who are at increased risk for health problems and health disparities.[1] **Health disparities** are health differences linked with social, economic, and/or environmental disadvantages. Health disparities adversely affect groups of people who often experience greater obstacles to health based on individual characteristics, such as socioeconomic status, age, gender, culture, religion, mental illness, disability, sexual orientation, or gender identity.[2]

Examples of vulnerable populations are[3,4]:

- The very young and the very old
- Individuals with chronic illnesses, disabilities, or communication barriers
- Veterans
- Racial and ethnic minorities
- Individuals who identify as lesbian, gay, bisexual, transgender, or queer (LGBTQ)
- Victims of human trafficking or sexual violence
- Individuals who are incarcerated and their family members
- Rural Americans
- Migrant workers
- Individuals with chronic mental health disorders
- Homeless people

Individuals typically have less access and use of health services, resulting in significant health disparities in life expectancy, morbidity, and mortality. They are also more likely to have one or more chronic physical and/or mental health illnesses.[5] Advancing health equity for all members of our society is receiving increased emphasis as a central goal of public health. **Health equity** is defined by the U.S. Department of Health and Human Services as the "attainment of the highest level of health for all people" and that "achieving health equity requires valuing everyone equally with focused and ongoing societal efforts to address avoidable inequities, historical and contemporary injustices, and the elimination of health and health care disparities."[6]

---

1 AJMC. (2006, November 1). Vulnerable populations: Who are they? *AJMC, 12*(1). https://www.ajmc.com/view/nov06-2390ps348-s352

2 HealthyPeople.gov. (2022, February 6). *Disparities.* Office of Disease Prevention and Health Promotion, U.S. Department of Health and Human Services. https://www.healthypeople.gov/2020/about/foundation-health-measures/Disparities

3 Joszt, L. (2018, July 20). 5 vulnerable populations in healthcare. *The American Journal of Managed Care.* https://www.ajmc.com/view/5-vulnerable-populations-in-healthcare

4 AJMC. (2006, November 1). Vulnerable populations: Who are they? *AJMC, 12*(1). https://www.ajmc.com/view/nov06-2390ps348-s352

5 AJMC. (2006, November 1). Vulnerable populations: Who are they? *AJMC, 12*(1). https://www.ajmc.com/view/nov06-2390ps348-s352

6 Liburd, L. C., Hall, J. E., Mpofu, J. J., Williams, S. M., Bouye, K., & Penman-Aguilar, A. (2020). Addressing health equity in public health practice: Frameworks, promising strategies, and measurement considerations. *Annual Review of Public Health, 41*(1), 417-432. https://www.annualreviews.org/doi/10.1146/annurev-publhealth-040119-094119

My Notes

Examples of vulnerable populations and associated resources available to promote health equity and reduce health disparities are further described in the following sections.

Age and Developmental Status

Developmental status and age are associated with vulnerability. Children have health and developmental needs that require age-appropriate care. Developmental changes, dependency on others, and different patterns of illness and injury require that attention be paid to the unique needs of children in the health system. The elderly population also has unique health care needs due to increased incidence of illness and disability, as well as the complex interactions of multiple chronic illnesses and multiple medications.[7]

Children and the elderly are also vulnerable to experiencing neglect and abuse. Nurses must be aware of signs of neglect and abuse and are legally mandated to report these signs. Read more about neglect, abuse, and mandatory reporting in the "Trauma, Abuse, and Violence" chapter.

Chronic Illness and Disability

Individuals with chronic illnesses and/or disabilities are more likely than the general population to experience problems in accessing a range of health care services. These vulnerable groups may also experience lack of coordination of care across multiple providers. In addition, individuals with specific chronic illnesses, such as individuals with mental illness or human immunodeficiency virus (HIV), may face social stigma that makes it challenging to seek and/or receive appropriate health care.[8] See Figure 17.1[9] for an image of a disabled individual who is considered a member of a vulnerable population.

---

7 Advisory Commision on Consumer Protection and Quality in the Health Care Industry. (n.d.). *Chapter eight: Focusing on vulnerable populations.* University of North Texas Libraries and U.S. Government Printing Office. https://govinfo.library.unt.edu/hcquality/meetings/mar12/papch08.htm

8 Advisory Commision on Consumer Protection and Quality in the Health Care Industry. (n.d.). *Chapter eight: Focusing on vulnerable populations.* University of North Texas Libraries and U.S. Government Printing Office. https://govinfo.library.unt.edu/hcquality/meetings/mar12/papch08.htm

9 "COVID-19_vaccination_center,_fair_grounds_Cologne,_1st_vaccination-8070.jpg" by Raimond Spekking is licensed under CC BY-SA 4.0

My Notes

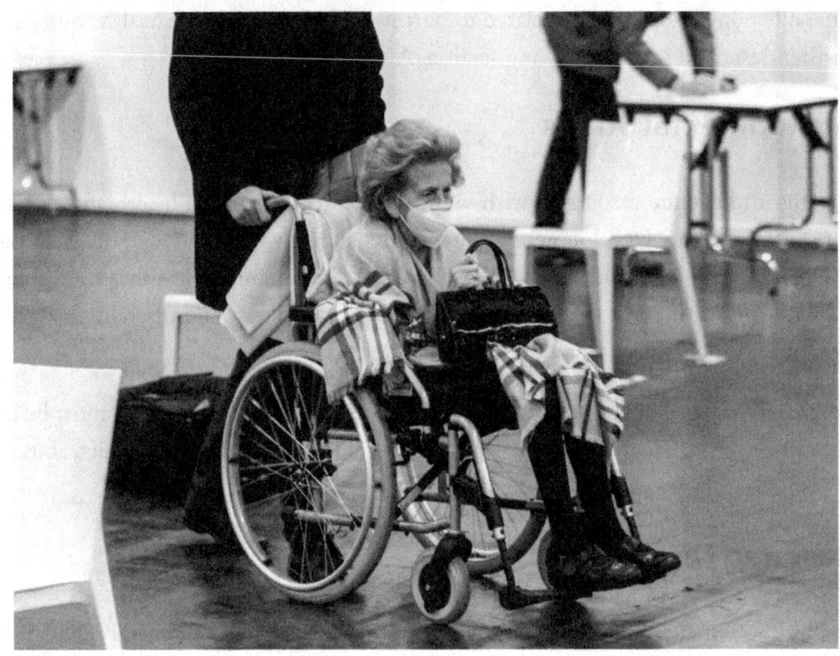

Figure 17.1 Member of a Vulnerable Population

In addition to experiencing challenges in accessing appropriate health care, adults with disabilities report experiencing more mental distress than the general population. In 2018 an estimated 17.4 million (32.9%) adults with disabilities experienced frequent mental distress, defined as 14 or more reported mentally unhealthy days in the past 30 days. Frequent mental distress is associated with poor health behaviors, mental health disorders, and limitations in daily life.[10] The National Center on Health, Physical Activity and Disability (NCHPAD) is a public health resource center that focuses on health promotion, wellness, and quality of life for people with disabilities.

The Barrier-Free Health Care Initiative is a national initiative by the American Disability Association and the Offices of the United States Attorneys that supports people with disabilities. It legally enforces appropriate access to health care services, such as effective communication for people who are deaf or have hearing loss, physical access to medical care for people with mobility disabilities, and equal access to treatment for people who have HIV/AIDS. This nationwide initiative sends a collective message that disability discrimination in health care is illegal and unacceptable.

Visit the Barrier-Free Health Care Initiative to learn more.

Visit the National Center on Health, Physical Activity and Disability (NCHPAD) for additional wellness resources.

---

10 Centers for Disease Control and Prevention. (2020, November 30). *The mental health of people with disabilities.* https://www.cdc.gov/ncbddd/disabilityandhealth/features/mental-health-for-all.html

Veterans

My Notes

A veteran is someone who has served in the military forces. Veterans have higher risks for mental health disorders, substance abuse, post-traumatic stress disorders, traumatic brain injuries, and suicide compared to their civilian counterparts. Medical records of veterans reveal that one in three clients was diagnosed with at least one mental health disorder.[11] Identifying and treating mental health disorders in veterans have the greatest potential for reducing suicide risk, but the reluctance in this population to seek treatment can make diagnosing and treating mental illness challenging. Nurses must be aware of their clients' military history, recognize risk factors for common disorders, and advocate for appropriate health care services.[12] See Figure 17.2[13] for an image of a veteran.

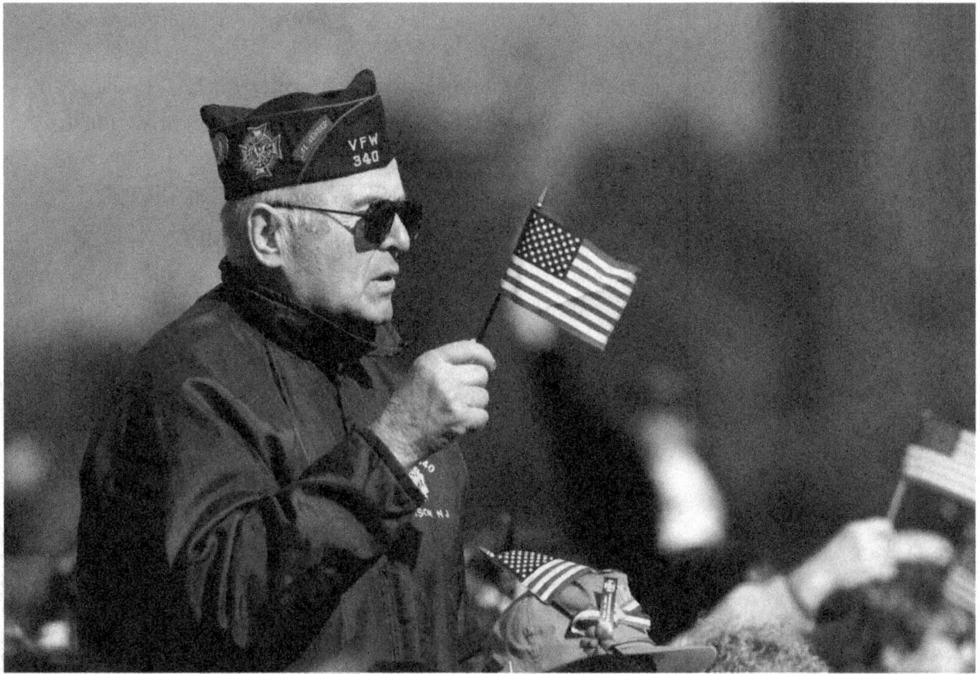

Figure 17.2 Armed Forces Veteran

Veterans Affairs (VA) provides health care and other benefits to individuals serving on active duty in the United States uniformed services. The Veterans Health Administration is the largest health care network in the United States with 1,255 health care facilities and serves nine million enrolled veterans each year. In addition to health care, benefits may include educational loans, home loans or housing grants, and life insurance. Nurses can refer clients who are veterans to the VA for more information about benefits.

Nurses can also refer veterans and their family members to the National Alliance on Mental Health (NAMI) Homefront course. NAMI Homefront is a class for families, caregivers, and friends of military service members

---

11 Olenick, M., Flowers, M., & Diaz, V. J. (2015). US veterans and their unique issues: Enhancing health care professional awareness. *Advances in Medical Education and Practice, 6*, 635–639. https://doi.org/10.2147/AMEP.S89479

12 Olenick, M., Flowers, M., & Diaz, V. J. (2015). US veterans and their unique issues: Enhancing health care professional awareness. *Advances in Medical Education and Practice, 6*, 635–639. https://doi.org/10.2147/AMEP.S89479

13 "DF-SD-03-05175" by Scott H. Spitzer, Civilian, USAF is in the Public Domain

My Notes

and veterans with mental health conditions. The course is designed specifically to help these individuals understand mental health disorders and improve their ability to support their service member or veteran.

Visit the Veterans Affairs (VA) website for additional information on health care and other benefits for military service members.

Visit the NAMI Homefront course to learn more about mental health conditions and resources available to military service members and their families.

Racial and Ethnic Minorities

Racial and ethnic minority populations in the United States experience significant health disparities.[14] See Figure 17.3[15] for an image of a child from a minority population. The U.S. Department of Health and Human Services Office of Minority Health provides Minority Population Profiles for Black/African Americans, American Indian/Alaska Natives, Asian Americans, Hispanic/Latinos, and Native Hawaiian/Pacific Islanders. Profiles include demographics, English language fluency, education, economics, insurance coverage and health status information, and full census reports. Nurses can access these profiles to view health care statistics regarding these populations and services available in their communities.

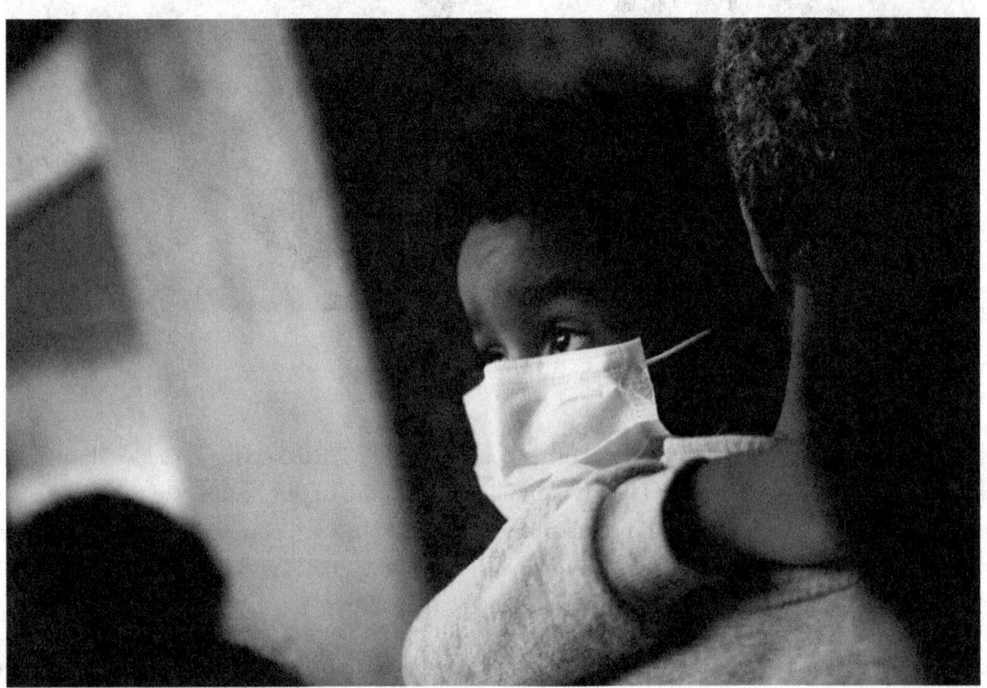

Figure 17.3 Child of a Minority Population

14 Olenick, M., Flowers, M., & Diaz, V. J. (2015). US veterans and their unique issues: Enhancing health care professional awareness. *Advances in Medical Education and Practice, 6*, 635–639. https://doi.org/10.2147/AMEP.S89479

15 "3678466365_da63d01385_b" by Xavier Donat is licensed under CC BY-NC-ND 2.0

My Notes

The Office of Minority Health is dedicated to improving the health of racial and ethnic minority populations through the development of health policies and programs that help eliminate health disparities.

Visit the Office of Minority Health to learn more about efforts to improve the health of racial and ethnic minority populations through health policy and program development. Examples of initiatives include the following[16]:

- COVID-19 Response
- Improving Cultural Competency for Behavioral Health Professionals
- Sickle Cell Disease Initiative

LGBTQ Population

The lesbian, gay, bisexual, transgender, and queer or questioning (LGBTQ) population encompasses all races and ethnicities, religions, and social classes. See Figure 17.4[17] for an image of a pride festival by an LGBTQ population. Research suggests that LGBTQ individuals experience health disparities linked to societal stigma, discrimination, and denial of their civil rights.[18] The LGBTQ population experiences high rates of mental health disorders. Substance abuse, suicide, and experiences of violence and victimization are frequent for LGBTQ individuals and can result in long-lasting effects.[19]

16 Olenick, M., Flowers, M., & Diaz, V. J. (2015). US veterans and their unique issues: Enhancing health care professional awareness. *Advances in Medical Education and Practice, 6*, 635–639. https://doi.org/10.2147/AMEP.S89479

17 "Pride_Festival_2013_On_The_Streets_Of_Dublin_(LGBTQ)_(9183775778).jpg" by infomatique is licensed under CC BY-SA 2.0

18 HealthyPeople.gov. (2022, February 6). *Lesbian, gay, bisexual, and transgender health.* Office of Disease Prevention and Health Promotion, U.S. Department of Health and Human Services. https://www.healthypeople.gov/2020/topics-objectives/topic/lesbian-gay-bisexual-and-transgender-health

19 HealthyPeople.gov. (2022, February 6). *Lesbian, gay, bisexual, and transgender health.* Office of Disease Prevention and Health Promotion, U.S. Department of Health and Human Services. https://www.healthypeople.gov/2020/topics-objectives/topic/lesbian-gay-bisexual-and-transgender-health

My Notes

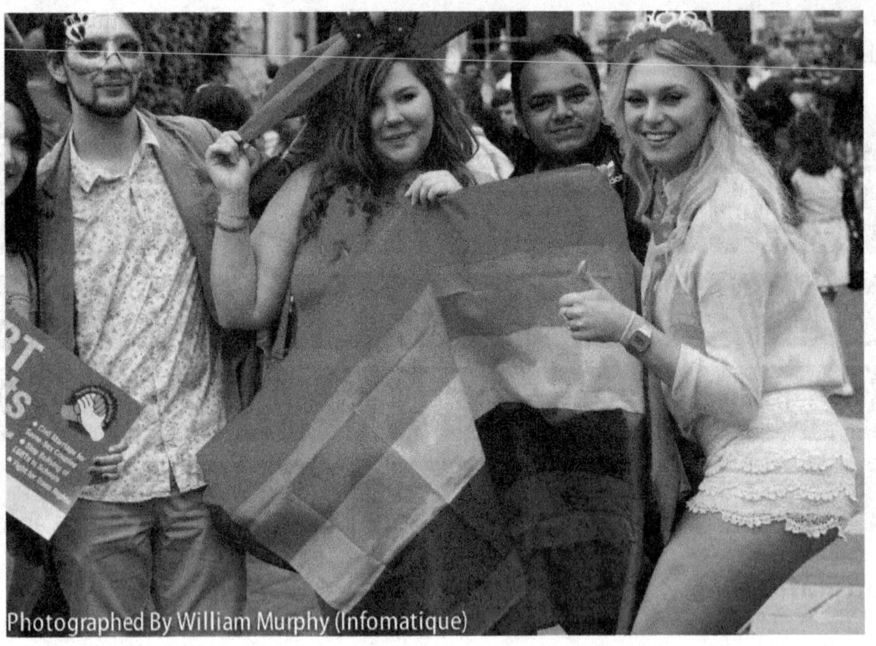
Photographed By William Murphy (Infomatique)

Figure 17.4 Pride Festival for the LGBTQ Population

Community efforts to improve the health of the LGBTQ population include these initiatives[20]:

- Training health professionals to appropriately inquire and support clients' sexual orientation and gender identity to promote regular use of health care services
- Training health professionals and students regarding culturally competent care
- Providing supportive social services to reduce suicide and homelessness among youth
- Curbing sexually transmitted infections and human immunodeficiency virus (HIV) transmission

Discover health services by state at CDC's LGBT Health website.

Human Trafficking Victims

Human trafficking victims are forced to work or provide commercial sex against their will in legal business settings and underground markets.[21] The International Labor Organization estimates there are 40.3 million victims of human trafficking globally. Victims include men, women, adolescents, and children.[22] Experts estimate that

20 HealthyPeople.gov. (2022, February 6). *Lesbian, gay, bisexual, and transgender health.* Office of Disease Prevention and Health Promotion, U.S. Department of Health and Human Services. https://www.healthypeople.gov/2020/topics-objectives/topic/lesbian-gay-bisexual-and-transgender-health

21 National Human Trafficking Hotline. (n.d.). *The victims.* https://humantraffickinghotline.org/what-human-trafficking/human-trafficking/victims

22 National Human Trafficking Hotline. (n.d.). *The victims.* https://humantraffickinghotline.org/what-human-trafficking/human-trafficking/victims

My Notes

100,000 incidents of sexual exploitation of minors occur each year in the United States.[23] Human trafficking victims have been identified in cities, suburbs, and rural areas in all 50 states and in Washington, D.C. See Figure 17.5[24] regarding human trafficking statistics reported by state in 2020.

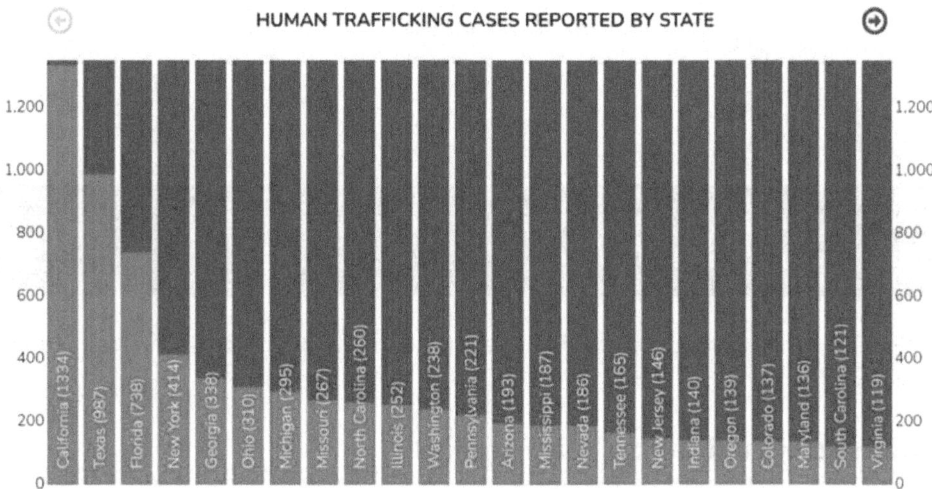

Figure 17.5 Human Trafficking Reported by State in 2020

Widespread lack of awareness and understanding of trafficking leads to low levels of victim identification. Individuals at risk include runaway and homeless youth, foreign nationals, and individuals with prior history of experiencing violence or abuse. A study in Chicago found that 56 percent of female prostitutes were initially runaway youth, and similar numbers have been identified for male populations.[25]

Foreign nationals who are trafficked within the United States face unique challenges. Recruiters located in home countries frequently require such large recruitment and travel fees that victims become highly indebted to the recruiters and traffickers.

Individuals who have experienced violence and trauma in the past are more vulnerable to future exploitation because the psychological effect of trauma is often long-lasting and challenging to overcome. Victims of domestic violence, sexual assault, war, or social discrimination may be targeted by traffickers who recognize the vulnerabilities left by these prior abuses.[26]

---

23 Office of the Attorney General for the District of Columbia. (n.d.). *Human trafficking initiatives.* https://oag.dc.gov/public-safety/human-trafficking-initiatives

24 This image is derived from Human Trafficking Hotline data and is in the Public Domain. Access for free at https://humantraffickinghotline.org/states

25 National Human Trafficking Hotline. (n.d.). *The victims.* https://humantraffickinghotline.org/what-human-trafficking/human-trafficking/victims

26 National Human Trafficking Hotline. (n.d.). *The victims.* https://humantraffickinghotline.org/what-human-trafficking/human-trafficking/victims

My Notes

These are some of the services victims of trafficking may need[27]:

- Emergency Services
- Crisis Intervention and Counseling
- Emergency Shelter and Referrals
- Urgent Medical Care
- Safety Planning
- Food and Clothing

For more information about the services available to victims of human trafficking, visit the National Human Trafficking Hotline Referral Directory.

See an example of a nurse providing care for victims of human trafficking in their community in the "Spotlight Application" section.

Incarcerated Individuals and Their Families

At the end of 2019, there were over 2 million people in U.S. prisons and jails with a nationwide incarceration rate of 810 inmates for every 100,000 adults. Higher rates of incarceration are seen among racial/ethnic minorities and people with lower levels of education. The United States incarcerates a larger share of its population than any other country in the world.[28] See Figure 17.6[29] for an illustration comparing worldwide incarceration rates.[30]

27 National Human Trafficking Hotline. (n.d.). *The victims.* https://humantraffickinghotline.org/what-human-trafficking/human-trafficking/victims

28 Gramlich, J. (2021, August 16). *America's incarceration rate falls to lowest level since 1995.* Pew Research Center. https://pewrsr.ch/2rfSmVL

29 "U.S. incarcerates a larger share of its population than any other country" by Pew Research Center, Washington, D.C. (August 13, 2021). Used under Fair Use. Access for free at https://www.pewresearch.org/fact-tank/2021/08/16/americas-incarceration-rate-lowest-since-1995/ft_21-08-12_incarceration_2/

30 Rich, J. D., & The Center for Prisoner Health and Human Rights, Miriam Hospital. *Incarceration and health.* [Working paper]. National Academies. https://sites.nationalacademies.org/cs/groups/dbassesite/documents/webpage/dbasse_083371.pdf

My Notes

U.S. incarcerates a larger share of its population than any other country

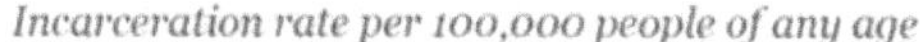

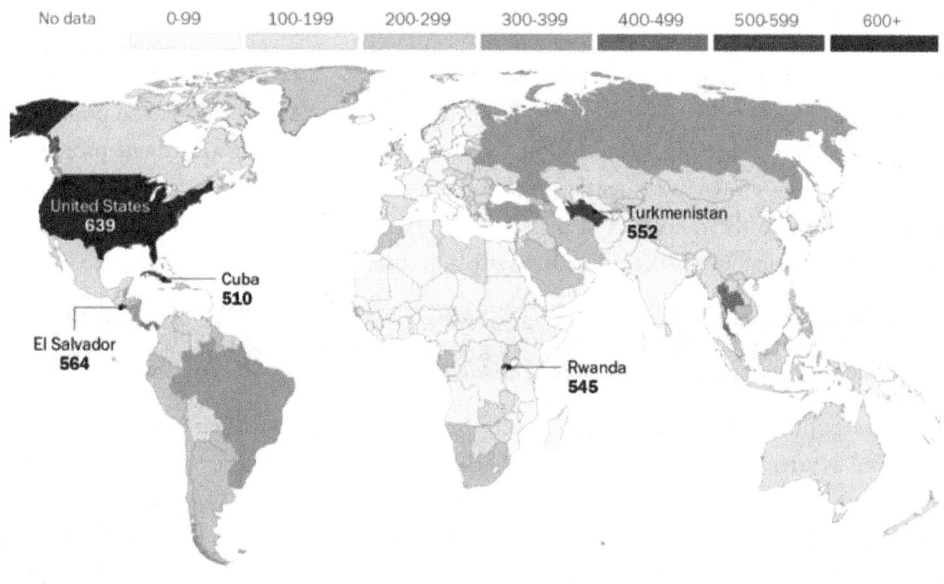

Note: Figures reflect most recent available data for each country. Territories are counted separately.
Data accessed Aug. 10, 2021.
Source: World Prison Brief, Institute for Crime & Justice Policy Research.

PEW RESEARCH CENTER

Figure 17.6 Comparison of Worldwide Incarceration Rates. Used under Fair Use.

Many individuals who are incarcerated have chronic health conditions, including mental illness and addiction. Over half of all inmates have a mental health disorder, and female inmates have higher rates of post-traumatic stress disorder (PTSD) than the general population. In fact, some experts believe that escalation of U.S. incarceration rates since the 1970s is associated with inadequate community-based health care for mental illness and addiction; left untreated, both conditions can lead to behaviors that result in incarceration.[31]

Health care is a constitutional right for prisoners. The 1976 Supreme Court decision in Estelle v. Gamble found that "deliberate indifference to serious medical needs of prisoners" constitutes a violation of the Eighth Amendment prohibition of cruel and unusual punishment. Nurses working in correctional facilities have a legal and ethical obligation to respond to requests for care. If an inmate's safety complaints are ignored, safety risks are not removed, or there is failure to provide proper medical attention, it is considered "deliberate indifference." Correctional nurses have a duty to evaluate prisoners' health needs and determine the level of care required. For example, the nurse determines if the prisoner should be moved to the medical unit or transferred to a health facility that can provide the level of care needed. In addition, all pertinent information of health encounters with prisoners must be thoroughly documented and include assessment finding, health needs, interventions taken, patient education, and evaluation of patient outcomes.[32]

---

31 Rich, J. D., & The Center for Prisoner Health and Human Rights, Miriam Hospital. *Incarceration and health.* [Working paper]. National Academies. https://sites.nationalacademies.org/cs/groups/dbassesite/documents/webpage/dbasse_083371.pdf

32 National Commission on Correctional Health Care. (n.d.). *Legal issues.* https://www.ncchc.org/legal-issues

My Notes

While the Supreme Court decision mandates health care provision for incarcerated populations in prisons and jails, it does not extend to those under supervision within the criminal justice system (e.g., on parole, probation, or home confinement).[33] However, the Patient Protection and Affordable Care Act (ACA) helps to ensure continuity of medical coverage and care when prisoners are released into the community.[34]

While mortality rates within prisons and jails are comparable to those of the general population, releasees are nearly 13 times more likely to die in the two weeks following their release than the general population. The most common cause of death is overdose. Interventions that follow in-prison drug treatment programs with post-release treatment have been shown to reduce drug use and associated recidivism (i.e., return to prison). There have also been efforts to improve the outcomes of prisoner reentry to society through assistance with employment, housing, and other transitional needs that ultimately affect health.[35,36]

The National Alliance on Mental Health (NAMI) provides several Re-Entry Planning resources.

Incarceration has a public health impact on prisoners' family members and their communities while they are incarcerated, as well as after their release. Community health is affected by incarceration due to economic impacts (i.e., consequences on families' well-being when income earners are removed) and long-term impacts on children's health and mental health (also referred to as adverse childhood events). For example, children of incarcerated parents are more likely to live in poverty, as well as have higher rates of learning disabilities, developmental delays, speech/language problems, attention disorders, aggressive behaviors, and drug and alcohol use. Additionally, children of incarcerated parents are up to five times more likely to enter the criminal justice system than children of nonincarcerated parents.[37,38]

Family-centered services for incarcerated parents and their children focus on parenting programs, family strengthening activities, nurturing of family relationships, and community support for families during incarceration and following release.

Read more about family-centered services at the U.S. Department of Health Services Child Welfare Information Gateway.

Read additional guidance and resources at CDC Correctional Health.

---

33 Gramlich, J. (2021, August 16). *America's incarceration rate falls to lowest level since 1995.* Pew Research Center. https://pewrsr.ch/2rfSmVL

34 Gramlich, J. (2021, August 16). *America's incarceration rate falls to lowest level since 1995.* Pew Research Center. https://pewrsr.ch/2rfSmVL

35 Rich, J. D., & The Center for Prisoner Health and Human Rights, Miriam Hospital. *Incarceration and health.* [Working paper]. National Academies. https://sites.nationalacademies.org/cs/groups/dbassesite/documents/webpage/dbasse_083371.pdf

36 Massoglia, M., & Pridemore, W. A. (2015). Incarceration and health. *Annual Review of Sociology, 41*, 291–310. https://doi.org/10.1146/annurev-soc-073014-112326

37 HealthyPeople.gov. (2022, February 6). *Incarceration.* Office of Disease Prevention and Health Promotion, U.S. Department of Health and Human Services. https://www.healthypeople.gov/2020/topics-objectives/topic/social-determinants-health/interventions-resources/incarceration

38 Massoglia, M., & Pridemore, W. A. (2015). Incarceration and health. *Annual Review of Sociology, 41*, 291–310. https://doi.org/10.1146/annurev-soc-073014-112326

Rural Americans

My Notes

Rural Americans are a population group that experiences significant health disparities. Rural risk factors for health disparities include geographic isolation, lower socioeconomic status, higher rates of health risk behaviors, limited access to health care specialists, and limited job opportunities. This inequality is intensified because rural residents are less likely to have employer-provided health insurance or Medicaid coverage.[39,40] See Figure 17.7[41] for an image of a small town in rural America.

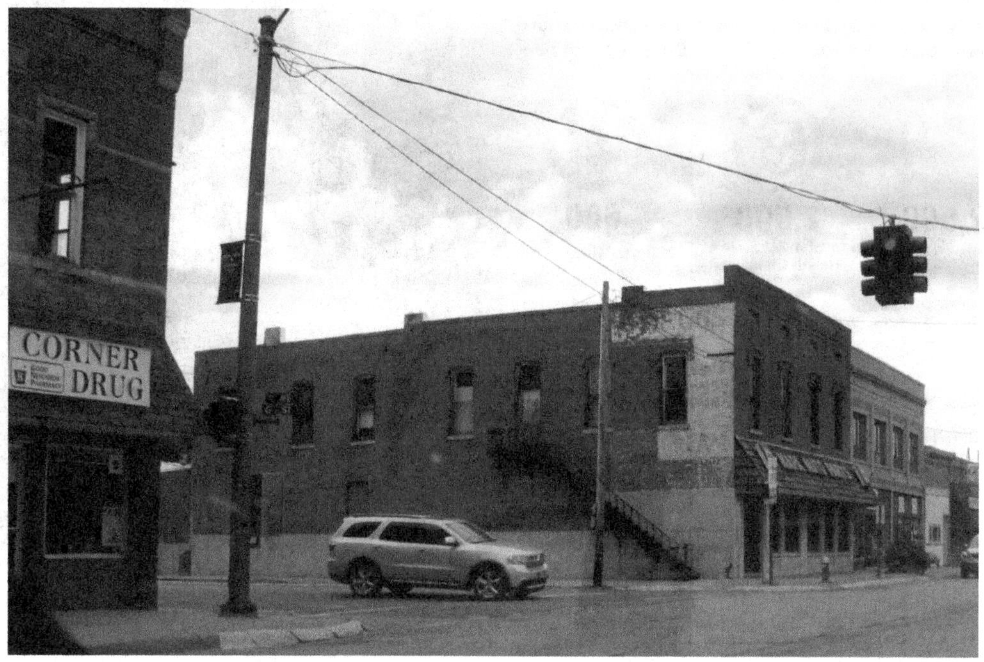

Figure 17.7 Rural America

For an in-depth look at rural health disparities, the Rural Health Information Hub Rural Health Series serves as a resource to examine rural mortality and preventable deaths, health-related behaviors, chronic disease, mental health services, and other related topics. The Federal Office of Rural Health Policy provides additional information regarding rural health policy, community health programs, and telehealth programs to increase access to health care for underserved people in rural communities. Two initiatives to improve rural health are the National Health Service Corps (NHSC) loan repayment program and telehealth.[42]

---

39 Rural Health Information Hub. (2019, April 22). *Rural health disparities.* https://www.ruralhealthinfo.org/topics/rural-health-disparities

40 United States Department of Agriculture. (2018). Rural America at a glance 2018 edition. *Economic Information Bulletin,* 200. https://www.ers.usda.gov/webdocs/publications/90556/eib-200.pdf?v=3360.9

41 "One_Light_Town"_Small_Town,_Nebraska_7-25-13a_(10784126756).jpg" by inkknife_2000 (7.5 million views +) is licensed under CC BY-SA 2.0

42 Health Resources & Services Administration. (n.d.). *Federal office of rural health policy.* https://www.hrsa.gov/rural-health/index.html

My Notes

NHSC builds healthy communities by supporting health care professionals dedicated to working in areas of the United States with limited access to care. NHSC offers educational loan repayment programs to health professionals who commit to working in underserved areas for specific lengths of time.[43]

See an infographic about NHSC in Figure 17.8.[44]

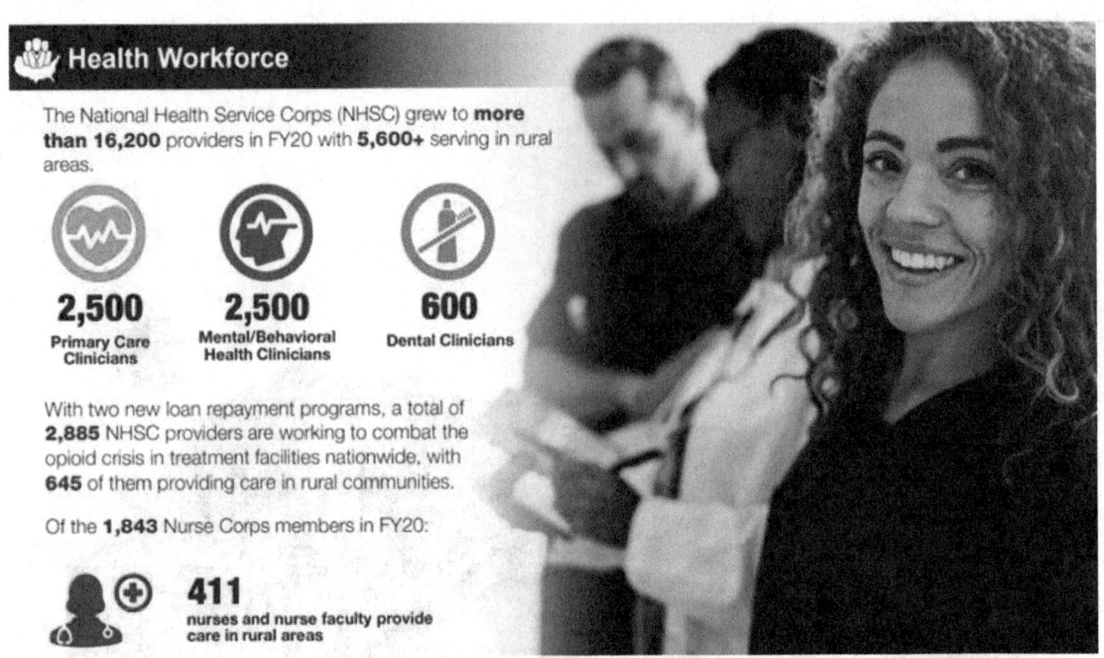

Figure 17.8 National Health Service Corps

Telehealth is a recent initiative to improve health care access to underserved communities. Telehealth is the use of digital technologies to deliver medical care, health education, and public health services by connecting multiple users in separate locations. See Figure 17.9[45] for an image of telehealth. Telehealth can improve health outcomes and access to care by delivering health services in underserved areas and remove barriers of time, distance, and provider scarcities.[46] Nurses support clients using telehealth and provide patient education.

However, telehealth can risk widening disparities for some socioeconomic groups with limited access to the resource necessary for effective telemedicine. Nurses can help ensure that health care systems tailor the use of technology to meet the needs of underserved populations.[47]

---

43 National Health Service Corps. *Health Resources & Services Administration.* https://nhsc.hrsa.gov

44 This image is derived from HRSA Programs Serve Rural Communities by Health Resources & Services Administration and is in the Public Domain

45 "Telemedicine_Consult.jpg" by Intel Free Press is licensed under CC BY-SA 2.0

46 Telligen & Great Plains Telehealth Resource & Assistance Center. (2014). *Telehealth: Start-up and resource guide.* https://www.healthit.gov/sites/default/files/telehealthguide_final_0.pdf

47 Ortega, G., Rodriguez, J. A., Maurer, L. R., Witt, E. E., Perez, N., Reich, A., & Bates, D. W. (2020). Telemedicine, COVID-19, and disparities: Policy implications. *Health Policy and Technology, 9*(3), 368–371. https://doi.org/10.1016/j.hlpt.2020.08.001

My Notes

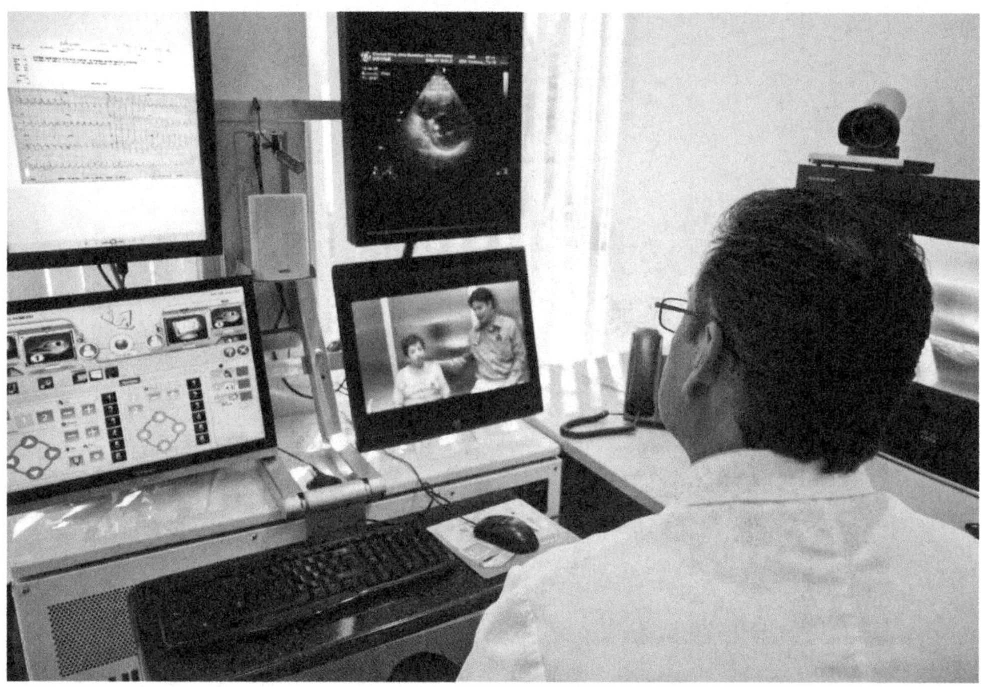

Figure 17.9 Telehealth

Visit the Rural Health Information Hub Rural Health Series to examine rural mortality and preventable deaths, health-related behaviors, chronic disease, mental health services, and other related topics.

Learn more about the NHSC and how it supports health care professionals to provide care in areas with limited access to health services.

Migrant Workers

A **migrant worker** is a person who moves within their home country or outside of it to pursue work. Migrant workers usually do not intend to stay permanently in the country or region in which they work. See Figure 17.10[48] for an image of migrant workers harvesting cabbage.

48 "5123728839_1b7ce92b5c_k" by Bob Jagendorf is licensed under CC BY-NC 2.0

My Notes

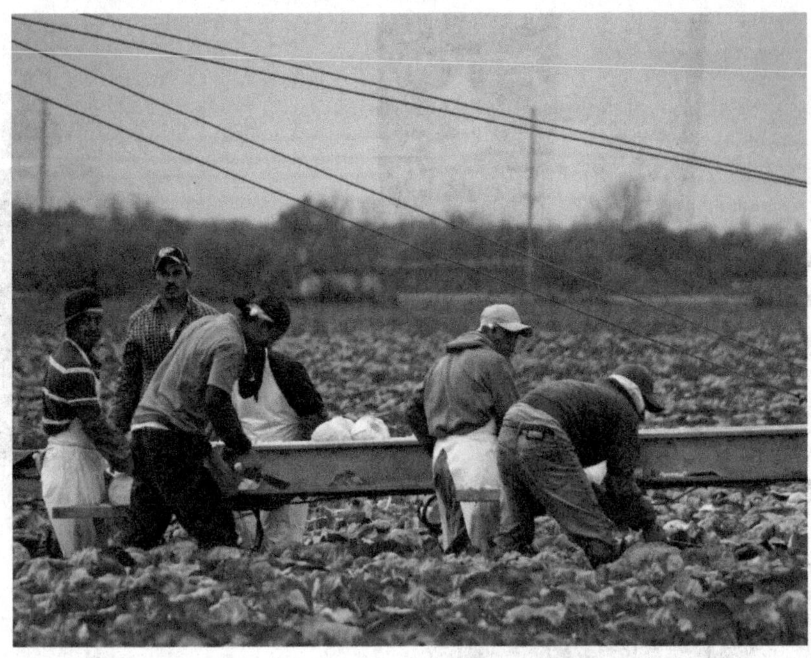

Figure 17.10 Migrant Workers Harvesting Cabbage

Migratory and seasonal agricultural workers (MASW) and their families face unique health challenges that can result in significant health disparities. Challenges can include the following[49]:

- Hazardous work environments
- Poverty
- Insufficient support systems
- Inadequate or unsafe housing
- Limited availability of clean water and septic systems
- Inadequate health care access and lack of continuity of care
- Lack of health insurance
- Cultural and language barriers
- Fear of using health care due to immigration status
- Lack of transportation

MSAW populations experience serious health problems including diabetes, malnutrition, depression, substance use, infectious diseases, pesticide poisoning, and injuries from work-related machinery. These critical health issues are exacerbated by the migratory culture of this population group that increases isolation and makes it difficult to maintain treatment regimens and track health records.[50]

---

49 Rural Health Information Hub. (2021, July 1). *Rural migrant health.* https://www.ruralhealthinfo.org/topics/migrant-health

50 Rural Health Information Hub. (2021, July 1). *Rural migrant health.* https://www.ruralhealthinfo.org/topics/migrant-health

My Notes

Successful strategies to support health services for migrant workers are as follows[51]:

- Culturally sensitive health education and outreach
- Educational materials at the appropriate literacy level
- Portable medical records and case management
- Mobile medical units
- Transportation services
- Translation services

Nurses can refer uninsured migrant farmworkers to Migrant Health Centers or other federally qualified health centers that are open to everyone. Individuals who do not have health insurance can pay for services based on a sliding-fee scale.

Read more about promoting migrant worker health at the Rural Migrant Health Information Hub.

Individuals with Mental Health Disorders

One in five American adults experiences some form of mental illness. Despite a recent focus on mental health in America, there are still many harmful attitudes and misunderstandings surrounding mental illness that can cause people to ignore their mental health and make it harder to reach out for help.[52]

Many individuals with mental health disorders go undiagnosed. Nurses must be aware of these common signs of mental health disorders[53]:

- Excessive worrying or fear
- Excessively sad feelings
- Confused thinking or problems concentrating and learning
- Extreme mood changes, including uncontrollable "highs" or feelings of euphoria
- Prolonged or strong feelings of irritability or anger
- Avoidance of friends and social activities
- Difficulties understanding or relating to other people
- Changes in sleeping habits or feeling tired and low energy
- Changes in eating habits, such as increased hunger or lack of appetite
- Changes in sex drive

---

51 Rural Health Information Hub. (2021, July 1). *Rural migrant health.* https://www.ruralhealthinfo.org/topics/migrant-health

52 Centers for Disease Control and Prevention. (2021, July 20). *Mental health.* https://www.cdc.gov/mentalhealth/index.htm

53 Centers for Disease Control and Prevention. (2021, July 20). *Mental health.* https://www.cdc.gov/mentalhealth/index.htm

My Notes

- Disturbances in perceiving reality (e.g., delusions and hallucinations)
- Inability to perceive changes in one's own feelings, behavior, or personality (i.e., lack of insight)
- Overuse of substances like alcohol or drugs
- Multiple physical ailments without obvious causes (such as headaches, stomachaches, or vague and ongoing "aches and pains")
- Thoughts of suicide
- Inability to carry out daily activities or handle daily problems and stress
- An intense fear of weight gain or overly concerned with appearance

Mental health conditions are also present in children. Because children are still learning how to identify and talk about thoughts and emotions, their most obvious symptoms are behavioral. Behavioral symptoms in children can include the following[54]:

- Changes in school performance
- Excessive worry or anxiety
- Hyperactive behavior
- Frequent nightmares
- Frequent disobedience or aggression
- Frequent temper tantrums

Nurses should recognize signs and symptoms of potentially undiagnosed mental health problems in all care settings and make appropriate referrals to mental health professionals and support organizations.

Visit the National Alliance on Mental Health (NAMI) website for resources on advocacy, education, support, and public awareness. NAMI's strategic goals are for people to get help early, get the best possible care, and be diverted from justice system involvement so that all individuals and families affected by mental illness can build better lives.[55]

Visit the web page, "Your Journey With Mental Illness" for several resources such as understanding your diagnosis, finding a health professional, understanding insurance, handling a crisis, and navigating finances and work.

NAMI Basics is an educational program for parents, family members, and caregivers who provide care for youth (ages 22 and younger) who are experiencing mental health symptoms. The program covers these topics:

- Impact mental health conditions can have on the entire family
- Different types of mental health care professionals and available treatment options and therapies

54 National Alliance on Mental Illness. (n.d.). *Warning signs and symptoms.* https://nami.org/About-Mental-Illness/Warning-Signs-and-Symptoms

55 National Alliance on Mental Health. (n.d.). *2020-2025 strategic plan.* https://nami.org/NAMInet/Board-of-Directors/Governance-Documents/NAMIStrategicPlan2020

My Notes

- Overview of the public mental health care, school, and juvenile justice systems and resources to help navigate these systems
- Child rights advocacy at school and in health care settings
- Preparation and response to crisis situations (self-harm, suicide attempts, etc.)
- Importance of self-care

Visit the NAMI Provider web page for an introduction of mental health professionals to the unique perspectives of people with mental health conditions and their families. It promotes empathy for their daily challenges and the importance of including them in all aspects of the treatment process.

Visit the NAMI In Our Own Voice web page to read about a program to promote a change in attitudes, assumptions, and ideas about people with mental health conditions. Presentations provide a personal perspective of mental health conditions, as leaders with lived experience talk openly about what it's like to have a mental health condition.

Homeless People

Homelessness can significantly affect an individual's health in three ways: health problems caused by homelessness, health problems that cause homelessness, and health conditions that are difficult to treat because of homelessness. As a result, the average age of death among homeless people is the mid-50s.[56]

Homeless people face multiple barriers to health care, including transportation, fragmentation of health care services, difficulty scheduling and keeping appointments, stigma of homelessness, lack of trust, social isolation, and significant basic physiological needs. Homeless people frequently have multiple needs resulting from exposure to violence or the elements, food insecurity, and untreated or undertreated physical and mental illnesses, resulting in frequent emergency department visits and hospitalizations.[57]

Effective health care for the homeless population addresses social determinants of health, such as housing, income, food, and social supports. The Medical Home Model developed by the Veterans Health Administration is an example of a proactive, primary care-based, interdisciplinary team model based on patient-centered, holistic care, and active communication and coordination among providers. This model is considered effective for patients with complex health care needs. See Figure 17.11[58] for an illustration of the Medical Home Model. As homeless veterans stabilize clinically and socially, as evidenced by their moving into permanent housing and demonstrating

---

56 O'Toole, T. P., Johnson, E. E., Aiello, R., Kane, V., & Pape, L. (2016). Tailoring care to vulnerable populations by incorporating social determinants of health: The veterans health administration's "homeless patient aligned care team" program. *Preventing Chronic Disease, 13*:150567. http://dx.doi.org/10.5888/pcd13.150567

57 O'Toole, T. P., Johnson, E. E., Aiello, R., Kane, V., & Pape, L. (2016). Tailoring care to vulnerable populations by incorporating social determinants of health: The veterans health administration's "homeless patient aligned care team" program. *Preventing Chronic Disease, 13*:150567. http://dx.doi.org/10.5888/pcd13.150567

58 This image is derived from O'Toole TP, Johnson EE, Aiello R, Kane V, Pape L. (2016). Tailoring care to vulnerable populations by incorporating social determinants of health: The veterans health administration's "homeless patient aligned care team" program. *Preventing Chronic Disease* 13:150567. http://dx.doi.org/10.5888/pcd13.150567

My Notes

appropriate self-care and health-seeking behaviors, they are transitioned to traditional care settings to continue their care.[59]

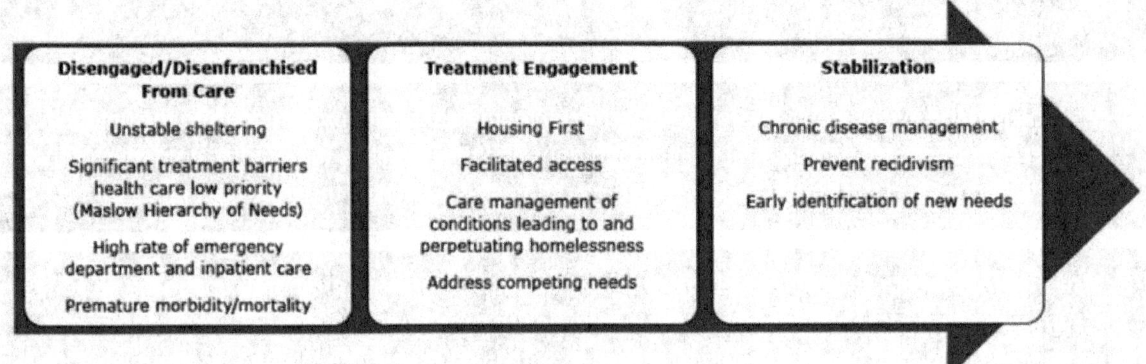

Figure 17.11 Medical Home Model

Medical Home Model

Core elements of the Medical Home Model distinguish it from traditional primary care with the following characteristics[60]:

- Low-threshold access to care
  - Open access with walk-in capacity and flexible scheduling (i.e., patients do not need an appointment to be seen by their care team)
  - Clinical outreach to homeless people on streets, in shelters, and in community locations such as soup kitchens
- Integrated services
  - Mental health services and primary care services are located close to each other, and providers from both services are involved in patients' health care plan
  - Sustenance needs (e.g., food or food vouchers, hygiene kits, clothes, bus passes, other transportation assistance) are available at the same location

59 O'Toole, T. P., Johnson, E. E., Aiello, R., Kane, V., & Pape, L. (2016). Tailoring care to vulnerable populations by incorporating social determinants of health: The veterans health administration's "homeless patient aligned care team" program. *Preventing Chronic Disease, 13*:150567. http://dx.doi.org/10.5888/pcd13.150567

60 O'Toole, T. P., Johnson, E. E., Aiello, R., Kane, V., & Pape, L. (2016). Tailoring care to vulnerable populations by incorporating social determinants of health: The veterans health administration's "homeless patient aligned care team" program. *Preventing Chronic Disease, 13*:150567. http://dx.doi.org/10.5888/pcd13.150567

My Notes

- Intensive health care management integrated with community agencies with an emphasis on ongoing, continuous care
- Ongoing staff training focused on development of homeless care skills

Research indicated the Medical Home Model reduced emergency department visits and hospitalizations of the homeless population by integrating supports that addressed social determinants of health into a clinical care model.[61]

61 O'Toole, T. P., Johnson, E. E., Aiello, R., Kane, V., & Pape, L. (2016). Tailoring care to vulnerable populations by incorporating social determinants of health: The veterans health administration's "homeless patient aligned care team" program. *Preventing Chronic Disease, 13*:150567. http://dx.doi.org/10.5888/pcd13.150567

17.3 SPOTLIGHT APPLICATION

This section will apply the tools from the "Community Assessment" chapter to providing care for victims of human trafficking as an example of a nurse generalist caring for a member of a vulnerable population. See Figure 17.12[1] regarding human trafficking initiatives.

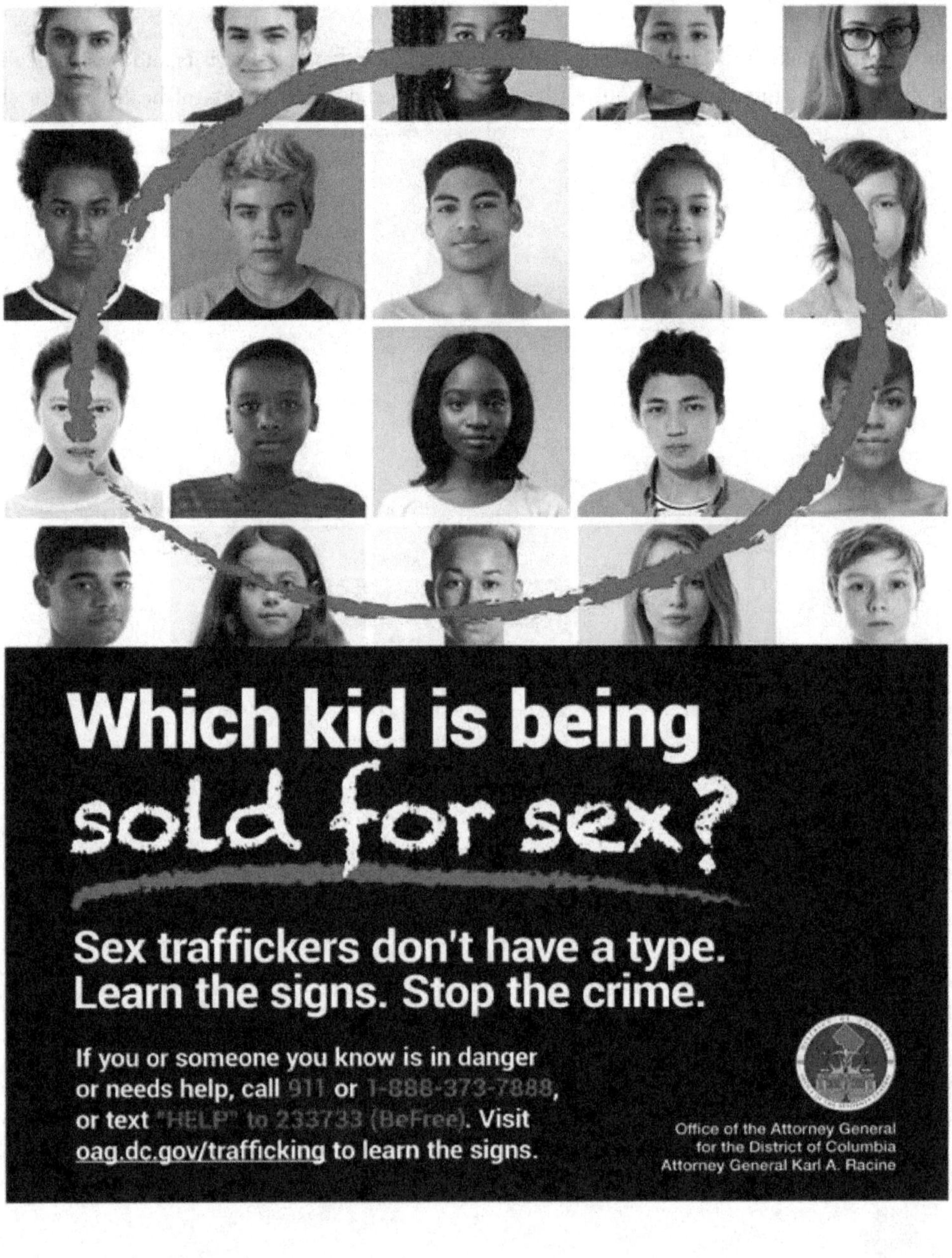

Figure 17.12 Human Trafficking Initiatives

1 "OAG-2020-Sex-Trafficking-Poster-English" by Office of Attorney General for the District of Columbia is in the Public Domain

My Notes

After hearing about a sexual trafficking arrest at a local hotel in the news, a nurse who works in the emergency department reads more information on the National Human Trafficking Hotline. Because the community is located near a major national interstate, the nurse realizes there are likely many unidentified victims of human trafficking passing through the community. The nurse develops a goal to improve the identification and support of individuals experiencing human trafficking in the community. The nurse begins a community health needs assessment by reading statistics on the National Human Trafficking Hotline, as well as additional information in the Adult Human Trafficking Screening Tool and Guide PDF by the U.S. Department of Health and Human Services' Administration for Children and Families. Based on this research, the nurse keeps the following tips in mind when conducting an assessment with a potential victim of trafficking[2,3]

- **Lack of self-identification.** Many victims do not self-identify as human trafficking victims due to lack of knowledge about the crime, as well as power and control dynamics involved in trafficking situations.
- **Being conscious of verbal and nonverbal messages.** When speaking with a potential victim of trafficking, the nurse plans on adopting open, nonthreatening body positioning; maintaining a calm tone of voice; displaying a warm, natural facial expression; using active listening skills; and mirroring the language the potential victim uses. For example, if the potential victim refers to her controller as her boyfriend, referring to that person as a "pimp" or a "sex trafficker" can negatively impact a therapeutic nurse-client relationship.
- **Being aware of power dynamics.** If a third party accompanies or interprets for the potential victim, the nurse plans on trying to speak to the potential victim alone or in a secure area with an official interpreter.
- **Being aware of canned stories.** Scripted stores are common, and the true story may not emerge until trust has been built with the potential victim.
- **Meeting the person's physical needs by offering a snack or beverage.** Most individuals experiencing human trafficking have been deprived of basic necessities, such as food, fluids, sleep, and urgent medical needs. Hunger is a very common problem for individuals who have been trafficked; a person who is hungry will have difficulty focusing and may be irritable.
- **Never allow confidential data to leave the office.** Ensure secure mechanisms to maintain privacy of client data (e.g., use effective passwords and/or locked file cabinets).
- **Being empathetic.** The decision to disclose trafficking can be mentally challenging, emotionally draining, and potentially physically unsafe for the victim. If the victim does not feel prepared to disclose during the immediate clinical visit, disclosure may occur at a future visit.[4]

---

2 National Human Trafficking Resource Center. (2011). *Human trafficking assessment for domestic violence & sexual assault programs.* https://humantraffickinghotline.org/sites/default/files/Assessment%20-%20Domestic%20Violence-Sexual%20Assault%20Programs.pdf

3 Macias-Konstantopoulos, W., & Owens, J. (2018). *Adult human trafficking screening tool and guide.* Administration for Children & Families and National Human Trafficking. https://www.acf.hhs.gov/sites/default/files/documents/otip/adult_human_trafficking_screening_tool_and_guide.pdf

4 Tracy, E. E., & Macias-Konstantopoulos, W. (2021). Human trafficking: Identification and evaluation in the health care setting. *UpToDate.* Retrieved March 16, 2022, from www.update.com

My Notes

Assessment

The nurse is aware of the warning signs an individual who is a victim of human trafficking or sexual violence may exhibit[5]:

- Shares a scripted or inconsistent history
- Is unwilling or hesitant to answer questions about an injury or illness
- Is accompanied by an individual who does not let the patient speak for themselves, refuses to let the patient have privacy, or who interprets for them
- Shares information about controlling or dominating relationships
- Demonstrates fearful or nervous behavior or avoids eye contact
- Is resistant to accept assistance or demonstrates hostile behavior
- Is unable to provide their address
- Is not aware of their location, the current date, or time
- Is not in possession of their identification documents
- Is not in control of his or her own money
- Is not being paid or wages are withheld

Sex trafficking victims may exhibit the following[6]:

- Patient is under the age of 18 and is involved in the commercial sex industry
- Has tattoos or other forms of branding, such as tattoos that say "Daddy," "Property of . . . ," "For sale," etc.
- Reports an unusually high number of sexual partners
- Does not have appropriate clothing for the weather or venue
- Uses language common in the commercial sex industry
- Experiences multiple sexually transmitted infections, pregnancies, miscarriages, or terminations

If concerning assessment findings are noted, the nurse plans on using a screening tool found in the Adult Human Trafficking Screening Tool and Guide PDF. Before beginning any conversation with the client, the nurse plans to assess for potential safety risks that may result from asking the client sensitive questions and to ensure privacy. The nurse also plans on being transparent about the limits of confidentiality regarding mandated reporting.[7]

---

5 Tracy, E. E., & Macias-Konstantopoulos, W. (2021). Human trafficking: Identification and evaluation in the health care setting. *UpToDate*. Retrieved March 16, 2022, from www.update.com

6 Tracy, E. E., & Macias-Konstantopoulos, W. (2021). Human trafficking: Identification and evaluation in the health care setting. *UpToDate*. Retrieved March 16, 2022, from www.update.com

7 Tracy, E. E., & Macias-Konstantopoulos, W. (2021). Human trafficking: Identification and evaluation in the health care setting. *UpToDate*. Retrieved March 16, 2022, from www.update.com

My Notes

Diagnosis

Several nursing diagnoses may apply to individuals experiencing human trafficking or sexual violence. Examples of diagnoses include the following[8]:

- *Post-Trauma Syndrome* related to insufficient social support
- *Powerlessness* related to insufficient sense of control
- *Chronic Low Self-Esteem* related to inadequate belonging
- *Risk for Impaired Emancipated Decision-Making* as manifested by insufficient privacy to openly discuss health care options

Outcomes Identification

The overall goal of the nurse is to identify and support victims of human trafficking or sexual violence. Individual SMART goals can be established for clients based on their circumstances. Some examples of SMART outcomes are as follows:

- The client will remain safe from injury and death.
- The client will verbalize local resources and support before the end of the visit.
- The client will acknowledge the traumatic experience and begin to work through the trauma by verbalizing feelings of fear, anger, anxiety, or helplessness during the visit.

Planning Interventions

The nurse prepares to respond quickly based on the client's circumstances by doing the following:

- Knowing how to contact law enforcement if the client or staff are in immediate danger.
- Being prepared to complete mandatory reporting requirements for minors and other circumstances according to state law.
- Creating a list of local services and resources to provide to human trafficking victims.

The nurse plans on sharing these resources regarding human trafficking with local community representatives associated with urgent care centers, clinics, primary care providers, and emergency departments.

Implementation

The nurse implements interventions with individuals seeking care based on assessment findings. Individualized interventions may include these steps:

- Contact law enforcement if the client or staff are in immediate danger.
- Create a safety plan by identifying the current level of risk and safety concerns. Outline concrete options for responding when the individual's safety is threatened.
- Refer the victim to local services and resources, such as food, shelter, and legal services.

---

8 Ackley, B., Ladwig, G., Makic, M. B., Martinez-Kratz, M., & Zanotti, M. (2020). *Nursing diagnosis handbook: An evidence-based guide to planning care* (12th ed.). Elsevier.

My Notes

- Share referral options. For assistance with finding referrals or other resources, contact the National Human Trafficking Hotline at 1–888–373–7888.
- Be prepared to respond to a potential trauma reaction. Encourage relaxation breathing and grounding techniques for immediate de-escalation. (Review crisis intervention in the "Stress, Coping, and Crisis Intervention" chapter and grounding techniques in the "Anxiety Disorders" chapter.)
- Perform mandatory reporting for minors and other circumstances according to state law. Read more about mandatory reporting in the box below.
- Report the case confidentially to appropriate authorities trained on human trafficking.
- Document assessment findings and referrals. Maintain client privacy and ensure the documentation is secure electronically or on paper.

Mandatory Reporting

Mandatory reporting is required for minors. Read more about mandatory reporting in the "Legal and Ethical Considerations in Mental Health Care" chapter. If reporting human trafficking of adults is not a component of your state's mandatory reporting statutes, certain circumstances may be considered reportable. Some of these "reportable" circumstances may include domestic violence, injuries caused in violation of criminal law, or injuries caused by a deadly weapon (e.g., firearm, knife, or machete). Some professionals hesitate to report potential victims of trafficking due to fears of violating the rules of the Health Insurance Portability and Accountability Act (HIPAA). HIPAA was written to protect patient confidentiality but was not designed to prevent the reporting of trauma and crimes. If you're unsure about whether HIPAA permits the reporting of patient information in a specific situation, human trafficking can still be reported without divulging individually identifiable patient health information. For example, you could report the gender, age of patient, and type of trafficking.[9]

Evaluation

The nurse plans on evaluating the success of achieving the overall goal to improve the identification and support of individuals experiencing human trafficking in the community in a variety of ways:

- Reviewing statistics reported by local law enforcement agencies regarding human trafficking cases.
- Reviewing statistics reported by the National Human Trafficking Hotline.
- Informally interviewing local community representatives associated with urgent care centers, clinics, primary care providers, and emergency departments regarding human trafficking cases.

9 Macias-Konstantopoulos, W., & Owens, J. (2018). Adult human trafficking screening tool and guide. *Administration for Children & Families and National Human Trafficking.* https://www.acf.hhs.gov/sites/default/files/documents/otip/adult_human_trafficking_screening_tool_and_guide.pdf

17.4 LEARNING ACTIVITIES

My Notes

Interactive Activities

An interactive H5P element has been excluded from this version of the text. You can view it online here: https://wtcs.pressbooks.pub/nursingmhcc/?p=806#h5p-56

An interactive H5P element has been excluded from this version of the text. You can view it online here: https://wtcs.pressbooks.pub/nursingmhcc/?p=806#h5p-58

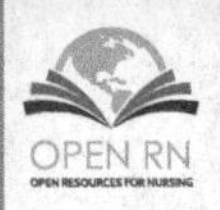

My Notes

XVII GLOSSARY

Health disparities: Health differences that are linked with social, economic, and/or environmental disadvantages. Health disparities adversely affect groups of people who often experience greater obstacles to health based on individual characteristics, such as socioeconomic status, age, gender, culture, religion, mental illness, disability, sexual orientation, or gender identity.

Health equity: The attainment of the highest level of health for all people.

Human trafficking victims: Individuals forced to work or provide commercial sex against their will in legal business settings and underground markets.

Migrant worker: A person who moves within their home country or outside of it to pursue work. Migrant workers usually do not intend to stay permanently in the country or region in which they work.

Telehealth: The use of digital technologies to deliver medical care, health education, and public health services by connecting multiple users in separate locations.

Vulnerable population: A group of individuals who are at increased risk for health problems and health disparities.

Chapter 18

Environmental Health and Emergency Preparedness

18.1 INTRODUCTION

My Notes

Learning Objectives

- Describe the nurse's role in promoting environmental health
- Identify environmental hazards and risks in the community and globally
- Explain nursing roles in disaster planning, emergency preparedness, and emergency response
- Apply principles of triage
- Outline tips for preventing and managing stress for disaster responders

Since the early years of the profession, nursing leaders such as Florence Nightingale and Lillian Wald have recognized the role of nurses in controlling the influence of environmental factors on health. Nurses have long appreciated that a healthy environment impacts the physical and mental health of individuals, families, communities, and populations.[1]

At some point during their career, nearly every nurse finds themselves caring for individuals affected by exposure to an environmental hazard or disaster. Disasters have environmental, physical, and psychological effects on individuals and communities. The increasing impacts of natural, man-made, and infectious disease disasters have changed health care and nursing perspectives around the world. Nurses are on the front lines in supporting individuals and communities affected by disasters. This chapter will review nurses' roles in promoting environmental health and treating individuals exposed to environmental hazards, as well as participating in emergency preparedness and disaster response and recovery.

1 American Nurses Association. (2007). *ANA's principles of environmental health for nursing practice with implementation strategies.* Nursesbooks.org. https://www.nursingworld.org/~4afaf8/globalassets/practiceandpolicy/work-environment/health--safety/principles-of-environmental-health-online_final.pdf

My Notes

18.2 ENVIRONMENTAL HEALTH

The American Nurses Association (ANA) established an *Environmental Health* standard defined as, "The registered nurse practices in a manner that advances environmental safety and health."[1] Review the competencies for this standard in the following box.

ANA's Environmental Health Competencies[2]

The registered nurse:

- Creates a safe and healthy workplace and professional practice environment
- Fosters a professional environment that does not tolerate abusive, destructive, and oppressive behaviors
- Promotes evidence-based practices to create a psychologically and physically safe environment
- Assesses the environment to identify and address the impact of social determinants of health on risk factors
- Reduces environmental health risks to self, colleagues, health care consumers, and the world
- Integrates environmental health concepts in practice
- Communicates information about environmental health risks and exposure risk strategies
- Advocates for the implementation of environmental health principles in communities in which they work and live
- Incorporates technologies to promote safe practice environments
- Uses products or treatments consistent with evidence- based practice to reduce environmental threats and hazards
- Examines how the health care consumer's biography affects their biology, resultant health issues, and the ecosystem
- Analyzes the impacts of social, political, and economic influences on the human health experience and global environment
- Advances environmental concerns and complaints through advocacy and appropriate reporting mechanisms
- Promotes sustainable global environmental health policies and conditions that focus on prevention of hazards to people and the natural environment

---

1 American Nurses Association. (2021). *Nursing: Scope and standards of practice* (4th ed.). American Nurses Association.

2 American Nurses Association. (2021). *Nursing: Scope and standards of practice* (4th ed.). American Nurses Association.

My Notes

The environment is the air we breathe, the water we drink, the food we eat, and the places where we live, work, and play. There is a connection between the environment and the health of individuals and communities. An environmental health hazard is a substance or pathogen that has the ability to cause an adverse health event in individuals or communities. Examples of environmental hazards are air contaminants, toxic waste, radiation, disease-causing microorganisms and plants, pesticides, heavy metals, chemicals in consumer products, and extreme temperatures and weather events.[3]

Environmental health hazards can be divided into five main categories: housing, occupational, atmosphere, foodborne diseases, and waterborne diseases. View examples of environmental hazards by category in Table 18.2.

Table 18.2 Environmental Hazards

Category	Environmental Hazards
Housing	**Building Contaminants:** Radon, asbestos, carbon monoxide, and lead **Personal Chemicals:** Nail polish remover, spray deodorant, and rubbing alcohol **Household Chemicals:** Kerosene, coal or wood-burning stoves, burning pine cones or wax candles, burning incense, chlorinated water in swimming pools, cleaning products, household detergents, plastic cement, acrylic paints, furniture wax, rubber-based paints, gasoline, white-out solvents, and pesticides (used in gardening chemicals and lawn care) **Electromagnetic Pollution:** Electric blankets, electrically heated water beds, fluorescent lighting, cathode ray tubes (computer terminals), microwave ovens, television sets, radio or TV transmission towers, short-wave radio transmitters, and high-voltage electrical power lines **Natural Contaminants:** Mold and pollen **Human Contaminants:** Second-hand smoke
Occupational	**Medical Chemicals:** Injectable phenol (found in allergy shots) and silver amalgam (found in some dental fillings) **Occupational Chemicals:** Radioactivity from direct radiation or decay from nuclear waste **Construction Materials & Industry:** Urea-formaldehyde foam insulation, asbestos insulation, fiberglass & particleboard, treated lumber, and silica air pollution **Noise Pollution:** Traffic, loud music, workplace equipment noise, and airports **Ergonomics:** Physical injuries due to positioning or lack of physical assistance **Communicable Infectious Disease:** Exposure to infections despite transmission precautions (i.e., airborne, droplet, or contact precautions). Read more about the chain of infection and transmission precautions in the "Infection" chapter of Open RN *Nursing Fundamentals.*
Atmosphere	**Air pollution** **Greenhouse Gasses:** Carbon dioxide, methane, nitrous oxide, and fluorinated gasses **Ultraviolet Radiation**

3 Centers for Disease Control and Prevention. (2019, January 3). *Introduction to environmental public health tracking.* https://www.cdc.gov/nceh/tracking/tracking-intro.html

My Notes

Category	Environmental Hazards
Waterborne Illness (Recreational or drinking water contaminated by disease-causing microbes or pathogens)	**Chemical and Metal Contaminants:** Chlorine, fluorine, mercury, lead, and nitrates **Common Microbes:** Cryptosporidiosis, cyclosporiasis, Escherichia, giardiasis, legionellosis, norovirus, shigellosis, blue-green algae, schistosome parasites (swimmer's itch), pseudomonas (hot tub rash), and cholera Read more about waterborne illness at the Wisconsin Department of Health or the Minnesota Department of Health. *Report waterborne illness to the state Department of Health.
Foodborne Illness (Consuming foods or beverages contaminated with bacteria, viruses, parasites, toxins, or chemicals)	**Common Pathogens:** Clostridium botulinum, listeria, campylobacter, norovirus, clostridium perfringens, cryptosporidiosis cyclosporiasis, Escherichia, giardiasis, salmonellosis, shigellosis, toxoplasmosis, yersiniosis, and hepatitis A Read more about foodborne illness at the Wisconsin Department of Health or Minnesota Department of Health. *Report foodborne illness to the state Department of Health.

Recognizing environmental hazards can help community health nurses provide information to community members and implement prevention strategies that promote positive outcomes. See Figure 18.1[4] for an example of prevention strategies related to the environmental hazard of lead poisoning.

4 "preventable.jpg" by unknown author for National Center for Environmental Health, Division of Environmental Health Science and Practice is in the Public Domain

My Notes

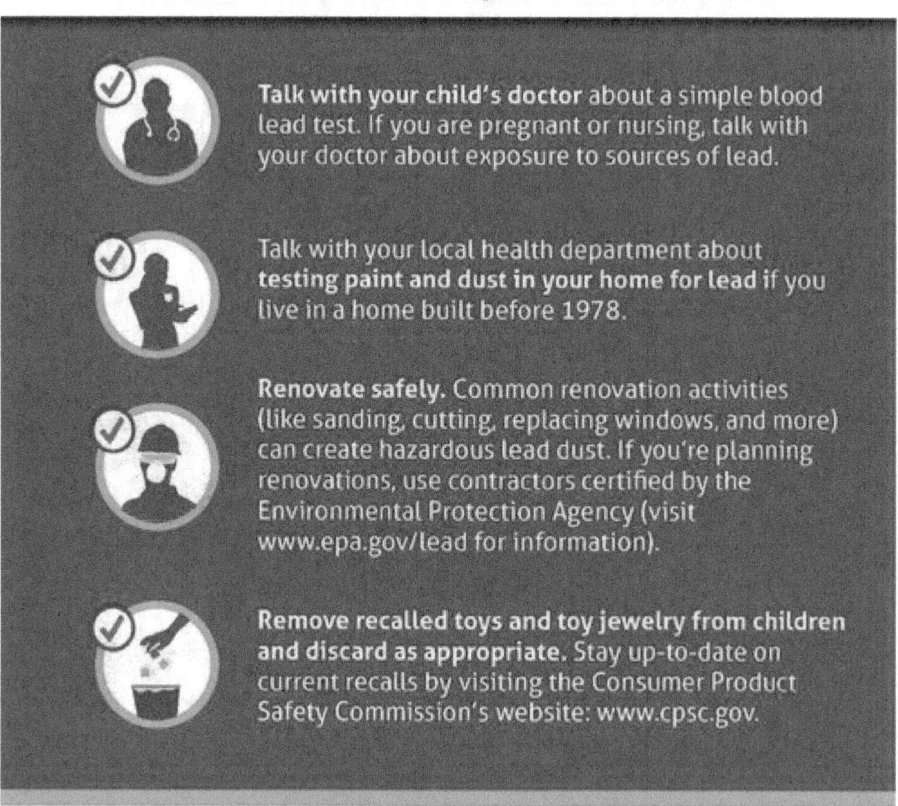

Figure 18.1 Lead Poisoning

Caring for individuals exposed to environmental hazards will be discussed in the following "Emergency Preparedness, Response, and Recovery" section.

Read more information about promoting environmental health and safety in nursing in the following box.

> Read a free e-book titled *Environmental Health in Nursing* published by the Alliance of Nurses for Healthy Environments (ANHE).

> Review the "Environmental Safety" section of the "Safety" chapter in Open RN *Nursing Fundamentals*.

My Notes

18.3 EMERGENCY PREPAREDNESS, RESPONSE, AND RECOVERY

A **disaster** is defined as a serious disruption of the functioning of a community or a society at any scale due to hazardous events interacting with conditions of exposure, vulnerability, and capacity that lead to human, material, economic, and environmental losses and impacts.[1] Every community must prepare to respond to disasters that include natural events (e.g., tornadoes, hurricanes, floods, wildfires, earthquakes, or disease outbreaks), man-made events (e.g., harmful chemical spills, mass shootings, or terrorist attacks), or infectious disease outbreaks. See Figure 18.2[2] for an image of the effects of the natural disaster Hurricane Katrina.

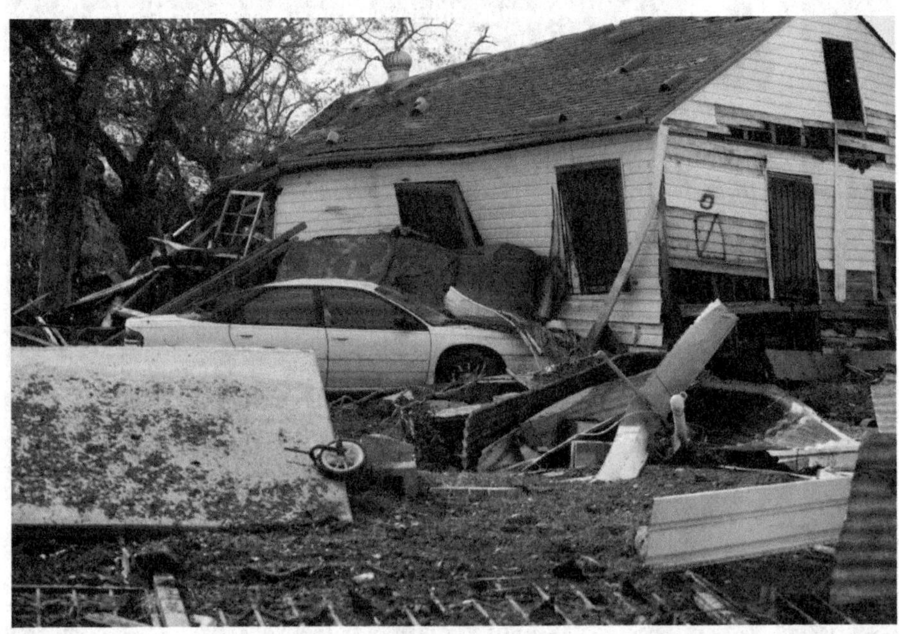

Figure 18.2 Effects of Hurricane Katrina

Emergency preparedness is the planning process focused on avoiding or reducing the risks and hazards resulting from a disaster to optimize population health and safety. **Disaster management** refers to the integration of emergency response plans throughout the life cycle of a disaster event. Because disasters cause physical and psychological effects in a community, emergency preparedness and disaster management emphasize collaboration and cooperative aid among health care institutions and community agencies to ensure a coordinated and effective response.[3]

Read the American Nurses Association resource regarding Disaster Preparedness.

1 National Academies of Sciences, Engineering, and Medicine. (2021). *The future of nursing 2020-2030: Charting a path to achieve health equity*. National Academies Press. https://doi.org/10.17226/25982

2 "LA_1603_9thDistDam121.jpg" by Booher, Andrea, Photographer is in the Public Domain

3 Savage, C. L. (2020). *Public/community health and nursing practice: Caring for populations* (2nd ed.). FA Davis.

My Notes

Emergency preparedness and disaster management are based on four key concepts: preparedness, mitigation, response, and recovery. This process guides decision-making when an emergency or disaster occurs in a community.[4] After the disaster event has concluded, evaluation of the effectiveness of the response occurs as part of planning emergency preparedness. See Figure 18.3[5] for a diagram that illustrates this theoretical framework for emergency preparedness. Each of these concepts is further discussed in the following subsections.

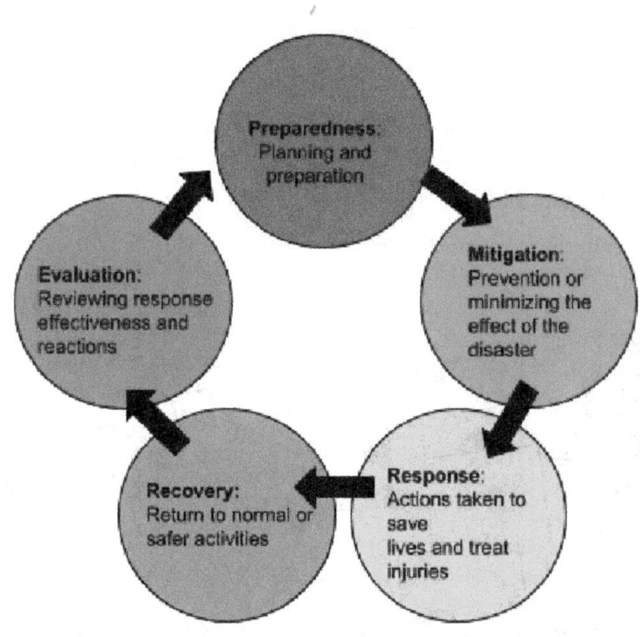

Figure 18.3 Key Concepts in Emergency Preparedness and Response

Preparedness

Preparedness includes planning, training personnel, and providing educational activities regarding potential disastrous events. Planning includes evaluating environmental risks and social vulnerabilities of a community. Environmental risk refers to the probability and consequences of an unwanted accident in the environment in which community members live, work, or play. Risk assessment also includes assessing social vulnerabilities that affect community resilience.[6]

Social vulnerability refers to the characteristics of a person or a community that affect their capacity to anticipate, confront, repair, and recover from the effects of a disaster.[7] Populations living in a disaster-stricken area are not

4 Emergency Management Institute. (2013). *ISS-111.A: Livestock in disasters.* Federal Emergency Management Agency. https://training.fema.gov/emiweb/downloads/is111_unit%204.pdf

5 "Environmental Health and Emergency Preparedness" by Dawn Barone for Open RN is licensed under CC BY 4.0

6 Flanagan, B. E., Hallisey, E. J., Adams, E., & Lavery, A. (2018). Measuring community vulnerability to natural and anthropogenic hazards: The Centers for Disease Control and Prevention's social vulnerability index. *Journal of Environmental Health, 80*(10). 34–36. https://www.ncbi.nlm.nih.gov/pmc/articles/PMC7179070/

7 Flanagan, B. E., Hallisey, E. J., Adams, E., & Lavery, A. (2018). Measuring community vulnerability to natural and anthropogenic hazards: The Centers for Disease Control and Prevention's social vulnerability index. *Journal of Environmental Health, 80*(10). 34–36. https://www.ncbi.nlm.nih.gov/pmc/articles/PMC7179070/

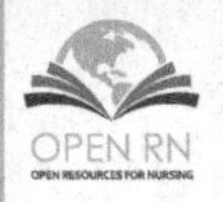

My Notes

affected equally. Many factors can weaken community members' ability to respond to disasters, including poverty, lack of access to transportation, and crowded housing. Evidence indicates that those living in poverty are more vulnerable at all stages of a catastrophic event, as are racial and ethnic minorities, children, elderly, and disabled people.[8] Socially vulnerable communities are more likely to experience higher rates of mortality, morbidity, and property destruction and are less likely to fully recover in the wake of a disaster compared to communities that are less socially vulnerable. Community health nurses must plan emergency responses to disasters that address these social vulnerabilities to decrease human suffering and financial loss.

The Centers for Disease Control and Prevention (CDC) and the Agency for Toxic Substances and Disease Registry (ATSDR) created a Social Vulnerability Index database and mapping tool designed to assist state, local, and tribal disaster management officials in identifying the locations of their most socially vulnerable populations. Geographic patterns of social vulnerabilities can be used in all phases of emergency preparedness and disaster management. See Figure 18.4[9] for an image of social vulnerability mapping.

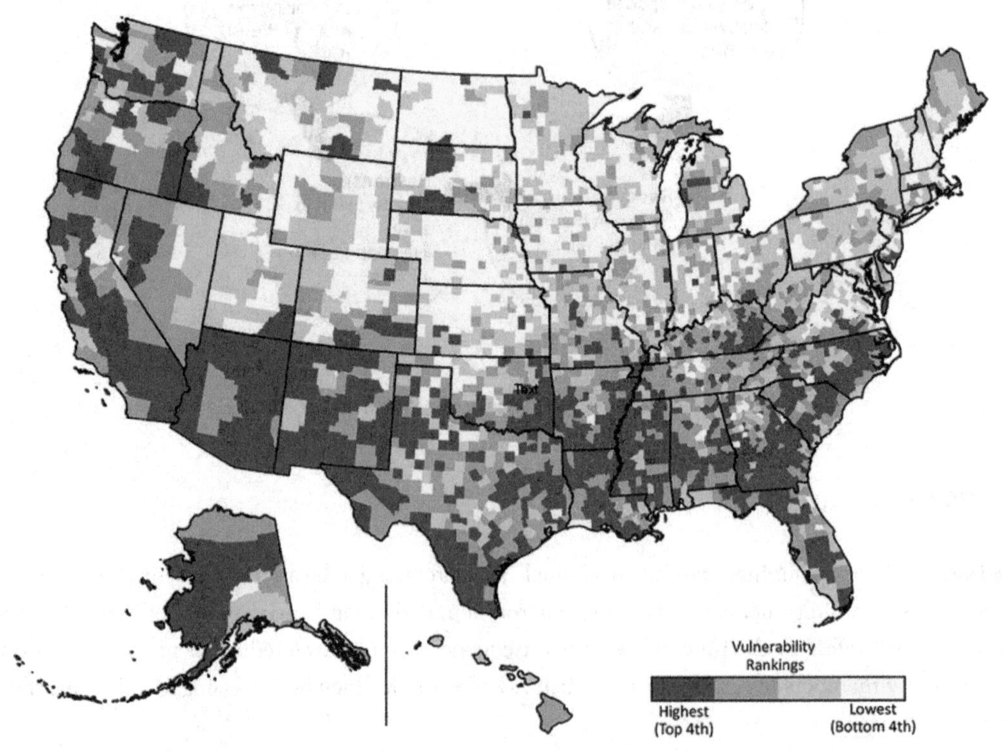

Figure 18.4 Social Vulnerability Mapping

View the CDC/ATSDR Social Vulnerability Index Interactive Map.

8 Flanagan, B. E., Hallisey, E. J., Adams, E., & Lavery, A. (2018). Measuring community vulnerability to natural and anthropogenic hazards: The Centers for Disease Control and Prevention's social vulnerability index. *Journal of Environmental Health, 80*(10). 34–36. https://www.ncbi.nlm.nih.gov/pmc/articles/PMC7179070/

9 Flanagan, B. E., Hallisey, E. J., Adams, E., & Lavery, A. (2018). Measuring community vulnerability to natural and anthropogenic hazards: The Centers for Disease Control and Prevention's social vulnerability index. *Journal of Environmental Health, 80*(10). 34–36. https://www.ncbi.nlm.nih.gov/pmc/articles/PMC7179070/

Mitigation

My Notes

Mitigation refers to actions taken to prevent or reduce the cause, impact, and consequences of disasters. Health care institutions and community health agencies plan three Cs to mitigate the effects of a disaster:

- **Communication:** An emergency communication plan identifies tools, resources, teams, and strategies to ensure effective actions during emergencies.
- **Coordination:** Coordination plays a crucial role in efficiency and effectiveness of disaster management by providing a big picture of an emergency and reducing uncertainty levels among responders.
- **Collaboration:** Collaboration allows responders to act together smoothly and helps reduce impact of the disaster.

Response

The **response** phase occurs in the immediate aftermath of a disaster. When a disaster occurs, actions are taken to save lives, treat injuries, and minimize the effect of the disaster. Immediate needs are addressed, such as medical treatment, shelter, food, and water, as well as psychological support of survivors. Personal safety and well-being in an emergency and the duration of the response phase depend on the level of a community's preparedness. Examples of response activities include implementing disaster response plans, conducting search and rescue missions, and taking actions to protect oneself, family members, pets, and other community members.[10]

While the immediate actions of responding to a disaster are treating physical injuries, psychological effects must be addressed as well. To minimize psychological effects, nurses and first responders can provide support to victims of the disaster by following these tips from the Substance Abuse and Mental Health Services Administration (SAMHSA)[11]:

- **Promote safety:** Ensure basic needs are met and provide simple instructions about how to receive these basic needs.
- **Promote calm:** Listen to people express their feelings and provide empathy and compassion even if they are angry, upset, or acting out. Offer objective information about the situation and efforts being made to help those affected by the disaster.
- **Promote connectedness:** Help people connect with friends, family members, and other loved ones. Keep families and family units together as best as possible, especially by keeping children with those whom they feel safe.
- **Promote self-efficacy:** Give suggestions about how people can help themselves and guide them toward the resources available. Encourage families and individuals to help meet their own needs.
- **Promote help and hope:** Know what services are available and direct people to those services and continue to update people about what is being done. When people are worried or scared, remind them that help is on the way.

---

10 Emergency Management Institute. (2013). *ISS-111.A: Livestock in disasters.* Federal Emergency Management Agency. https://training.fema.gov/emiweb/downloads/is111_unit%204.pdf

11 Substance Abuse and Mental Health Services Administration. (2005). *Psychological first aid for first responders.* [Handout]. U.S. Department of Health & Human Services. https://store.samhsa.gov/product/Psychological-First-Aid-for-First-Responders/NMH05-0210

My Notes

Disaster Response Protocols

When thinking about responding to a disaster, first responders and emergency personnel come to mind such as law enforcement, fire departments, and emergency medical technicians (EMTs). However, nurses are also called upon to assist in emergencies or disasters and must be competent in responding. Nurses may be involved in triaging individuals for treatment.

To respond effectively when a disaster occurs, emergency responders perform **triage** by prioritizing treatment for individuals affected by the disaster or emergency. **Field triage** sorts victims affected by the event and ranks victims based on the severity of their symptoms. **Disaster triage** determines the severity of injuries suffered by victims and then systematically distributes them to local health care facilities based on their severity.

Simple Triage and Rapid Treatment (START) is an example of a triage system established by the U.S. Department of Health and Human Services that prioritizes treatment of victims by using standard colors indicating the severity of symptoms and prognosis. See Figure 18.5[12] for the START algorithm. The following colors indicate severity of injury and prognosis:

- **RED:** Emergent needs
  - Life-threatening needs, such as alterations in airway, breathing, and circulation; impairment in neurological systems; or severe, life-threatening injuries.
  - They may have less than 60 minutes to survive.
  - These patients will be seen first or immediately.
- **YELLOW:** Urgent, but delayed needs
  - Life-threatening needs; status is not anticipated to change quickly or significantly in the next hours, so transport can be delayed.
- **GREEN:** Non-urgent needs, often referred to as the "walking wounded"
  - Minor injuries; status is not likely to deteriorate over the next several days.
  - Many individuals can assist with obtaining their own care.
- **BLACK:** The person has died or is expected to die soon
  - This person is unlikely to survive given the severity of their injuries, level of available care, or both.
  - Palliative care and pain relief should be provided.

12 "StartAdultTriageAlgorithm.png" by unknown author at CHEMM is in the Public Domain

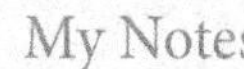

START Adult Triage

Able to walk? — Yes → MINOR → SECONDARY TRIAGE

No ↓

Spontaneous breathing — No → Position airway — Spontaneous breathing → IMMEDIATE

Position airway — APNEA → EXPECTANT

Yes ↓

Respiratory Rate — >30 → IMMEDIATE

<30 ↓

Perfusion — Radial pulse absent[1] or capillary refill > 2 sec → IMMEDIATE

Radial pulse present or capillary refill < 2 sec ↓

Mental status — Doesn't obey commands → IMMEDIATE

Obeys commands ↓

DELAYED

Triage Categories

EXPECTANT — Black Triage Tag Color
- Victim unlikely to survive given severity of injuries, level of available care, or both
- Palliative care and pain relief should be provided

IMMEDIATE — Red Triage Tag Color
- Victim can be helped by immediate intervention and transport
- Requires medical attention within minutes for survival (up to 60)
- Includes compromises to patient's Airway, Breathing, Circulation

DELAYED — Yellow Triage Tag Color
- Victim's transport can be delayed
- Includes serious and potentially life-threatening injuries, but status not expected to deteriorate significantly over several hours

MINOR — Green Triage Tag Color
- Victim with relatively minor injuries
- Status unlikely to deteriorate over days
- May be able to assist in own care: "Walking Wounded"

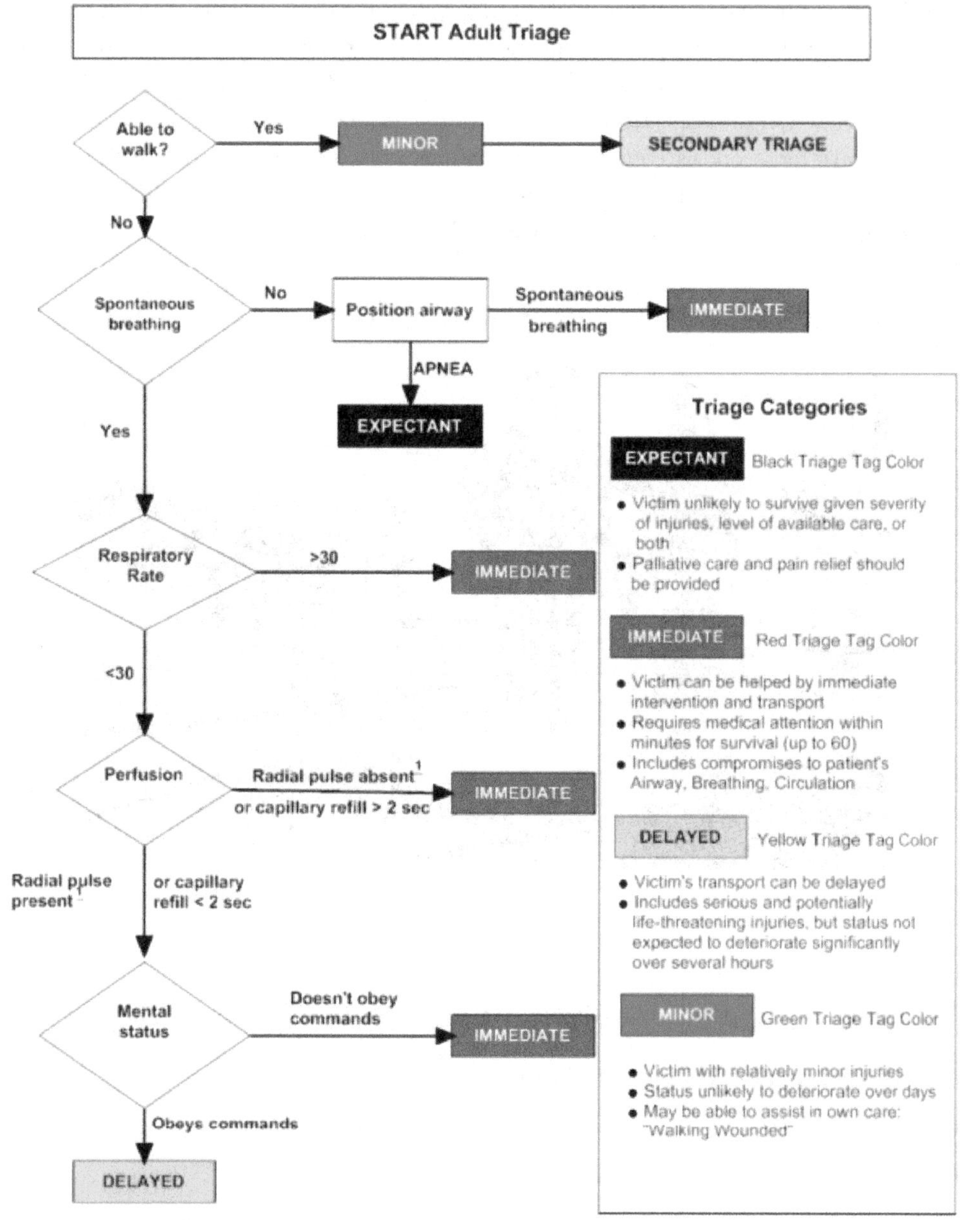

Adopted from http://www.start-triage.com

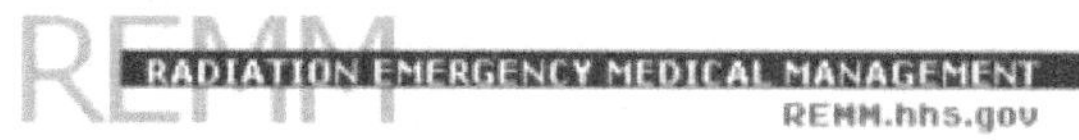

Figure 18.5 START Adult Triage

Providing Care for Those Exposed to Environmental Hazards

Nurses may be involved in caring for clients who have been exposed to chemicals or other environmental hazards. See Table 18.3 for assessment findings and interventions for a variety of exposures. **Chelation therapy** is a treatment indicated for heavy metal poisoning such as mercury, arsenic, and lead. Chelators are medications that bind to the metals in the bloodstream to increase urinary excretion of the substance.

My Notes

Some chemical exposures require decontamination to treat the individual, as well as to protect others around them, including first responders, nurses, and other patients. **Decontamination** is any process that removes or neutralizes a chemical hazard on or in the patient to prevent or mitigate adverse health effects to the patient; protect emergency first responders, health care facility first receivers, and other patients from secondary contamination; and reduce the potential for secondary contamination of response and health care infrastructure. For example, if a farmer enters a rural hospital's emergency department after chemical exposure to an insecticide spray, decontamination may be required. See Figure 18.6[13] for an image of decontamination.

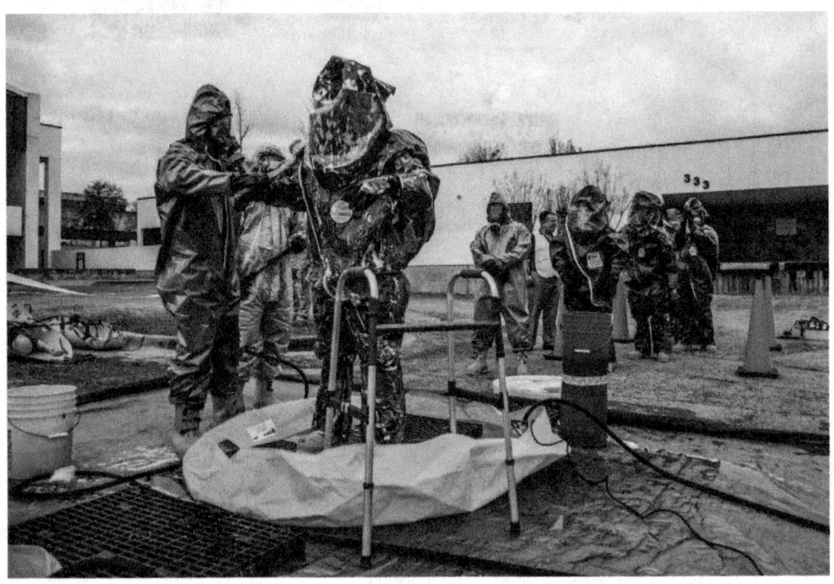

Figure 18.6 Decontamination

The decision to decontaminate an individual should take into account a combination of these key indicators[14]:

- Signs and symptoms of exposure displayed by the patient
- Visible evidence of contamination on the patient's skin or clothing
- Proximity of the patient to the location of the chemical release
- Contamination detected on the patient using appropriate detection technology
- The chemical and its properties
- Request by the patient for decontamination, even if contamination is unlikely

13 "decontamination26.jpg" by Benjamin Crossley CDP/FEMA is in the Public Domain

14 U.S. Department of Homeland Security, & U.S. Department of Health & Human Services. (2014). *Patient decontamination in a mass chemical exposure incident: National planning guidance for communities.* http://www.phe.gov/Preparedness/responders/Documents/patient-decon-natl-plng-guide.pdf

My Notes

Table 18.3 Assessment Findings and Interventions for Exposure to Various Environmental Hazards

Chemical or Hazard	Assessment Findings	Interventions
Carbon Monoxide (CO) Poisoning (Auto exhaust and improperly vented or malfunctioning furnaces or fuel-burning devices)[15]	Primarily decreased mental status from confusion to coma May have cherry-red appearance of the lips and skin *Note: Pulse oximetry does not reflect accurate oxygenation levels because CO binds to hemoglobin.	■ Remove from source of exposure ■ Provide fresh air ■ Administer high-flow oxygen by face mask; may require intubation and mechanical ventilation ■ Obtain arterial blood gas (ABG) sample of carboxyhemoglobin ■ Administer hyperbaric oxygen, if necessary
Lead Poisoning (Lead-contaminated paint dust, water, or food and bullets in wild game)[16,17]	Abdominal pain, constipation, fatigue, joint pain, muscle pain, headache, anemia, memory deficits, psychiatric symptoms, elevated blood pressure, decreased kidney function, decreased sperm count, increased mortality *Note: Some symptoms may be irreversible.	■ Remove source of exposure ■ Monitor blood lead level (toxic effects occur if > 10 mcg) ■ Monitor hemoglobin and hematocrit for anemia ■ Monitor urinary output ■ Administer chelation therapy with ethylenediaminetetraacetic acid (EDTA) ■ Educate about lead-related health risks and removal of lead-based paint and other sources of exposure using safe OSHA practices

15 Clardy, P. F., & Manaker, S. (2021, June 17). Carbon monoxide poisoning. *UpToDate.* Accessed April 3, 2022, from www.update.com

16 World Health Organization. (2021, October 11). *Lead poisoning.* https://www.who.int/news-room/fact-sheets/detail/lead-poisoning-and-health

17 Goldman, R. H., & Hu, H. (2021, November 4). Lead exposure and poisoning in adults. *UpToDate.* Accessed April 3, 2022, from www.update.com

My Notes

Chemical or Hazard	Assessment Findings	Interventions
Formaldehyde Poisoning (Construction and agriculture products and disinfectants)[18]	Eye and skin irritation, abdominal pain, bronchospasm, shortness of breath, decreased respiratory rate, acute kidney failure	■ Remove from source of exposure ■ Provide fresh air (fumes are toxic) ■ Decontaminate ■ Flush eyes with water ■ Shower to cleanse skin ■ Administer oxygen as needed ■ If swallowed, don't induce vomiting ■ Administer activated charcoal or gastric lavage
Arsenic Poisoning (Contaminated groundwater, tobacco smoke, hide tanning, and pressure treated wood)[19,20]	Nausea/vomiting, abdominal pain, diarrhea, paresthesias, muscle cramping, skin pigmentation changes, skin lesions and cancers, cardiac dysrhythmias, death	■ Decontaminate skin and hair ■ Test urine for arsenic (it is rapidly cleared from blood) ■ Test hair follicles, fingernails, and skin for long-term exposure ■ Administer activated charcoal ■ Administer chelation therapy with dimercaprol or DMSA ■ Administer IV fluids to maintain urine output ■ Provide continuous cardiac monitoring ■ Identify and remove source of exposure
Mercury (Thermometers, sphygmomanometers, fluorescent light bulbs, amalgam tooth fillings, and contaminated fish)[21]	Acute inhalation exposure in occupational settings may cause cough, dyspnea, chest pain, excessive salivation, inflammation of gums, severe nausea/vomiting, diarrhea, dermatitis	■ Remove from source of exposure ■ Blood or urine mercury tests ■ If inhaled, oxygenation, bronchodilators, chelation treatment ■ If ingested, administer chelation therapy ■ If consume fish, fish with 0.3 to 0.49 ppm of mercury can be safely consumed three times per month but those with greater than 0.5 ppm should be avoided

18 Agency for Toxic Substances and Disease Registry. (2014, October 21). *Medical management guidelines for formaldehyde.* Centers for Disease Control and Prevention. https://www.cdc.gov/TSP/MMG/MMGDetails.aspx?mmgid=216&toxid=39

19 World Health Organization. (2018, February 15). *Arsenic.* https://www.who.int/news-room/fact-sheets/detail/arsenic

20 Goldman, R. H. (2020, October 8). Arsenic exposure and poisoning. *UpToDate.* Accessed April 3, 2022, from www.update.com

21 Beauchamp, G., Kusin, S., & Elinder, C. (2022, February 1). *Mercury toxicity. UpToDate.* Accessed April 3, 2022, from www.update.com

My Notes

Chemical or Hazard	Assessment Findings	Interventions
Radon Gas (Naturally occurring gas resulting from the decay of trace amounts of uranium found in the earth's crust)[22]	Persistent cough, hoarseness, wheezing, shortness of breath, coughing up blood, chest pain, frequent respiratory infections like bronchitis and pneumonia, loss of appetite, weight loss, fatigue, lung cancer	■ Measure levels of radon in the home (testing kits available) ■ Install radon mitigation system in home ■ Provide public education
Infectious Disease (HIV, hepatitis, sexually transmitted diseases, and COVID-19)	Symptoms are based on disease process	■ Blood tests for HIV, hepatitis, syphilis ■ Quarantine and contact trace as indicated by health department ■ Implement transmission-based precautions based on route of transmission ■ Provide public education about the disease and how it is spread ■ Report communicable disease based on state reporting requirements. Each state has requirements for reporting communicable disease to the Department of Health. For example, see Wisconsin's Department of Health Communicable Disease Reporting Requirements or Minnesota's Department of Health Communicable Disease Reporting Requirements.
Frostbite (Overexposure of skin to cold)[23]	White or grayish color of exposed skin, may be hard or waxy to touch; lack of sensitivity to touch or numbness and tingling; clear or blood-filled blisters after thawing; cyanosis after rewarming indicates necrosis	■ Remove wet clothing ■ Warm skin slowly in warm (not hot) water or with body heat ■ Do not rub area or allow walking on frostbitten feet because of potential tissue damage ■ May administer tPA for severe injury with thrombosis

22 National Radon Defense. (n.d.). *Radon symptoms.* https://www.nationalradondefense.com/radon-information/radon-symptoms.html

23 Zafren, K., & Mechem, C. C. (2021, February 1). Frostbite: Emergency care and prevention. *UpToDate.* Accessed April 3, 2022, from www.update.com

My Notes

Chemical or Hazard	Assessment Findings	Interventions
Organophosphates (Insecticides and bioterrorism nerve agents)[24]	Acute onset of symptoms related to cholinergic excess: bradycardia, increased salivation, tearing, urination, vomiting and diarrhea, diaphoresis, paralysis, respiratory failure, hypotension, seizures Intermediate syndrome: neck flexion weakness, cranial nerve abnormalities, muscle weakness	■ Remove from source of exposure ■ Aggressively decontaminate ■ Administer 100% oxygen (may require endotracheal intubation) ■ Monitor RBC acetylcholinesterase ■ Administer atropine (prevents cholinergic activation) ■ Administer IV fluids for hypotension ■ Administer benzodiazepines for seizures
Bioterrorism (Anthrax, smallpox, nerve agents, and ricin)[25]	Symptoms are based on the agent	■ Activate 911 ■ Decontaminate as indicated ■ Manage ABCs ■ Coordinate with emergency management officials

Access up-to-date, evidence-based information for suspected poisoning at the Poison Control Center or call 1-800-222-1222.

Read more about Patient Decontamination in a Mass Chemical Exposure Incident by the U.S. Department of Homeland Security and the U.S. Department of Health and Human Services.

Recovery

During the recovery period, restoration efforts occur concurrently with regular operations and activities. The recovery period from a disaster can be prolonged. Examples of recovery activities include the following[26]:

- Preventing or reducing stress-related illnesses and excessive financial burdens
- Rebuilding damaged structures
- Reducing vulnerability to future disasters

When people are affected by a disaster, they may respond in a variety of different ways. It is natural and expected to respond to a disaster with emotions such as fear, worry, sadness, anxiety, depression, and despair. Many people

24 Bird, S. (2021, September 23). Organophosphate and carbamate poisoning. *UpToDate.* Accessed April 3, 2022, from www.update.com

25 Adalja, A. A. (2022, January 10). Identifying and managing casualties of biological terrorism. *UpToDate.* Accessed April 3, 2022, from www.update.com

26 Emergency Management Institute. (2013). *ISS-111.A: Livestock in disasters.* Federal Emergency Management Agency. https://training.fema.gov/emiweb/downloads/is111_unit%204.pdf

My Notes

exhibit **resiliency**, the ability to cope with adversity and recover emotionally from a traumatic event.[27] However, the mental health of the population must be considered and monitored during recovery from any disastrous event. For example, some people may relive previous traumatic experiences or revert to using substances to cope. Behavioral health responses such as post-traumatic stress disorder (PTSD), substance use disorder, and increased risk for suicide should always be considered when assessing individuals' responses to a disaster.

Effects from trauma extend beyond the physical damages from any disaster. It may take time for individuals to recover physically and emotionally. Survivors of a community disaster should be encouraged to take steps to support each other to promote adaptive coping. Use the following box to read additional information in the "Tips for Survivors of a Traumatic Event" handout by the Substance Abuse and Mental Health Services Administration (SAMHSA).

Read the SAMHSA handout on "Tips for Survivors of a Traumatic Event" PDF.

Review concepts related to loss and the stages of grief in the "Grief and Loss" chapter of Open RN *Nursing Fundamentals.*

Agencies Providing Emergency Assistance

Many federal, state, and local agencies provide support to communities during disasters. The Federal Emergency Management Agency (FEMA) is the agency that promotes disaster mitigation and readiness and coordinates response and recovery following the declaration of a major disaster. FEMA defines a disaster as an event that results in large numbers of deaths and injuries; causes extensive damage or destruction of facilities that provide and sustain human needs; produces an overwhelming demand on state and local response resources and mechanisms; causes a severe long-term effect on general economic activity; and severely affects state, local, and private sector capabilities to begin and sustain response activities.[28] FEMA employees represent every U.S. state, local, tribal, and territorial area and are committed to serving our country before, during, and after disasters.

Disasters are declared using established guidelines and procedures. Because all disasters are local, they are initially declared at the local level. This declaration is typically made by the local mayor. When the mayor determines that capabilities of local resources have been or are expected to be exceeded, state assistance is requested. If the state chooses to respond to a disaster, the governor of the state will direct implementation of the state's emergency plan. If the governor determines that the resource capabilities of the state are exceeded, the governor can request that the president declare a major disaster in order to make federal resources and assistance available to qualified state and local governments. This ordered sequence is important to ensure appropriate financial assistance.[29]

A **state of emergency** is declared when public health or the economic stability of a community is threatened, and extraordinary measures of control may be needed. For example, an infectious disease outbreak like COVID-19 can cause the declaration of a state of emergency. A county or municipal agency is designated as the local emergency

---

27 Substance Abuse and Mental Health Services Administration. (2022, March 23). *Disaster preparedness, response, and recovery*. U.S. Department of Health & Human Services. https://www.samhsa.gov/disaster-preparedness

28 Emergency Management Institute. (2013). *ISS-111.A: Livestock in disasters.* Federal Emergency Management Agency. https://training.fema.gov/emiweb/downloads/is111_unit%204.pdf

29 Emergency Management Institute. (2013). *ISS-111.A: Livestock in disasters.* Federal Emergency Management Agency. https://training.fema.gov/emiweb/downloads/is111_unit%204.pdf

My Notes

management agency, and local law specifies the chain of command in emergencies. Use the following box to access more information about federal and local agencies that provide emergency assistance.

Examples of Organizations That Provide Emergency Assistance

Federal

- *Federal Emergency Management Agency (FEMA)*
- *Strategic National Stockpile*
- *Cybersecurity and Infrastructure Security Agency (CISA)*

Local

- *Local FEMA agencies (each state)*
- *American Red Cross*
- *Local county emergency management divisions*

18.4 NURSES' ROLES IN EMERGENCY RESPONSE

My Notes

Together with emergency personnel, community organizations, health care providers, and other members of the health care team, nurses play a key role in carrying out emergency response plans. Before, during, and after disasters, nurses provide education and health promotion interventions to protect the community and keep people safe from environmental hazards. During the emergency response, nurses assist in first aid, triage patients' needs, direct victims to resources and community support, and continuously assess and monitor patients' physical and psychological needs. Nurses also assist with community organization through logistical organization of response and prevention needs, such as coordination of blood drives, clothing drives, management of shelters, and other social needs that exist in the community. When disaster strikes, nurses are challenged to use their skills and scope of practice to the fullest to provide the best care for their community.[1]

See an example Disaster Nursing Timeline on page 250 of *The Future of Nursing 2020-2030: Charting a Path to Achieve Health Equity* ebook.

The ability to care for and protect vulnerable citizens depends substantially on the preparedness of the nursing workforce. The nursing workforce available to participate in U.S. disaster and public health emergency response includes all licensed nurses (licensed practical/vocational nurses [LPNs/LVNs] and registered nurses [RNs]), civilian and uniformed services nurses at the federal and state levels, nurses who have recently retired, and nurses who volunteer in organizations (e.g., National Disaster Medical System, Medical Reserve Corps, National Voluntary Organizations Active in Disasters, and the American Red Cross). Each of these entities plays a critical role in the nation's ability to respond to and recover from disasters and large-scale public health emergencies such as the COVID-19 pandemic.[2] The increasing frequency of natural and environmental disasters, along with public health emergencies such as the COVID-19 pandemic, highlights the critical importance of having a national nursing workforce prepared with the knowledge, skills, and abilities to respond.[3]

Nurses' Roles in Pandemics and Other Infectious Disease Outbreaks

When infectious disease outbreaks occur, nurses are called to the front lines to care for patients very quickly. In the past few decades, infectious disease outbreaks have been occurring more frequently and with more intensity, and nurses, along with health care agencies, must be prepared to respond to such emergencies. Some of the ways nurses respond are by doing the following[4]:

- Tracking disease prevalence and epidemiology of diseases
- Assisting with screening and testing, along with vaccine distribution
- Providing direct care to affected individuals in hospitals and outpatient clinics

---

1 National Academies of Sciences, Engineering, and Medicine. (2021). *The future of nursing 2020-2030: Charting a path to achieve health equity.* National Academies Press. https://doi.org/10.17226/25982

2 National Academies of Sciences, Engineering, and Medicine. (2021). *The future of nursing 2020-2030: Charting a path to achieve health equity.* National Academies Press. https://doi.org/10.17226/25982

3 National Academies of Sciences, Engineering, and Medicine. (2021). *The future of nursing 2020-2030: Charting a path to achieve health equity.* National Academies Press. https://doi.org/10.17226/25982

4 National Academies of Sciences, Engineering, and Medicine. (2021). *The future of nursing 2020-2030: Charting a path to achieve health equity.* National Academies Press. https://doi.org/10.17226/25982

My Notes

- Educating the public and community about disease prevention and treatment
- Providing psychological support to those fearful of the emergency

New infectious diseases require nurses to receive continuing education regarding infection prevention, diagnosis, treatment, and health promotion. This may include gaining new knowledge about medications, transmission precautions, personal protective equipment (PPE), and evidence-based nursing interventions and medical treatments. Nurses must use critical thinking and apply new evidence-based practices to provide quality care to individuals in their community affected by disease.

The Impact of the COVID-19 Pandemic on Nurses

In December 2019 the novel coronavirus, known as COVID-19, was first detected in China. By March 2020 the World Health Organization declared a worldwide pandemic for what has been called the worst public health emergency in the past 100 years. By March 2022 almost 80 million cases were identified in the United States, with over 977,000 deaths. Worldwide, over 488 million cases were diagnosed, with over 6 million deaths.[5,6]

View the CDC's Covid Data Tracker or Our World in Data's Data Tracker for up-to-date COVID information.

The COVD-19 pandemic created a health care environment never before seen in modern times. Nurses were called upon to care for patients, often lacking proper personal protective equipment (PPE) and medical equipment, to properly support patient health. They cared for patients above and beyond the acuity that they normally managed in their area of expertise and provided frequent end-of-life care. They communicated regularly by phone with loved ones of patients who were dying due to quarantine guidelines and visitor limitations. Staffing shortages became critical as illness spread to nurses and their family members.[7]

As a result, thousands of nurses were still stressed, frustrated, and overwhelmed two years into the pandemic. In October 2021 the American Nurses Association found the following in a mental health and wellness survey of nurses[8]:

- Over 34% rated their emotional health as not, or not at all, emotionally healthy.
- 42% reported having an extremely stressful, disturbing, or traumatic experience due to COVID-19.
- Among nurses who said they intend to leave their position in the next six months, 48% cited the top reason as work negatively affecting their health and well-being, followed closely by insufficient staffing (41%).

The American Nurses Foundation Executive Director, Kate Judge stated, "The COVID-19 pandemic is not over yet, and its impact will persist for a long time. Its challenges have left the nursing profession in a particularly

---

5 Centers for Disease Control and Prevention. (n.d.). *COVID data tracker.* https://covid.cdc.gov/covid-data-tracker/#datatracker-home

6 "Daily new confirmed COVID-19 feathers per million people" by Our World in Data is licensed under CC BY 4.0

7 National Academies of Sciences, Engineering, and Medicine. (2021). *The future of nursing 2020-2030: Charting a path to achieve health equity.* National Academies Press. https://doi.org/10.17226/25982

8 American Nurses Foundation. (2021, October 26). *New survey data: Thousands of nurses are still stressed, frustrated, and overwhelmed almost 2 years into the pandemic.* [News release]. https://www.nursingworld.org/news/news-releases/2021/new-survey-data-thousands-of-nurses-are-still-stressed-frustrated-and-overwhelmed-almost-2-years-into-the-pandemic/

My Notes

vulnerable state, exacerbating nurse staffing shortages, and negatively impacting nurses' quality of life. Nurses are playing a pivotal role in efforts to end this pandemic, so we must ensure nurses are physically and psychologically safe and healthy to function optimally in caring first for themselves, their families, patients, and communities. A robust nursing workforce is essential to our nation's health and, therefore, nurses' well-being and mental health must be a top priority. The data collected from this survey overwhelmingly demonstrate the need to provide consistent and comprehensive support for our nation's nurses."[9]

The American Psychiatric Nurses Association provides COVID resources to support nurses as they address concerns and promote mental health as a result of the COVID-19 pandemic.

Preventing and Managing Stress in Disaster Responders

Engaging in disaster and emergency response work is stressful for nurses and first responders. Depending on the nature of the event, sources of stress may include exposure to scenes of human suffering, risk for personal harm, life-and-death decision-making, intense workloads, limited resources, and separation from family members who may also be in harm's way. Responders can take actions to protect themselves and to manage stress before a disaster or other traumatic event, as well as during the response and recovery phases. These actions can also help when returning home after a particularly traumatic shift.[10]

Read the Tips for Disaster Responders: Preventing and Managing Stress handout from the SAMHSA on tips for preventing and managing stress for disaster responders.

Read more information about stress in the health care system and self-care in the "Burnout & Self-Care" chapter of Open RN *Nursing Management and Professional Concepts.*

9 American Nurses Foundation. (2021, October 26). *New survey data: Thousands of nurses are still stressed, frustrated, and overwhelmed almost 2 years into the pandemic.* [News release]. https://www.nursingworld.org/news/news-releases/2021/new-survey-data-thousands-of-nurses-are-still-stressed-frustrated-and-overwhelmed-almost-2-years-into-the-pandemic/

10 Substance Abuse and Mental Health Services Administration. (2014). *Tips for disaster responders: Preventing and managing stress.* [Handout]. U.S. Department of Health & Human Services. https://store.samhsa.gov/sites/default/files/d7/priv/sma14-4873.pdf

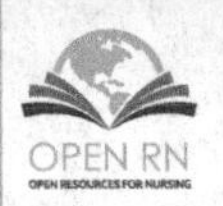

My Notes

18.5 SPOTLIGHT APPLICATION

Sam, a nurse who works at the local hospital, hears about a flooding disaster in a nearby community. Major roads are flooded, and grocery stores have been destroyed. Power lines were knocked down during the storm, and cell phone service is not working. Sam starts to wonder, "What if?" . . . "What if a disaster happens here and I'm not home with my family – how will I know if they are safe? How will I stay safe? What obligations will I have at work?"

As a compassionate nurse, Sam feels a need to respond to others in a crisis but also has a concern about ensuring the well-being of his family members. A Google search reveals the American Nurses Association document "Who Will Be There?" PDF. He realizes the discomfort he is feeling about responding to a potential future disaster event is due to the conflict of ethical principles regarding the nurse's obligation to care for others, as well as the obligation to care for oneself.[1] He decides to respond to this ethical dilemma by preparing his personal response should a disaster occur.

Sam reads additional information called "Make a Plan" provided by the U.S. Department of Homeland Security's website "Ready.gov."[2] Several questions come to mind as Sam reflects on his anticipated response to a disaster:

1. How will I receive alerts and warnings about a disaster in my community?
2. Are there any laws in my state that require my participation as a nurse in disaster response?
3. What is my employer's emergency response plan? What is my expected role as an employed nurse?
4. What state and local disaster preparedness plans currently exist in my community?
5. How will I get to work safely if a disaster occurs?
6. How will I communicate with my family members and ensure their safety if a disaster occurs?

Sam reads additional information provided by the Federal Emergency Management Agency (FEMA) and starts to create his personal and family disaster plan.[3]

Reflective Questions

1. Consider the questions Sam posed as he considered his potential disaster response. What additional questions do you have about your role in a disaster response? What are the answers to these questions in your community and at your place of employment?
2. Create your own personal and family disaster plan.

---

1 American Nurses Association. (2017). *Who Will Be There? Ethical, the law, and a nurse's duty to respond in a disaster.* https://www.nursingworld.org/~4ad845/globalassets/docs/ana/who-will-be-there_disaster-preparedness_2017.pdf

2 U.S. Department of Homeland Security. (2022, May 18). *Make a plan.* https://www.ready.gov/plan

3 FEMA. (2018). *Create your family emergency communication plan.* https://www.ready.gov/sites/default/files/2021-04/family-emergency-communication-plan.pdf

18.6 LEARNING ACTIVITIES

My Notes

Interactive Activities

An interactive H5P element has been excluded from this version of the text. You can view it online here: https://wtcs.pressbooks.pub/nursingmhcc/?p=1074#h5p-59

An interactive H5P element has been excluded from this version of the text. You can view it online here: https://wtcs.pressbooks.pub/nursingmhcc/?p=1074#h5p-60

My Notes

XVIII GLOSSARY

Chelation therapy: Treatment for heavy metal poisoning such as mercury, arsenic, and lead. Chelators are medications that bind to the metals in the bloodstream to increase urinary excretion of the substance.

Decontamination: Any process that removes or neutralizes a chemical hazard on or in the patient in order to prevent or mitigate adverse health effects to the patient; protect emergency first responders, health care facility first receivers, and other patients from secondary contamination; and reduce the potential for secondary contamination of response and health care infrastructure.

Disaster: A serious disruption of the functioning of a community or a society at any scale due to hazardous events interacting with conditions of exposure, vulnerability, and capacity that lead to human, material, economic, and environmental losses and impacts.

Disaster management: Response to a disaster with integration of emergency response plans throughout the life cycle of a disaster event.

Emergency preparedness: The planning process focused on avoiding or ameliorating the risks and hazards resulting from a disaster to optimize population health and safety. The process includes four key concepts: preparedness, mitigation, response, and recovery. Evaluation occurs after a disaster event as the planning process continues.

Environmental health hazard: A substance or pathogen that has the ability to cause an adverse health event in individuals or communities.

Mitigation: Actions taken to prevent or reduce the cause, impact, and consequences of disasters. When a disaster occurs, actions are taken to save lives, treat injuries, and minimize the effect of the disaster. Immediate needs are addressed, such as medical treatment, shelter, food, and water, as well as psychological support.

Preparedness: Planning, training personnel, and providing educational activities regarding potential disastrous events. Planning includes evaluating environmental risks and social vulnerabilities of a community.

Recovery: Restoration efforts occur concurrently with regular operations and activities, such as preventing or reducing stress-related illnesses and excessive financial burdens.

Resiliency: The ability to cope with adversity and recover emotionally from a traumatic event.

Response: Actions taken in the immediate aftermath of a disaster, such as saving lives, treating injuries, and minimizing the effects of the disaster. Immediate needs are addressed, such as medical treatment, shelter, food, and water, as well as psychological support of survivors.

Simple Triage and Rapid Treatment (START): A triage system from the U.S. Department of Health and Human Services that prioritizes victims by color (red, yellow, green, and black) for efficient and effective treatment.

Social vulnerability: The characteristics of a person or a community that affect their capacity to anticipate, confront, repair, and recover from the effects of a disaster.

State of emergency: Status that is declared when the public health or the economic stability of a community is threatened, and extraordinary measures of control may be needed.

Triage: Prioritizing care for individuals affected by a disaster or emergency.

Answer Key

CHAPTER 1

My Notes

Answers to interactive elements are given within the interactive element.

My Notes

CHAPTER 2

Answers to interactive elements are given within the interactive element.

CHAPTER 3

My Notes

Answers to interactive elements are given within the interactive element.

My Notes

CHAPTER 4

Answers to interactive elements are given within the interactive element.

CHAPTER 5

My Notes

Answers to interactive elements are given within the interactive element.

My Notes

CHAPTER 6

Answers to interactive elements are given within the interactive element.

CHAPTER 7

My Notes

Answers to interactive elements are given within the interactive element.

My Notes

CHAPTER 8

Answers to interactive elements are given within the interactive element.

CHAPTER 9

My Notes

Answers to interactive elements are given within the interactive element.

My Notes

CHAPTER 10

Critical Thinking Questions

1. *DSM-5* lists these as unique mental health illness diagnoses, but the symptoms of each may cross over. In obsessive-compulsive personality disorder, the client exhibits orderliness and perfectionism. However, in personality disorders, the behaviors do not come and go or fluctuate, and there is no insight that the behavior is abnormal. In fact, clients typically believe their behavior is normal and beneficial. Additionally, the client does not perform repetitive actions that are classic to OCD. In contrast, OCD is caused by anxiety, and the severity of the obsessions and compulsions vary according to the level of anxiety. Clients with OCD exhibit repetitive actions such as excessive handwashing or repeatedly checking the door is locked or counting items. Clients have insight into the behavior and view it as abnormal and distressing, so they are more likely to seek treatment.
2. Name that personality disorder:
    a. Histrionic
    b. Paranoid
    c. Borderline
    d. Schizoid
    e. Dependent
    f. Antisocial
    g. Avoidant
    h. Narcissistic
    i. Obsessive-Compulsive
    j. Schizotypal
3. Check your medication knowledge:
    a. Low-dose antipsychotics
    b. Mood stabilizers and low-dose antipsychotics
    c. Mood stabilizers and omega-3
4. Compare normal adolescent development with trait similarities of personality disorders:

    Cluster A: May not trust others, prefers to be alone, and may have magical thinking (imagination)

    Cluster B: Disregards right from wrong, lies, gets into trouble, impulsive, overreactive, emotional, and easily influenced by others

    Cluster C: Social discomfort, shy, fearful, and lacks self-confidence

Answers to interactive elements are given within the interactive element.

CHAPTER 11

My Notes

Answers to interactive elements are given within the interactive element.

My Notes

CHAPTER 12

Answers to interactive elements are given within the interactive element.

CHAPTER 13

Questions:

1. What symptoms of an eating disorder is Tiffany demonstrating? Tiffany is exhibiting symptoms of anorexia nervosa.
2. What other assessment findings does the nurse anticipate? See Table 13.3a – Chapter 13.
3. What laboratory tests will likely be ordered during this visit? Laboratory tests may include a complete blood count, electrolyte levels, glucose level, thyroid function tests, erythrocyte sedimentation rate (ESR), and creatine phosphokinase (CPK).
4. What type of psychotherapy would be helpful for Tiffany? Cognitive behavioral therapy and family-based therapy would be useful psychotherapy treatments for Tiffany.
5. What conditions would cause Tiffany to be hospitalized? Tiffany would be hospitalized if her vital signs are unstable, laboratory findings present acute health risk, and she has rapidly worsening symptoms or suicidal ideation with a plan and is unable to contract for safety.
6. Tiffany is hospitalized. Create a brief nursing care plan for Tiffany including a nursing diagnosis, SMART goal, and 3-5 nursing interventions.

Diagnosis: Imbalanced Nutrition: Less Than Body Requirements

SMART Goal: Client will gain at least one pound weekly until reaching healthy weight classification according to her BMI.

Sample Interventions:

- The client will be weighed on Mondays, Wednesdays, and Fridays and progress determined based on a target weight established by the dietician.
- A pleasant, calm atmosphere will be provided at mealtimes.
- The client will be observed during meals to prevent hiding or throwing away food and at least one hour after eating to prevent purging.
- The client will be encouraged to make her own menu choices as she approaches her goal weight.
- Knowledge and skills gained from individual, family, and group therapy sessions will be reinforced with the client and her family.

Answers to interactive elements are given within the interactive element.

My Notes

CHAPTER 14

Answers to interactive elements are given within the interactive element.

CHAPTER 15

My Notes

Answers to interactive elements are given within the interactive element.

My Notes

CHAPTER 16

Answers to interactive elements are given within the interactive element.

CHAPTER 17

My Notes

Answers to interactive activities are provided within the activity.

My Notes

CHAPTER 18

Answers to interactive elements are given within the interactive element.